Human Reproductive Biology

Human Reproductive Biology

Edited by Francisco Armstrong

hayle medical

New York

Hayle Medical,
750 Third Avenue, 9th Floor,
New York, NY 10017, USA

Visit us on the World Wide Web at:
www.haylemedical.com

ISBN: 978-1-63241-758-9

The publisher's policy is to use permanent paper from mills that operate a sustainable forestry policy. Furthermore, the publisher ensures that the text paper and cover boards used have met acceptable environmental accreditation standards.

Printed in China.

Cataloging-in-Publication Data

Human reproductive biology / edited by Francisco Armstrong.
p. cm.
Includes bibliographical references and index.
ISBN 978-1-63241-758-9
1. Human reproduction. 2. Human biology. 3. Reproduction. 4. Reproductive health.
5. Fertility, Human. I. Armstrong, Francisco.
QP251 .H86 2019
612.6--dc23

Table of Contents

Preface

In my initial years as a student, I used to run to the library at every possible instance to grab a book and learn something new. Books were my primary source of knowledge and I would not have come such a long way without all that I learnt from them. Thus, when I was approached to edit this book; I became understandably nostalgic. It was an absolute honor to be considered worthy of guiding the current generation as well as those to come. I put all my knowledge and hard work into making this book most beneficial for its readers.

The branch of biology which includes the study of reproduction, reproductive systems, sexual development, sexual maturity, endocrinology and fertility is known as reproductive biology. Human reproductive biology is mainly controlled through the hormones. They are responsible for the growth and maturation of the human reproductive structures as they send signals to the body. The female reproductive system and the male reproductive system are the two main components of human reproductive biology. The female reproductive system consists of the ovaries, oviducts, vagina, uterus and mammary glands, whereas, the male reproductive system consists of the sex accessory glands, testes, sex accessory ducts and external genitalia. The topics included in this book on human reproductive biology are of utmost significance and bound to provide incredible insights to readers. It studies, analyzes and upholds the pillars of human reproductive biology and its utmost significance in modern times. Students, researchers, experts and all associated with human reproductive biology will benefit alike from this book.

I wish to thank my publisher for supporting me at every step. I would also like to thank all the authors who have contributed their researches in this book. I hope this book will be a valuable contribution to the progress of the field.

Editor

1

Modulatory effects of trophoblast-secreted CXCL12 on the migration and invasion of human first-trimester decidual epithelial cells are mediated by CXCR4 rather than CXCR7

Jiayi Zheng, Haiping Wang and Wenhui Zhou*

Abstract

Background: Maternal-fetal crosstalk during embryo implantation is complex and regulated by local signaling molecules. Chemokines and their receptors are critical signaling components required for implantation and the process of pregnancy. This study aimed to explore whether human first-trimester trophoblast cells (TCs) were capable of modulating the migration and invasion of human first-trimester decidual epithelial cells (DECs) via CXCL12/CXCR4/CXCR7 signaling.

Method: The expression of CXCR4 and CXCR7 in DECs was examined by immunohistochemistry, immunocytochemistry, immunofluorescence, flow cytometry, real-time polymerase chain reactions and western blotting. The effects of recombinant human CXCL12 (rhCXCL12) and TC-conditioned medium (TC-CM) on DEC viability in vitro were explored using a viability assay. The modulatory effects of rhCXCL12 and TC/DEC co-cultures on DEC migration and invasion were examined with migration/invasion assays.

Result: CXCR4 and CXCR7 were co-expressed in human first-trimester DECs. Human rhCXCL12 and TC-CM had no effects on DEC viability in vitro ($P > 0.05$). Both exogenous CXCL12 and co-culture with TCs significantly increased the migration and invasion of DECs ($P < 0.05$). Neutralizing antibodies against CXCR4 ($P < 0.05$) or CXCL12 ($P < 0.05$), but not CXCR7 ($P > 0.05$), significantly blocked the enhanced migration and invasion of DECs induced by exogenous CXCL12 or TC co-culture.

Conclusions: CXCR4 and CXCR7 were co-expressed in human first-trimester DECs. TC-derived CXCL12 promoted the migration and invasion of DECs via CXCR4, but not CXCR7, in a paracrine manner during early pregnancy.

Keywords: CXCL12/CXCR4/CXCR7, Decidual epithelial cell (DEC), Trophoblast (TC), Maternal-fetal crosstalk

Background

The application of assisted reproductive technology (ART) in the clinic has made great achievements in infertility treatment. However, even when embryos/blastocysts estimated to be top grade are transferred, the occurrence of pregnancy failure is still inevitable, suggesting the importance of implantation [1, 2].

Successful implantation requires the perfect coordination between the fetal-derived trophoblasts (TCs) and maternal-derived decidual cells via a complex network of molecules signaling in an autocrine and paracrine manner. Decidual epithelial cells (DECs), serving as a critical modulator for conceptus attachment, have been ignored for many years. In addition to providing nutrition and energy for the fetus, decidual epithelial cells have gradually been shown to be involved in immune regulation, TC invasion, protection against infections, and the production of growth

* Correspondence: 77305875@qq.com
Medical Center for Human Reproduction, Beijing Chaoyang Hospital, Capital Medical University, Beijing 100020, People's Republic of China

factors and cytokines [3–8]. Deficient glandular activity has been observed in some recurrent miscarriages, further implying an important role for endometrial glands in pregnancy [6].

DECs have gradually attracted increasing attention in recent years. However, due to the difficulty in isolating and culturing primary cells, there is limited information available about the interaction between TCs and decidual glands. The motility of DECs during implantation and early pregnancy is still an open question.

Chemokine (C-X-C motif) ligand 12 (CXCL12) is a small cytokine. CXCL12 and its receptors CXCR4/CXCR7 are involved in several crucial reproductive biology processes, including uterine natural killer cell recruitment, placentation, implantation and embryogenesis [9–12].

Our team focuses on the roles of chemokines and chemokine receptors in the maternal-fetal dialogue. We have confirmed that human first-trimester TCs not only modulate their own invasiveness via the CXCL12/CXCR4 axis but also promote the motility of DSCs via CXCR4 ligation [12, 13]. Our recent research further revealed the expression of CXCR7 (another high affinity receptor for CXCL12) in human first-trimester TCs and DSCs [14, 15]. Moreover, steroid hormones showed priming effects on CXCR4 and CXCR7 expression in human cycling and early pregnant DSCs before the emergence of an embryo [14, 15]. These results indicate the potential importance of the CXCL12/CXCR4/CXCR7 axis in implantation and early pregnancy. With the discovery of CXCR7, researchers may need to re-examine the role of the CXCL12/CXCR4 signaling pathway. Our knowledge of the expression and function of CXCR7 at the maternal-fetal interface and its relation to CXCL12/CXCR4 signaling remains to be elucidated.

The aims of this study are first, to examine CXCR4 and CXCR7 expression in human first-trimester DECs, and second, to determine the effects of TC-derived CXCL12 on DEC functions. We hope this study improves our understanding of the detailed mechanisms underlying the maternal-fetal dialogue during implantation and early pregnancy and provides new clues for the diagnosis and treatment of implantation failure-related infertility and early miscarriage.

Methods

Tissue collection

As previously described, [12, 13, 15] human decidual and villous tissues were collected from patients who underwent an elective surgical abortion in first-trimester pregnancies (gestational age 6–10 weeks) for non-medical reasons at Beijing Chaoyang Hospital from 2015 to 2016. Samples were collected in ice-cold DMEM (Dulbecco's Modified Eagle's Medium; Gibco), then immediately transported to the laboratory and separated for paraffin embedding or cell isolation [12, 13, 15]. This study was approved by the Human Research Ethics Committee of Beijing Chaoyang Hospital. All participants completed an informed consent form prior to the collection of tissue samples.

Immunohistochemistry

The method for IHC was previously established in the laboratory [12, 16, 17]. Briefly, the decidual tissues were routinely fixed with 4% formalin and embedded in paraffin. Antigen retrieval was performed by microwave heating in 0.01 M sodium citrate buffer (pH 6.0) at 800 W for 3 min to initiate boiling and then for 7 min at 400 W to continue boiling. After cooling down to the room temperature, the 10 min heating procedure was repeated with fresh buffer. H_2O_2 (0.3%) in phosphate-buffered saline (PBS) was employed to block endogenous peroxidase activity in the sections. After treatment with a protein blocking solution containing 5% bovine serum albumin to block non-specific binding, sections were incubated with mouse anti-human CXCR4 (25 μg/ml), CXCR7 (20 μg/ml) monoclonal antibody (Catalogue number MAB172/MAB4227, R&D Systems, Abingdon, UK) or mouse immunoglobulin (Ig)G isotype control (20 μg/ml, Sino-America Co. Ltd., Shanghai, China) overnight at 4 °C. A streptavidin/biotin detection reagent kit (ZSGB-BIO Co. Ltd., Beijing, China) with 3, 30-diaminobenzidine tetrahydrochloride (DAB) was employed to detect signals, and Harris hematoxylin was used as counter-stain. The expression of CXCL12, CXCR4 and CXCR7 in human first-trimester TCs has been confirmed in our previous study [12–14]. According to an ELISA, the concentration of accumulated CXCL12 in TC-CM increased constantly in vitro [12]. In the present study, human first-trimester TCs were used as positive control. Mouse isotype IgG was used as negative controls. The experiments were perform using ten independent samples.

Isolation and culture of human first-trimester DECs

DECs were isolated according to the method established in our laboratory [18]. Endometrial tissues were digested independently with 0.1% collagenase IV for 1 h at 37 °C on the shaker. The resulting digest was passed through a 38 μm sieve. Then, the reverse side of the 38 μm sieve was washed with DMEM, which was collected and centrifuged at 1000 g for 15 min. The pellet was diluted with DMEM containing 15% heat-inactivated fetal bovine serum (FBS) and seeded in a culture flask. After 4 h of culture, the suspension containing non-attached cells was collected and seeded on 6-well plates pre-coated with extracellular matrix (ECM; Sigma, St. Louis, MO, USA). With this method, the purity of the cultured

DECs can reach to 90% according to ICC identification (positive for CK7 and negative for vimentin) [18].

Isolation and culture of human first-trimester TCs

Villus tissue was treated by repeated trypsin digestions according to the method previously established [12–14]. Briefly, placental tissues were collected and digested with 0.25% trypsin (Amresco) and 2.5 K units/ml DNase type I (Sigma, St. Louis, MO, USA) for 10 min at 37 °C with gentle agitation. The digested cell suspension was collected and the residual tissue was subjected to two to three additional cycles of 10 min digestions. Cell suspensions obtained from each digestion were mixed, carefully layered over a discontinuous Percoll gradient (65–20%, in 5% step), and thereafter centrifuged at 1000 g for 20 min. Cells sedimenting at densities between 1.048 and 1.062 g/ml were collected and washed with DMEM. These cells were then diluted at a density of 5×10^5 cells/well, and maintained in complete DMEM (2 mM glutamine, 25 mM HEPES, 100 IU/ml penicillin and 100 mg/ml streptomycin), supplemented with 15% FBS and incubated in a 5% CO_2 incubator at 37 °C. This method yields 95% pure TCs, the characterization of TCs is reported in a previous publication [12].

Immunocytochemistry

The method for ICC was previously established in the laboratory [12, 14]. Briefly, the isolated DECs and TCs were cultured for 24–48 h, before being fixed with 4% paraformaldehyde and washed with PBS. After treatment with 0.3% H_2O_2 in PBS to block endogenous peroxidase activity, cells were blocked with 7% horse serum in PBS and incubated with mouse anti-human CXCR4 and CXCR7 monoclonal antibodies. The antibodies used, as well as the other procedures, were identical to the described above for IHC. Experiments were performed using five independent TC and DEC preparations in each.

Immunofluorescence

Immunofluorescence was used to detect the expression and position of CXCR7 and CXCR4 in DECs. The isolated DECs were seeded on 6-well plates which were pre- coated with cover glasses at a density of 2×10^6 cells/ml × 2 ml per well. At 80–90% confluence, the cells were fixed in 4% paraformaldehyde and treated with 0.2% Triton X-100. After blocking with goat serum for 2 h at room temperature, the cells were incubated with mouse anti-human CXCR4 (25 μg/ml, catalogue number MAB172, R&D Systems, Abingdon, UK) and rabbit anti-human CXCR7 monoclonal antibodies (20 μg/ml, catalogue number ab72100, Abcam, Cambridge, MA,). After three washes with PBS, the cells were incubated with fluoresce-in isothiocyanate (FITC) conjugated donkey anti-rabbit immunoglobulin (Ig) G (1:100, 10 μg/L) or Texas Red conjugated donkey anti-mouse IgG (1:100, 10 μg/L) (Rockland) at room temperature for 60 min in darkness and then incubated with DAPI (Santa Cruz Biotechnology) for 5 min at 37 °C. Images were captured with an Olympus fluorescence microscope (Olympus, Tokyo, Japan). The experiments were perform using three samples.

Enzyme-linked immunosorbent assay

As previously described, [12] purified TCs were seeded in a 24-well plate pre-coated with matrigel at a density of 5×10^5 cells/ml. Trophoblast supernatants were collected after 24, 48 and 72 h of culture. Each supernatant was centrifuged at 2000 g and stored at − 70 °C. A human CXCL12 Quantikine enzyme-linked immunosorbent assay (ELISA) kit (Quantikine, R&D Systems, DSA00) was used to measure chemokine levels in each supernatant, according to the manufacturer's instructions. The intra-assay coefficient of variation is 3.5%, inter-assay coefficient of variation is 9.6%. The average value of each sample was used for statistical analysis. The ELISA was conducted in duplicate in three separate experiments.

Real-time PCR

Total cellular RNA was extracted from primary DEC cultures and reverse transcribed, according to our previously described method [12, 15]. Brifly, Total RNA was extracted from cells by Trizol (Invitrogen). The reverse transcription reaction was performed using Fast Quant RT Kit (with gDNAase) (TIANGEN), according to the manufacturer's instructions. Then, cDNAs were amplified with a fluorescence ratio PCR instrument (Roche 96) in a reaction with a final volume of 20 μl containing cDNAs (1 μl), YBR FAST qPCR Master Mix (10 μl), and primers (0.6 μl). A 5 min precycle at 95 °C was followed by 40 cycles of 15 s at 95 °C, 20 s at 60 °C and 15 s at 72 °C. The primer pairs for cDNA amplification were: 5'-CCG AGG CCC TAG CTT TCT TC-3′(forward) and 5′-GAG GAT CTT GAG GCT GGA CC-3′(reverse) for human CXCR4 (128 bp); 5'-GGC TTG CCT GGA CTT CTG TA-3′ (forward) and 5'-GTC AGC ACT ATG CCT CCC AA (reverse) for human CXCR7 (168 bp); 5′-CAT CAC CAT CTT CCA GGA GCG A-3′ (forward) and 5′-GTC TTC TGG GTG GCA G TG ATG G -3′ (reverse) for GAPDH(341 bp). Human first-trimester villi were used as a positive control. RNase-Free ddH_2O was used as negative control. The housekeeping gene GAPDH was served as internal control. The experiments were performed on six samples by Beijing Yuan Quan Yi Ke Bio-Tech Co., Ltd.

Western blotting

Proteins were extracted with pre-cooled RIPA buffer. After protein concentrations were measured using a BCA protein assay kit (SaiNuoBo-BIO, Beijing, China), cell lysates containing 10 μg of total protein were mixed with loading buffer, boiled at 95 °C for 5 min and loaded onto polyacrylamide-bisacrylamide gels (5% stacking gel and 12% separating gel). After the sodium dodecyl sulfate-polyacrylamide gel electrophoresis (SDS-PAGE), proteins were transferred to nitrocellulose membranes (Millipore Corporation, USA). Membranes were blocked with 5% fatty acid-free milk-TBST solution (Tris-buffered saline containing 0.1% Tween 20, pH 7.4) for 30 min at room temperature, and then incubated with rabbit anti-human CXCR4 (Abcam, Cambridge, UK, ab124824, diluted 1:500 in 5% fatty acid-free milk-TBST) or CXCR7 (diluted 1:500 in 5% fatty acid-free milk-TBST) antibodies overnight at 4 °C. After 5 washes with TBST solution, membranes were incubated with a peroxidase-conjugated goat anti-rabbit IgG secondary antibody (Beijing TDY BioTech Co. Ltd., diluted 1:10000 in fatty acid-free milk 5% in TBST) for 40 min at room temperature. β-actin antibody (Beijing TDY BioTech Co. Ltd., diluted 1:5000 in fatty acid-free milk 5% in TBST) was used as control. Proteins were revealed by Immobilon Western chemiluminescent HRP substrate (Millipore, MA, USA). Integrated optical densities of protein bands were measured using the Image Master VDS software. Experiments were performed on six samples at SINOBLE Biotechnology Center.

Flow cytometry

Freshly isolated DECs were collected for the FCM analysis as previously described [13]. Briefly, cells were washed with phosphate-buffered saline (PBS) three times. After blocking with 10% FBS, cells were mixed with mouse anti-human CXCR4-PE-CY5 (5 μL/100 μL, catalogue number 15–9999-42, eBioscience, CA, USA,) or CXCR7-PE monoclonal antibody (5 μL/100 μL; clone 8F11-M16, Biolegend, San Diego, CA, USA). The corresponding mouse immunoglobulin (Ig) G2a-PE-CY5 or (Ig) G2a-PE isotype control was used as a negative control. After 30 min incubation in the dark at room temperature, the number of CXCR4, CXCR7 positive cells were measured using FACS flow cytometry system (BD FACS Canto II USA). The experiments were run duplicate in five different samples.

Cell viability assay

The CCK-8 kit (Cell Counting Kit, DOJINDO Laboratories, Japan) assay was applied to evaluate the effects of CXCL12 on cell viability, as described previously [12]. Briefly, freshly isolated TCs were seeded in 6-well plates pre-coated with ECM at a density of 1×10^6 cell/ml per well and cultured continuously for 48 h. Supernatants, namely TC-CM, were collected, centrifuged at 2000 g, and then stored at − 70 °C. The isolated DECs were re-suspended in DMEM supplemented with 15% FBS and seeded in 96-well flat-bottom microplates at a density of 2×10^4 cells/well. After reaching 70–80% confluence, cells were starved with DMEM containing 1% FBS for 12 h before treatment. The medium was removed once again, and cells were treated with rh CXCL12 (100 ng/ml, catalogue number 300-28A-100, PeproTech, USA,) or TC-CM for 48 h. Before this stimulation, some of the wells with cells were pre-incubated with CXCL12 (25 μg/ml, catalogue number AF-351-NA, R&D Systems, Abingdon, UK), CXCR4 (20 μg/ml, catalogue number MAB172, R&D Systems, Abingdon, UK) or CXCR7 (10 μg/ml, catalogue number K0223–3, MBL international, Japan) neutralizing antibodies. Then, CCK-8 reagent (1:10) was added to the wells and incubated at 37 ° C for 1 h. Absorbance was measured at a wavelength of 450 nm using an automatic microplate reader. Samples were run in triplicate and experiments were performed using three different samples.

Migration and invasion assays

The migration and invasion of DECs were evaluated objectively with transwell plates, according to a previous study [12, 13]. For the migration assay, isolated DECs were directly seeded on the upper chamber (8 mm pore size, 6.5 mm diameter; Corning, NY, USA). For the invasion assay, isolated DECs were plated on the cell inserts pre-coated with 20 μl ECM (BD Matrigel™, Basement Membrane Matrix, USA) and two sets of experiments were performed as described below.

First, freshly isolated DECs (2×10^5 cells in 200 μl of DMEM) were treated with rh CXCL12 (100 ng/ml). Before this stimulation, some of the wells with cells were pre-incubated with CXCR4 (20 μg/ml, catalogue number MAB172, R&D Systems, Abingdon, UK), CXCL12 (25 μg/ml, catalogue number AF-351-NA, R&D Systems, Abingdon, UK) or CXCR7 (10 μg/ml, catalogue number K0223–3, MBL international, Japan) neutralizing antibodies. The lower chamber was filled with 800 μl of DMEM supplemented with 10–15% FBS. Cells were then incubated at 37 °C for 48 h. Cultures of DECs alone were used as control.

Second, the TC and DEC co-culture invasion model was established to observe whether the invasiveness of DECs was regulated by TC-derived signals. Briefly, isolated TCs (2×10^5 cells in 800 μl of DMEM supplemented with 15% FBS) were pre-seeded in the lower chambers and cultured for 24 h at 37 °C. Then, freshly isolated DECs (2×10^5 in 200 μl DMEM) that had been pre-blocked with CXCR4 (20 μg/ml), CXCL12 (25 μg/ml) or CXCR7 (10 μg/ml) neutralizing antibodies were plated in the upper chamber. Cells were then incubated at 37 °C for an additional 48 h. Cultures of DECs alone were used as control.

The inserts were removed, washed with PBS and the non-invading cells and ECM were removed from the upper surface of the filter by wiping it with a cotton bud. The inserts were then fixed with 4% paraformaldehyde for 24 h and treated with 0.1% Triton X-100 for 40 min at room temperature. After blocking with goat serum for 2 h at room temperature, the inserts were incubated with primary anti-human keratin 7 antibody (1: 50, catalogue number 15539–1-AP, Protein Tech, Chicago, IL, USA,) overnight at 4 °C. After three washes with PBS, the inserts were incubated with biotinylated secondary antibody for 30 min at 37 °C and then incubated with DAPI (Santa Cruz Biotechnology) for 5 min at 37 °C. Images were captured with an Olympus fluorescence microscope (Olympus, Tokyo, Japan). The number of cells that had migrated to the lower surface was counted at a magnification of 200. Results were assessed by two independent researchers to eliminate inter-individual variability, and the invasive index was calculated as the proportion of the migrated cells of the experiment group relative to its own control. Each group was performed in duplicate and the experiment was repeated by 3 samples.

Statistical analysis

Statistical comparisons of the data from the various groups were performed using one-way ANOVA followed by Dunnett's post hoc t-test, when appropriate. Data are expressed as means ± SEM. Differences between groups were considered statistically significant at $P < 0.05$.

Results

Expression of CXCR4/CXCR7 in human first-trimester DECs

The immunochemical staining shown in Figs 1 and 2 revealed a brown-colored staining specific for CXCR4 or CXCR7 in the cytomembrane, cytoplasm and nucleus of human first-trimester DECs in vivo and in vitro.

The immunofluorescence results in Fig. 3 showed that CXCR4 and CXCR7 protein were co-expressed in

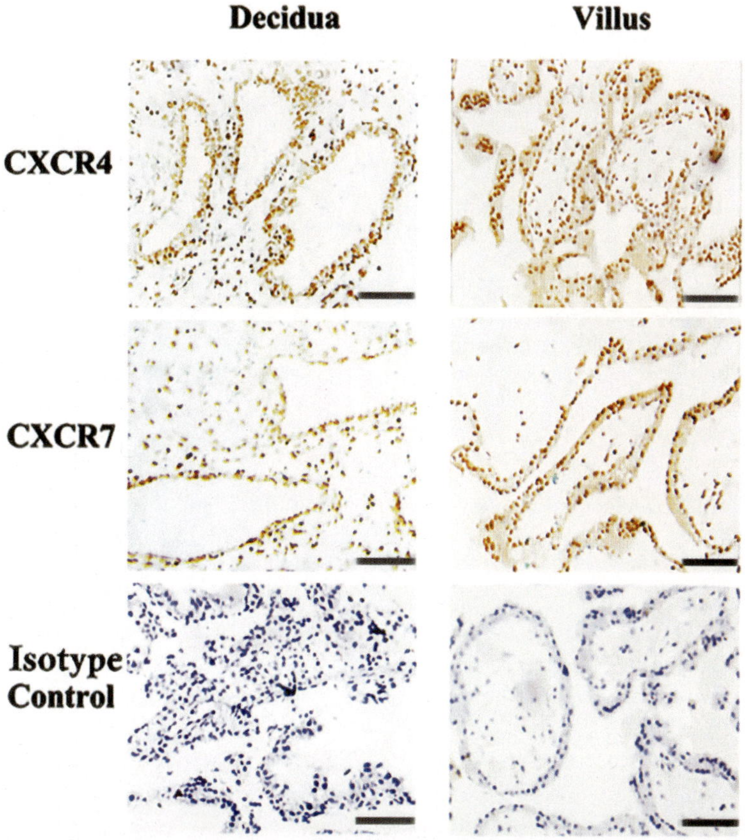

Fig. 1 CXCR4 and CXCR7 were co-expressed in human first-trimester decidual epithelial cells in vivo. Immunohistochemistry expression of CXCR4 and CXCR7 molecules in first-trimester human decidual epithelial cells (DECs). Specific brown-colored staining for CXCR4 and CXCR7 were observed in the membrane, cytoplasm and nucleus of the primary-cultured DECs ($n = 10$). No staining was observed in cells stained with murine isotype control antibodies. Human first-trimester villi were used as positive controls. Murine isotype represents a negative control. Experiments were performed using ten independent endometrial samples.—— —200 μm

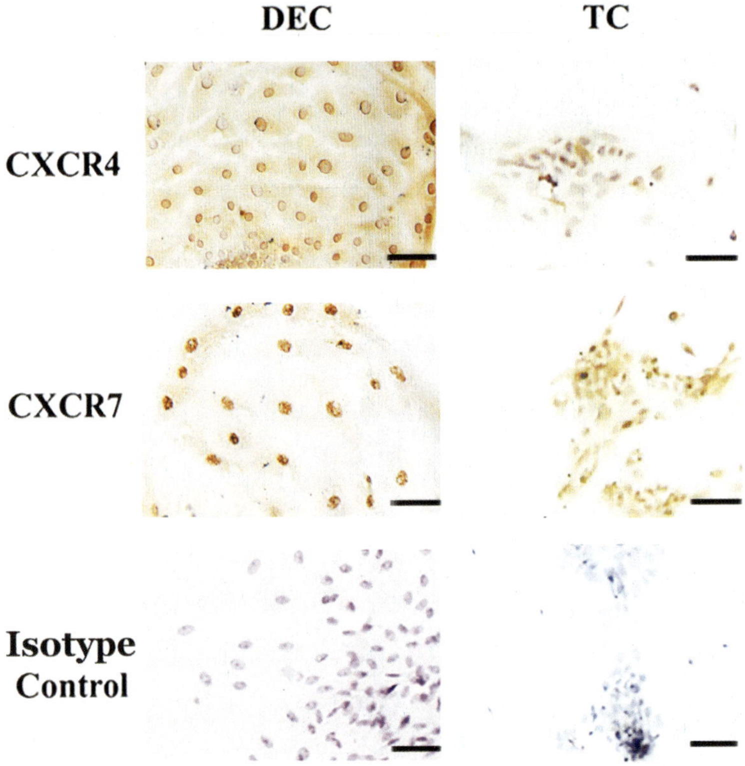

Fig. 2 CXCR4 and CXCR7 were co-expressed in primary human first-trimester decidual epithelial cell cultures in vitro. Immunocytochemistry detection of CXCR4 and CXCR7 expression in first-trimester human primary cultured decidual epithelial cells (DECs). Specific staining against CXCR4 or CXCR7 was observed in the membrane, cytoplasm and nucleus of the DECs ($n = 5$). No staining was observed in cells stained with murine isotype control antibodies. Human first-trimester cultured cytotrophoblasts were used as positive controls. Magnification: × 200. Experiments were performed using five independent endometrial samples. ——50 μm

human in vitro cultured DECs. Both the red fluorescence (CXCR7) and green fluorescence (CXCR4) was clearly recognized in the same area of the cells, including the cytomembrane, cytoplasm and nucleus.

As shown in the real-time PCR results presented in Fig. 4a, both the CXCR4 and CXCR7 genes were transcribed in human first-trimester DECs in vitro, and the mean levels of the CXCR4 and CXCR7 mRNAs in DECs were 15.0877 and 0.6158, respectively, changed from positive control.

The expression of the CXCR4 and CXCR7 proteins in DECs was detected by western blotting. As shown in Fig. 4b, the CXCR4 and CXCR7 proteins were co-expressed in human first-trimester DECs. The relative intensities of the CXCR4 and CXCR7 proteins were 0.4135 ± 0.1538 and 0.1222 ± 0.0219, respectively.

We used flow cytometry to detect the expression of CXCR4 and CXCR7 on the membranes of human first-trimester DECs from 5 independent samples. CXCR4 and CXCR7 proteins were detected in all of the analyzed samples. The the percentage of CXCR4-positive cells varied from 10.5% to 16.0%, with an average of 14.26 ± 1.00%, while the percentage of CXCR7-positive cells ranging between 1.2 and 1.8%, with an average of 1.50 ± 0.11% (Fig. 4c).

The soluble CXCL12 content in TC-CM

The primary cultured human first-trimester TCs secreted CXCL12 spontaneously in vitro, as shown in ELISA assays (Fig. 5). The concentration of CXCL12 increased with time in culture: it was 49.57 ± 2.42 ng/ml, 173.80 ± 6.22 ng/ml and 240.77 ± 10.83 ng/ml at 24, 48 and 72 h in culture.

The CXCL12/CXCR4/CXCR7 axis had no effect on the viability of human first-trimester DECs in vitro

As shown in Fig. 6, neither CXCL12 (1.04 ± 0.04, $P > 0.05$) nor TC-CM (1.02 ± 0.05, $P > 0.05$) increased the viability of DECs in vitro. Likewise blocking the CXCL12, CXCR4 or CXCR7 also failed to affect DEC viability ($P > 0.05$).

TC-derived CXCL12 promoted the migration and invasion of human first-trimester DECs by binding to CXCR4, rather than CXCR7

In the migration assay (Fig. 7), both exogenous CXCL12 (1.79 ± 0.05, $P < 0.01$) and co-culture with TC (1.53 ±

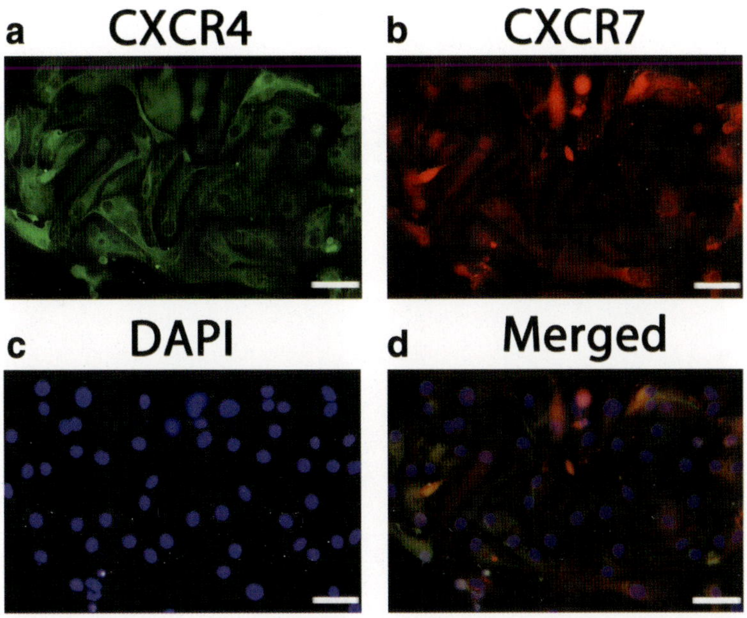

Fig. 3 CXCR4 and CXCR7 were co-expressed in primary human first-trimester DECs cultures in vitro. Immunofluorescence detection of both CXCR4 and CXCR7 protein were expressed in the membrane, cytoplasm and nucleus of DECs. **a** Expression of CXCR4 (green fluorescence) in DECs; **b** Expression of CXCR7 (red fluorescence) in DECs; **c** DAPI staining in DECs; **d** The merged picture. Magnification: × 400. Experiments were performed using three independent endometrial samples. —50 μm

0.08, $P < 0.05$) significantly increased the migration of human first-trimester DECs in vitro compared to the corresponding control. CXCL12 (1.79 ± 0.05 vs 1.02 ± 0.06 and 1.01 ± 0.07, respectively for control, $P < 0.01$) or TC co-culture-induced migration (1.53 ± 0.08 vs 1.14 ± 0.05 and 1.11 ± 0.02, respectively for control, $P < 0.05$) was decreased after treatment with neutralizing antibodies against CXCR4 or CXCL12. However, the blockade of CXCR7 failed to inhibit the CXCL12 (1.79 ± 0.05 vs 1.64 ± 0.05, $P > 0.05$) or TC co-culture-induced (1.53 ± 0.08 vs 1.46 ± 0.07, $P > 0.05$) increase in migration.

The results of the invasion assay (Fig. 8) were similar to the migration assay. The number of invaded DECs was significantly increased after treatment with exogenous CXCL12 (1.96 ± 0.09 vs 1.00, $P < 0.01$) or co-culture with TC (1.67 ± 0.09 vs 1.00, $P < 0.01$) compared with the corresponding controls. Addition of antibodies against CXCR4 or CXCL12 effectively blocked the CXCL12- stimulated invasion of DECs (1.96 ± 0.09 vs 1.13 ± 0.04 and 1.09 ± 0.03, $P < 0.01$) as did the TC co-culture (1.67 ± 0.09 vs 1.08 ± 0.06 and 1.10 ± 0.05, $P < 0.01$). Treatment with the CXCR7 neutralizing antibody alone was unable to block the increased invasion induced by exogenous CXCL12 (1.96 ± 0.09 vs 1.61 ± 0.10, $P > 0.05$) or TC co-culture (1.67 ± 0.09 vs ± 1.48 ± 0.10, $P > 0.05$). Although the invasive index of the CXCR4 + CXCR7 combination group was significantly lower than the CXCL12 group (1.96 ± 0.09 vs 1.15 ± 0.04, $P < 0.01$) or TC co-culture group (1.67 ± 0.09 vs 1.10 ± 0.07, $P < 0.01$), no significant differences in invasion were observed between the CXCR4 alone and CXCR4 + CXCR7 combination groups [1.13 ± 0.04 vs 1.15 ± 0.04, $P > 0.05$ (CXCL12 treatment); 1.08 ± 0.06 vs 1.10 ± 0.07, $P > 0.05$ (TC co-culture)].

Discussion

In the present study, we confirmed the co-expression of CXCR4 and CXCR7 in human DECs in situ and in in vitro cultures at both the mRNA and protein levels. Fetal-derived TCs are the main sources of CXCL12 [12, 13, 19, 20]. Thus, it is reasonable to infer that at maternal-fetal interface, the co-expression of two receptors for a common fetal-derived chemokine in DECs might be an important mechanism by which the maternal endometrium can better coordinate with the embryo/fetus during implantation and early pregnancy via the timely "sensing" of some fetal-derived signals by maternal-derived cells.

The in vitro viability of DECs was not affected by treatment with CXCL12 or TC-CM, supporting previous findings from our team showing that the CXCL12/CXCR4 axis had no effect on the viability or PCNA expression of DSCs in vitro [12, 13]. However, in contrast to DECs and DSCs, TCs increase their own viability in vitro through CXCL12/CXCR4 binding [21]. CXCL12/CXCR4/CXCR7 signaling has also been shown to mediate the growth of several types of tumors [22–24]. Thus, a question is raised: why is the

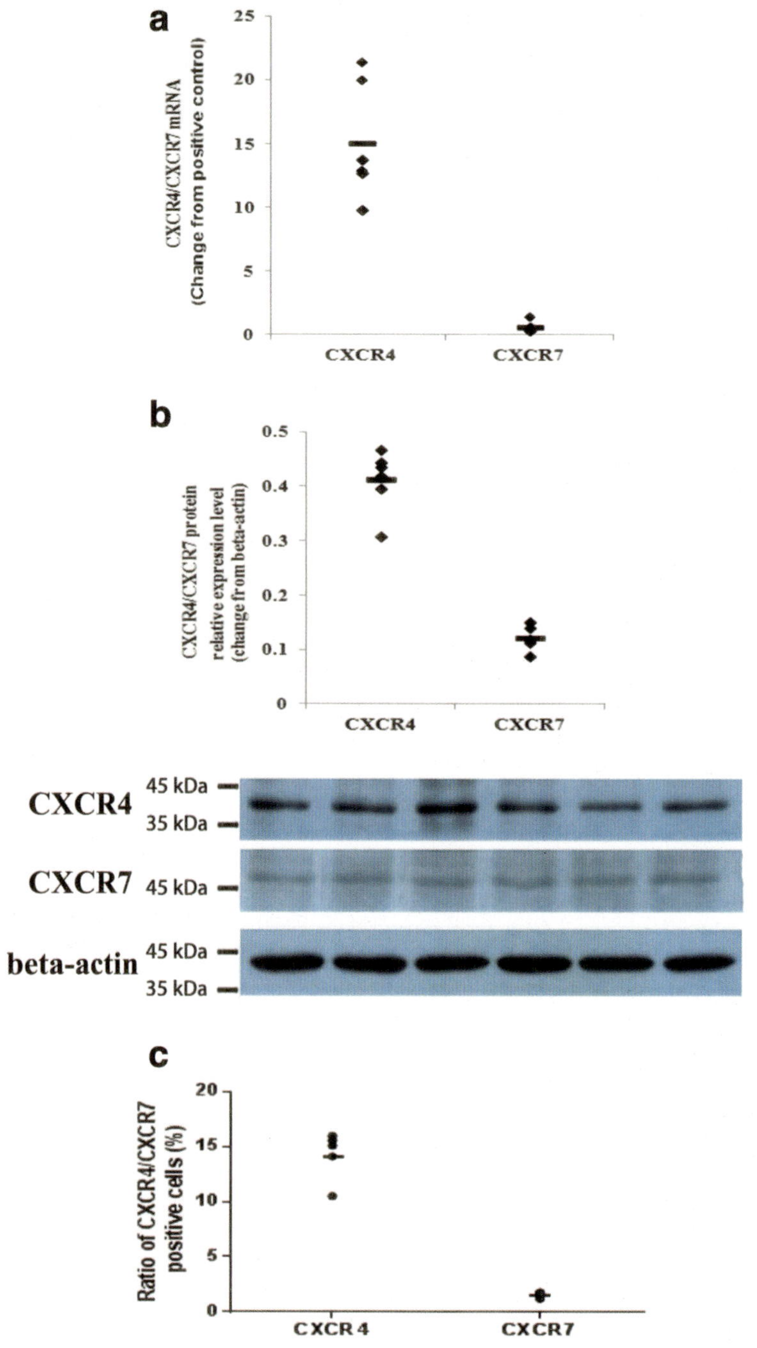

Fig. 4 Expression levels of CXCR4 and CXCR7 in primary human first-trimester decidual epithelial cell cultures. Expression of the CXCR4 and CXCR7 mRNAs and proteins was detected in primary human first-trimester decidual epithelial cell (DEC) cultures. **a** The expression of the CXCR4 and CXCR7 genes in DECs was examined by real-time PCR. The level of the CXCR4 or CXCR7 gene was equal to the ratio of the absorbance of the target gene to the control. The transverse line represents the average CXCR4 and CXCR7 levels in DECs. (n = 6). **b** The expression of CXCR4 and CXCR7 proteins in DECs was detected by western blotting. (n = 6). **c** Flow cytometry results of the expression of CXCR4 and CXCR7 on the membranes human first-trimester DECs (n = 5). The transverse line represents mean percentage of CXCR4 or CXCR7 positive cells

CXCL12/CXCR4/CXCR7 axis not required for the viability of DECs or DSCs, when they are stably co-expression in these two cell types? We postulate that this signaling pathway might exert different effects on different types of cells. During implantation and placentation, other biological functions of the maternal-derived cells rather than proliferation and viability might be more important for the crosstalk with the

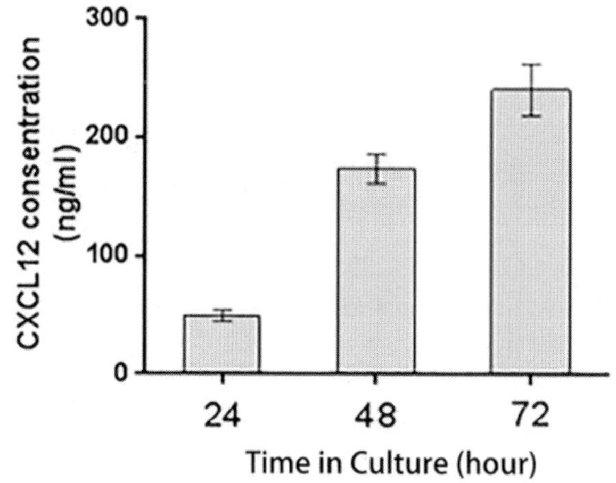

Fig. 5 Primary human first-trimester trophoblast cultures spontaneously secreted CXCL12 in vitro. Spontaneous CXCL12 secretion in supernatants of in vitro cultured TCs measured at 24, 48 and 72 h in culture.($n = 3$)

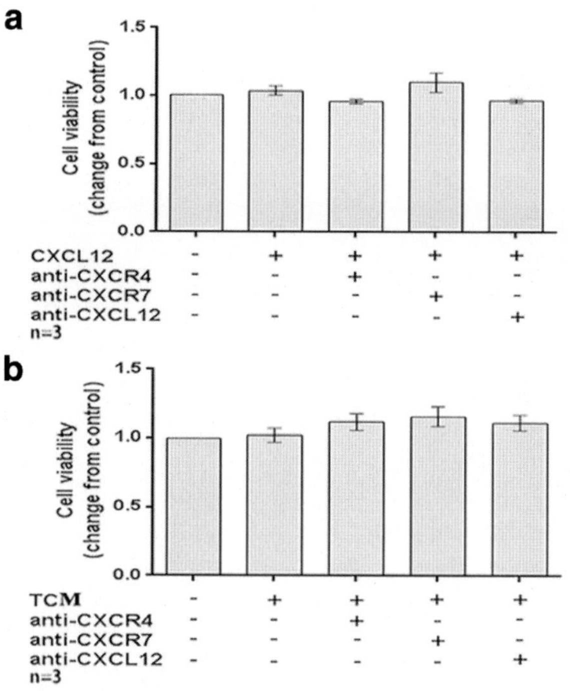

Fig. 6 The CXCL12/CXCR4/CXCR7 axis had no effect on the viability of human first-trimester DECs in vitro. The CCK-8 assay was used to explore the effects of the CXCL12/CXCR4/CXCR7 axis on decidual epithelial cell (DEC) viability. The viability index was changed compared to the corresponding control. **a** The rhCXCL12 treatment had no detectable effect on the viability of human first-trimester DECs in vitro. **b** Effects of TCM from trophoblasts on DEC viability in vitro. CXCL12: treated with 100 ng/ml recombinant human CXCL12; anti-CXCR4, treated with 20 μg/ml CXCR4 neutralizing antibody; anti-CXCR7, treated with 10 μg/ml CXCR7 neutralizing antibody; anti-CXCL12, treated with 25 μg/ml CXCL12 neutralizing antibody; TCM: trophoblast-conditioned medium. Data are presented as average ± SEM. ($n = 3$)

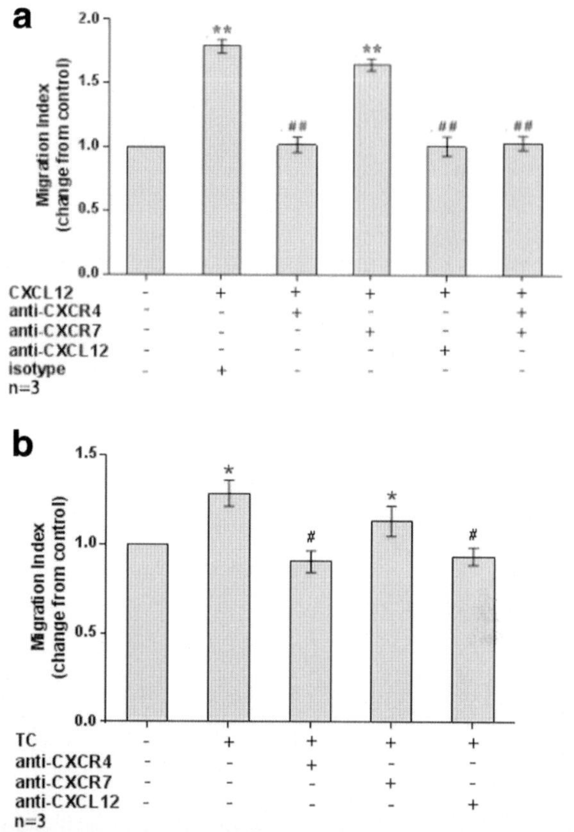

Fig. 7 TC-derived CXCL12 induced DEC migration by binding to CXCR4 rather than CXCR7. **a** The addition of CXCL12 significantly increased DECs migration in vitro, while neutralizing antibodies to CXCR4 or CXCL12 effectively inhibited the CXCL12-stimulated DEC invasiveness. The CXCR7 antibody failed to block the CXCL12-induced increase in DEC migration. ($n = 3$). **b** Co-culture with TCs significantly increased the DECs migration in vitro, and a neutralizing antibody against CXCR4 or CXCL12 effectively inhibited the CXCL12-stimulated DEC migration. The CXCR7 antibody failed to block the TC co-culture-induced increase in DEC migration. * $P < 0.05$, ** $P < 0.01$, compared to the control; # $P < 0.05$, ## $P < 0.01$, compared to the CXCL12-treated group or TC co-culture group. Data are presented as average ± SEM. ($n = 3$)

fetal-derived TCs. Of course, this assumption requires further study.

A unique strength of this study is the investigation into the modulatory effects of TCs on the motility of DECs via the CXCL12/CXCR4/CXCR7 axis. An enormous amount of research effort has examined the invasion of TCs but has neglected the motile characteristics of other type of cells at the maternal-fetal interface [25, 26]. Our knowledge of the characteristics of DEC, particularly whether DECs have the ability to migrate or invade during early pregnancy, has remained an open question until now. In the present study, DECs from early pregnancy are capable of spontaneously migrating and invading in vitro, and these abilities are further increased after stimulation with a TC-derived signal (CXCL12) and CXCR4

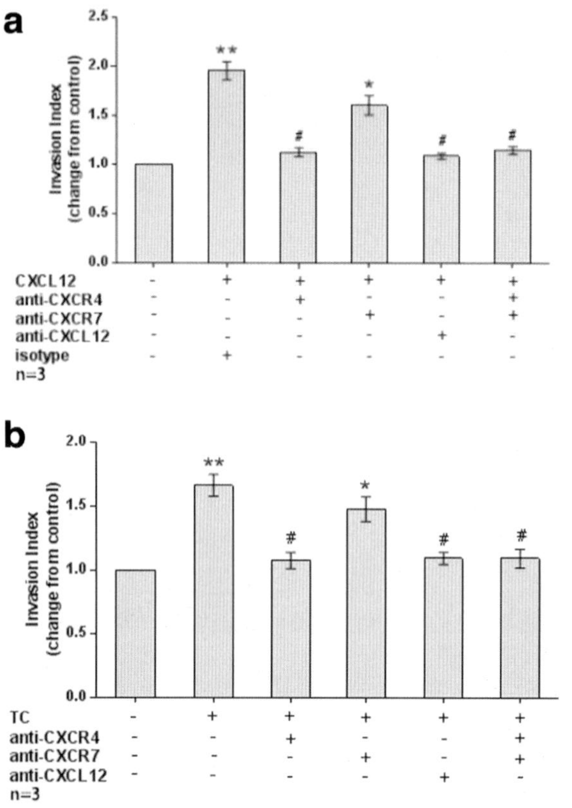

Fig. 8 TC-derived CXCL12 increased DEC invasion by binding to CXCR4 rather than CXCR7. **a** The addition of CXCL12 significantly increased the DECs invasion in vitro, while neutralizing antibody against CXCR4 or CXCL12 effectively inhibited the CXCL12-stimulated DEC invasion. The CXCR7 antibody failed to block the CXCL12-induced increase in DEC invasion. ($n = 3$). **b** Co-culture with TCs significantly increased DEC invasion in vitro, and a neutralizing antibody against CXCR4 or CXCL12 effectively inhibited the TC co-culture-stimulated DEC invasion. The CXCR7 antibody failed to block the TC co-culture-induced increase in DEC invasion. * $P < 0.05$, ** $P < 0.01$, compared to the control; # $P < 0.01$, compared to the CXCL12-treated group or TC co-culture group. Data are presented as average ± SEM. ($n = 3$)

binding. According to our previous study, human first-trimester DSCs also migrate after activation of the CXCL12/CXCR4 signaling pathway [12, 13]. Obviously, as the main maternal-derived cells at the maternal-fetal interface, both DECs and DSCs initially display motile potential after "sensing" the signal released by TCs (CXCL12) via the co-expression of the same receptor, CXCR4.

Recently, several researchers have begun to focus on the regulation of the decidua and control of TC invasion [4, 25, 27]. In animal studies, focal adhesion proteins undergo dynamic changes in their distributions in uterine luminal epithelial cells that disassembled from the site of focal adhesions at the time of implantation, facilitating the removal of uterine luminal epithelial cells for embryo invasion [28, 29]. Together with these studies, our results have caused us to re-examine some previous views on the role of the endometrium and have provided a new perspective of maternal-fetal interactions during implantation: the decidual cells, to some degree, can make way for the invading trophoblast cells.

In our opinion, the endometrium might be dynamically motile and make positive adjustments rather than merely passively waiting for the embryo to better accept the arrival of the embryo. The ability of DECs to migrate is important for obtaining a better understanding of endometrial receptivity, implantation and clinical treatments for recurrent implantation failure.

As a newly identified second receptor for CXCL12, the biological function of CXCR7 is much more complicated and controversial than CXCR4 [19, 23, 24, 30–33]. Some researchers have postulated that CXCR7 acts as a decoy receptor because of its inability to induce calcium mobilization, cell migration or integrin activation upon binding to CXCL12, [20, 23, 30] whereas others argue against this hypothesis due to the observed roles of CXCR7 in signaling activity and migration, particularly in tumor growth and metastasis [23, 31–33]. In the present work, the addition of CXCR7 neutralizing antibody failed to block the TC-induced increase in DEC invasion. However, treatment with CXCR4 or CXCL12 neutralizing antibody significantly decreased the invasive index, but no differences in the blocking effects were observed among the CXCR4 alone, CXCL12 alone and CXCR4 + CXCR7 combination groups. Thus, despite the co-expression of CXCR4 and CXCR7 in DECs, the effects of TC-derived CXCL12 on promoting DEC migration and invasion are mainly mediated by CXCR4, rather than CXCR7. The lack of CXCR7 function in CXCL12/CXCR4-mediated DEC invasion suggests that CXCR7 has a decoy function at the maternal-fetal interface. Thus, the cell type may determine whether CXCR7 activates signaling or sequesters CXCL12 upon binding.

Notably, unlike CXCR4, CXCR7 is also a receptor for CXCL11 (IFN-inducible T cell alpha chemoattractant (I-TAC), [20] and CXCL11 has been confirmed to be expressed in the uterus during the peri-implantation period [33, 34]. Moreover, CXCR3, another receptor for CXCL11, is also expressed at the maternal-fetal interface, and CXCL11/CXCR3 signaling mediates the migration of TCs and T cells [33, 34]. Therefore, we cannot exclude the possibility that CXCL12/CXCR7-mediated responses are potentially modulated by CXCL11/CXCR3 signaling. The complexity of the chemokine network at the maternal-fetal interface might be beyond our imagination, and more research is required to elucidate the interaction between the fetus and endometrium during implantation and early pregnancy. Additionally, it is very difficult for us to obtain sufficient number of abortion tissues and the sample size limits the data analysis and the soundness of the present results. Thus, there is still a long way to unveil the role of chemokine and chemokine receptor at the mateo-fetal interface.

Conclusions

As shown in the present study, CXCR4 and CXCR7 are co-expressed in human first-trimester DECs and TC-derived CXCL12 promotes the migration and invasion of DECs by binding to CXCR4, rather than CXCR7. The discovery that TC-released signals are capable of modulating the migratory and invasive behaviors of DECs contributes to a better understanding of the crosstalk in different type of cells at the maternal-fetal interface during implantation and early pregnancy, and provides new clues for the clinical treatment for recurrent implantation failure and early miscarriage.

Abbreviations

CXCL12: C-X-C motif chemokine ligand 12; CXCR4: C-X-C chemokine receptor type 4; CXCR7: C-X-C chemokine receptor type 7; DAB: 3, 30-diaminobenzidine tetrahydrochloride; DEC: Decidual epithelial cell; DMEM: Dulbecco's Modified Eagle's Medium; DSC: Decidual stroma cells; ELISA: Enzyme-linked immunosorbent assay; FBS: Fetal bovine serum; ICC: Immunocytochemistry; IHC: Immunohistochemistry; PBS: Phosphate-buffered saline; PCR: Polymerase chain reaction; rhCXCL12: Recombinant human CXCL12; TBST: Tris-buffered saline with Tween 20; TC: Trophoblast cell; TC-CM: TC-conditioned medium

Acknowledgements

We thank Professor Wei Ma in Gamete and Embryo Department Laboratory of Capital Medical University for his technical assistance. We also thank Dr. Xiaoxi Huang of Medical Research Center of Beijing Chaoyang Hospital for his help with revising the article.

Funding

This work was supported by grants from the National Natural Science Foundation of China (81471511, 81270753), the Personnel Training Plan of The Health Care System of Beijing (2013-3-021) and the Talent Development Program of Beijing Chaoyang Hospital (to Wenhui Zhou).

Authors' contributions

JYZ was responsible for performing the experiments, conducting interviews with the patients and statistically analyzing the data. HPW participated in performing the experiments. WHZ was responsible for the study design, analyzing the results, drafting the manuscript, critical discussions, and communications to the editor. All authors read and approved the manuscript.

Competing interests

The authors declare that they have no competing interests.

References

1. Valdes CT, Schutt A, Simon C. Implantation failure of endometrial origin: it is not pathology, but our failure to synchronize the developing embryo with a receptive endometrium. Fertil Steril. 2017;108(1):15–8.
2. Karizbodagh MP, Rashidi B, Sahebkar A, Masoudifar A, Mirzaei H. Implantation Window and Angiogenesis. J Cell Biochem. 2017. https://doi.org/10.1002/jcb.26088.
3. Hirota Y, Osuga Y, Hasegawa A, Kodama A, Tajima T, Hamasaki K, Koga K, Yoshino O, Hirata T, Harada M, Takemura Y, Yano T, Tsutsumi O, Taketani Y. Interleukin (IL)-1beta stimulates migration and survival of first-trimester villous cytotrophoblast cells through endometrial epithelial cell-derived IL-8. Endocrinology. 2009;150:350–6.
4. Salamonsen LA, Evans J, Nguyen HP, Edgell TA. The Microenvironment of Human Implantation: Determinant of Reproductive Success. Am J Reprod Immunol. 2016;75(3):218–25. https://doi.org/10.1111/aji.12450.
5. Hempstock J, Cindrova-Davies T, Jauniaux E, Burton GJ. Endometrial glands as a source of nutrients, growth factors and cytokines during the first trimester of human pregnancy: a morphological and immunohistochemical study. Reprod Biol Endocrinol. 2004;20:2–58.
6. Burton GJ, Jauniaux E, Charnock-Jones DS. Human early placental development: potential roles of the endometrial glands. Placenta. 2007;(Suppl A):S64–9.
7. Aplin JD, Ruane PT. J. Embryo-epithelium interactions during implantation at a glance. Cell Sci. 2017;130(1):15–22. https://doi.org/10.1242/jcs.175943.
8. Jones CJ, Choudhury RH, Aplin JD. Tracking nutrient transfer at the human maternofetal interface from 4 weeks to term. Placenta. 2015;36(4):372–80.
9. Tao Y, Li YH, Piao HL, Zhou WJ, Zhang D, Fu Q, Wang SC, Li DJ, Du MR. CD56(bright)CD25+ NK cells are preferentially recruited to the maternal/fetal interface in early human pregnancy. Cell Mol Immunol. 2015;12(1):77–86.
10. Ashley RL, Antoniazzi AQ, Anthony RV, Hansen TR. The chemokine receptor CXCR4 and its ligand CXCL12 are activated during implantation andplacentation in sheep. Reprod Biol Endocrinol. 2011;9:148.
11. Mithal DS, Ren D, Miller RJ. CXCR4 signaling regulates radial glial morphology and cell fate during embryonic spinal corddevelopment. Glia. 2013;61(8):1288–305.
12. Zhou WH, Du MR, Dong L, Yu J, Li DJ. Chemokine CXCL12 promotes the cross-talk between trophoblasts and decidual stromal cells in human first-trimester pregnancy. Hum Reprod. 2008;23:2669–79.
13. Ren L, Liu YQ, Zhou WH, Zhang YZ. Trophoblasts derived chemokine CXCL12 promotes CXCR4 expression and invasion of human first-trimester decidual stromal cells. Hum Reprod. 2012;27:366–74.
14. Zhou WH, Ren L, Liu Y, Zhang YZ. Expression of chemokine receptor CXCR7 in human first-trimester trophoblasts and decidual stromal cells. Chinese J Clin (Electronic Edition). 2013;7:1436–40.
15. Zhou WH, Wu X, Hu WD, Du MR. Co-expression of CXCR4 and CXCR7 in human endometrial stromal cells is modulated by steroid hormones. Int J Clin Exp Pathol. 2015;8:2449–60.
16. Hu W, Liu Y, Zhou W, Si L, Ren L. CXCL16 and CXCR6 are coexpressed in human lung cancer in vivo and mediate the invasion of lung cancer cell lines in vitro. Plos one. 2014;9(6):e99056.
17. Hu W, Zhen X, Xiong B, Wang B, Zhang W, Zhou W. CXCR6 is expressed in human prostate cancer in vivo and is involved in the in vitro invasion of PC3 and LNCap cells. Cancer Science. 2008 (IF:3.471);99(7):1362–1369
18. Liu YQ, Ren L, Zhou WH, Zhang YZ. Isolation, culture and identification of decidual stromal cells and decidual epithelial cells of human first-trimester pregnancy. Medical J Wuhan University. 2012;33:195–8.
19. Hanna J, Wald O, Goldman-Wohl D, Prus D, Markel G, Gazit R, Katz G, Haimov-Kochman R, Fujii N, Yagel S, Peled A, Mandelboim O. CXCL12 expression by invasive trophoblasts induces the specific migration of CD16-human natural killer cells. Blood. 2003;102:1569–77.
20. Burns JM, Summers BC, Wang Y, Melikian A, Berahovich R, Miao Z, Penfold ME, Sunshine MJ, Littman DR, Kuo CJ, Wei K, McMaster BE, Wright K, Howard MC, Schall TJ. A novel chemokine receptor for SDF-1 and I-TAC involved in cell survival, cell adhesion, and tumor development. J Exp Med. 2006;203:2201–13.
21. Wu X, Li DJ, Yuan MM, Zhu Y, Wang MY. The expression of CXCR4/ CXCL12 in first-trimester human trophoblast cells. Biol Reprod. 2004;70:1877–85.

22. Hattermann K, Mentlein R. An infernal trio: the chemokine CXCL12 and its receptors CXCR4 and CXCR7 in tumor biology. Ann Anat. 2013;195:103–10.
23. Sánchez-Martín L, Sánchez-Mateos P, Cabañas C. CXCR7 impact on CXCL12 biology and disease. Trends Mol Med. 2013;19:12–22.
24. Singh AK, Arya RK, Trivedi AK, Sanyal S, Baral R, Dormond O, Briscoe DM, Datta D. Chemokine receptor trio: CXCR3, CXCR4 and CXCR7 crosstalk via CXCL11 and CXCL12. Cytokine Growth Factor Rev. 2013;24:41–9.
25. Sharma S, Godbole G, Modi D. Decidual control of trophoblast invasion. Am J Reprod Immunol. 2016;75:341–50.
26. Baines KJ, Renaud SJ. Transcription factors that regulate trophoblast development and function. Prog Mol Biol Transl Sci. 2017;145:39–88.
27. Grewal S, Carver JG, Ridley AJ, Mardon HJ. Implantation of the human embryo requires Rac1-dependent endometrial stromal cell migration. Proc Natl Acad Sci USA. 2008;105:16189–94.
28. Diao H, Paria BC, Xiao S, Ye X. Temporal expression pattern of progesterone receptor in the uterine luminal epithelium suggests its requirement during early events of implantation. Fertil Steril. 2011;95(6):2087–93.
29. Kaneko Y, Lecce L, Day ML, Murphy CR. ß (1) and ß (3) integrins disassemble from basal focal adhesions and ß (3) integrin is later localised to the apical plasma membrane of rat uterine luminal epithelial cells at the time of implantation. Reproduction, Fertility, and Development. 2011;23(3):481–95.
30. Hartmann TN, Grabovsky V, Pasvolsky R, Shulman Z, Buss EC, Spiegel A, Nagler A, Lapidot T, Thelen M, Alon R. A crosstalk between intracellular CXCR7 and CXCR4 involved in rapid CXCL12-triggered integrin activation but not in chemokine-triggered motility of human T lymphocytes and CD34+ cells. J Leukoc Biol. 2008;84:1130–40.
31. Chen Q, Zhang M, Li Y, Xu D, Wang Y, Song A, Zhu B, Huang Y, Zheng JC. CXCR7 Mediates Neural Progenitor Cells Migration to CXCL12 Independent of CXCR4. Stem Cells. 2015;33(8):2574–85.
32. Yamada K, Maishi N, Akiyama K, Towfik Alam M, Ohga N, Kawamoto T, Shindoh M, Takahashi N, Kamiyama T, Hida Y, Taketomi A, Hida K. CXCL12-CXCR7 axis is important for tumor endothelial cell angiogenic property. Int J Cancer. 2015;137(12):2825–36.
33. Hirota Y, Osuga Y, Koga K, Yoshino O, Hirata T, Morimoto C, Harada M, Takemura Y, Nose E, Yano T, Tsutsumi O, Taketani Y. The expression and possible roles of chemokine CXCL11 and its receptor CXCR3 in the human endometrium. J Immunol. 2006;177:8813–21.
34. Nancy P, Tagliani E, Tay CS, Asp P, Levy DE, Erlebacher A. Chemokine gene silencing in decidual stromal cells limits T cell access to the maternal-fetal interface. Science. 2012;336(6086):1317–21.

2

Whether vitamin D was associated with clinical outcome after IVF/ICSI

Jing Zhao, Xi Huang, Bin Xu, Yi Yan, Qiong Zhang and Yanping Li*

Abstract

Background: There exist contradictive views on whether the vitamin D has association with clinical outcome of in vitro fertilization (IVF) and/or intracytoplasmic sperm injection (ICSI). The present meta-analysis aim to establish whether vitamin D was associated with clinical outcomes of IVF/ICSI.

Methods: MEDLINE, Google Scholar and the Cochrane Library from database inception to March 2017 were searched. Clinical studies, which evaluated the association of vitamin D level and the clinical outcomes after IVF/ICSI, were included. The Main Outcome Measures were clinical pregnancy, ongoing pregnancy, and live birth.

Results: In the analysis of clinical pregnancy, 9 cohort studies were included. Of which, 2 studies and 3 studies were identified in analyzing ongoing pregnancy and live birth, respectively. Meta-analysis showed trends toward lower clinical pregnancy [RR 0.91, (95% CI 0.77–1.07)] and higher ongoing pregnancy [RR 1.06, (95% CI 0.95–1.19)] for women with deficient level of vitamin D. The probability of live birth for women with deficient level of vitamin D was significantly lower than cases with sufficient level of vitamin D [RR 0.74, (95% CI 0.58–0.90)].

Conclusions: Deficient vitamin D was associated with decreased probability of live birth after IVF/ICSI. So vitamin D should be supplied to women with deficient level vitamin D.

Keywords: Vitamin D, Clinical pregnancy, Live birth, Assisted reproduction technology

Background

As a steroid hormone, Vitamin D exerts effect by binding with vitamin D receptor, which is a member of the nuclear receptors families [1, 2]. It was established that many tissues have vitamin D receptor, such as ovarian, endometrium, fallopian tube epithelial cells, placenta, decidual cells, hypothalamus, and pituitary [3–6]. Vitamin D plays critical role in the system of female reproduction, such as oocyte development, production of anti-Mullerian (AMH), ovarian steroidogrnrsis, endometrial receptivity, et al. It was supposed that vitamin D is associated with clinical pregnancy outcome of IVF/ICSI cycles.

So far, there were myriads of studies evaluating the association between vitamin D level and the clinical outcomes after ART. Some studies have indicated that deficient vitamin D was associated with pregnancy rate [7–13]. In contrast, some researchers found no association between vitamin D statuses with outcomes after IVF/ICSI cycles [14–18].

At present, two meta-analysis studies have evaluated the association between vitamin D level and outcomes of IVF/ICSI. One was done by Vanni et al., including three studies with 353 women. The study only compared the one outcome that is–clinical pregnancy rate, and found that deficient vitamin D was associated with lower probability of clinical pregnancy without statistically significance compared with vitamin D sufficient women [19]. The other meta-analysis, including five studies with 1238 women, compared both clinical pregnancy rate and

* Correspondence: LYP7798@126.com
Reproductive Medicine Center, Xiangya Hospital, Central South University, 87 Xiang Ya Road, Changsha, Hunan 410008, People's Republic of China

live birth rate. The results displayed that deficient vitamin D was uncorrelated with clinical pregnancy rate, but related to decreased probability of live birth [20]. Although the design of the previous meta-analysis was suitable, the samples size of some studies was small.

So, it is necessary to conduct a systematic review and meta-analysis including more suitable studies to evaluated further whether deficient level vitamin D have effect on clinical pregnancy, ongoing pregnancy, and live birth after IVF/ICSI.

Methods

Identification of the literature

MEDLINE, Google Scholar and the Cochrane Library from inception until March 2017 were searched. The terms used to search literatures were as follows: one including terms on vitamin D (vitamin D, 25-hydroxy vitamin D, 25(OH) D, 1,25-$(OH)_2D$), the other one including terms on reproductive techniques (in vitro fertilization, IVF, intracytoplasmic sperm injection, ICSI, assisted reproduction technologies, ART). Related citations were generated by combining the above terms with "AND". Only papers fully published in English were covered. These included papers were reviewed by two investigators independently, and group discussion was needed if there was any discrepancies.

Study selection and data extraction

Studies evaluated the association between serum vitamin D levels and clinical outcomes after ART were selected. The primary outcomes of interest were clinical pregnancy and/or ongoing pregnancy, and /or live birth. For studies to be eligible, outcome data (with pregnancy rate and/or ongoing pregnancy rate and/or live birth rate in women with deficient or sufficient vitamin D levels) were extracted in 2×2 tables. We also recorded the study design, treatment protocol, threshold for deficient vitamin D, number of pregnant / live birth cycles with deficient or sufficient vitamin D levels. Newcastle–Ottawa Quality Assessment Scales was used to evaluate the quality of the observational studies [21]. Two reviewers completed the quality assessment, Group discussion was needed when there was any disagreements about inclusion.

Statistical analysis

We applied the meta-analysis method to complete the comparisons of study-by-study with the risk ratios (RRs) of the individual 2×2 tables. Forest plots were used to evaluate the heterogeneity of the included studies and the I^2 value quantified heterogeneity between studies. Mantel- Haenszel Random effect models were implied according to the heterogeneity to calculate an overall RR and its 95% CI. A P-value of 0.10 rather than conventional level of 0.05 was considered to have statistical significance because of the low power of the X^2 test for heterogeneity when studies have small sample size. The meta-analysis was conducted with RevMan 5.0 (Cochrane Collaboration, Oxford, UK).

Results

Studies selection and characteristics

The search strategy yielded 52 citations, 17 of which are excluded after reviewing the titles and abstracts. Five of the 35 remaining publications were not suitable because either pregnancy or live birth data were not reported, and three papers were excluded because a 2×2 table was not extracted from the results. The remained 18 papers were reviews, meta-analysis or animal experiments. (Fig. 1).

The total number of eligible trails included in the present study was 9 (three IVF study, one ICSI study, three IVF/ICSI studies, and two oocyte donation studies) comprising 2254 couples reported clinical pregnancy rate after IVF/ICSI with 1112 pregnant cycles. 2 papers involved 784 couples also reported ongoing pregnancy rate and 3 studies involved 655 pregnant women with 238 live birth cycles.

The characteristics of included studies were depicted in Table 1. Of these 9 studies, 5 were retrospective studies and 4 were prospective studies. All the studies evaluated the vitamin D level in the serum, one study by Firouzabadi et al. [14] also examined the follicular fluid. The threshold for deficient vitamin D was 20 ng/ml in seven studies, 10 ng/ml in one study and 75 nmol/l in another study.

Meta-analysis

The present meta-analysis included 9 studies to evaluate the association between deficient level vitamin D and the clinical pregnancy outcomes after ART treatments. We found that there was a trend (without significance) toward lower in clinical pregnancy in women with deficient level of vitamin D compared with those with sufficient level of vitamin D. As the Q statistic P-value was below 0.1, there were heterogeneity of the studies ($I^2 = 68\%$, $P = 0.002$). The random effects model was implied and the combined RR was 0.91 (95% CI, 0.77, 1.07; $P = 0.26$) (Fig. 2).

Among these studies, 2 papers evaluated the association between deficient vitamin D and on ongoing pregnancy at the same time. The results indicated that a similar ongoing pregnancy rate in patients with deficient and sufficient level vitamin D. The Q statistic P-value was above 0.1, indicating homogeneity of the studies ($I^2 = 0\%$, $P = 0.39$). The fixed effects model was implied and the combined RR was 1.06 (95% CI, 0.95, 1.19; $P = 0.32$) (Fig. 3).

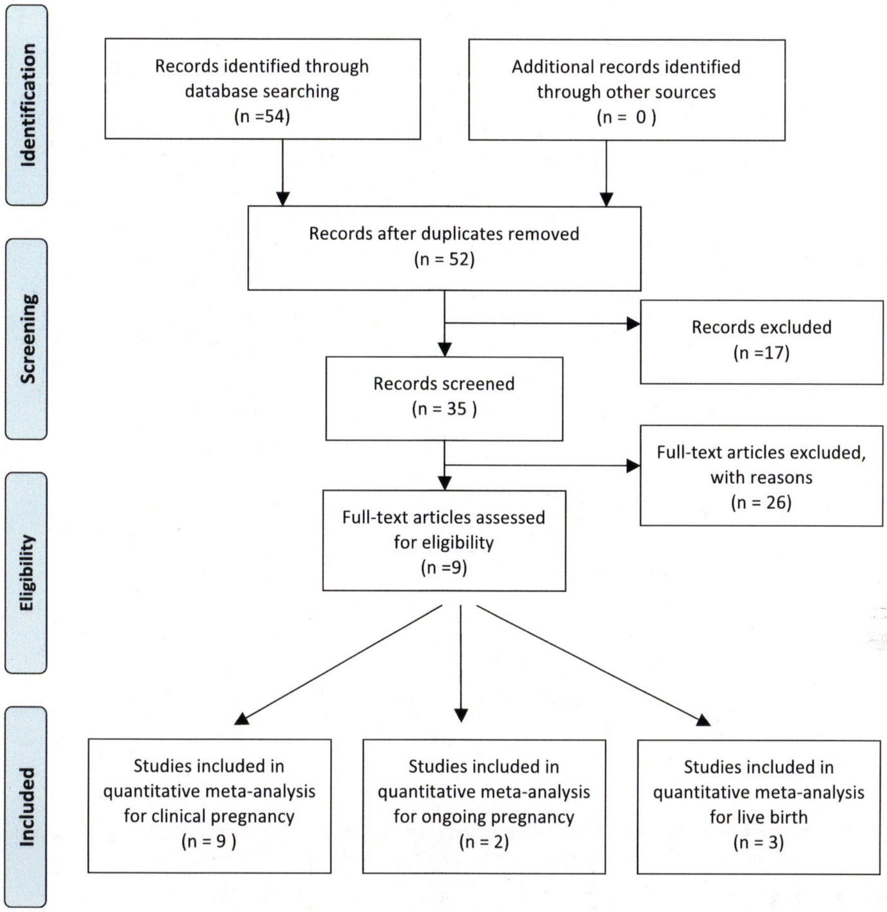

Fig. 1 Flow chart showing study selection process

Additionally, live birth rate was also evaluated and 3 studies were included. The results of meta-analysis showed a significantly lower live birth rate in women with deficient level vitamin D compared with ones with sufficient level vitamin. There was little heterogeneity in the results ($I^2 = 0\%$, $P = 0.74$). The fixed effects model combined RR was 0.72 (95% CI, 0.58, 0.90; $P = 0.004$) (Fig. 4).

The studies got high score on the Newcastle-Ottawa Quality Assessment Scale (not shown). The funnel plots of meta-analysis evaluating the association between vitamin D levels and the ongoing pregnancy and live birth after IVF/ICSI showed symmetrical shapes, indicating no publication bias (Additional file 1: Figure S1 and Additional file 2: Figure S2). However, a modest publication bias was seen when the clinical pregnancy was evaluated (Additional file 3: Figure S3).

Discussion

So far, only two systematic reviews and meta-analyses have evaluated the association between vitamin D level and the clinical outcomes of IVF/ICSI cycles. To our knowledge, the present study is the largest in regard to sample size with 3693 IVF/ICSI cycles. In the present review, 9 studies, 2 studies and 3 studies were included to evaluate the association between vitamin D and clinical pregnancy, ongoing pregnancy and live birth, respectively. Vitamin D level was statistically associated with live birth (RR 0.74; 95%CI 0.58–0.90) and was not related to clinical pregnancy (RR 0.91; 95% CI 0.77–1.07) and ongoing pregnancy (RR 1.06; 95% CI 0.95–1.19). The three RR value demonstrated that deficient vitamin D was associated with a decreased chance of live birth, while had similar probability in clinical pregnancy and ongoing pregnancy with women with sufficient vitamin D. The conclusion was agreement with the systematic reviews by Valeria et al. and Lv et al. [19, 20], but we included additional several publications and evaluated not only clinical pregnancy but also ongoing pregnancy and live birth after IVF/ICSI.

As mentioned above, Vitamin D plays an important role in the female reproductive system [3, 6]. Therefore, a woman's vitamin D level is supposed to be related to reproductive health and pregnant outcomes. The effect

Table 1 Characteristic of studies included in our meta-analysis

Studies	Country	Study design	Protocol	Sample size	The time of sample collection	Vd grouping criteria	Outcome measures	Main result	Main confounding factors
Anifandis et al. 2010 [8]	Greece	Retrospective cohort study	Short agonist protocol IVF/ICIS	101	During oocyte retrieval	< 20 ng/ml; 20.1-30 ng/ml; > 30 ng/ml	Clinical pregnancy rate (CPR)	Higher FF levels of 25(OH)D are associated with lower FF glucose levels and with lower CPR	Age BMI Oocytes retrieved (n)
Rudick et al. 2012 [10]	USA	Retrospective cohort study	Long agonist Flare-up GnRH-ant IVF/ICSI	188	After hCG administration	< 20 ng/ml; 20-30 ng/ml; > 30 ng/ml	ou	Opposite relation between 25(OH)D levels and IVF outcomes by race	Age BMI Embryos transferred (n, quality) Poor ovarian reserve
Firouzabadi et al. 2013 [14]	Iran	Prospective cohort study	Long GnRH-a protocol IVF	221	On the day of ovum pick-up	< 10 ng/ml 10-29 ng/ml 30-100 ng/ml	CPR	No significant association between FF or serum levels of 25(OH)D and CPR	None
Garbedian et al. 2013 [9]	USA	Prospective cohort study	Long GnRH-a Flare-up GnRH-ant IVF	162	Before oocyte retrieval	< 75 nmol/l ≥75 nmol/l	CPR	High vitamin D level was related to higher CPR	Age BMI Day 5[v. day3] embryo transfer
Fabris et al. 2014 [17]	Spain	Retrospective cohort study	Egg donation recipients	267	After 2 weeks of HRT	< 20 ng/ml; 20-30 ng/ml; > 30 ng/ml	CPR; Ongoing pregnancy rate	Low vitamin D level was not related to decreased CPR with egg donation.	BMI
Paffoni et al. 2014 [12]	Italy	Prospective cohort study	Long GnRH-a Flare-up GnRH-ant IVF	335	Prior to to initiation of COH	< 20 ng/ml; ≥20 ng/ml	CPR; Implantation rate	High vitamin D level was related to higher CPR	Race BMI
Polyzos et al. 2014 [13]	Belgium	Retrospective cohort study	Irrespective of the protocol Single, blastocyst IVF/ICSI	368	On the day of hCG administration	< 20 ng/ml; ≥20 ng/ml	Chemical PR CPR; Live birth rate (LBR)	Low vitamin D level was related to lower clinical pregnancy rate and live birth rate	Season of embryo transfer
Rudick et al. 2014 [11]	USA	Retrospective cohort study	Egg donation recipients	99	At the time of down-regulation	< 20 ng/ml; 20-30 ng/ml; > 30 ng/ml	CPR; LBR	Higher 25(OH)D levels associated with higher CPR and LBR	Recipient age Recipient BMI Embryos transferred (n, quality)
Franasiak et al. 2015 [18]	Canada	Retrospective cohort study	Long GnRH-a Flare-up GnRH-ant FET/ICSI	517	On the day of ovulation trigger	< 20 ng/ml; 20-30 ng/ml; > 30 ng/ml	CPR Ongoing PR	Vitamin D had no relationship with IVF outcomes	Age No. of embryo transferred Race

of deficient vitamin D level on reproduction has been investigated since the 1970s. Some studies believed that deficient vitamin D might have detrimental effect on the women infertility and pregnant outcomes of IVF [7–10]. However, other studies found that vitamin D deficiency did not play a critical role in the outcome of ART [14–16]. These discrepancies may be attributed to differences in patients' mean age, ethnicity, race, BMI, countries, social economic status, the season, exposure categorization, analysis methods, and study design [22].

Although the discrepancies between studies, the combined results indicated that vitamin D deficiency may bring negative effect on the outcome of ART. The possible mechanism may be as follows:

Firstly, it was reported that vitamin D might have effect on the development of follicle and embryo. Mice, in which the VDR genes have been knocked out, showed damaged folliculogenesis and underdevelopment of uterine in a previous animal experiments [23]. Vitamin D brought beneficial effect on the ovarian steroidogenesis and stimulated the production of Insulin-like growth factor-binding protein-1 (IGFBP-1) in ovary. Vitamin D promotes the production of estradiol, estrone, and progesterone [24]. Vitamin D level of reproductive age women was correlated with their serum AMH levels

Study or Subgroup	deficient group Events	deficient group Total	sufficient group Events	sufficient group Total	Weight	Risk Ratio M-H, Random, 95% CI
Anifandis 2010	10	25	19	61	5.4%	1.28 [0.70, 2.36]
Fabris 2014	68	92	122	175	17.0%	1.06 [0.91, 1.24]
Firouzabadi 2013	23	50	51	171	9.7%	1.54 [1.06, 2.25]
Franasiak 2015	144	206	215	311	18.2%	1.01 [0.90, 1.14]
Garbedian 2013	36	95	42	78	11.1%	0.70 [0.51, 0.98]
Paffoni 2014	30	154	56	181	9.5%	0.63 [0.43, 0.93]
Polyzos 2014	98	239	70	129	14.8%	0.76 [0.61, 0.94]
Rudick 2012	14	39	63	149	7.8%	0.85 [0.54, 1.34]
Rudick 2014	10	26	41	73	6.6%	0.68 [0.40, 1.16]
Total (95% CI)		**926**		**1328**	**100.0%**	**0.91 [0.77, 1.07]**
Total events	433		679			

Heterogeneity: $Tau^2 = 0.04$; $Chi^2 = 24.78$, df = 8 (P = 0.002); $I^2 = 68\%$
Test for overall effect: Z = 1.12 (P = 0.26)

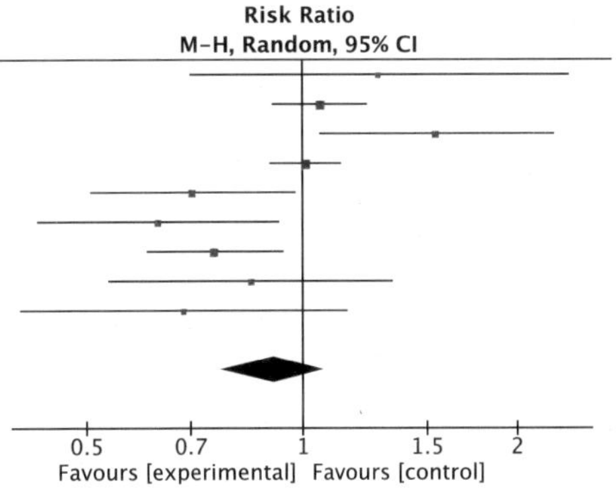

Fig. 2 Forest plot showing the results of meta-analysis of studies comparing the effect of deficient vitamin D and sufficient vitamin D on clinical pregnancy after IVF/ICSI

[25], so vitamin D may involved in the production of AMH in adults.

Secondly, Vitamin D was identified with influence upon endometrial receptivity. It was identified that vitamin D receptor was expressed in the endometrium of mice [26], whereas vitamin D receptor mutant female mice have an underdeveloped uterus and were infertile [27]. One study demonstrated the 1,25(OH) $_2D_3$ administration could up-regulate the expression of HOXA10 mRNA and protein by combining with its receptor in the endometrial stromal cells, and HOXA10 is essential for female fertility and embryo implantation [28]. This view was further supported by a vitro cell experiments with human endometrial cells lines, indicating that the 1a–hydroxylase enzyme was up-regulated in the endometrial stromal cells of early pregnancy [29]. In an oocyte donor study, adjusted clinical pregnancy rates and live birth rate were lower in VD-deficient recipients than those of vitamin D sufficient recipients. This study suggested that vitamin D might affect the reproduction through mediating the endometrium, not the follicular or oocytes [11].

Thirdly, recent researches demonstrated that vitamin D is significant not only for embryo implantation but also for gestation as well. Clinical studies have shown that pregnant women with deficient vitamin D are more likely to be with preeclampsia, gestational diabetes, and cesarean section [30–32]. Varying levels expression of vitamin D and HOXA10 were tested in the endometrium, decidua and placenta throughout pregnancy [33]. Therefore, it was suggested that vitamin D plays a crucial role in keeping healthy pregnancy [34]. These may be the possible explanations for higher ongoing pregnancy rate while lower live birth rate.

Additionally, vitamin D affects the implantation and early pregnancy by involving the immune-modulating effect. Some studies showed that vitamin D may inhibit the activity of decidual T-cell and reduce the production of some cytokines such as interleukin 1 (IL-1), IL-6 and TNF-a, which are considered to be essential for embryo implantation and endometrial receptivity [29, 35]. The vitamin leads to a transition from T helper 1(TH-1) to the more tolerant TH-2. Endometrial cells produce 1a hydroxylase, which activates 25-OH vitamin D and is up-regulated by IL-1β produced by the blastocyst. Lower level of vitamin D has a tendency to increase the percentage of B cells, INF-a producing Th cells and NK cytotoxicity, all of these were factors for RM [36].

With regard to strength, the present study leads to a more accurate evaluation with the pooled RRs rather than individual study. The pooled results of included studies indicated that deficient vitamin D was associated with decreased chance of live birth after IVF/ICSI cycles. While evaluating the association between vitamin D and clinical pregnancy and ongoing pregnancy, the combined RRs showed a decreased trend in clinical pregnancy [RR

Study or Subgroup	deficient group Events	deficient group Total	sufficient group Events	sufficient group Total	Weight	Risk Ratio M-H, Fixed, 95% CI
Fabris 2014	56	92	93	175	29.4%	1.15 [0.92, 1.42]
Franasiak 2015	131	206	193	311	70.6%	1.02 [0.90, 1.17]
Total (95% CI)		**298**		**486**	**100.0%**	**1.06 [0.95, 1.19]**
Total events	187		286			

Heterogeneity: $Chi^2 = 0.74$, df = 1 (P = 0.39); $I^2 = 0\%$
Test for overall effect: Z = 1.00 (P = 0.32)

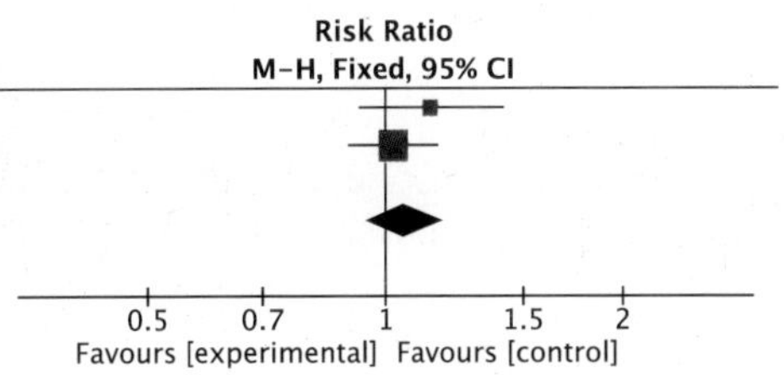

Fig. 3 Forest plot showing the results of meta-analysis of studies comparing the effect of deficient vitamin D and sufficient vitamin D on ongoing pregnancy after IVF/ICSI

Study or Subgroup	deficient group Events	Total	sufficient group Events	Total	Weight	Risk Ratio M-H, Fixed, 95% CI
Polyzos 2014	78	239	61	129	68.3%	0.69 [0.53, 0.89]
Rudick 2012	11	39	48	149	17.2%	0.88 [0.50, 1.52]
Rudick 2014	8	26	32	73	14.5%	0.70 [0.37, 1.32]
Total (95% CI)		**304**		**351**	**100.0%**	**0.72 [0.58, 0.90]**
Total events	97		141			

Heterogeneity: Chi² = 0.60, df = 2 (P = 0.74); I² = 0%
Test for overall effect: Z = 2.88 (P = 0.004)

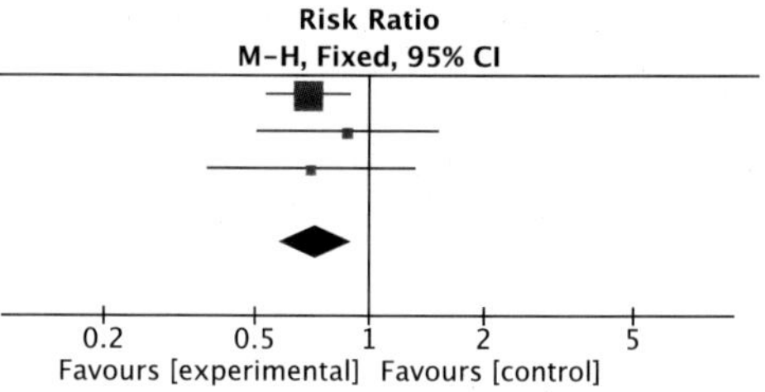

Fig. 4 Forest plot showing the results of meta-analysis of studies comparing the effect of deficient vitamin D and sufficient vitamin D on live birth after IVF/ICSI

0.91; 95% CI 0.77–1.07] and an increased trend in ongoing pregnancy [RR 1.06; 95% CI 0.94–1.19] but the differences had no significances.

Certainly, the present meta-analysis still has its limitations. A major limitation was the obvious heterogeneity among these included studies' characteristics, including varied study designs (retrospective/retrospective studies), different ovarian stimulation protocols (GnRH-a long or short protocol/GnRH-ant protocol), different treatment types (IVF / ICSI) and different threshold for deficient vitamin D level (20 ng/ml, 10 ng/ml or 75 nmol/L). In addition, small sample size of some included studies and short of meaningful confounders adjustment were also the limitations of the present study. In spite of these shortcomings, the present systematic review and meta-analysis reviewed and summarized the results of relative publications with valuable summary.

Conclusion

This systematic review showed that deficient vitamin D has negative effect on the pregnancy after IVF/ICSI treatment. As the sample sizes of some studies were small and the study characteristics were different, further random cohort studies are needed to observe the effect of vitamin D supplementation and explore the possible effect mechanisms.

Abbreviations

ART: Assisted reproductive technology; CI: Confidence interval; ICSI: Intracytoplasmic sperm injection; IR: Implantation rate; IVF: In vitro fertilization; OR: Odds ratio; PR: Pregnancy rate

Acknowledgments

Not applicable

Funding

This project was supported by the National Natural Science Foundation of China (Grant No. 81401269).

Authors' contributions

ZJ contributed to the study design and acquisition of data, article drafting and revising as well as organization of the final approval of the version to be published. HX contributed substantially to the interpretation of the data and helped with drafting and revision of the article. LY contributed to conception and design, acquisition of data and analysis and interpretation of data. YY and XB contributed significantly to the acquisition, analysis and interpretation of the data. ZQ helped with revision of the article. All authors read and approved the final manuscript.

Competing interests

The authors declare that they have no competing interests.

References

1. Halloran BP, DeLuca HF. Effect of vitamin D deficiency on fertility and reproductive capacity in the female rat. J Nutr. 1980;110:1573–80.
2. Johnson LE, HF DL. Vitamin D receptor null mutant mice fed high levels of calcium are fertile. J Nutr. 2001;131:1787–91.
3. Kinuta K, Tanaka H, Moriwake T, Aya K, Kato S, Seino Y. Vitamin D is an important factor in estrogen biosynthesis of both female and male gonads. Endocrinology. 2000;141:1317–24.
4. Hurley WL, Doane RM. Recent developments in the roles of vitamins and minerals in reproduction. J Dairy Sci. 1989;72:784–804.
5. Halhali A, Acker GM, Garabedian M. 1,25-Dihydroxyvitamin D_3 induces in vivo the decidualization of rat endometrial cells. J Reprod Fertil. 1991;91:59–64.
6. Harkness LS, Bonny AE. Calcium and vitamin D status in the adolescent: key roles for bone, body weight, glucose tolerance, and estrogen biosynthesis. J Pediatr Adolesc Gynecol. 2005;18:305–11.
7. Ozkan S, Jindal S, Greenseid K, Shu J, Zeitlian G, Hickmon C, et al. Replete vitamin D stores predict reproductive success following in vitro fertilization. Fertil Steril. 2010;94:1314–9.
8. Anifandis GM, Dafopoulos K, Messini CI, Chalvatzas N, Liakos N, Pournaras S, et al. Prognostic value of follicular fluid 25-OH vitamin D and glucose levels in the IVF outcome. Reprod Biol Endocrinol. 2010;8:91.
9. Garbedian K, Boggild M, Moody J, Liu KE. Effect of vitamin D status on clinical pregnancy rates following in vitro fertilization. CMAJ Open. 2013;1:E77–82.
10. Rudick B, Ingles S, Chung K, Stanczyk F, Paulson R, Bendikson K. Characterizing the influence of vitamin D levels on IVF outcomes. Hum Reprod. 2012;27:3321–7.
11. Rudick BJ, Ingles SA, Chung K, Stanczyk FS, Paulson RJ, Bendikson KA. Influence of vitamin D levels on in vitro fertilization outcomes in donor-recipient cycles. Fertil Steril. 2014;101:447–52.

12. Paffoni A, Ferrari S, Vigano P, Pagliardini L, Papaleo E, Candiani M, Tirelli A, Fedele L, Somigliana E. Vitamin D deficiency and infertility insights from in vitro fertilization cycles. J Clin Endocrinol Metal. 2014;99:1–9.
13. Polyzos NP, Anckaert E, Guzman L, Schiettecatte J, Landuyt LV, Camus M, Smitz J, Tournaye H. Vitamin D deficiency and pregnancy rates in women undergoing single embryo, blastocyst stage, transfer (SET) for IVF/ICSI. Hum Reprod. 2014;29:2032–40.
14. Firouzabadi RD, Rahmani E, Rahsepar M, Firouzabadi MM. Value of follicular fluid vitamin D in predicting the pregnancy rate in an IVF program. Arch Gynecol Obstet. 2014;289:201–6.
15. Aleyasin A, Hosseini MA, Mahdavi A, Safdarian L, Fallahi P, Mohajeri MR, et al. Predictive value of the level of vitamin D in follicular fluid on the outcome of assisted reproductive technology. Eur J Obstet Gynecol Reprod Biol. 2011;159:132–7.
16. Van de Vijver A, Drakopoulos P, Van Landuyt L, Vaiarelli A, Blockeel C, Santos-Ribeiro S, et al. Vitamin D deficiency and pregnancy rates following frozen–thawed embryo transfer: a prospective cohort study. Hum Reprod. 2016;31:1749–54.
17. Fabris A, Pacheco A, Cruz M, Puente JM, Fatemi H, Garcia-Velasco JA. Impact of circulating levels of total and bioavailable serum vitamin D on pregnancy rate in egg donation recipients. Fertil Steril. 2014;102:1608–12.
18. Franasiak JM, Molinaro TA, Dubell EK, Scott KL, Ruiz AR, Forman EJ, et al. Vitamin D levels do not affect IVF outcomes following the transfer of euploid blastocysts. Am J Obstet Gynecol. 2015;212:315e1–6.
19. Vanni VS, Vigano P, Somigliana E, Papaleo E, Paffoni A, Pagliardini L, et al. Vitamin D and assisted reproduction technologies: current concepts. Reprod Biol Endocrinol. 2014;12:47.
20. Lv SS, Ji YW, Wang XQ, Wang Y, Yong X. Serum vitamin D status and in vitro fertilization outcomes: a systematic review and meta-analysis. Arch Gynecol Obstet. 2016;293:1339–45.
21. Wells G, SBOD. The Newcastle-Ottawa Scale (NOS) for Assessing the Quality of non-randomised Studies in Meta-analysis, Improving Quality and Impact. Oxford: Proceedings or the Third Symposium on Systematic Reviews beyond the Basics; 2000.
22. Nesby-O'Dell S, Scanlon KS, Cogswell ME, Gillespie C, Hollis BW, Looker AC, et al. Hypovitaminosis D prevalence and determinants among African American and white women of reproductive age: third National Health and nutrition examination survey, 1988-1994. Am J Clin Nutr. 2002;76:187–92.
23. Yoshizawa T, Handa Y, Uematsu Y, Takeda S, Sekine K, Yoshihara Y, et al. Mice lacking the vitamin D receptor exhibit impaired bone formation, uterine hypoplasia and growth retardation after weaning. Nat Genet. 1997;16:391–6.
24. Parikh G, Varadinova M, Suwandhi P, Araki T, Rosenwaks Z, Poretsky L, et al. Vitamin D regulates steroidogenesis and insulin-like growth factor binding protein-1 (IGFBP-1) production in human ovarian cells. Horm Metab Res. 2010;42:754.
25. Aflatoonian A, Mashayekhy M, Mohamadian F, Moghaddam FM. The correlation between follicular fluid anti-mullerian hormone levels and fertilization and embryo quality in ART cycles. Iran J Reprod Med. 2010;8:157–60.
26. Zarnani AH, Shahbazi M, Salek-Moghaddam A, Zareie M, Tavakoli M, Ghasemi J, et al. Vitamin D(3) receptor is expressed in the endometrium of cycling mice throughout the estrous cycle. Fertil Steril. 2010;93:2738–43.
27. Johnson LE, Deluca HF. Vitamin D receptor null mutant mice fed high levels of calcium are fertile. J Nutrition. 2001;131:1787–91.
28. Lerchbaum E, Obermayer-Pietsch B. Mechanisms in endocrinology: vitamin D and fertility: a systematic review. Eur J Endocrinol. 2012;166:765–78.
29. Vigano P, Lattuada D, Mangioni S, Ermellino L, Vignali M, Caporizzo E, et al. Cycling and early pregnant endometrium as a site of regulated expression of the vitamin D system. J Mol Endocrinol. 2006;36:415–24.
30. Merewood A, Mehta SD, Chen TC, Bauchner H, Holick MF. Association between severe vitamin D deficiency and primary caesarean section. J Clin Endocrinol Metab. 2009;94:940–5.
31. Shand AW, Nassar N, Von Dadelszen P, Innis SM, Green TJ. Maternal vitamin D status in pregnancy and adverse pregnancy outcomes in a group at high risk for pre-eclampsia. BJOG. 2010;117:1593–8.
32. Soheilykhah S, Mojibian M, Rashidi M, Rahimi-Saghand S, Jafari F. Maternal vitamin D status in gestational diabetes mellitus. Nutr Clin Pract. 2010;25:524–7.
33. Evans KN, Nguyen L, Chan J, Innes BA, Bulmer JN, Kilby MD, et al. Effects of 25-hydroxyvitamin D3 and 1,25-dihydroxyvitamin D3 on cytokine production by human decidual cells. Biol Reprod. 2006;75:816–22.
34. Bodnar LM, Catov JM, Simhan HN, Holick MF, Powers RW, Roberts JM. Maternal vitamin D deficiency increases the risk of preeclampsia. J Clin Endocrinol Metab. 2007a;92:3517–22.
35. Pasco JA, Wark JD, Carlin JB, Ponsonby A-L, Vuillermin PJ, Morley R. Maternal vitamin D in pregnancy may influence not only offspring bone mass but other aspects of musculoskeletal health and adiposity. Med Hypothes. 2008;71:266–9.
36. Chen X, Yin B, Lian R-C, Zhang T, Zhang H-Z, Diao L-H, et al. Modulatory effects of vitamin D on peripheral cellular immunity in patiens with recurrent miscarriage. Am J Reprod Immunol. 2016;76:432–8.

Maternal physical activity before IVF/ICSI cycles improves clinical pregnancy rate and live birth rate

Meng Rao[1], Zhengyan Zeng[2] and Li Tang[1*]

Abstract

Objective: This meta-analysis was aimed to evaluate the association between maternal physical activity before IVF/ICSI cycles and reproductive outcomes.

Methods: We searched databases of PubMed, EMBASE and Web of Science electronic databases, and ongoing trials up to November 2017 to identify studies that focused on the relationship between maternal physical activity before IVF/ICSI cycles and reproductive outcomes, including implantation rate, clinical pregnancy rate, miscarriage rate and live birth rate. Odds ratio (OR) with 95% confidence intervals, were calculated to assess the results of each outcome.

Results: Eight published studies encompassing 3683 infertile couples undergoing IVF/ICSI treatment were included into the analysis. There was an increasing, but not statistically significant, trend in implantation rate for physically active women when compared with physically inactive women (OR = 1.95, 95% CI 0.99–3.83, $I^2 = 77\%$). No significant difference was found in miscarriage rate between physically active women and physically inactive women (OR = 0.76, 95% CI 0.41–1.44, $I^2 = 49\%$). However, rates of clinical pregnancy and live births in physically active women were significantly higher than those in physically inactive women (OR = 1.96, 95% CI 1.40, 2.73, $I^2 = 42\%$ and OR = 1.95, 95% CI 1.06–3.59, $I^2 = 82\%$, respectively). Subgroup analysis helped to confirm these results.

Conclusions: Female physical activity before IVF/ICSI cycles was associated with increased rates of clinical pregnancy and live births, whereas only a small but not statistically significant increase was found in implantation rate, and no effect was shown on miscarriage rate.

Keywords: Physical activity, ART, IVF/ICSI, Reproductive outcome

Background

The prevalence of infertility is estimated to be 12–15% in couples of childbearing age [1, 2]. Even though the development of assisted reproductive technology (ART) has helped many couples achieve pregnancies, the rates of pregnancy and live births among all ART-treated couples is still not satisfactory. How to improve assisted reproductive outcome has become a critical topic for both infertile couples and clinicians.

Physical activity is generally considered to be a health promoting behaviour as it is associated with reduced risks of cardiovascular disease, diabetes and cancers [3, 4]. A number of epidemiological studies have focused on the effects of physical activity on fertility, but no consensus has been reached until now [5–7]. Most of the investigators reported that moderate physical activity benefits female fertility [5–7], whereas high intensity and frequency of physical activity increase subfertility and infertility, mainly ovulatory infertility [6], and increasing vigorous physical activity is associated with delayed time to spontaneous pregnancy [7]. Similar conclusions were also reached in athletes, who have been shown to have a higher

* Correspondence: tanglikm@163.com
[1]Department of reproduction and genetics, the First Affiliated Hospital of Kunming Medical University, No. 295 Xi Chang road, Kunming 650032, China
Full list of author information is available at the end of the article

prevalence of reproductive dysfunction compared with non-athletes [8, 9].

Physical activity during pregnancy has been shown to improve reproductive outcome [10, 11]. However, no consensus has been reached regarding the effect of physical activity before ART on pregnancy outcome [12–14]. A population-based cohort study [12] showed that women engaged in physical activity for ≥4 h/week had a 40% decreased likelihood of live birth in in vitro fertilization (IVF) cycles compared with women not regularly engaged in physical activity. This conclusion was supported by some other investigations focusing on IVF or intracytoplasmic sperm injection (ICSI) cycles [13, 15, 16]. Whereas a randomized controlled trial (RCT) [17] showed no differences in pregnancies or live births between the physical activity intervention and control groups. Gaskins et al. [14] also found that time spent in moderate to vigorous physical activities and total metabolic equivalent task hours before IVF were not associated with probability of implantation, clinical pregnancy or live birth.

Therefore, in this systemic review and meta-analysis, we aimed to evaluate the association between maternal physical activity before IVF/ICSI cycles and reproductive outcomes, to provide a comprehensive analysis of the current data and a context for how to counsel infertile couples and physicians trying to improve the success rate of assisted reproductive treatment.

Methods

Literature search

A systematic literature review was performed to identify all published studies on PubMed, EMBASE and Web of Science electronic databases, and Clinicaltrails.gov up to November 2017. The search was limited to human studies published in English. The following terms were used to search the databases: ("physical activity OR physical active OR physical non-active OR exercise") AND ("assisted reproductive OR IVF OR ICSI"). The reference lists of the relevant publications were also manually searched for related studies. Two researchers independently completed the literature search and identified the eligible studies. Conflicting decisions were resolved through consensus with a third researcher. The studies were included if they satisfied the following criteria: 1) infertile couples treated with ART, 2) pregnancy outcomes were compared between physical active and non-active women, or women with different levels of physical activity, and 3) pregnancy outcomes included implantation rate, clinical pregnancy rate, miscarriage rate or live birth rate. The implantation rate should be calculated as the ratio of the number of gestational sacs/number of transferred embryos; the clinical pregnancy should be diagnosed by ultrasonography 4 weeks after embryo transfer; the miscarriage rate was defined as the number of miscarriages in the first 20 weeks of gestation per clinical pregnancy; and the live birth rate was defined as the number of deliveries that resulted in at least one live-born baby per initiated cycle. The studies were excluded if 1) the subjects were athletes; 2) they were published as an abstract, letter to editor, case report or review; and 3) they failed to provided enough data for data analysis.

Data extraction

Two reviewers independently extracted the data from the included articles according to the following information: first author, year of publication, country, number of patients, age, body mass index (BMI), physical activity intensity, treatment and pregnancy outcomes. We needed the data to be expressed as the odds ratio (OR) and 95% confidence interval (CI). If not, the data were extracted and then transferred to this form according to specific statistical methods. In addition, data from different subgroups were extracted for possible synthesis if necessary. The corresponding author was contacted for more information if the data presented in the article was inadequate for analysis.

Quality assessment of included studies

A total of 8 studies were eligible and enrolled into the meta-analysis, 7 of which were cohort studies, so the Newcastle-Ottawa Quality Assessment Scale (NOS) was used for the quality assessment [18]. The NOS evaluates a high quality study from the three aspects: selection of participants, comparability of study groups, and the ascertainment of outcomes of interest. A score of 6–9 is considered to suggest a high quality and low risks of bias. Discrepancies were resolved through consensus. For another randomised controlled trial (RCT) published by Moran et al. [17], the Cochrane risk of bias tool was applied to evaluate the quality based on randomization, blinding of outcome assessment, completeness of outcome assessment, selective reporting, and other bias [19]. Each domain was categorized as low, high, or unclear.

Quality of evidence

The quality of the evidence for all outcomes were assessed using the criteria of the Grading of Recommendations Assessment, Development and Evaluation (GRADE) system (study limitations, consistency of effect, imprecision, indirectness, and publication bias), which specifies four levels of evidence: high, moderate, low, and very low quality evidence [20, 21]. The quality of evidence could be downgraded by one or two levels if serious or very serious deficiencies in these criteria were considered.

Statistical analysis

All analyses were performed with Review Manager version 5.2 software (The Cochrane Collaboration). A standard meta-analytic method was used to compare the studies included in this study, and the odds ratio (OR) with its 95% CI was applied to express the combined result. A random-effects model was used. The degree of heterogeneity was also measured by the I^2 statistic, where $I^2 > 50\%$ was regarded as an indicator of significant heterogeneity [22]. Evaluation of inter-study variance was performed by calculating Tau^2, which represents the estimated standard deviation of underlying effects across studies. Subgroup analysis was also conducted to further analyze the effect of physical activity on pregnancy outcome based on the following aspects: controlling for important potential confounders, principally age and BMI (Yes or No) and whether the intensity of exercise in physically active women was > 2.5 h/week in each study (Yes or No/Not clear). The level of statistical significance was set at $P < 0.05$.

Results

Literature search

The literature search resulted in 273 articles for review, including 2 additional studies identified by manual search. After removing duplicate studies and reviewing titles and abstracts, 19 full-text articles were screened and assessed for eligibility. Thereafter, another 11 articles were excluded because these studies either focused on male but not female physical activity ($n = 3$), or they did not provide data on implantation rate, pregnancy rate, miscarriage rate or live birth rate ($n = 8$). Finally, 8 full-text studies comprising 3683 infertile couples were included in this meta-analysis [12–17, 23, 24]. Figure 1 shows the flow diagram of the selection process. Morris et al. [12] collected the data on physical activity by using a simple questionnaire described in the text. Ferreira et al. [23] used a validated lifestyle questionnaire reported elsewhere [25]. Both Kucuk et al. [16] and Ramezanzadeh et al. [24] used the original International Physical Activity Questionnaires in their studies (http://uacc.arizona.edu/sites/default/files/ipaq_english_telephone_short.pdf). The physical activity in the Moran et al. [17] study was a home-based physical conditioning and walking program as described elsewhere [26]. Evenson et al. [15] used a modified Kaiser Physical Activity Survey [27] that was described in detail in another study [28]. The questionnaire used in the Palomba et al. [13] study was formulated on the basis of the well-validated Global Physical Activity Questionnaire (www.who.int/chp/steps/GPAQ%20Instrument%20and%20Analysis%20 Guide%20v2.pdf). In the Gaskins et al. [14] study, another validated questionnaire was used for data collection [29]. The characteristics of these studies are summarized in Table 1.

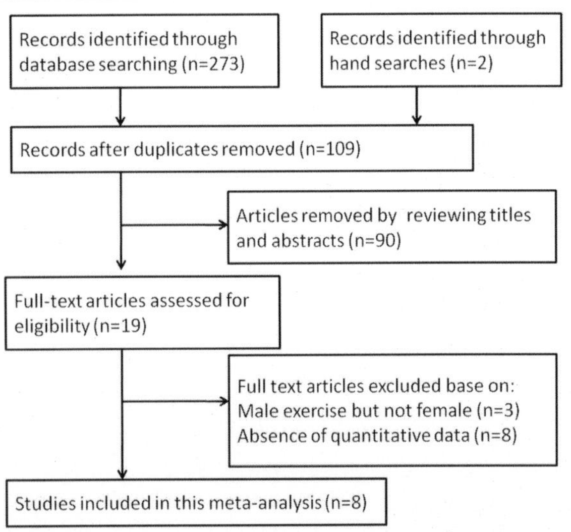

Fig. 1 Flow chart for selection of eligible studies

Quality assessment

As shown in Table 2, the observational studies had a Newcastle-Ottawa Scale score ranging from 7 to 8, suggesting a low risk of bias. The category most often missed by studies was comparability because only age and/or BMI were adjusted for confounding in all included studies, many other factors like duration of infertility, male factors etc. were also critical for the outcomes of ART. The RCT had low risk of bias in the domains of random sequence generation, blinding of outcome assessment, incomplete outcome data and selective reporting, and had high risk of bias in allocation concealment. Whereas there was unclear risk of bias in the aspect of blinding of participants and personnel.

Implantation rate

Only three of the eight included studies reported the implantation rate [13, 16, 24], of which two showed improvement of the implantation rate, and the other presented no obvious association. As a group, the studies in this meta-analysis did not show a significant difference in implantation rate for women performing regular physical activity; however, there was a trend toward the association of physical activity before IVF/ICSI cycles with implantation rate (OR = 1.95, 95% CI 0.99–3.83, $n = 583$, $I^2 = 77\%$, low quality evidence), even though heterogeneity existed (Fig. 2).

Clinical pregnancy rate

Seven of the included studies presented data on clinical pregnancy rate [13–17, 23, 24]. Five of the studies showed a significant increase in clinical pregnancy rate among women who undertook regular physical activity, and the remaining articles failed to find any association.

Table 1 Summary of included studies

Author/year	No. of infertile couples	Treatment	Study type	Contrast	Evaluation of physical activity	Controlling for confounders	Pregnancy outcomes
Morris/2006	2232	IVF	Prospective	Regular exercise > 1 h/week versus no regular exercise	Simple questionnaires	Age, BMI	Miscarriage rate; Live birth rate
Ferreira/2010	436	ICSI	Prospective	Regular exercise at least 1 h for 3 times/week versus no regular exercise	Validated lifestyle questionnaire	Age	Miscarriage rate; Clinical pregnancy rate
Kucuk/2010	131	ICSI	Prospective	Moderate physical activity versus low physical activity	IPAQ [a]	Age, BMI	Implantation rate; Clinical pregnancy rate; Miscarriage rate; Live birth rate
Moran/2011	38	IVF	Prospective	Exercise and diet intervention versus control	Patients participated in the Comprehensive Lifestyle Intervention Program (CLIP)	Age, BMI	Clinical pregnancy rate; Miscarriage rate; Live birth rate
Ramezanzadeh /2012	236	IVF/ICSI	Prospective	More than 3 h/week moderate-intensity exercise or 5 h/week low-intensity exercise versus not	IPAQ [a]	None	Implantation rate; Clinical pregnancy rate
Evenson/2014	121	IVF	Prospective	Total activity index ≥10.6 versus < 10.6	Modified Kaiser Physical Activity Survey	Age, BMI	Clinical pregnancy rate; Live birth rate
Palomba/2016	216	IVF/ICSI	Prospective	Regular physical activity versus no regular physical activity	Self-administered semiquantitative general health questionnaires formulated on the basis of Global Physical Activity Questionnaire	Age, BMI	Implantation rate; Clinical pregnancy rate; Miscarriage rate; Live birth rate
Gaskins/2016	273	IVF	Prospective	Total physical activity> 2.5 h/week versus ≤2.5 h/week	A validated questionnaire	None	Clinical pregnancy rate; Miscarriage rate; Live birth rate

[a]*IPAQ* International Physical Activity Questionnaires

Meta-analysis of all 7 of these studies showed an overall increase in clinical pregnancy rate among those undertaking regular exercise compared with no regular exercise (OR = 1.96, 95% CI 1.40–2.73, $n = 1451$, $I^2 = 42\%$, moderate quality evidence), with non-significant heterogeneity (Fig. 2). In 4 of the 7 studies, age and BMI were controlled between the physically active and inactive women. When combining these studies, subgroup meta-analysis showed an increase in the clinical pregnancy rate among physically active women when compared with physically inactive women (OR = 2.92, 95% CI 1.89–4.52). The other three studies, which were not well controlled for age and BMI, also showed a significant increase in clinical pregnancy rate when the subjects undertook regular physical activity (OR = 1.50, 95% CI 1.04–2.15). In three of the seven studies, physically active women exercised for more than 2.5 h/week, and when we combined these studies, the results showed a 1.49-fold increase in clinical pregnancy rate for physically active women in comparison with control subjects (95% CI 1.04–2.15). In the other four studies, the authors did not clearly present the intensity of physical activity, or the exercise intensity in the physically active women was not more than 2.5 h/week. Nevertheless, the combination of these studies still showed an increase in the clinical pregnancy rate for physically active women (OR = 2.92, 95% CI 1.89–4.52), as shown in Table 3.

Table 2 Quality assessment of included studies

Author/year	Selection	Exposure	Comparability	Total score
Morris/2006	3	3	1	7
Ferreira/2010	4	3	1	8
Kucuk/2010	4	3	1	8
Ramezanzadeh/2012	4	3	0	7
Evenson/2014	4	3	1	8
Palomba/2016	4	3	1	8
Gaskins/2016	4	3	0	7

Newcastle-Ottawa Quality Assessment Scale (NOS) was used for the quality assessment

Miscarriage rate

Six articles included data on miscarriage rate, and all showed no significant difference in miscarriage rate between physically active and inactive women [12–14, 16, 17, 23]. The meta-analysis showed no significant association of

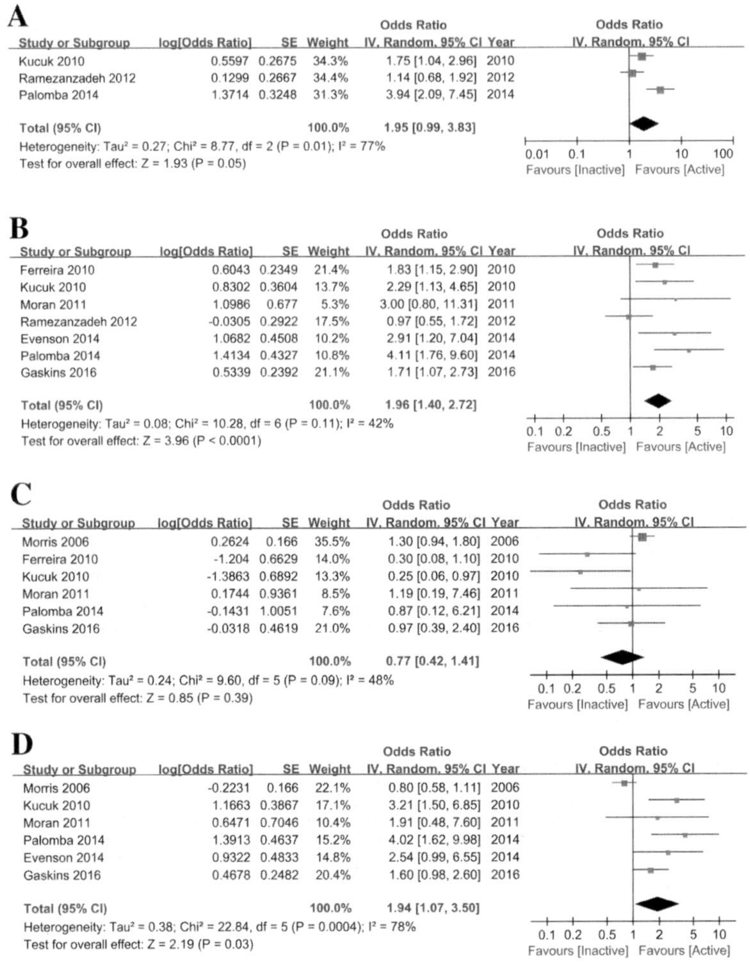

Fig. 2 Forest plot (random-effects model) of physical activity before IVF/ICSI cycles and pregnancy outcome following IVF/ICSI cycles. **a** implantation rate; (**b**) clinical pregnancy rate; (**c**) miscarriage rate and (**d**) live birth rate

physical activity with miscarriage rate (OR = 0.76, 95% CI 0.41–1.44, n = 3326, I^2 = 49%, low quality evidence), with an acceptable heterogeneity (Fig. 2). In subgroup analysis, the combined results were very similar between the studies controlled for age and BMI and those in which age and BMI were not well controlled (OR = 0.85, 95% CI 0.37–1.92 and OR = 0.59, 95% CI 0.19–1.84, respectively). Combined results for age and BMI were also very consistent when the studies were stratified by exercise intensity in the physically active women (OR = 0.60, 95% CI 0.19–1.85 and OR = 0.83, 95% CI 0.34–2.06, respectively), as shown in Table 3.

Live birth rate

Six studies reported data on live birth rate [12–17], among which 2 studies showed a significant increase in live birth rate for women who exercised regularly when compared with those who did not. Two other studies presented an increasing, but not statistically significant, trend for live birth rate. Additionally, another population-based study indicated a decreasing trend in live birth rate for physical active women even though the decrease was not statistically significant. The meta-analysis showed a positive association between physical activity and live birth rate (OR = 1.95, 95% CI 1.06–3.59, n = 3011, I^2 = 82%, low quality evidence), but heterogeneity existed (Fig. 2). In the subgroup analysis, combination of the results of the 5 studies controlled for age and BMI showed no obvious effect of physical activity on the live birth rate (OR = 2.10, 95% CI 0.90–4.86, I^2 = 85%), whereas the pooled results changed significantly when the study by Morris et al. [12] was removed (OR = 3.03, 95% CI 1.90–4.84, I^2 = 0). The combined results showed an increase in live birth rate among women undertaking regular exercise (OR = 1.63, 95% CI 1.03–2.58, I^2 = 0) for those studies in which exercise intensity was > 2.5 h/week. Nevertheless, the live birth rate was not significantly affected in the studies in which exercise intensity was not > 2.5 h/week or not clearly described (OR = 2.16, 95% CI 0.84–5.54, I^2 = 88%), as shown in Table 3.

Table 3 Subgroup analysis for the effect of maternal physical activity on pregnancy outcome following IVF/ICSI

Subgroup	No. of studies	OR (95% CI)	Tau^2	I^2	$P_{subgroup}$
Age, BMI controlling					
Clinical pregnancy rate					
Yes	4	2.92 (1.89–4.52)	0	0	
No	3	1.50 (1.04–2.15)	0.04	38	0.02
Miscarriage rate					
Yes	4	0.85 (0.37–1.92)	0.32	46	
No	2	0.59 (0.19–1.84)	0.36	52	0.62
Live birth rate					
Yes	5	2.10 (0.90–4.86)	0.72	85	
No	1	1.60 (0.98–2.60)	N/A	N/A	0.58
Exercise > 2.5 h/week in physical active women					
Clinical pregnancy rate					
Yes	4	1.56 (1.11–2.21)	0.03	27	
NO/ Not clear[a]	3	2.91 (1.83–4.62)	0	0	0.03
Miscarriage rate					
Yes	3	0.71 (0.32–1.55)	0.09	16	
NO/ Not clear[a]	3	0.70 (0.19–2.56)	0.77	64	0.99
Live birth rate					
Yes	2	1.65 (1.07–2.56)	0	0	
NO/ Not clear[a]	4	2.16 (0.84–5.54)	0.79	88	0.62

The subgroup analysis was not conducted on implantation rate since there were only 3 studies reported this data

OR odds ratio, *CI* confidence interval, *N/A* not applicable

[a]Intensity of physical activity was not > 2.5 h/week in physical active women in these studies, or the data was not clearly described

Discussion

To our knowledge, this is the first meta-analysis to evaluate the relationship between female physical activity before IVF/ICSI cycles and ART outcomes. We found that physical activity before IVF/ICSI cycles is associated with better assisted reproductive outcomes, mainly based on the increase in the rates of clinical pregnancy and live birth, and also a small but not statistically significant increase in the implantation rate, whereas the miscarriage rate was not associated with physical activity in women before ART cycles. These results suggested that exercise before IVF/ICSI cycles may clearly help physically inactive women to improve their chance of a successful pregnancy.

The effect of exercise on fertility and IVF outcomes has been a subject of considerable dispute. A recent population-based cohort study indicated that moderate exercise is associated with better clinical outcomes, regardless of BMI [7]. In 2008, the (United States Department of Health and Human Services (USDHHS) released in the "Physical Activity Guidelines for Americans" which recommended at least 150 min of moderate-intensity physical activity per week for pregnant women without obstetric/medical complications [30]. However, until now, no population-based RCT was conducted to show whether moderate physical activity prior to IVF/ICSI was beneficial to ART outcomes. The only RCT enrolled 38 overweight/obese women who received lifestyle intervention (exercise and weight-loss diet) or standard treatment for 5–9 weeks before oocyte pick-up. The results showed no significant improvement of clinical pregnancy and live birth in intervention patients compared with control. However, the small sample size in that study may be insufficient to draw a solid conclusion. In this meta-analysis, we provided a comprehensive analysis of the current data and found a 1.96-fold and 1.94-fold increase of clinical pregnancy rate and live birth rate, respectively, in physical active women compared with physical inactive women. Whereas no significant differences were found in implantation rate and miscarriage rate. According to the GRADE criteria, the combined results were assessed with moderate to low quality evidence, since most included studies were prospective cohort studies, and cofounders like dietary pattern, duration of physical activity as well as male factors in patients would affect clinical outcomes. Additionally, heterogeneity among studies existed in every clinical outcome. Considering that the following two aspects may affect the combined results: 1) age and BMI were critical confounders affecting IVF/ICSI outcomes [27–29], but were not controlled in some of included studies; 2) Intensity of physical activity was not consistent among included studies, we performed sub-group analysis to further evaluate the relationship between physical activity before IVF/ICSI cycles and clinical outcomes. As a result, we found very similar pooled effects in comparison with the overall results, suggesting that the effect of physical activity on pregnancy outcome was independent of age and weight loss. Additionally, in most of the included studies, patients reduced their physical activity when pregnancy was achieved. This may help to exclude the effect of physical activity during pregnancy on assisted reproductive outcomes, and this has been shown in several studies [31–33].

The mechanisms by which physical activity prior to IVF/ICSI cycles improves pregnancy outcome may be very complex, and no molecular pathway has been identified. The most relevant determinants of regular physical activity on reproductive outcome seem to be mainly related to its effect on the clinical pregnancy rate. This may be due to the following reasons: First, physical activity performed to improve health status may promote changes in energy balance, which, in turn, is tightly correlated with the reproductive system [34]. Second, physical activity may improve the assisted reproductive outcome through insulin sensitization, restore ovarian function [35] and sensitize the ovary to clomiphene citrate during simple ovulation induction [36]. Many infertile women are characterized by obesity, which is positively associated with insulin resistance, for instance, in polycystic ovary syndrome [37, 38]. Regular physical activity is also known to be an effective therapeutic intervention to improve glucose homeostasis and insulin sensitivity [39]. Endometrial insulin resistance should also be noted because studies have proved that a reduction in insulin resistance at the endometrial level induced by insulin-sensitizing agents leads to changes in the expression of glucose transporter endometrial protein [40] and is associated with a declining risk for miscarriage and implantation failure in IVF cycles during clinical observation [41]. Additionally, regular physical activity can help relieve stress and anxiety, which have been shown to be important risk factors affecting the assisted reproductive outcome [33, 42].

The strength of this review is that we focused on the effect of a very common lifestyle choice on assisted reproductive outcome, and the conclusion is very critical when providing consultation to infertile couples. All included studies established a good contrast between no regular physical activity and regular physical activity, and the intensity of physical activity was within a normal range. This excluded the effect of high-intensity physical activity (e.g., that performed by athletes) on pregnancy outcome. This study also has several limitations. First, the number of included studies was limited. The information on physical activity was based on the memories of the infertile couples. However, all physical activity information of the participants was recorded before the IVF/ICSI cycles, and they did not know whether they would become pregnant, which suggests the truthfulness of the results. Second, the questionnaires in the included studies differed from each other and bias cannot be excluded, even though all studies established a reliable contrast regarding different levels of physical activity. Third, we could not eliminate the effects from other confounders, such as etiology of infertility, dietary habits and psychological factors, which may also affect assisted reproductive outcomes.

To provide better evidence regarding the relationship between physical activity before ART and clinical outcomes, carefully controlled and sufficiently powered intervention studies are needed, frequency, intensity and duration of physical activity and potential confounders like dietary pattern, male factor etc. should be considered.

Conclusion

From this meta-analysis, we conclude that physical activity before IVF/ICSI cycles is associated with increased rates of clinical pregnancy and live births, whereas only a small but not statistically significant increase was found in the implantation rate and no effect was shown on the miscarriage rate following IVF/ICSI cycles. It is necessary to determine the status of physical activity in women when they come to the clinic for infertility treatment, and suggesting to physically inactive women that they do more exercise is expected to improve the pregnancy outcome. However, the conclusions reached from this meta-analysis are based primarily on observational studies, and population-based randomized clinical trials will be needed to confirm the results.

Abbreviations

ART: Assisted reproductive technology; BMI: Body mass index; ICSI: Intracytoplasmic sperm injection; IVF: In vitro fertilization; OR: Odds ratio; RCT: Randomized controlled trial

Acknowledgements

We acknowledge the professional manuscript editing services of Armstrong-Hilton Ltd.

Funding

This study was not supported by any funding.

Capsule

The findings of this meta-analysis suggested that physical activity before ART is very helpful in improving clinical outcomes. This may be important for the treatment of infertility, especially for physically inactive women.

Authors' contributions

MR and LT participated in the conception and design of the study. MR and ZZ searched and collected the data, performed the analysis and wrote the manuscript. LT revised the manuscript and gave final approval of this manuscript. All authors read and approved the final manuscript.

Competing interests

The authors declare that they have no competing interests.

Author details

[1]Department of reproduction and genetics, the First Affiliated Hospital of Kunming Medical University, No. 295 Xi Chang road, Kunming 650032, China. [2]Department of Neurology, the First Affiliated Hospital of Kunming Medical University, Kunming 650032, China.

Reference

1. JF ML. Infertility evaluation. Obstet Gynecol Clin N Am. 2012;39:453–63.
2. Rooney KL, Domar AD. The impact of lifestyle behaviors on infertility treatment outcome. Curr Opin Obstet Gynecol. 2014;26:181–5.
3. Rasiah R, Thangiah G, Yusoff K, Manikam R, Chandrasekaran SK, Mustafa R, Bakar NB. The impact of physical activity on cumulative cardiovascular disease risk factors among Malaysian adults. BMC Public Health. 2015;15:1242.
4. Hardefeldt PJ, Penninkilampi R, Edirimanne S, Eslick GD. Physical activity and weight loss reduce the risk of breast cancer: a meta-analysis of 139 prospective and retrospective studies. Clin Breast Cancer. 2017;S1526-8209:30429-3.

6. Gudmundsdottir SL, Flanders WD, Augestad LB. Physical activity and fertility in women: the north-Trondelag health study. Hum Reprod. 2009;24:3196–204.
7. Wise LA, Rothman KJ, Mikkelsen EM, Sorensen HT, Riis AH, Hatch EE. A prospective cohort study of physical activity and time to pregnancy. Fertil Steril. 2012;97:1136–42. e1131-1134
8. Otis CL, Drinkwater B, Johnson M, Loucks A, Wilmore J. American College of Sports Medicine position stand. The female athlete triad. Med Sci Sports Exerc. 1997;29:i–ix.
9. Warren MP, Perlroth NE. The effects of intense exercise on the female reproductive system. J Endocrinol. 2001;170:3–11.
10. Kramer MS, SW MD. Aerobic exercise for women during pregnancy. Cochrane Database Syst Rev. 2006:CD000180. https://doi.org/10.1002/14651858.CD000180.pub2..
11. Gavard JA, Artal R. Effect of exercise on pregnancy outcome. Clin Obstet Gynecol. 2008;51:467–80.
12. Morris SN, Missmer SA, Cramer DW, Powers RD, McShane PM, Hornstein MD. Effects of lifetime exercise on the outcome of in vitro fertilization. Obstet Gynecol. 2006;108:938–45.
13. Palomba S, Falbo A, Valli B, Morini D, Villani MT, Nicoli A, La Sala GB. Physical activity before IVF and ICSI cycles in infertile obese women: an observational cohort study. Reprod BioMed Online. 2014;29:72–9.
14. Gaskins AJ, Williams PL, Keller MG, Souter I, Hauser R, Chavarro JE, Team ES. Maternal physical and sedentary activities in relation to reproductive outcomes following IVF. Reprod BioMed Online. 2016;33:513–21.
15. Evenson KR, Calhoun KC, Herring AH, Pritchard D, Wen F, Steiner AZ. Association of physical activity in the past year and immediately after in vitro fertilization on pregnancy. Fertil Steril. 2014;101:1047–54. e1045
16. Kucuk M, Doymaz F, Urman B. Effect of energy expenditure and physical activity on the outcomes of assisted reproduction treatment. Reprod BioMed Online. 2010;20:274–9.
17. Moran L, Tsagareli V, Norman R, Noakes M. Diet and IVF pilot study: short-term weight loss improves pregnancy rates in overweight/obese women undertaking IVF. Aust N Z J Obstet Gynaecol. 2011;51:455–9.
18. Stang A. Critical evaluation of the Newcastle-Ottawa scale for the assessment of the quality of nonrandomized studies in meta-analyses. Eur J Epidemiol. 2010;25:603–5.
19. Higgins J, Green S. Cochrane handbook for systematic reviews of interventions. Version 5.1.0. The Cochrane Collaboration. 2011. http://training.cochrane.org/handbooks. Accessed 4 Feb 2018.
20. Atkins D, Best D, Briss PA, Eccles M, Falck-Ytter Y, Flottorp S, Guyatt GH, Harbour RT, Haugh MC, Henry D, et al. Grading quality of evidence and strength of recommendations. BMJ. 2004;328:1490.
21. Guyatt G, Oxman AD, Akl EA, Kunz R, Vist G, Brozek J, Norris S, Falck-Ytter Y, Glasziou P, DeBeer H, et al. GRADE guidelines: 1. Introduction-GRADE evidence profiles and summary of findings tables. J Clin Epidemiol. 2011;64:383–94.
22. Higgins JPT, Cochrane Green S. Cochrane handbook for systematic reviews of interventions. Version 5.1.0 [updated March 2011]. Oxford: The Cochrane Collaboration; 2011.
23. Ferreira RC, Halpern G, Figueira Rde C, Braga DP, Iaconelli A Jr, Borges E Jr. Physical activity, obesity and eating habits can influence assisted reproduction outcomes. Womens Health (Lond). 2010;6:517–24.
24. Ramezanzadeh F, Kazemi A, Yavari P, Nasr-Esfahani MH, Nejat S, Rahimi-Foroshani A, Saboor-Yaraghi A. Impact of body mass index versus physical activity and calorie intake on assisted reproduction outcomes. Eur J Obstet Gynecol Reprod Biol. 2012;163:52–6.
25. Ribeiro AC, Sávioll KEO, MLCF R, THM C, Schmitz BA. Validation of a food frequency questionnaire for the adult population. Rev Nutr. 2006;19:10–6.
26. Cleanthous X, Noakes M, Brinkworth GD, Keogh JB, Williams G, Clifton PM. A pilot comprehensive lifestyle intervention program (CLIP)–comparison with qualitative lifestyle advice and simvastatin on cardiovascular risk factors in overweight hypercholesterolaemic individuals. Nutr Metab Cardiovasc Dis. 2011;21:165–72.
27. Ainsworth BE, Sternfeld B, Richardson MT, Jackson K. Evaluation of the kaiser physical activity survey in women. Med Sci Sports Exerc. 2000;32:1327–38.
28. Evenson KR, Chasan-Taber L, Symons Downs D, Pearce EE. Review of self-reported physical activity assessments for pregnancy: summary of the evidence for validity and reliability. Paediatr Perinat Epidemiol. 2012;26:479–94.
29. Wolf AM, Hunter DJ, Colditz GA, Manson JE, Stampfer MJ, Corsano KA, Rosner B, Kriska A, Willett WC. Reproducibility and validity of a self-administered physical activity questionnaire. Int J Epidemiol. 1994;23:991–9.
30. U.S Department of Health and Human Services, & physical activity guidelines advisory committee. Physical activity guidelines advisory committee report, 2008. Washington; 2008. Retrieved from: http://www.health.gov/PAguidelines/Report/. Accessed 4 Feb 2018.
31. Matthiesen SM, Frederiksen Y, Ingerslev HJ, Zachariae R. Stress, distress and outcome of assisted reproductive technology (ART): a meta-analysis. Hum Reprod. 2011;26:2763–76.
32. An Y, Sun Z, Li L, Zhang Y, Ji H. Relationship between psychological stress and reproductive outcome in women undergoing in vitro fertilization treatment: psychological and neurohormonal assessment. J Assist Reprod Genet. 2013;30:35–41.
33. Frederiksen Y, Farver-Vestergaard I, Skovgard NG, Ingerslev HJ, Zachariae R. Efficacy of psychosocial interventions for psychological and pregnancy outcomes in infertile women and men: a systematic review and meta-analysis. BMJ Open. 2015;5:e006592.
34. Redman LM. Physical activity and its effects on reproduction. Reprod BioMed Online. 2006;12:579–86.
35. Yusuf S, Anand S. Body-mass index, abdominal adiposity, and cardiovascular risk. Lancet. 2011;378:226–7. author reply 228
36. Palomba S, Falbo A, Russo T, Orio F, Tolino A, Zullo F. Systemic and local effects of metformin administration in patients with polycystic ovary syndrome (PCOS): relationship to the ovulatory response. Hum Reprod. 2010;25:1005–13.
37. Honnma H, Endo T, Kiya T, Shimizu A, Nagasawa K, Baba T, Fujimoto T, Henmi H, Kitajima Y, Manase K, et al. Remarkable features of ovarian morphology and reproductive hormones in insulin-resistant Zucker fatty (fa/fa) rats. Reprod Biol Endocrinol. 2010;8:73.
38. Wang Y, Qu J, Wu X, Hou L, Erkkola R, Wang Y. Different phenotypes of polycystic ovary syndrome by Rotterdam criteria are differently steroidogenic but similarly insulin resistant. Fertil Steril. 2010;93:1362–5.
39. Helmrich SP, Ragland DR, Leung RW, Paffenbarger RS Jr. Physical activity and reduced occurrence of non-insulin-dependent diabetes mellitus. N Engl J Med. 1991;325:147–52.
40. Zhai J, Liu CX, Tian ZR, Jiang QH, Sun YP. Effects of metformin on the expression of GLUT4 in endometrium of obese women with polycystic ovary syndrome. Biol Reprod. 2012;87:29.
41. Palomba S, Falbo A, La Sala GB. Effects of metformin in women with polycystic ovary syndrome treated with gonadotrophins for in vitro fertilisation and intracytoplasmic sperm injection cycles: a systematic review and meta-analysis of randomised controlled trials. BJOG. 2013;120:267–76.
42. Hammerli K, Znoj H, Barth J. The efficacy of psychological interventions for infertile patients: a meta-analysis examining mental health and pregnancy rate. Hum Reprod Update. 2009;15:279–95.

4

Circulating osteopontin and its association with liver fat content in non-obese women with polycystic ovary syndrome

Yuying Wang[1†], Wei Zhou[2†], Chunhua Wu[3], Yi Zhang[1], Tzuchun Lin[1], Yun Sun[4], Wei Liu[1,4*] and Tao Tao[1*]

Abstract

Background: Osteopontin (OPN) plays an important role in inflammatory processes and insulin resistance. Polycystic ovary syndrome (PCOS) is a reproductive metabolic disease associated with insulin resistance and metabolic abnormalities, including high levels of liver fat content (LFC). The objective of this study was to explore whether circulating OPN independently contributes to elevated LFC in non-obese PCOS patients.

Methods: This study included 61 non-obese PCOS patients and 56 age-matched healthy women from Shanghai, China. After an overnight fast, all participants underwent anthropometric measurements, oral glucose tolerance tests, lipid profile and sex hormone measurements. Quantitative measurement of LFC by ultrasonography was performed. OPN concentrations were measured using ELISA. An independent samples t-test and the Mann-Whitney U test were performed to compare variables between the two groups; one-way ANOVA and Kruskal-Wallis test were performed to compare four subgroups of patients. Correlations were determined by Spearman's correlation tests. Stepwise multiple linear regression analyses were performed to assess for independent contributors. A receiver operating characteristic curve with the maximum Youden index was calculated for the optimal cut-off value.

Results: In non-obese PCOS women, circulating OPN levels were increased in the subgroups with a higher body mass index (BMI) and free androgen index (FAI), and the LFC levels were increased in the elevated OPN subgroups. Moreover, increased OPN was associated with increased FAI and LFC in PCOS women, and the association between OPN and LFC was independent of triglyceride, HOMA-IR and FAI after adjusting for PCOS status in all participants. OPN combined with FAI and hsCRP may better predict NAFLD than WHR in this study cohort. However, there was no significant difference in circulating OPN levels between non-obese PCOS and normal control women.

Conclusions: Increased OPN levels may be related to FAI and elevated LFC in non-obese women with PCOS.

Keywords: Polycystic ovary syndrome, Osteopontin, Liver fat content, Hyperandrogenism

Background

Polycystic ovary syndrome (PCOS) is a complex reproductive and metabolic disorder related to insulin resistance with a 5–10% morbidity in women of fertile age [1]. As PCOS is characterized by insulin resistance and hyperandrogenism, it is often accompanied by metabolic syndrome and an increased risk of cardiovascular events [2]. It is believed that the occurrence and progression of metabolic disorders in PCOS patients are closely related to the chronic low-level inflammation of intra-abdominal adipose tissue [3, 4]. Among the metabolic disorders in PCOS patients, nonalcoholic fatty liver disease (NAFLD), which is considered the hepatic expression of metabolic syndrome [5], leads to a significant increase in the morbidity and pathology scores in PCOS patients, independent of obesity and other coexisting metabolic disorders [6–9].

* Correspondence: sue_liuwei@163.com; taotaozhen@hotmail.com
Yuying Wang and Wei Zhou are joint co-authors.
†Equal contributors
[1]Department of Endocrinology and Metabolism, Renji Hospital, School of Medicine, Shanghai Jiaotong University, 160 Pujian Road, Shanghai 200127, China
Full list of author information is available at the end of the article

NAFLD is an important manifestation of metabolic syndrome in the liver characterized by the presence of hepatic steatosis on imaging or histology in the absence of secondary causes of hepatic fat accumulation such as significant alcohol consumption, use of steatogenic medication or hereditary disorders [10]. A liver biopsy is the gold standard for the detection of liver fat content (LFC) in humans, but this invasive test is not routinely used in clinical practice; proton magnetic resonance ([1H]-MRS) [11, 12] and chemical shift-encoded magnetic resonance imaging (MRI) [13] are also accurate methods for assessing hepatic fat deposition, but they are not routinely performed due to high cost. A quantitative ultrasound method was recently established for detecting LFC and is proven to be a noninvasive method that provides results that are highly consistent with [1H]-MRS and histological liver steatosis grade ($r = 0.85$ and 0.79, respectively) [14]. Studies have shown that computer-aided measurements of the US hepatic/renal echo-intensity ratio (H/R) are highly correlated with liver fat content determined by histology and [1H]-MRS [15, 16]. The method used in this study was established based on a standardized H/R and the ultrasound hepatic echo-intensity attenuation rate (HA), which are reported to be positively correlated with the LFC measured by [1H]-MRS ($r = 0.884$, and 0.711, respectively) [17]. The ultrasound H/R can independently predict 78% of LFC detected by [1H]-MRS, and the addition of ultrasound HA improves the adjusted explained variance to 79.8% [17]. Compared to liver biopsy, MRS and MRI, the quantitative ultrasound method is non-invasive, time-saving, and relatively cheap; therefore, we chose to use the quantitative ultrasound method to assess the levels of LFC in this study population.

Osteopontin (OPN) is a glycoprotein that is involved in multiple biological and pathological conditions including immunity, inflammation, insulin resistance, reproduction, and steatosis and fibrosis of various tissues. OPN plays a role in immunomodulatory functions as an early T lymphocyte activator [18]. Studies demonstrate a significant increase of OPN levels in chronic low-grade inflammation and insulin resistance-related diseases such as obesity. Furthermore, OPN can induce inflammatory signalling from human adipocytes and adipose tissue macrophage infiltration, and impair differentiation and insulin sensitivity of primary adipocytes [19–22]. Growing evidence suggests that OPN is also involved in the regulation of female reproductive functions, such as follicular growth and ovulation regulation [23]. Recent studies have also found that plasma OPN levels are closely related to the degree of liver fibrosis in alcoholic liver disease [24]. Furthermore, previous studies suggest that OPN deficiency can reduce hepatic steatosis and inflammation in obese mice fed a high fat diet [21, 25]. In these studies, OPN expression was found to be essential for NAFLD progression, involving hepatic steatosis, inflammation and fibrosis. Therefore, it is now recognized that OPN is closely related to metabolic and reproductive disorders, as well as NAFLD. However, research on the correlation between serum OPN levels and LFC has not been evaluated in non-obese PCOS patients in the Chinese population.

The aim of this study was to assess whether OPN levels in non-obese PCOS patients are higher than that of age- and BMI-matched non-PCOS patients and the relationship between OPN levels and LFC.

Methods

Participants

Sixty-one women with PCOS and fifty-six control women were enrolled in the study from Shanghai, China. The age of the subjects ranged from 18 to 45 years old, and they were normal weight or overweight with a BMI < 28 kg/m^2 according to the Cooperative Meta-Analysis Group of the Working Group on Obesity in China Criteria [26]; normal weight was defined as body mass index (BMI) < 24 kg/m^2, overweight was defined as 24 kg/m^2 $\leq$ BMI < 28 kg/m^2, and obesity was defined BMI of $\geq$28 kg/m^2. The diagnosis of PCOS was based on the National Institutes of Health 1990 Criteria [27]. Control women were screened by medical history, physical examination, laboratory evaluation and transvaginal ultrasound to select those with normal cycles, those who are non-hirsute, and those who do not have hyperandrogenaemia (serum testosterone below 0.6 ng/mL). All women that were pregnant (diagnosed by a urine pregnancy test) or had abnormal thyroid function and prolactin levels were excluded [27]. Women who received glucocorticoids, anti-androgen agents, oral contraceptives, anti-inflammatory agents, ovulation induction agents, anti-obesity medications, steatogenic medications, or insulin sensitizing agents within the previous 3 months were excluded. All women with history of significant alcohol consumption and hereditary disorders that might cause secondary hepatic fat accumulation were excluded.

All evaluations and procedures in this study were conducted according to the Declaration of Helsinki for Medical Research involving Human Subjects. This study was approved by the ethics committee of Shanghai Renji Hospital and written consent was obtained from each subject after full explanation of the purpose and nature of all study procedures.

Quantitative measurement of LFC by ultrasonography

Quantitative measurement of LFC was determined by ultrasonography described in a previously study [14, 17]. All instrument settings were calibrated using a tissue-mimicking phantom (Model 057; Computerized Imaging Reference Systems, Norfolk, VA) and fixed before measurements were obtained to maintain consistency among the ultrasound machines. The phantom contains abdominal organ models that display as ultrasound images. The ultrasonographists were trained to obtain ultrasound images, including one image with both the liver and the right kidney clearly visualized in the sagittal liver/kidney view in the lateral position and another image with the liver in the right intercostal view at the anterior axillary line in the supine position [14, 17].

All images were transferred to a personal computer and analysed using the NIH image software (ImageJ 1.41, National Institutes of Health, Bethesda, MD). In the sagittal liver/right kidney view, a region of interest (ROI) of 1.5 * 1.5 cm^2 in the liver parenchyma without blood vessels, bile ducts, and other focal hypo/hyperechogenic structures was selected. Another ROI of 0.5 * 0.5 cm^2 was identified in the right renal cortex with no large vessels or renal sinus or medulla at the same depth as the liver ROI. In the right intercostal view at the anterior axillary line, two ROIs of 1.5 * 1.5 cm^2 were selected in homogeneous regions of the liver along the same ultrasound transmission line near the liver's anterior and posterior margins. The linear distance between the two ROIs was also measured. The grey scale mean value of the pixels within the ROIs was used as the measurement of echo intensity. We then divided the average hepatic grey scale by the average renal cortex grey scale to obtain the ultrasound hepatic/renal echo-intensity ratio. We obtained the standardized ultrasound hepatic/renal ratio and standardized hepatic attenuation rate using the phantom. The LFC was obtained according to the following predictive formula: LFC (%) = 62.592 * standardized ultrasound hepatic/renal ratio + 168.076* standardized hepatic attenuation rate – 27.863 [14, 17].

Anthropometric measurements

The height and weight of each subject in light clothing were measured to the nearest 1 cm and 0.1 kg, respectively, using a digital scale and stadiometer. BMI was calculated as body weight (kg) divided by height (m) squared. Waist circumference (WC) and hip circumference (HC) were measured by a single individual. WC was determined by measuring the circumference at the narrowest point between the lower border of the rib cage and the iliac crest. HC was determined by measuring the circumference at the level of the symphysis pubis and the greatest gluteal protuberance. The waist-to-hip ratio (WHR) was then calculated by dividing the WC by the HC. Body fat percentage (FAT%) was assessed by foot-to-foot measures of bioelectrical impedance obtained using a TBF-300 body composition analyser (TANITA, U.K. Ltd., Middlesex, UK).

Laboratory analyses

All laboratory evaluations were performed at 0800 h after an overnight fast during the early follicular phase (days 2–5) of a spontaneous menstrual cycle, except in subjects with amenorrhoea > 3 months who were examined randomly. All women underwent a standard oral glucose tolerance test (OGTT) with 75 g of glucose. Blood samples were drawn before the glucose load (t = 0 min) and after the glucose load (t = 30, 60, 120, and 180 min). Glucose and insulin samples were stored at 4 ° C and analysed the day of sampling. All serum samples for OPN were stored at – 70 °C until assayed.

Competitive electrochemiluminescence immunoassays on the Elecsys Autoanalyser 2010 (Roche Diagnostics, Indianapolis, IN) were used to quantify serum total testosterone. Sex hormone binding globulin (SHBG) levels were measured by the chemiluminescent immunoassay (Elecsys autoanalyser 2010, Roche Diagnostics) validated for plasma SHBG. The coefficient of variation (CV) for SHBG using this methodology was 6%. FAI was calculated as the percentage ratio of total testosterone to SHBG [28]. A normal androgen level was defined as FAI < 7 [29]. Plasma glucose was determined using the glucose oxidase methodology. All measurements were performed with Roche reagents (D 2400 and E 170 Modular Analytics modules with Roche/Hitachi analysers; Roche Diagnostics, Indianapolis, USA). Insulin levels were measured by radioimmunoassay (RIA). The intra-assay CV of insulin and steroid hormone assays were 5.5% and < 10%, respectively. To estimate insulin resistance, the homeostasis assessment insulin resistance index (HOMA-IR) was calculated according to the equation fasting serum insulin (μU/ml) * fasting plasma glucose (mmol/ l)/22.5 [30]. The Matsuda Index was calculated using the eqs. 10,000/square root of [(fasting glucose x fasting insulin) x (mean glucose x mean insulin during OGTT)] [31]. The deposition index (DI) was calculated to estimate the β-cell response relative to the prevailing insulin sensitivity using the eq. $DI = \Delta I_{30}/\Delta G_{30}$ (mIU/mmol)/HOMA-IR = $(I_{30}-I_0)/(G_{30}-G_0)/$ HOMA-IR [32]. Analysis of high-sensitivity C-reactive protein (hsCRP) was performed using immunonephelometric methods and a BN-II analyser (Dade Behring, Deerfeld, Germany). The inter- and intra-assay coefficients of variation were 4.9% and 6.8%, respectively.

The plasma OPN level was measured using an enzyme-linked immunosorbent assay (ELISA) kit (R&D Systems, Minneapolis, MN, USA) according to the manufacturer's instructions. The intra-assay CV was < 4.1% and the inter-assay CV was < 6.7%. All samples were analysed in duplicate. The assays have < 0.5% cross-reactivity observed with available related molecules and a < 50% cross-species reactivity observed with species tested.

Statistical analyses

All statistical analyses were performed using SPSS version 23 (SPSS Inc., Chicago, IL, USA). The results are reported as the mean with the standard deviation for variables with a normal distribution and median with the interquartile range (25–75%) for variables with a skewed distribution. For variables with a normal distribution, an independent samples t-test was performed to compare variables between two groups; one-way ANOVA followed by the LSD test was performed for the four subgroups. For variables with a skewed distribution, the Mann-Whitney U test was performed to compare variables between the two groups; the Kruskal-Wallis test followed by the Mann-Whitney U test was performed for the four subgroups. The relationships between levels of OPN, LFC and other variables were evaluated by the Spearman's correlation test. Stepwise multiple linear regression analyses were performed to assess the independent contributors of OPN and LFC. To determine the optimal threshold to predict LFC, the point on the receiver operating characteristic (ROC) curve with the maximum Youden index [sensitivity-(1-specificity)] was calculated. $P < 0.05$ was considered statistically significant.

Results

Clinical, hormonal and metabolic features of PCOS and non-PCOS women

The clinical characteristics and biochemical variables of PCOS and non-PCOS women are summarized in Table 1. The age, BMI, FAT%, HOMA-IR, DI, TG, and high-density lipoprotein cholesterol (HDL-C) and low-density lipoprotein cholesterol (LDL-C) levels were comparable between the PCOS and non-PCOS groups (all $P > 0.05$). However, compared to the non-PCOS group, the PCOS group had much higher WHR, AUCglucose, AUCinsulin, TC, hsCRP, T, FAI and A_2, while the Matsuda Index and SHBG were lower in the PCOS group (all $P < 0.05$).

The PCOS and non-PCOS women were divided into four subgroups according to their BMI. Lean PCOS and lean non-PCOS women did not differ except in levels of TC and sex hormones (T and FAI) ($P < 0.05$ for all). When we compared overweight non-PCOS and overweight PCOS women, there were similarities in metabolic parameters, while their sex hormones including T, SHBG, A_2 and FAI, were quite different ($P < 0.05$ for all). Other clinical, metabolic and hormonal parameters are shown in Additional file 1: Table S1.

Comparison of OPN levels in different subgroups

The mean value of OPN was moderately higher in PCOS patients compared to non-PCOS women, but this finding was not statistically significant (13.65 ng/mL vs 11.78 ng/mL, $P = 0.160$, Fig. 1a). Furthermore, we divided all participants into four subgroups according to PCOS and BMI status and compared the mean values of OPN. We observed that the mean value of OPN in overweight PCOS patients was significantly higher than that of lean PCOS patients (15.09 vs 10.31 ng/mL, $P = 0.01$, Fig. 1b), while there was no difference between lean control women and overweight control women (11.15 vs 12.81 ng/mL, $P = 0.229$, Fig. 1b). Similar levels of OPN were also found between lean control women and lean PCOS patients and between overweight control women and overweight PCOS women (both $P > 0.05$, Fig. 1b). Since hyperandrogenism is an important characteristic of PCOS patients, we explored whether androgen has an impact on the OPN level. We compared OPN levels and FAI to identify whether OPN levels change with bioactive testosterone estimated by FAI. In PCOS patients, the OPN levels were higher in those with FAI > 7 compared to those with FAI < 7 (9.61 ng/mL vs 15.22 ng/mL, $P = 0.007$, Fig. 1c). The baseline data according to FAI in PCOS women are shown in Additional file 1: Table S2.

Comparison of LFC levels in different subgroups by PCOS status, BMI and OPN

The mean value of LFC was significantly higher in PCOS patients compared to age- and BMI- matched non-PCOS women (14.47% vs 8.93%, $P = 0.002$, Fig. 2a). All participants were then divided into different subgroups according to BMI and diagnosis. In the PCOS group, the mean value of LFC in overweight patients was significantly higher than that of lean patients (19.61% vs 8.32%, $P < 0.001$, Fig. 2b). In the non-PCOS group, the mean value of LFC in overweight women was significantly higher than that of lean women (11.95% vs 7.47%, $P = 0.001$, Fig. 2b). The mean value of LFC was significantly higher in overweight PCOS patients compared to that of overweight non-PCOS patients (19.61% vs 11.95%, $P = 0.021$, Fig. 2b). However, lean PCOS patients and lean non-PCOS women were observed to have similar LFC levels ($P = 0.348$, Fig. 2b).

To explore whether OPN affects LFC in PCOS women, we further divided the subjects into subgroups according to the quartiles of OPN levels and compared LFC levels among these four subgroups. In PCOS subjects, LFC was higher in women with OPN levels in the second (6.6% vs 17.14% $P = 0.002$), third (6.6% vs 18.58% $P < 0.001$) and fourth quartiles (6.6% vs 12.59% $P = 0.004$, Fig. 2c) compared to those with OPN levels in the lowest quartile. The baseline data of the four subgroups according to OPN levels in PCOS women are shown in Additional file 1: Table S3.

Correlation between OPN and LFC with clinical/biochemical parameters in PCOS patients

Given the association between high OPN levels and increased adiposity, correlations between OPN and anthropometric/metabolic parameters were investigated (Table 2). In PCOS women, the OPN level had a positive linear relationships with LFC ($P = 0.004$). Moreover, OPN

Table 1 Clinical characteristics and biochemical variables in women with and without PCOS

Parameters	PCOS			non-PCOS			P value
	Total	Lean	Overweight	Total	Lean	Overweight	(PCOS vs non-PCOS)
N	61	30	31	56	38	18	
Age, yrs	26(21–31)	24.5(21–31.25)[d]	26(23–31)	26(24–29)	25.5(24–27)	29.5(26.75–34)[a]	0.415
BMI, kg/m^2	24.98(21.7–26.98)	21.7(19.41–23.3)[d]	26.89(25.63–27.77)[c,f]	22.06(21–24.91)	21.59(20.41–22.11)	27.48(24.91–27.85)[a]	0.062
WHR	0.87 ± 0.07	0.83 ± 0.07[d]	0.91 ± 0.06 [c,f]	0.85 ± 0.07	0.82 ± 0.06	0.9 ± 0.07[a]	0.043
FAT%	32.5(28.5–37.3)	28.8(22.85–31.6)[d]	37.55(35.88–41.55)[c,f]	31.2(23.7–38.6)	24.25(21.3–27.3)	38.6(36.5–41.4)[a]	0.772
AUCglucose	10.69(9.38–12.54)	9.77(7.89–11.79)	11.63(10.49–13.06)[c,f]	9.69(8.1–11.66)	8.79(7.51–10.74)	10.73(9.73–12.6)[a]	0.018
AUCinsulin	107.57(54.18–161.07)	81.25(48.38–130.12)	137.51(91.62–193.94)[c,f]	73.46(45.57–114.58)	68.93(44.48–98.54)	83.72(43.96–137.69)	0.017
HOMA-IR	2.21(1.39–4.2)	1.62(0.92–2.31)[d]	3.47(2.14–4.96)[c]	1.93(1.19–2.69)	1.61(1–2.25)	3.22(1.85–4.46)[a]	0.066
Matsuda Index	65.61(40.35–105.8)	101.18(69.86–152.44)	49.8(37.46–63.53)[c,f]	100.13(63.46–154.98)	110.19(86.21–166.93)	70.21(42.8–113.74)[a]	0.008
DI	8.67(4.55–16.1)	14.17(7.23–20.69)[d]	6.14(2.37–9.79)[c,f]	10.94(5.48–22.47)	18.09(8.81–23.94)	5.49(1.98–7.43)[a]	0.213
TG, mmol/L	1.17(0.8–1.53)	0.87(0.72–1.18)[d]	1.26(1.09–1.78)[f]	1.29(0.77–1.6)	1.07(0.66–1.6)	1.48(1.15–1.93)[a]	0.704
TC, mmol/L	4.42(4.01–4.88)	4.14(3.91–4.75)[b,d]	4.6(4.01–5.18)[c]	4.2(3.41–4.89)	3.56(3.34–4.6)	4.66(4.34–5.16)[a]	0.024
HDL-C, mmol/L	1.25(1.08–1.54)	1.45(1.27–1.67)[d]	1.18(1.02–1.25)[c,f]	1.44(1.21–1.57)	1.47(1.34–1.65)	1.18(1.04–1.31)[a]	0.218
LDL-C, mmol/L	2.77 ± 0.83	2.49 ± 0.68[d]	3.04 ± 0.89[c,f]	2.55 ± 0.58	2.35 ± 0.53	2.96 ± 0.48[a]	0.101
hsCRP, mg/L	1.09(0.33–3.03)	0.54(0.22–1.35)[d]	2.04(0.55–4.15)[c,f]	0.37(0.17–1.65)	0.27(0.17–0.44)	1.82(0.74–3.91)[a]	0.014
T, nmol/	2.36(1.66–2.75)	2.36(1.4–2.83)[b,d]	2.4(1.83–2.63)[c,e]	1.63(1.39–1.87)	1.6(1.4–1.79)	1.73(1.02–2.03)	< 0.001
SHBG, nmol/L	23.3(14.6–45.7)	35.05(20.58–66.28)	18.7(11.3–29.7)[c,e,f]	41.75(30.73–60.05)	50.2(38.7–62.75)	32.85(18.58–39.6)[a]	< 0.001
FAI	9.29(4.46–15.25)	5.57(2.81–11.43)[b]	12.54(7.27–19.73)[c,e,f]	3.61(2.48–5.2)	3.19(2.45–4.44)	5.4(2.61–7.73)[a]	< 0.001
A_2, μg/dL	5.9(4.22–7.98)	4.52(2.14–6.97)	6.49(4.83–9.5)[c,e]	2.85(2.24–5.52)	2.97(2.26–5.64)	2.73(2.11–5.83)	0.019

Data are shown as the mean ± SD for variables with a normal distribution and median with the interquartile range (25–75%) for skewed variables. For variables with a normal distribution, an independent samples t-test was performed to compare variables between two groups; a one-way ANOVA followed by the LSD test was performed among the four subgroups of women (lean control, overweight control, lean PCOS, and overweight PCOS). For variables with a skewed distribution, the Mann-Whitney U test was performed to compare variables between the two groups; the Kruskal-Wallis test followed by the Mann-Whitney U test was performed for the four subgroups of women

BMI Body mass index, *WC* Waist circumference, *WHR* Waist hip ratio, *FAT%* Body fat percentage, *AUCglucose* Area under curve for OGTT glucose, *AUCinsulin* Area under curve for OGTT insulin, *HOMA-IR* Homeostasis model assessment of insulin resistance, *DI* Disposition index, *TG* Triglyceride, *TC* Total cholesterol, *HDL-C* High-density lipoprotein cholesterol, *LDL-C* Low-density lipoprotein cholesterol, *hsCRP* high sensitivity C reactive protein, *T* Total testosterone, *SHBG* Sex hormone binding globulin, *FAI* Free androgen index A_2 androstenedione

To convert testosterone to ng/ml, divide by 3.467; To convert cholesterol to mg/dL, divide by 0.02586; to convert triglycerides to mg/dL, divide by 0.01129; to covert glucose to mg/dL, divide by 0.05551; to convert total testosterone to ng/ml, divide by 3.467

[a] $P < 0.05$ for lean non-PCOS women vs overweight non-PCOS women
[b] $P < 0.05$ for lean non-PCOS women vs lean PCOS women
[c] $P < 0.05$ for lean non-PCOS women vs overweight PCOS women
[d] $P < 0.05$ for overweight non-PCOS women vs lean PCOS women
[e] $P < 0.05$ for overweight non-PCOS women vs overweight PCOS women
[f] $P < 0.05$ for lean PCOS women vs overweight PCOS women

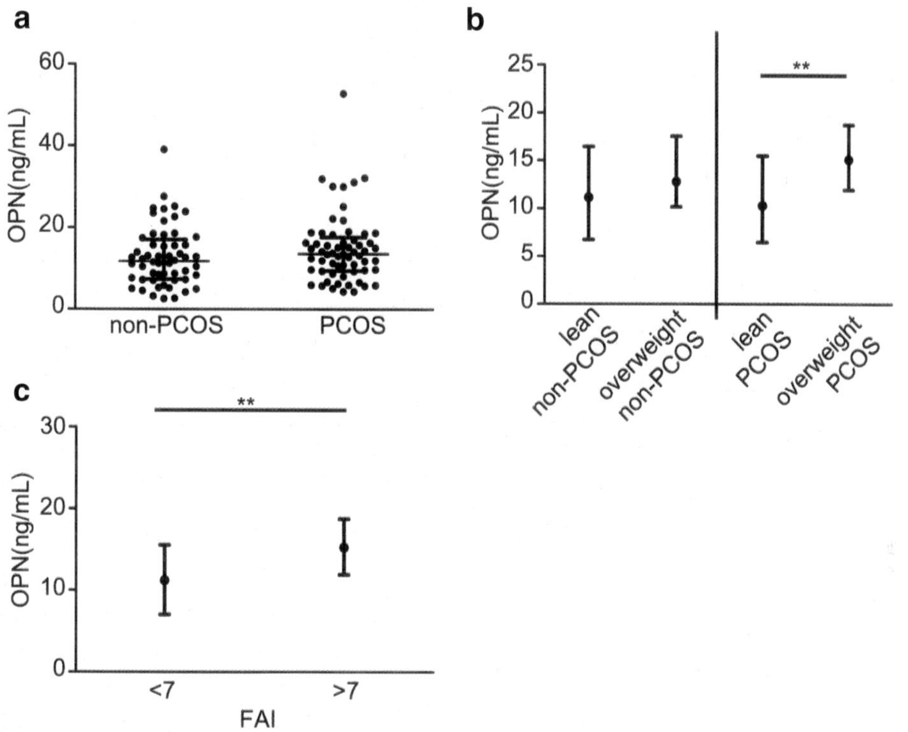

Fig. 1 OPN levels in the lean/overweight non-PCOS and PCOS groups and in FAI quartile groups. (**a**) OPN levels in the non-PCOS group and PCOS group. (**b**) OPN levels in lean and overweight non-PCOS groups and lean and overweight PCOS groups. (**c**) OPN levels by FAI in the PCOS group. For comparison between two groups, the Mann-Whitney U test was performed. The Kruskal-Wallis test followed by the Mann-Whitney U test was performed to test the differences among the four subgroups. Data are displayed as median with interquartile range. *$P < 0.05$, **$P < 0.01$. FAI: free androgen index.

level positively correlated with AUCinsulin ($P = 0.016$), HOMA-IR ($P = 0.02$), and FAI ($P = 0.016$). Furthermore, there were strong inverse linear correlations between OPN level and SHBG ($P = 0.027$) and the Matsuda Index ($P = 0.037$). However, we did not find a correlation between OPN level and anthropometry parameters, lipid profile, hsCRP, AUCglucose, or DI (Table 2).

Given the association between high LFC levels and increased adiposity, correlations between LFC and anthropometric/metabolic parameters were investigated (Table 2). In PCOS women, the LFC level had positive linear relationships with BMI, FAT% and WHR ($P < 0.01$ for all). LFC level also had positive linear relationships with AUCglucose ($P < 0.001$), AUCinsulin ($P < 0.001$), HOMA-IR ($P < 0.001$), TG ($P < 0.001$), LDL-C ($P = 0.041$), hsCRP ($P = 0.003$), and FAI ($P < 0.001$). Furthermore, strong inverse linear correlations were found between LFC level and the Matsuda Index ($P < 0.001$), DI ($P = 0.01$), SHBG ($P < 0.001$) and HDL-C ($P < 0.001$, Table 2).

Determinants of LFC

To investigate the independent determinants of LFC among all women studied, we performed a stepwise multiple regression analysis on LFC with OPN, HOMA-IR, FAI, TG and PCOS status as potential contributors. We observed that FAI, HOMA-IR, TG and OPN, but not PCOS status, explained 33.5% of the variance in LFC (adjusted $R^2 = 0.335$, $P < 0.001$) with FAI ($\beta = 0.347$, $P < 0.001$), HOMA-IR ($\beta = 0.201$, $P = 0.013$), TG ($\beta = 0.236$, $P = 0.004$) and OPN ($\beta = 0.178$, $P = 0.023$, Table 3) being significant independent contributors. Therefore, FAI, HOMA-IR, TG and OPN were all found to be independent predictors of LFC.

ROC analysis for LFC

To further elucidate the relationship between OPN and LFC, we used the ROC curve to find potential contributors of elevated LFC risk for NAFLD diagnosis (LFC > 5%). In all participants, the area under the curve (AUC) in the ROC analysis was 0.606 for OPN, 0.615 for FAI and 0.691 for hsCRP. We combined the three potential contributors of LFC and found that the AUC increased to 0.71 from 0.622 for WHR, indicating that the combination of OPN, FAI and hsCRP are optimal predictors for the diagnosis for NAFLD (Table 4).

Discussion

In this study, we investigated circulating OPN levels in non-obese women with PCOS compared to normal control women and determined the correlation between

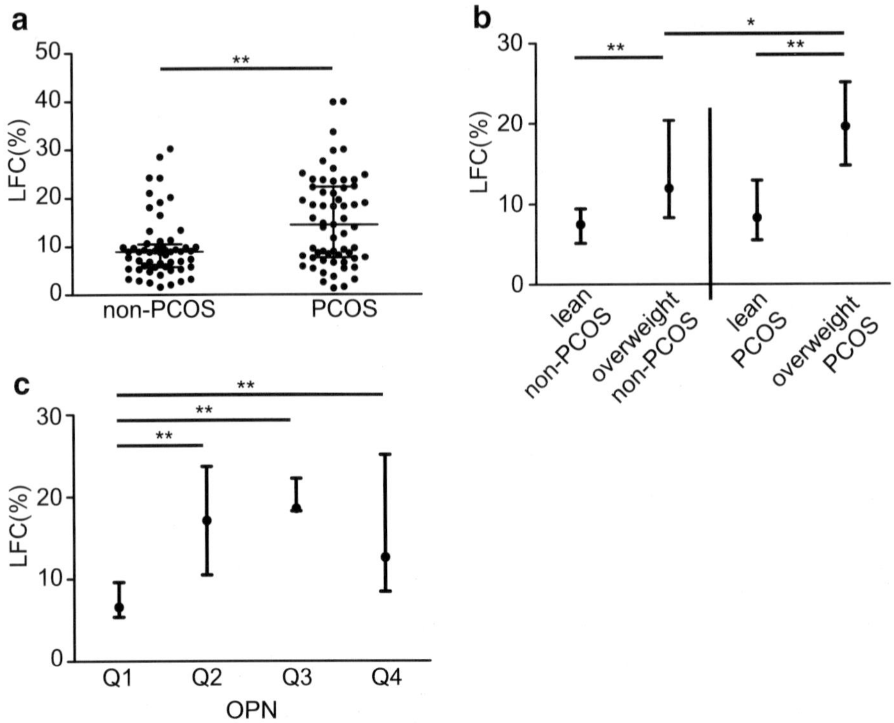

Fig. 2 LFC levels in lean/overweight non-PCOS and PCOS groups and in OPN quartile groups. (**a**) LFC levels in non-PCOS and PCOS groups. (**b**) LFC levels in lean and overweight non-PCOS groups and lean and overweight PCOS groups. (**c**) LFC levels by OPN quartiles in the PCOS group For comparison between PCOS and non-PCOS groups, the Mann-Whitney U test was performed. The Kruskal-Wallis test followed by the Mann-Whitney U test was performed to test the differences among the four subgroups. Data are displayed as median with interquartile range. *$P < 0.05$, **$P < 0.01$. LFC: liver fat content.

OPN and LFC. The main finding of this study was that the circulating OPN level is associated with the degree of FAI in non-obese PCOS women and the OPN is an independent contributor of LFC. OPN combined with FAI and hsCRP was an optimal predictor of NAFLD in this study cohort. However, there was no significant difference in circulating OPN levels between non-obese PCOS and normal control women.

There is an increasing number of studies investigating the relationship between OPN and metabolic diseases, but there have been no definitive conclusions to date. Whether OPN independently contributes to the development of metabolic disturbance in PCOS patients is also unknown. Because OPN has multiple functions in adipose tissue, we hypothesized that OPN may be involved in the insulin resistance in PCOS patients. Although differences in insulin resistance estimated by HOMA-IR were not readily apparent between PCOS and non-PCOS women in this non-obese cohort, the level of SHBG, a potential alternative index of insulin resistance, was significantly decreased in non-obese women with PCOS. Our study also suggests that OPN levels are negatively correlated with SHBG levels.

Since hyperandrogenism is one of the most important features of PCOS pathogenesis, we analysed the differences in OPN levels in different FAI subgroups of PCOS patients. We found that an increased circulating OPN level was more common in higher FAI groups and associated with high degree of FAI in non-obese PCOS patients. This finding is consistent with a recent study that showed that OPN levels are associated with free testosterone levels [33]. In the BMI subgroup analysis, OPN levels were significantly higher in the overweight PCOS group compared to the lean PCOS group, while this difference was not found in control women. This suggests that hyperandrogenism may play an important role in elevating OPN levels, for there is only a small BMI difference among patients with hyperandrogenaemia.

In the present study, there was no significant difference in serum OPN levels between non-obese PCOS and control women. This finding is inconsistent with that of a recent study showing that PCOS is associated with increased serum OPN levels [33]. The major discrepancy may be due to the relatively low BMI and comparable HOMA-IR in our cohort. However, given the observational design of our study and Saklamaz's study, causality cannot be established. The precise mechanisms of the potential role of OPN in PCOS must be further investigated.

While there is growing evidence with regard to OPN playing a crucial role in metabolic disorders, particularly

Table 2 Correlation of OPN and LFC with clinical and biochemical parameters in PCOS women

	OPN		LFC	
	r	*P*	*r*	*P*
OPN	/	/	0.36	0.004
liver	0.360	0.004	/	/
BMI	0.246	0.056	0.621	< 0.001
WHR	0.118	0.372	0.514	< 0.001
FAT%	0.239	0.273	0.569	0.005
AUCglucose	0.203	0.116	0.495	< 0.001
AUCinsulin	0.321	0.016	0.488	< 0.001
HOMA-IR	0.300	0.02	0.474	< 0.001
Matusda index	−0.282	0.037	− 0.569	< 0.001
DI	−0.082	0.546	−0.337	0.01
TG	0.067	0.607	0.464	< 0.001
HDL-C	−0.208	0.107	−0.514	< 0.001
LDL-C	−0.093	0.476	0.263	0.041
hsCRP	0.137	0.291	0.375	0.003
SHBG	−0.283	0.027	−0.533	< 0.001
FAI	0.308	0.016	0.443	< 0.001

Associations between OPN and LFC with other variables were determined by the Spearman correlation analysis
LFC Liver fat content, *BMI* Body mass index, *WHR* Waist-to-hip ratio, *FAT%* Body fat percentage, *AUCglucose* Area under curve for OGTT glucose, *AUCinsulin* Area under curve for OGTT insulin, *HOMA-IR* Homeostasis model assessment of insulin resistance, *DI*: disposition index, *TG* Triglyceride, *HDL-C* High-density lipoprotein cholesterol, *LDL-C* Low-density lipoprotein cholesterol, *hsCRP* High sensitive C reaction protein, *SHBG* Sex hormone binding globulin, *FAI* Free androgen index

focusing on NAFLD and obesity, data on OPN and LFC in PCOS are rather limited. To our knowledge, this is the first report describing the increased circulating OPN levels associated with a high degree of LFC in non-obese PCOS women. In line with a previous study, despite differences in BMI of the patient cohorts, OPN was observed to be correlated with several metabolic parameters such as BMI, WHR (waist circumference in a previous study), glucose and insulin levels, HOMA-IR, TG, HDL-C, LDL-C, and hsCRP [34]. Moreover, PCOS patients with OPN levels in the third quartile showed a 2.82 times greater LFC than those in the PCOS group with OPN levels in the lowest quartile (18.58% vs 6.6%). Interestingly, compared to those in the second and third quartiles, subjects with OPN levels in the highest quartile had a lower LFC. Since OPN is elevated in the progression of simple steatosis to nonalcoholic steatohepatitis and fibrosis [34], the change in LFC levels may account for this decline in OPN. In this study, we excluded fibrosis using the BMI, age, ALT and triglycerides (BAAT) index because of the relatively low BMI and age in this cohort. In addition, a stepwise linear regression analysis showed that the serum OPN level is a predictor of LFC independent of TG, HOMA-IR and FAI, indicating that the effect of changes in OPN levels on the metabolic phenotype of PCOS may be the result of a mechanism that is independent of insulin sensitivity.

Table 3 Effects of OPN and clinical parameters on LFC in all participants adjusted for PCOS status

		95%CI		*P* value
	β	Lower Bound	Upper Bound	
FAI	0.326	0.178	0.473	< 0.001
TG	3.199	1.068	5.33	0.004
HOMA-IR	0.671	0.146	1.197	0.013
OPN	0.189	0.026	0.352	0.023

Stepwise multiple linear regression analyses were performed to evaluate the effects of FAI, TG, HOMA-IR and OPN on LFC adjusted for PCOS status
LFC Liver fat content, *FAI* Free androgen index, *TG* Triglyceride, *HOMA-IR* Homeostasis model assessment of insulin resistance

Table 4 ROC curve analysis of LFC risk (> 5%) in all participants

	Cut-off point	AUC	Sensitivity	Specificity
WHR	0.905	0.622	0.35	1
OPN	13.005	0.606	0.51	0.8
hsCRP	0.77	0.691	0.51	0.867
FAI	6.155	0.615	0.441	0.8
OPN + FAI + hsCRP		0.71	0.667	0.8

WHR Waist-hip ratio, *hsCRP* High sensitive C reaction protein, *FAI* Free androgen index

There are several limitations in this study. First, the observational design cannot prove causality. Second, we quantitatively determined the LFC levels by ultrasonography. Although [1H]-MRS is the most accurate, noninvasive and quantitative LFC detection method based on a large-scale population study, there is sufficient correlation in LFC detection between quantitative ultrasonography and MRS. In addition, we detected serum OPN levels by ELISA, which has been found to be consistent with the results of western blot analyses [35].

Conclusions

In conclusion, the levels of circulating OPN in non-obese Chinese women positively correlated with the FAI and LFC levels. Furthermore, OPN is an independent predictor of LFC in PCOS women and may contribute to the metabolic phenotypes of PCOS through mechanisms independent of insulin resistance. In addition, OPN combined with FAI and hsCRP may be an optimal predictor for NAFLD in PCOS. Further studies are needed to elucidate the mechanism of OPN in the development of NAFLD in PCOS patients.

Acknowledgements
We thank all the women enrolled in the study and gratefully acknowledge the assistance of the nursing staff at Renji Hospital.

Funding
This work was supported by the National Natural Science Foundation of China (grant number 81200628), the Natural Science Foundation of Shanghai (grant number 12ZR1417800), and the Shanghai Science and Technology Development Fund (grant number 08411953000).

Authors' contributions
YW contributed to acquisition of data, analysis of data, and drafting the manuscript and approved the final version of the manuscript. WZ contributed to analysis of data and drafting the manuscript and approved the final version of the manuscript. CW contributed to acquisition of data and drafting the manuscript and approved the final version of the manuscript. YZ and TL contributed to the experimental work and approved the final version of the manuscript. YS contributed to the study design and acquisition of data and approved the final version of the manuscript. WL contributed to the study design, drafting the manuscript and critical discussion and approved the final version of the manuscript. TT contributed to the study design, drafting the manuscript, analysis of data and critical discussion and approved the final version of the manuscript.

Competing interests
The authors declare no competing interests.

Author details
[1]Department of Endocrinology and Metabolism, Renji Hospital, School of Medicine, Shanghai Jiaotong University, 160 Pujian Road, Shanghai 200127, China. [2]Department of Emergency, South Campus, Renji Hospital, School of Medicine, Shanghai Jiaotong University, Shanghai, China. [3]Division of Ultrasonography, Department of Radiology, Renji Hospital, School of Medicine, Shanghai Jiaotong University, 160 Pujian Road, Shanghai 200127, China. [4]Shanghai Key laboratory for Assisted Reproduction and Reproductive Genetics, Center for Reproductive Medicine, Renji Hospital, School of Medicine, Shanghai Jiaotong University, 160 Pujian Road, Shanghai 200127, China.

References
1. Diamanti-Kandarakis E, Kouli CR, Bergiele AT, Filandra FA, Tsianateli TC, Spina GG, et al. A survey of the polycystic ovary syndrome in the Greek island of lesbos: hormonal and metabolic profile. J Clin Endocrinol Metab. 1999; 84(11):4006.
2. Hahn S, Tan S, Sack S, Kimmig R, Quadbeck B, Mann K, et al. Prevalence of the metabolic syndrome in German women with polycystic ovary syndrome. Exp Clin Endocrinol Diabetes. 2007;115:130–5.
3. Legro RS, Arslanian SA, Ehrmann DA, Hoeger KM, Murad MH, Pasquali R, et al. Diagnosis and treatment of polycystic ovary syndrome: an Endocrine Society clinical practice guideline. J Clin Endocrinol Metab. 2013;98:4565–92.
4. Azziz R. PCOS: a diagnostic challenge. Reprod BioMed Online. 2004;8:644–8.
5. Uchil D, Pipalia D, Chawla M, Patel R, Maniar S. Narayani, et al. non-alcoholic fatty liver disease (NAFLD)–the hepatic component of metabolic syndrome. J Assoc Physicians India. 2009;57:201–4.
6. Qu Z, Zhu Y, Jiang J, Shi Y, Chen Z. The clinical characteristics and etiological study of nonalcoholic fatty liver disease in Chinese women with PCOS. Iran J Reprod Med. 2013;11:725–32.
7. Cerda C, Perez-Ayuso RM, Riquelme A, Soza A, Villaseca P, Sir-Petermann T, et al. Nonalcoholic fatty liver disease in women with polycystic ovary syndrome. J Hepatol. 2007;47:412–7.
8. Gambarin-Gelwan M, Kinkhabwala SV, Schiano TD, Bodian C, Yeh HC, Futterweit W. Prevalence of nonalcoholic fatty liver disease in women with polycystic ovary syndrome. Clin Gastroenterol Hepatol. 2007;5:496–501.
9. Karoli R, Fatima J, Chandra A, Gupta U, Islam FU, Singh G. Prevalence of hepatic steatosis in women with polycystic ovary syndrome. J Hum Reprod Sci. 2013;6:9–14.
10. Haas JT, Francque S, Staels B. Pathophysiology and mechanisms of nonalcoholic fatty liver disease. Annu Rev Physiol. 2016;78:181–205.
11. McPherson S, Jonsson JR, Cowin GJ, O'Rourke P, Clouston AD, Volp A, et al. Magnetic resonance imaging and spectroscopy accurately estimate the severity of steatosis provided the stage of fibrosis is considered. J Hepatol. 2009;51:389–97.
12. Marchesini G, Day CP, Dufour JF, Canbay A, Nobili V, Ratziu V, et al. EASL-EASD-EASO clinical practice guidelines for the management of non-alcoholic fatty liver disease. J Hepatol. 2016;64:1388–402.
13. Kuhn JP, Hernando D, Mensel B, Kruger PC, Ittermann T, Mayerle J, et al. Quantitative chemical shift-encoded MRI is an accurate method to quantify hepatic steatosis. J Magn Reson Imaging. 2014;39:1494–501.
14. Xia MF, Bian H, Yan HM, Lin HD, Chang XX, Li XM, et al. Assessment of liver fat content using quantitative ultrasonography to evaluate risks for metabolic diseases. Obesity (Silver Spring). 2015;23:1929–37.
15. Webb M, Yeshua H, Zelber-Sagi S, Santo E, Brazowski E, Halpern Z, et al. Diagnostic value of a computerized hepatorenal index for sonographic quantification of liver steatosis. AJR Am J Roentgenol. 2009;192:909–14.
16. Mancini M, Prinster A, Annuzzi G, Liuzzi R, Giacco R, Medagli C, et al. Sonographic hepatic-renal ratio as indicator of hepatic steatosis: comparison with H-1 magnetic resonance spectroscopy. Metabolism. 2009;58:1724–30.
17. Xia MF, Yan HM, He WY, Li XM, Li CL, Yao XZ, et al. Standardized ultrasound hepatic/renal ratio and hepatic attenuation rate to quantify liver fat content: an improvement method. Obesity (Silver Spring). 2012;20:444–52.
18. Ashkar S, Weber GF, Panoutsakopoulou V, Sanchirico ME, Jansson M, Zawaideh S, et al. Eta-1 (osteopontin): an early component of type-1 (cell-mediated) immunity. Science. 2000;287:860–4.
19. Nomiyama T, Perez-Tilve D, Ogawa D, Gizard F, Zhao Y, Heywood EB, et al. Osteopontin mediates obesity-induced adipose tissue macrophage infiltration and insulin resistance in mice. J Clin Invest. 2007;117:2877–88.
20. Zeyda M, Gollinger K, Todoric J, Kiefer FW, Keck M, Aszmann O, et al. Osteopontin is an activator of human adipose tissue macrophages and directly affects adipocyte function. Endocrinology. 2011;152:2219–27.
21. Kiefer FW, Zeyda M, Gollinger K, Pfau B, Neuhofer A, Weichhart T, et al. Neutralization of osteopontin inhibits obesity-induced inflammation and insulin resistance. Diabetes. 2010;59:935–46.
22. Gomez-Ambrosi J, Catalan V, Ramirez B, Rodriguez A, Colina I, Silva C, et al. Plasma osteopontin levels and expression in adipose tissue are increased in obesity. J Clin Endocr Metab. 2007;92:3719–27.
23. Kuwabara Y, Katayama A, Tomiyama R, Piao H, Kurihara S, Ono S, et al. Gonadotropin regulation and role of ovarian osteopontin in the periovulatory period. J Endocrinol. 2015;224:49–59.
24. Patouraux S, Bonnafous S, Voican CS, Anty R, Saint-Paul MC, Rosenthal-Allieri MA, et al. The osteopontin level in liver, adipose tissue and serum is correlated with fibrosis in patients with alcoholic liver disease. PLoS One. 2012;7:e35612.
25. Kiefer FW, Neschen S, Pfau B, Legerer B, Neuhofer A, Kahle M, et al. Osteopontin deficiency protects against obesity-induced hepatic steatosis and attenuates glucose production in mice. Diabetologia. 2011;54:2132–42.
26. Zhou BF, Cooperative Meta-Analysis Group of the Working Group on Obesity in China. Predictive values of body mass index and waist circumference for risk factors of certain related diseases in Chinese adults–study on optimal cut-off points of body mass index and waist circumference in Chinese adults. Biomed Environ Sci. 2002;15:83–96.
27. Lane DE. Polycystic ovary syndrome and its differential diagnosis. Obstet Gynecol Surv. 2006;61:125–35.
28. Carter GD, Holland SM, Alaghbandzadeh J, Rayman G, Dorringtonward P. Wise PH. Investigation of hirsutism - testosterone is not enough. Ann Clin Biochem. 1983;20:262–3.

29. Jones H, Sprung VS, Pugh CJA, Daousi C, Irwin A, Aziz N, et al. Polycystic ovary syndrome with Hyperandrogenism is characterized by an increased risk of hepatic steatosis compared to Nonhyperandrogenic PCOS phenotypes and healthy controls, independent of obesity and insulin resistance. J Clin Endocr Metab. 2012;97:3709–16.
30. Matthews DR, Hosker JP, Rudenski AS, Naylor BA, Treacher DF, Turner RC. Homeostasis model assessment: insulin resistance and beta-cell function from fasting plasma glucose and insulin concentrations in man. Diabetologia. 1985;28:412–9.
31. Seltzer HS, Allen EW, Herron AL Jr, Brennan MT. Insulin secretion in response to glycemic stimulus: relation of delayed initial release to carbohydrate intolerance in mild diabetes mellitus. J Clin Invest. 1967;46:323–35.
32. Kahn SE, Prigeon RL, McCulloch DK, Boyko EJ, Bergman RN, Schwartz MW, et al. Quantification of the relationship between insulin sensitivity and beta-cell function in human subjects. Evidence for a hyperbolic function. Diabetes. 1993;42:1663–72.
33. Saklamaz A, Calan M, Yilmaz O, Kume T, Temur M, Yildiz N, et al. Polycystic ovary syndrome is associated with increased osteopontin levels. Eur J Endocrinol. 2016;174:415–23.
34. Nagoshi S. Osteopontin: versatile modulator of liver diseases. Hepatol Res. 2014;44:22–30.
35. Sreekanthreddy P, Srinivasan H, Kumar DM, Nijaguna MB, Sridevi S, Vrinda M, et al. Identification of potential serum biomarkers of glioblastoma: serum osteopontin levels correlate with poor prognosis. Cancer Epidemiol Biomark Prev. 2010;19:1409–22.

5

Integration analysis of microRNA and mRNA paired expression profiling identifies deregulated microRNA-transcription factor-gene regulatory networks in ovarian endometriosis

Luyang Zhao[1,2†], Chenglei Gu[1,3†], Mingxia Ye[1], Zhe Zhang[1], Li'an Li[1], Wensheng Fan[1*] and Yuanguang Meng[1*]

Abstract

Background: The etiology and pathophysiology of endometriosis remain unclear. Accumulating evidence suggests that aberrant microRNA (miRNA) and transcription factor (TF) expression may be involved in the pathogenesis and development of endometriosis. This study therefore aims to survey the key miRNAs, TFs and genes and further understand the mechanism of endometriosis.

Methods: Paired expression profiling of miRNA and mRNA in ectopic endometria compared with eutopic endometria were determined by high-throughput sequencing techniques in eight patients with ovarian endometriosis. Binary interactions and circuits among the miRNAs, TFs, and corresponding genes were identified by the Pearson correlation coefficients. miRNA-TF-gene regulatory networks were constructed using bioinformatic methods. Eleven selected miRNAs and TFs were validated by quantitative reverse transcription-polymerase chain reaction in 22 patients.

Results: Overall, 107 differentially expressed miRNAs and 6112 differentially expressed mRNAs were identified by comparing the sequencing of the ectopic endometrium group and the eutopic endometrium group. The miRNA-TF-gene regulatory network consists of 22 miRNAs, 12 TFs and 430 corresponding genes. Specifically, some key regulators from the miR-449 and miR-34b/c cluster, miR-200 family, miR-106a-363 cluster, miR-182/183, FOX family, GATA family, and E2F family as well as CEBPA, SOX9 and HNF4A were suggested to play vital regulatory roles in the pathogenesis of endometriosis.

Conclusion: Integration analysis of the miRNA and mRNA expression profiles presents a unique insight into the regulatory network of this enigmatic disorder and possibly provides clues regarding replacement therapy for endometriosis.

Keywords: Endometriosis, Endometrium, MicroRNAs, Transcription factors, Integrative analysis

Background

Endometriosis is characterized by the presence of endometrial tissue (endometrial glandular and stromal) abnormally outside the uterine cavity [1]. In women of reproductive age, there is a 6–10% incidence rate, which may even reach 35–50% in women who are enduring pelvic pain and/or infertility [2, 3]. Despite its high prevalence, the etiology and pathophysiology of endometriosis are still not fully understood. It is widely accepted that endometriosis is a multifactorial, polygenic disorder [4]. A large amount of molecular aberrations exist between the ectopic endometrium (EC) (endometriotic lesions) and the eutopic endometrium (EU), which could potentially explain the mechanism of the abnormal growth of EU outside the uterus.

microRNAs (miRNAs) are endogenous, single-stranded, 18–22 nucleotide RNAs that mainly inhibit gene

* Correspondence: fanwensheng99@sina.com; meng6512@vip.sina.com
†Equal contributors
[1]Department of Gynecology and Obstetrics, People's Liberation Army (PLA) Medical School, Chinese PLA General Hospital, Beijing 100853, China
Full list of author information is available at the end of the article

expression at the post-transcriptional level [5]. They negatively regulate the translation of target messenger RNAs (mRNAs) via the sequence specific recognition of the "seed sequence" and repress translation and/or degrade the target mRNAs according to the degree of complementary nucleotides [6]. Transcription factors (TFs) are a group of proteins that regulate gene expression by binding to specific DNA sequences at the transcriptional level [7]. Depending on its function, the transcription of an adjacent gene is either activated or repressed [8]. As two vital gene regulatory molecules, miRNAs and TFs can share common target genes and exert effects on each other [9]. As such, the miRNA expression levels can be regulated by TFs, and the mRNAs encoding TFs can be inhibited by miRNAs [10]. In addition, miRNAs and TFs can form a feed-back loop (FBL) or feed-forward loop (FFL) in cooperation to fine tune gene expression [11]. The combinatorial regulation of TFs and miRNAs is suggested to play vital roles in various biological processes and disease pathogenesis [12–15].

Accumulating evidence suggests that aberrant miRNA and TF expression may be involved in the pathogenesis and development of endometriosis [16–25]. Although differences in miRNA expression profiling between EC and EU from women with endometriosis have previously been reported, almost no previous studies have focused on the integrative analysis of miRNA-mRNA interactions and solved the complex problem of the identification of miRNA-TF-gene regulatory networks. With the aim of further understanding the abnormal molecule changes in the occurrence and development of endometriosis, we used high-throughput sequencing techniques to detect miRNA and mRNA expression profiling in paired EC and EU. Joint analysis of the miRNA-TF-gene regulatory network can help us survey the key genomic factors and understand the mechanism of endometriosis at the molecular level.

Methods

Patient samples

The study protocol was approved by the Local Ethical Committee of the Chinese PLA General Hospital, and each patient was required to provide written consent.

Sixty tissue samples (30 paired EC and EU) from 30 patients with ovarian endometriosis were obtained from the Chinese PLA general hospital. Among them, eight paired EC and EU samples were selected and prepared for small RNA sequencing and mRNA sequencing. The remaining samples were used for validation. All of the patients were confirmed to have endometriosis by histological examination and diagnosed as being at a moderate to severe (III-IV) stage by the revised American Fertility Society (r-AFS) classification during laparoscopic surgery [26]. EC samples were obtained during laparoscopy, and EU samples were obtained through curettage before the laparoscopic procedure. Only patients in the secretory phase of the menstrual cycle, which was confirmed by the method of Noyes et al. [27], and without any hormonal treatment history, were included in the study. Clinical characteristics of the patients are listed in Additional file 1.

Tissue processing, RNA extraction and quality control

All tissue samples were divided into two parts: one half was fixed and prepared for pathological examination and the other half was placed in RNA-later solution (Sigma Aldrich, Poland) at 4 °C for 24 h and subsequently transferred to −80 °C until further use. Total RNA was extracted using a single-step acid guanidinium thiocyanate-phenol-chloroform method [28]. The quality and purity of RNA were examined by a Nanodrop 8000 spectrophotometer (Thermo Scientific, Waltham, MA, USA). RNA integrity was analyzed using the RNA 6000 Nano Kit and Small RNA Kit with the Bioanalyzer 2100 (Agilent, Santa Clara, CA). Samples with an absorbance wavelength ratio (A260/A280) ≥ 1.9 and an RNA integrity number ≥ 8 were included.

Small RNA sequencing (small RNA-seq) and data analysis

For small RNA sequencing, 3 μg of total RNA was used for library preparation as previously reported with little modification [29]. The purified libraries were sequenced on an Illumina HiSeq 2000 platform by Annoroad Genome (Beijing, China). The detailed protocol is described in Additional file 2. In brief, the raw data were processed with Python scripts to ensure its quality and were then filtered by Q30 statistics. The clean data were mapped to the Ensemble database (GRCh37) (http://grch37.ensembl.org/index.html) [30] using Bowtie (v1.01) [31] and compared with miRBase (Release 21) [32] to identify mature miRNAs. For each sample, the count and RPM (reads per million total reads) value of the miRNAs were collected. DEGseq (v1.18.0) [33] was used for differential expression analysis with the parameters of differentially expressed miRNAs (DEM) set with a false discovery rate (FDR) < 0.05 and |log2 fold change (FC)| ≥ 1.

mRNA sequencing (mRNA-seq) and data analysis

For mRNA sequencing, 3 μg of RNA per sample was prepared for library preparation. The Ribo-Zero Gold Kit (Epicentre, USA) and NEB Next Ultra RNA Library Prep Kit (NEB, Ipswich, USA) were used for rRNA removal and library construction following the manufacturer's protocols. For high-throughput sequencing, paired-end 150-bp sequencing of the cDNAs was performed on an Illumina HiSeq4000 system (Illumina, USA) conducted by Annoroad Genome (Beijing, China). The raw data were processed with Perl scripts to ensure the quality of the data used in subsequent analyses (details in Additional file 2).

Bowtie2 (v2.2.3) [34] was used to build the genome index, and clean data were mapped to the human genome (GRCh37) (http://grch37.ensembl.org/index.html) using TopHat (v2.0.12) [35]. The read counts of each gene were counted by HTSeq (v0.6.0) [36], and the reads per kilobase of one gene per million reads (RPKM) were calculated to estimate the expression level of genes in each sample. DEGseq (v1.18.0) [33] was used to analyze differentially expressed genes (DEGs) with parameters of FDR < 0.05 and |log2FC| ≥ 1.

Identification of miRNA/TF/gene interactions and a regulatory network

The miRNA and mRNA expression profiles were analyzed by MAGIA2 (http://gencomp.bio.unipd.it/magia2/) to identify miRNA-TF-gene binary interactions and circuits [37]. The miRNA-target interactions were predicted by the TargetScan database [38] with a z-score ≥ 0.7. TF-miRNA interactions were identified from the mirGen2.0 [39] and TransmiR [40] databases, and TF-gene interactions were obtained from the 'TFBS conserved' track of the UCSC genome annotation for human (version hg19) (http://genome.ucsc.edu/) database, restricting the z-score to ≥ 3. Two types of mixed regulatory circuits were also identified: (i) FFL, which is a TF that regulates both a given miRNA and their common target gene and (ii) FBL, which is a miRNA that regulates both a given TF and their common regulated gene. The Pearson correlation coefficient (PCC) was used to measure the relationships with a PCC > 0.6 and a *P*-value < 0.05. The integrative miRNA-TF-gene regulatory network was visualized by Cytoscape (v3.2) [41].

Functional analysis

To explore the functional roles of DEGs in the miRNA-TF-gene networks, we used DAVID, which integrates the Gene Ontology (GO) and Kyoto Encyclopedia of Genes and Genomes (KEGG) databases to analyze biological functions [42]. The enrichment values of GO terms and KEGG pathways were implemented by the hypergeometric test, and q (adjusted as *p*-value) < 0.05 was considered to be significantly enriched.

Quantitative reverse transcription-polymerase chain reaction (qRT-PCR) validation

Six miRNAs (miR-34c-5p, miR-106a-5p, miR-182-5p, miR-200a-3p, miR-449b-5p, and miR-615-3p) and five TFs (CEBPA, FOXC1, E2F1, GATA1, and HNF4A) were selected for validation analysis. U6 was selected as the miRNA endogenous control, and GAPDH was used as the mRNA endogenous control. Primer sequences are listed in Additional file 3. miRNA cDNA synthesis was conducted with the miRNA cDNA Kit (ComWin Biotech, Beijing), and total cDNA synthesis was conducted by a RevertAid™ First Strand cDNA Synthesis Kit (Thermo, USA). Relative miRNA expression was determined according to the miRNA Real-Time PCR Assay Kit (ComWin Biotech, Beijing), and relative mRNA expression was determined according to the THUNDERBIRD™ SYBR qPCR Mix (TOYOBO, Japan). qRT-PCR was performed on an ABI PRISM 7500 (Applied Biosystems, CA, USA). Relative expression was calculated using the ABI PRISM 7500 version 2.0.6 software (Applied Biosystems, CA, USA) with the $2^{-\Delta\Delta Ct}$ method [43].

Results

Small RNA-seq analysis and DEM profiling

The small RNA-seq generated 216,333,583 reads with an average of 13,520,849 reads per sample. The FastQC quality test showed that 182,420,380 of the reads had a Q-score ≥ 30; these reads were considered in further analyses. A proportion of clean reads was mapped to the miRBase database (v21.0) for each sample and is listed in Additional file 4. Of the 1574 miRNAs analyzed by small RNA sequencing, 1163 with a normalized count value greater than 1 in at least one sample in both the EC and EU groups were further analyzed. Unsupervised hierarchical clustering showed that the overall miRNA profile of EC was wholly different from that of EU (Fig.1a). Using the selection criteria mentioned above, 107 DEMs were found, including 41 up-regulated miRNAs and 66 down-regulated miRNAs, between EC and paired EU. Among them, miR-514b-3p was the most up-regulated, with an FC of 330.31, whereas miR-375 was the most down-regulated, with an FC of 154.52 (Additional file 5).

mRNA-seq analysis and DEG profiling

mRNA-seq generated 1,748,534,484 reads with an average of 109,283,405 reads per sample. The FastQC quality test showed that 1,721,709,042 (98.46%) reads reached Q30; these reads were considered for further analyses. Of these reads, 93.17% were mapped to hg19, and 98.56% were uniquely aligned. The detailed filtering and mapping data are listed in Additional file 6. Unsupervised hierarchical clustering analysis showed that the transcriptome profiling of the EC group was significantly different from that of the EU group (Fig. 1b). Using the same criteria that were used for the miRNAs, a total of 6112 DEGs with 3228 up-regulated mRNA transcripts and 2884 down-regulated mRNA transcripts were identified. The most up- and down-regulated mRNAs were IGHV3–49 (ENSG00000211965) and FXYD4 (ENSG00000150201), with FCs of 3253.41 and 1024.16, respectively. Additional file 7 lists the top 25 up- and down-regulated mRNAs identified by our sequencing.

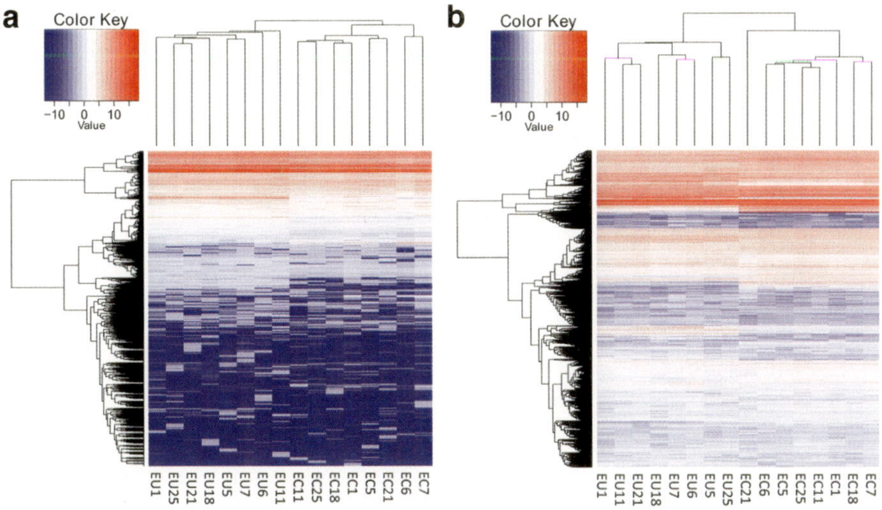

Fig. 1 Heat map showing differentially expressed miRNAs and mRNAs from ectopic endometria compared with paired eutopic endometria. Rows represent miRNAs (**a**) or mRNAs (**b**); columns represent profiled samples. The relative expression is depicted according to the color scale. Red indicates up-regulation; blue indicates down-regulation. EU means eutopic endometrium and EC means ectopic endometrium

Identification of miRNA/TF/gene interactions and regulatory networks

One hundred seven DEMs and 6112 DEGs identified in the previous steps were considered for the miRNA/TF/gene binary interaction and regulatory network analysis.

According to the standard of absolute PCC > 0.6, correlation analysis revealed 379 paired miRNA-target regulatory interactions between 15 miRNAs (miR-20b-5p, miR-30d-5p, miR-34c-5p, miR-106a-5p, miR-133b, miR-141-3p, miR-182-5p, miR-183-5p, miR-196b-5p, miR-200a-3p, miR-200b-3p, miR-200c-3p, miR-363-3p, miR-449a, and miR-449b-5p), five TFs (GATA6, GATA2, FOXO1, FOXC1, and CEBPA) and 223 genes. Although miRNAs usually suppress target mRNAs, positively paired miRNA-mRNA correlations are occasionally observed under certain conditions [44]. For this reason, we identified all of the differentially expressed miRNA-gene pairs, including 174 negative correlating pairs and 205 positive correlating pairs. In the case of TF-gene interactions, 310 regulatory pairs involving seven TFs (E2F1, CEBPA, FOXC1, FOXL1, FOXO1, GATA1, and SOX9) and 261 corresponding genes were identified. For TF-miRNA interactions, a total of 23 TF-miRNA pairs between seven TFs (E2F1, E2F2, FOXJ1, FOXL1, GATA1, HNF4A, and SOX9) and 19 miRNAs (miR-20b-5p, miR-34b-3p, miR-34b-5p, miR-34c-5p, miR-106a-5p, miR-133b, miR-182-5p, miR-183-5p, miR-196b-5p, miR-200a-3p, miR-200b-3p, miR-202-3p, miR-216a-5p, miR-224-5p, miR-363-3p, miR-449a, miR-449b-5p, miR-449c-5p, and miR-708-5p) were involved in the comparison. Moreover, we revealed five mixed circuits, including one FFL (FOXL1/miR-133b/PRDM1) and four FBLs (miR-182-5p/FOXO1/NUAK1, miR-182-5p/FOXO1/SCN9A, mi R-133b/FOXC1/EYA4, and miR-133b/FOXC1/LHFP).

Based on the relationships of binary interactions and circuits, we constructed the miRNA-TF-gene regulatory network. The final integrated network contained 22 miRNAs, 12 TFs and 430 genes (Table 1, Fig. 2). To identify key regulators in the integrated networks, we also calculated the node degree of the involved miRNAs and TFs. The node degree is a centrality measure method that directly counts the links of one node. The few nodes that have a high degree in the network are called hubs, which reflect their importance in a large number of interactions [45]. As a result, the node degrees of the selected miRNAs and TFs ranged from 1 to 117 in our data. The top five key regulators in the miRNA-TF-gene network of endometriosis were FOXC1, FOXO1, miR-182-5p, miR-106a-5p, and CEBPA, which were directly connected to 117, 64, 57, 49, and 49 corresponding targets, respectively (Table 1).

Functional analysis

Functional enrichment analysis of all of the target genes involved in the networks provided us with an overall clue regarding their functional roles in endometriosis. GO analysis revealed that the target genes in the GO cellular component (GO-CC) category were enriched in 16 terms, such as the plasma membrane, proteinaceous extracellular matrix and Z disc. The GO molecular function (GO-MF) category was enriched in six terms, including sequence-specific DNA binding, transcriptional activator activity and cell adhesion molecule binding. In the biological process category of GO terms (GO-BP), 20 terms included cell adhesion, whereas embryonic skeletal system morphogenesis, extracellular matrix organization and angiogenesis were significantly

Table 1 The key regulators and their targets identified in the integrated network in endometriosis

ID	Node degree	Fold change	Target
FOXC1	117	7.26	ZNF521, MKX, ENOX1, TENM4, CHN2, PLXDC2, ZFHX4, COLEC12, FAM19A2, ICAM5, DCN, DGKG, PTPN3, PDGFC, PBX3, EPHA3, C7orf10, NMNAT3, MDFI, SCG5, GPC6, FGF14, ADAMTSL3, F13A1, FIGN, SNAP25, BNC2, GPR1, ICA1, BOC, PLXNC1, NRK, VDR, OMG, CHL1, SYNDIG1, DRP2, EPHB2, SORCS2, RP4-794H19.2, SDK1, PLCB4, HS6ST3, NTM, FAM133A, HOXA11, NUGGC, SELP, TTC29, HOXA3, NKAIN3, SYTL2, HOXA11-AS, EN2, CNTN3, DNAJC15, GPC3, GALNTL6, LINC00922, CASZ1, COL11A1, RAB11FIP4, RAB3C, AMPD1, C9orf135, TWIST2, MAP3K19, C9orf171, FRMD5, GRM8, GJB2, MECOM, ETV1, ALCAM, DOCK2, REV3L, EYA4, CACNA1D, PLXNA4, GRB7, SCN9A, PDE7B, PAX2, DLGAP1, PCDHA4, KPNA2, KIRREL3, CCDC19, SLC14A2, KLHL13, COL28A1, MAOA, MARCH1, CACNA1I, NEBL, SGCD, MAFB, LHFP, DSCAML1, ADAMTS9, POU6F2, PHLPP1, EYA2, ERBB4PCLO, OPCML, SESTD1, MAFF, MPZL2, SOX30, PLCZ1, RP11-536O18.2, RGS6, GRIN2A, CYTIP, ITPR1
FOXO1	64	−3.56	HAND2-AS1, EFNA1, GRB7, RASD1, EN2, ICA1, SESTD1, CNKSR2, RP11-383H13.1, VSIG2, CP, RP11-792D21.2, MRC1, PDGFC, BARX2, KCNH1, NKAIN3, HS6ST3, CHST9, WDFY4, HOXC4, PPP1R9A, NUAK1, PTPRR, LHFPL3, CR1, SHROOM3, PLCB4, RGS6, HOXC8, TMPRSS2, LINGO2, AOAH, COLEC12, MASP1, MAP3K5, MLIP, SPTLC3, TENM4, SLC2A1-AS1, PLXNC1, ZFHX4, SLC6A7, RALGAPA2, SORCS1, EPHB2, DNAJC6, HOXC6, MAFF, NMNAT3, NALCN, SMPX, SCN9A, ST8SIA4, CAPN8, TTYH2, NBL1, CD83, GALNT16, NTM, COL24A1, ST6GALNAC5, CPNE5, FGF10
miR-182-5p	57	−5.34	RAB40B, SLC1A2, SCN1, APHYHIPL, FAT3, SLC2A8, **FOXO1**, **CEBPA**, PDE7B, RPH3A, ESRRG, CALCR, RHPN2, TP53INP2, SLITRK4, PTGER3, FN1, DENND2C, EPHA3, ZNF831, PIK3R1, SLC9A2, TCF19, SCN9A, GRIA1, FUT9, LDB3, PRRG3, PRDM16, SPRY3, ADRA2C, THBS2, SLC22A5, LIPG, FST, BNC2, ADAMTS18, GDNF, MPP1, FAM78A, KIAA1210, TMEM86A, RNF183, F13A1, ERBB4, NUAK1, IRF6, SEMA5A, LPPR4, AP1S3, MYO5B, KIAA1244, TPD52, GRHL2, CXADR, CELSR1, KIAA1324
miR-106a-5p	49	−3.72	VASH2, OSM, MYCN, JAZF1, ETV1, BCL11B, TP73, ITGB8, SV2B, CD274, ANKRD33B, GRHL2, DENND5B, CYP26B1, LIF, PKIA, ERBB3, RASL11B, RORC, VEGFA, NR4A2, SHANK2, PARD6B, BHLHE41, GPC6, RASD1, PDE3B, HEG1, RUNX1, SULF1, MYO5B, TTC9, CNGB3, ZFPM2, BNC2, SLC46A3, PBX3, EXPH5, ADAMTSL2, PCYT1B, APCDD1, FAM129A, SEMA5A, FAIM2, MTF1, KIF5A, NBL1, PTPN3, NRP2
CEBPA	49	5.73	VASH2, OSM, MYCN, JAZF1, ETV1, BCL11B, TP73, ITGB8, SV2B, CD274, ANKRD33B, GRHL2, DENND5B, CYP26B1, LIF, PKIA, ERBB3, RASL11B, RORC, VEGFA, NR4A2, SHANK2, PARD6B, BHLHE41, GPC6, RASD1, PDE3B, HEG1, RUNX1, SULF1, MYO5B, TTC9, CNGB3, ZFPM2, BNC2, SLC46A3, PBX3, EXPH5, ADAMTSL2, PCYT1B, APCDD1, FAM129A, SEMA5A, FAIM2, MTF1, KIF5A, NBL1, PTPN3, NRP2
GATA1	41	7.62	**miR-202-3p**, ATP10B, MATN3, PAPPA2, RAB31, PDE10A, FRMD5, ABCA6, PRR5L, TSPAN2, SLC8A3, SYNDIG1L, MDGA2, ENOX1, FOXC1, FGF14, CLIC6, RASGRF2, ANTXR1, ZNF469, PCYT1B, MAPK4, ENAM, NRP2, SYNPO, DRP2, CHN2, PDE7B, ZNF521, PPP2R2B, ITGA8, NTM, MKX, SLC14A2, GALNT5, COL8A1, BDNF, ADAMTSL2, DPYSL3, THSD7B, GPC6
miR-20b-5p	40	−4.16	TP73, LIF, CYP26B1, RASL11B, GRHL2, SV2B, RASD1, CD274, DENND5B, VEGFA, HEG1, BCL11B, PARD6B, PKIA, MYO5B, RUNX1, GPC6, BHLHE41, PDE3B, SULF1, SHANK2, TTC9, EXPH5, NR4A2, SLC46A3, ZFPM2, BNC2, PCYT1B, ADAMTSL2, NBL1, PBX3, APCDD1, FAM129A, FAIM2, KIF5A, MTF1, PTPN3, NRP2, SEMA5A, CNGB3
miR-200b-3p	37	−16.72	PLXNA4, CASR, ELK4, PARD3B, DCDC2, DENND5B, PARD6B, PKIA, KRT80, HOXA5, KLHL14, SGCE, NOG, PTCH1, **GATA2**, ST6GALNAC5, PRDM16, BNC2, SLC6A1, TP73, SCN3B, ANK3, HOOK1, PAG1, PVRL4, BAG5, GLIS2, JAZF1, DDIT4L, CNTFR, CHN2, CASZ1, NRP2, KIAA1456, OCLN, CECR2, PAK6
FOXL1	37	20.45	**miR-34c-5p, miR-34b-3p, miR-34b-5p, miR-133b**, PDE3A, SV2B, PRDM16, HOXD10, ZFHX4, PLXNC1, MSRB3, ZNF521, SEMA5A, HOXD11, ST18, SCN9A, MCF2, ENOX1, NTF3, FOXO1, OPCML, EPB41L4B, C7orf10, PPL, KLHL13, CASZ1, MME, POSTN, RUNX1, COL24A1, VEGFA, GPC6, ANKRD33B, HPSE2, GRIA3, NRXN1, PLCB1
miR-363-3p	36	−2.92	EN2, SLC12A5, NRK, BCL11B, SESTD1, PRKAR2B, DACT1, PTPRO, RHPN2, HEG1, BTG2, CACNA1H, B3GALT2, PPP1R9A, ZNF469, PRDM16, KLF2, HAND2, ZFHX4, ESRP1, WWC1, GRAMD1B, SLC6A1, MPP1, ZFPM2, **GATA6**, ADAMTSL3, TTC9, ADAMTS9, PDE10A, PCYT1B, MSRB3, HOXC8, HOXC4, MTF1, KCNH1
miR-200c-3p	36	−27.15	PPP1R12B, CASR, FAT3, STX1A, DCDC2, VEGFA, PLXNA4, VASH2, PARD3B, JAZF1, PKIA, KRT80, DENND5B, RIMKLB, HOXA5, KIAA1456, SGCE, SLC6A1, PAK6, PRDM16, SCN3B, ST6GALNAC5, BNC2, HOOK1, ELK4, EFNA1, CASZ1, GLIS2, DDIT4L, PVRL4, PAG1, NRP2, CHN2, CECR2, PARD6B, OCLN
miR-30d-5p	29	−3.93	CHL1, MFSD6, CLCF1, PLS1, COL9A3, BNC2, NRXN3, ME1, EPHB2, NUAK1, PAG1, NRP2, RGS6, HOXB8, GDNF, CORO2A, EPB41L4B, RASD1, PPP1R9A, GCNT2, HELZ, ATP2B2, CECR2, GPT2, IP6K3, SCARA5, DLG5, RNF165, FAM83F
miR-133b	19	9.16	BTBD3, FOXC1, ENPEP, JUP, ELF3, PTH1R, PRDM16, GPM6A, CTGF, BICC1, HOXD1, HOXA9, LHFP, CELF4, LTBP1, GDNF, PTPRZ1, LRRC2, ANK2
miR-449b-5p	14	−114.1	PKIA, FUT9, GAS1, NR4A2, RAB11FIP4, CSF1R, KIAA1045, ZDHHC23, GABRA3, SIDT1, ANK3, SPRY3, TPD52, PCLO
miR-449a	13	−70.83	CSF1R, ANK3, ZDHHC23, FUT9, SDK2, GNAO1, GABRA3, TPD52, SBK1, NR4A2, SPRY3, PCLO, DPYSL4
miR-196b-5p	13	−13.72	HMGA1, OPCML, COL1A1, NRK, IGDCC4, RGS6, ELK4, PARD6B, HOOK1, BNC2, PBX3, HOXA9, HOXC8
SOX9	13	−12.89	MELK, DCDC2, NTN1, DPP6, UNC93A, FOSL1, ASIC2, LINC00669, NPAS3, BRIP1, DMBT1, EN2, C20orf26
HNF4A	12	−9.63	**miR-20b-5p, miR-363-3p, miR-106a-5p, miR-196b-5p, miR-182-5p, miR-224-5p, miR-183-5p, miR-200a-3p, miR-708-5p, miR-200b-3p, miR-216a-5p, miR-449a**
	11	−15.91	SPRY3, KIAA1045, GABRA3, ANK3, STX1A, CSF1R, PARD6B, PCLO, RAP1GAP, TPD52

Table 1 The key regulators and their targets identified in the integrated network in endometriosis *(Continued)*

ID	Node degree	Fold change	Target
miR-34c-5p			
miR-200a-3p	9	−35.83	SCD5, PLXNA4, CYP26B1, PLXDC1, PAPPA, OSBPL6, MN1, RHPN2, GATA6
miR-141-3p	9	−56.69	PLXNA4, PLXDC1, SCD5, PAPPA, MN1, CYP26B1, GATA6, OSBPL6, RHPN2
miR-183-5p	7	−5.72	EZR, RAB11FIP4, KIAA0101, SLC1A2, MAL2, SLAIN1, SPRY3
E2F1	4	−3.74	**miR-449a, miR-449c-5p, miR-449b-5p**, MELK
FOXJ1	1	−98.82	**miR-449a**
E2F2	1	−3.56	**miR-196b-5p**

The identified miRNAs and TFs in "Target" were highlighted in bold type

enriched (Fig. 3a). KEGG pathway analysis demonstrated that the DEG targets were associated with 27 pathways, such as the calcium-signaling pathway, cAMP signaling pathway, and transcriptional misregulation in cancer pathway (Fig. 3b).

Validation by qRT-PCR

The qRT-PCR results were consistent with the sequencing results in that all six selected miRNAs (miR-34c-5p, miR-106a-5p, miR-182-5p, miR-200a-3p, miR-449b-5p, and miR-615-3p) and five TFs (CEBPA, FOXC1, E2F1, GATA1, and HNF4A) were differentially expressed with the same trend (up- or down-regulated) of sequencing and reached statistical significance (Fig. 4).

Discussion

Several microarray studies were conducted to obtain DEMs between EC and EU from women with endometriosis [18, 46, 47], but overlapping data are limited, which suggests that the molecular changes caused by endometriosis might be more complex than we assumed. Additionally, miRNA target prediction methods based on sequence complementarity have been used to annotate the functions of DEMs in these studies, which may contain a high false positive rate and false negative rate [48]. Therefore, the functions of most of the identified DE miRNAs in endometriosis remain unclear due to a lack of definite target genes and confounding downstream validations. Network analysis allows structured grouping of miRNAs, TFs and target genes; thus, network construction is essential for identifying critical molecular changes and understanding their functional roles. To our knowledge, this is the first study to establish concomitant miRNA-TF-gene binary interactions and regulatory networks between the EC and the EU from patients with endometriosis. At first, our study revealed 107 DEMs and 6112 DEGs by sequencing. The large differential expression profiling was refined by PCC to 22 functionally DE miRNAs, 12 TFs and 430 target genes. The network included some well-studied candidate miRNAs and genes (e.g., miR-183-5p, FOXO1, and VEGFA) but also identified many novel objects (e.g., the miR-449 family and miR-106a-363 cluster). Here, we discuss these key regulators in the network, with the hope of providing valuable information for understanding the molecular mechanism of endometriosis.

The highly conserved miR-449 family encoded by the CDC20B gene consists of three members: miR-449a, miR-449b, and miR-449c. Accumulating evidence suggests that the miR-449 family plays an important role in cell proliferation, migration and invasion and might serve as a tumor suppressor in miRNAs [49]. Consistently, miR-449 members were absent or down-regulated in various human malignancies, such as liver cancer [50], breast cancers [51], lung cancer [52], and ovarian clear cell carcinoma [53]. In the current study, we reported the first significant down-regulation of miR-449a, miR-449b-5p, and miR-449c-5p in ectopic endometrial tissue. Considering that endometriosis shares many characteristics with malignant diseases, such as invasion and immigration, it is very likely that the lower expression of miR-449 plays an important role in the pathogenesis of endometriosis. miR-34b and miR-34c are classified into the same cluster and share related functions with miR-449 due to their structural similarities [54, 55]. Much attention has been focused on miR-34 therapeutics for cancer [56, 57]. In addition, miR-34 mimics have been used in several preclinical studies and a phase I clinical trial, and they have shown potential as anticancer therapeutics [58]. Our study identified the down-regulation of miR-34b-3p, which is consistent with the results from Teague et al. [16]. Moreover, we also identified two down-regulated miRNAs, namely, miR-34b-5p and miR-34c-5p, which have been reported by Burney et al. in the eutopic endometrium compared with normal endometrium [17]. Their results suggested that down-regulation of miR-34b and miR-34c was involved in

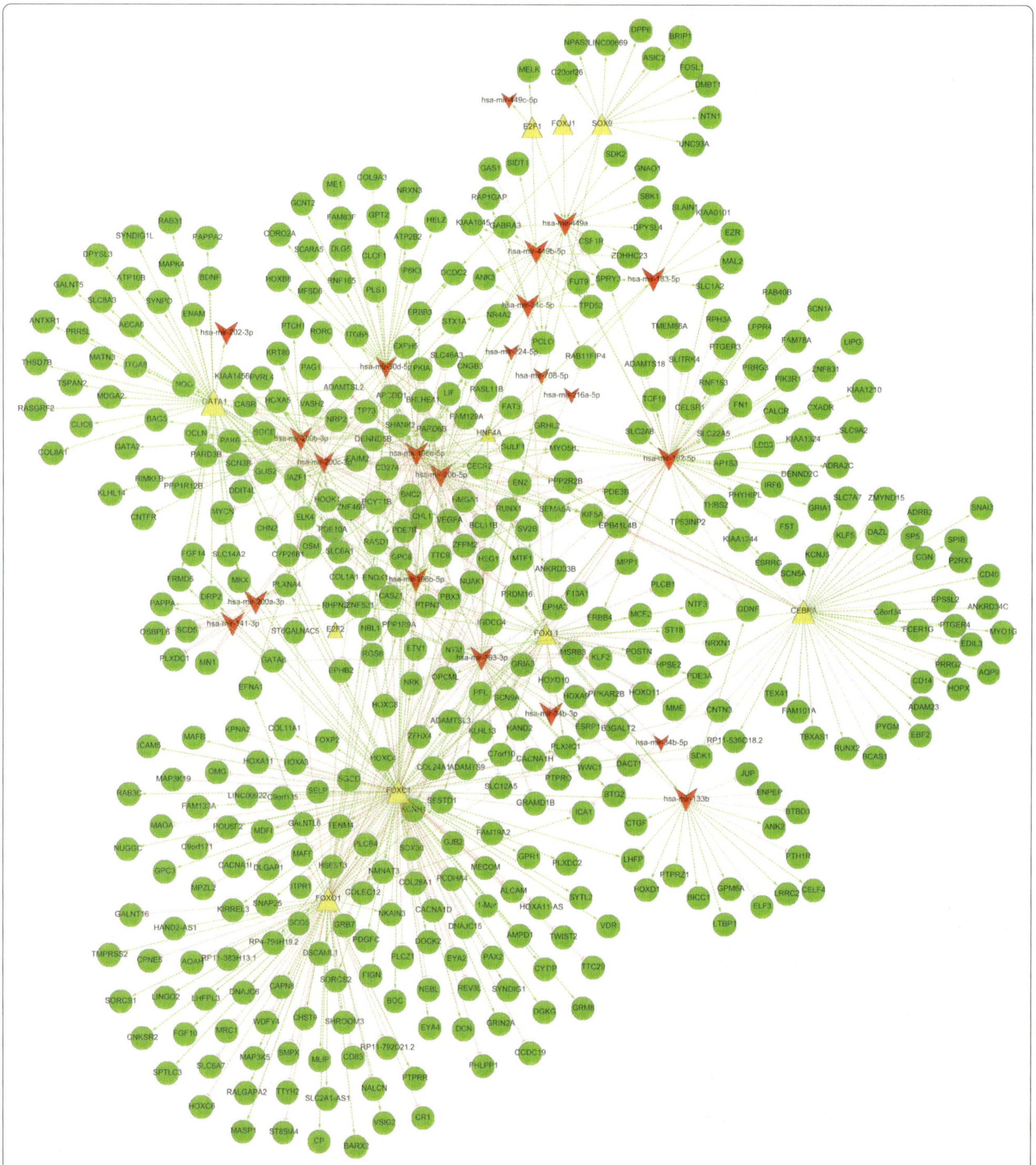

Fig. 2 The integrated endometriosis-related miRNA-transcription factor-gene regulation network. Red represents miRNA; yellow represents transcription factor; green represents target gene

the initiation and maintenance of endometriosis. Given the therapeutic role of miR-34 in cancer and its structural similarity to miR-449 [54], mimics from the miR-449 and miR-34b/c cluster could also be potential miRNA replacement therapies in endometriosis. We therefore suggest that further studies focus on both the miR-34 and miR-449 families by analyzing their function and target genes in endometriosis.

The miR-200 family is another important set of miRNAs that was down-regulated in the present study and has been reported to be reduced in many solid tumors [59]. The miR-200 family contains two groups, miR-

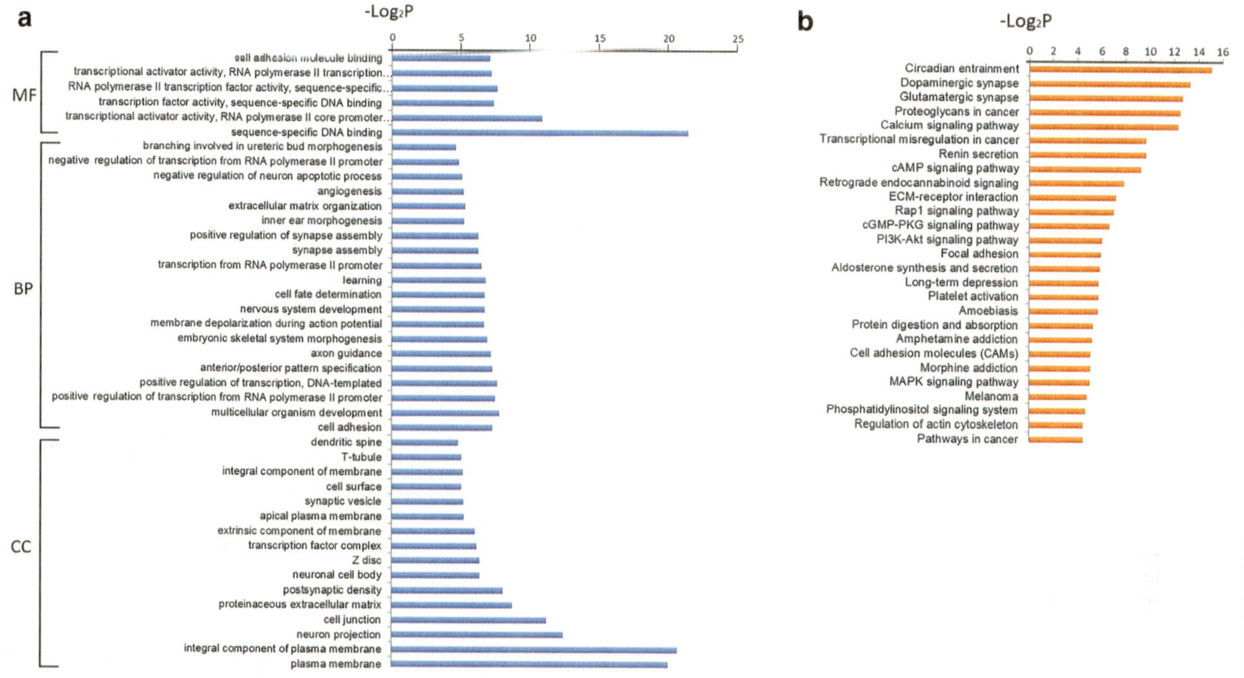

Fig.3 a GO terms enriched by differentially expressed genes that involved in regulatory network. BP represents biological processes; CC represents cellular components; MF represents molecular functions. b KEGG pathways enriched by differentially expressed genes that involved in regulatory network

200a/b/429 and miR-200c/141, that regulate a cohort of target genes involved in epithelial-mesenchymal transition, metastasis and angiogenesis [60], which are important events in the pathogenesis of endometriosis [61]. Previous studies revealed deregulated miR-200 family members in endometriotic lesions compared with eutopic endometrium [16, 18] and in eutopic endometrium compared with normal endometrium [19]. Circulating miR-200a and miR-141 have also been proposed as candidate biomarkers for endometriosis [62]. The present study is not the first to identify lower levels of miR-141-3p, miR-200a-3p, miR-200b-3p and miR-200c-3p in endometriosis. However, our report confirmed the previous results and identified a series of corresponding genes of these miRNAs, which may be involved in many physical or pathological processes in endometriosis. For example, JAZF1, which is regulated by miR-200b/c, is a proto-oncogene known to be affected by chromosomal translocation in endometrial stromal tumors [63]. In the study by Yotova et al., JAZF1 was hyper-methylated and down-regulated in stromal cells from ovarian ectopic endometria compared with normal endometria [25]. As another example, TP73, which is regulated by miR-200b, is part of the TP53 family and plays a role in the cell cycle, apoptosis and infertility [64], and no previous research has revealed its functions in endometriosis.

miR-363, miR-20b, and miR-106a are transcribed from the miR-106a-363 cluster [65]. All of these miRNAs were down-regulated in ectopic lesions according to our results. Intriguingly, these miRNAs have dual functions either as tumor suppressors or as oncogenic miRNAs. A high level of miR-363-3p suppresses the proliferation of human hepatocellular carcinoma cells [66] and decreases the metastasis of neuroblastoma cells [67], whereas the knock-down of miR-363-3p was reported to suppress carcinogenesis in gastric cancer cells [68]. Li et al. demonstrated that miR-20b acts as an oncogene by contributing to breast tumorigenesis [69], but Hong et al. found that miR-20b was markedly down-regulated and served as a tumor suppressor miRNA in papillary thyroid carcinoma [70]. Li et al. identified increased miR-106a as playing an oncogenic role in pancreatic cancer [71]. In contrast, Zhi et al. reported that miR-106a could inhibit proliferation and promote apoptosis in astrocytoma cells [72]. As no study has previously reported the functions of miR-363-3p, miR-20b and miR-106a in endometriosis, we infer that the decreased expression of these three miRNAs might have tumor suppressive-like functions in the initiation, progression, and metastasis of endometriotic lesions. Additionally, many corresponding target genes, such as ADAMTS family members, which are also known tumor suppressor genes, are down-regulated, consistent with the present study, which confirmed our inference indirectly.

miR-182-5p, which belongs to the miR-183/96/182 cluster, contains the highest node degree in the identified DEMs and shows a 5.3-fold down-regulation in EC versus EU. This finding is consistent with the results obtained

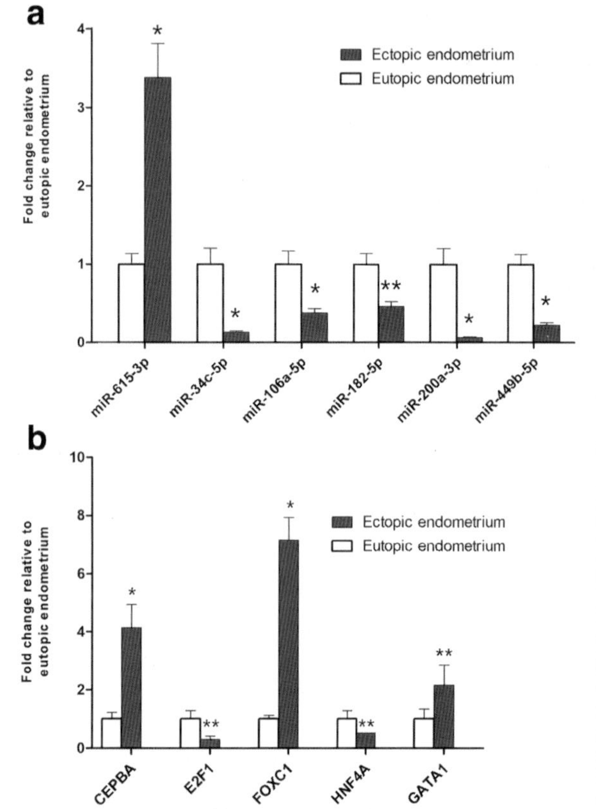

Fig. 4 qRT-PCR analysis of the six miRNAs expressions (**a**) and five transcription factors expressions (**b**) in ectopic endometria ($n = 22$) and paired eutopic endometria ($n = 22$). Grey column represents ectopic endometrium; white column represents eutopic endometrium. Significant fold changes in ectopic vs. eutopic endometrium are marked by *, $P \leq 0.01$; ** $P \leq 0.001$. The error bar denotes SEM (standard error of the mean)

from the microarray screening and qRT-PCR validation by Filigheddu et al. [18] Similar to miR-182-5p, miR-183-5p expression in ectopic endometrium was 5.7-fold down-regulated in our study and was confirmed by previously published reports [47, 73]. Additionally, functional analysis indicated that the down-regulation of miR-183 can inhibit apoptosis and enhance the invasive ability of endometrial stromal cells [47]. These findings indicate that aberrant miR-182/183 expression is part of the epigenetic mechanism of pathogenesis and the development of endometriosis.

Based on the integrative regulatory network, a series of TFs also attracted our attention, including FOX family members, GATA family members, and E2F family members, as well as CEBPA, SOX9 and HNF4A. FOX (fork-head box) proteins are a family of transcription factors involved in many pathologic and physiological processes, such as cell growth, proliferation, and longevity [74]. The FOX subfamilies, such as FOXO, FOXC and FOXP, play different roles in different types of diseases [75]. Here, we identified four important FOX subfamily members, FOXO1, FOXC1, FOXL1 and FOXJ1, which co-operatively regulate the integrative networks in endometriosis. FOXO1 serves as an anti-oncogene in various malignancies through diverse mechanisms, such as promoting apoptosis and facilitating DNA repair [76] and was decreased by 3.5-fold in endometriotic tissue in the present study. Previous data showed the same trend with lower FOXO1 levels expressed in endometriosis, which might contribute to an overactive PI3K/AKT pathway, but the underlying mechanisms are not well understood [77]. Additionally, two FBLs, miR-182-5p/FOXO1/NUAK1 and miR-182-5p/FOXO1/SCN9A, were observed and their functions are expected to be explored in the future. In recent years, an elevated expression of FOXC1 has been detected in different tumors, such as esophageal cancer [78], hepatocellular carcinoma [79] and osteosarcoma [80]. The current views on its function and molecular mechanisms reveal that FOXC1 as an oncogene plays multiple roles in cancer progression and metastasis by affecting different targets [78–81]. The present study evaluated FOXC1 expression by high-throughput sequencing and qRT-PCR, and both results indicated that FOXC1 increased approximately sevenfold in EC compared with EU. Furthermore, FOXC1 was identified as a direct target of miR-133b and shares the same targets including EYA4 and LHFP.

GATA1, GATA2 and GATA6 belong to the GATA family, which mainly plays roles in morphogenesis and organogenesis [82]. Our study observed that GATA1 could increase the miR-202-3p expression level and act on 40 targets in the endometriotic lesion. Although the cause of the high expression of GATA1 is not yet clear, Hawkins et al. reported that miR-202-3p was up-regulated in EC compared to normal endometria [19]. Moreover, we suggest that GATA2 and GATA6, as target TFs of the miR-200 family, might be involved in the pathogenesis of endometriosis together with the miR-200 family.

E2F1 is the most important TF in the E2F family, which is known to integrate cell cycle progression with DNA repair, replication, and multiple checkpoints [83]. Interestingly, the function of E2F1 in tumors is a paradox; both positive and negative effects of E2F1 on tumorigenesis have been observed [84]. The present study showed down-regulation of the E2F1 target miR-449 family members, which suggests that their combination possibly initiates endometriosis. E2F2, another important family member of E2F, is also involved in regulating the cell cycle and is associated with cancer growth [85]. A previous study reported that E2F2 can promote the development of liver cancer [86] and can also inhibit the proliferation of prostate cancer cell lines [87]. In our joint analysis, we observed that the down-regulated E2F2 is consistent with a lower expression of miR-196b-5p. Before our research,

Abe et al. found that miR-196b-5p was down-regulated in ectopic endometria compared with normal endometria by microarray. Their subsequent functional experiments revealed that miR-196b can inhibit proliferation and induce apoptosis in endometriotic stromal cells [21], which led us to hypothesize that E2F2 might also play important roles in endometriosis by targeting miR-196b.

CEBPA is an important TF controlling hematopoietic differentiation and homeostasis, gene mutation and aberrant expression, which may contribute to hematological system diseases [88]. We observed that highly expressed CEBPA in EC targets 49 corresponding genes and that like FOXO1, was targeted by miR-182-5p. In a recent study, Wang et al. reported that miR-182 can repress CEBPA in hepatocellular carcinoma and is involved in the AKT signaling pathway [89]. This negative correlation between miR-182 and CEBPA is consistent with our result; however, their specific mechanism and involvement in the downstream signaling pathway in endometriosis need to be further confirmed.

Notably, the integrative data revealed that HNF4A targets 12 miRNAs and thus might be a miRNA "hub" in endometriosis. HNF4A is a critical factor in liver function and digestive diseases [90]. The mechanisms of HNF4A and its target miRNAs have not been fully elucidated yet; it is known that HNF4A can directly up-regulate some specific miRNAs to stabilize the hepatocyte phenotype [91]. This unexpected finding requires further validation to identify the underlying mechanism mediated by HNF4A in endometriosis.

GO and KEGG enrichment analysis delineated 42 functional terms and 27 important signaling pathways, most of which are consistent with the current knowledge on endometriosis. For example, the most significant term and pathway are plasma membrane (GO: 0005886) and the PI3K-Akt signaling pathway, which enriched 145 and 17 DEGs, respectively. Ectopic lesions are exposed to a unique peritoneal microenvironment that is characterized by elevated levels of hormones, inflammation, oxidative stress and iron [92]. These abnormal molecules can influence cell survival and regulate cellular functions through binding to cell membrane receptors, and then lead to the subsequent cascading activation of kinase signaling pathways [93]. Therefore, the plasma membrane term and PI3K-Akt signaling pathway are clearly relevant for endometriosis. The PI3K-Akt pathway, which integrates a variety of extracellular signals and regulates various cellular functions, including cell growth, differentiation, transformation and survival, is being investigated as a therapeutic target in other diseases and thus may also represent a target for endometriosis treatment [94, 95]. In addition, our enrichment analysis revealed some novel dysregulated signaling pathways, such as the Rap1 signaling pathway and the retrograde endocannabinoid signaling pathway, and their functions should be further investigated.

Despite our novel results, the limitations of this study should also be mentioned. First, the number of sequenced samples was relatively inadequate, and only non-hormonal treated patients with moderate to severe stage disease within the secretory phase were enrolled. Endometriosis is a complex disease that is influenced by multiple factors, such as the menstrual cycle, CA125 levels and various subtypes. These differences might impact the expression profile. Although normalized samples are helpful to determine the key pathogenic molecules, our study was most likely underpowered in discovering DEMs and DEGs with subtle expression differences due to the limited sample size. Second, the present results are preliminary and descriptive. Integrative analysis of paired miRNA and mRNA profiling data cannot entirely exclude false positive results. In addition, only some of the identified miRNAs and TFs were validated by qRT-PCR. Therefore, other experiments, such as cross-linking immunoprecipitation or functional experimental validation, are needed to holistically validate the interactions identified by our method. Furthermore, the positive findings that were not included in the network might contain valuable information and are worthy of further discussion. Third, various computational methods have been devised to measure the miRNA-mRNA regulatory relationships in recent years, such as correlation analysis, regression models, Bayesian network learning and causal inference techniques [96]. However, which one is the best method remains an open question in practical use. Here, we used the typical Pearson correlation coefficient to analyze the relationship between DEMs and DEGs, which might lead to some differences from other methods and an inevitable loss of information.

Conclusion

In summary, we provide the first characterization of miRNA-TF-gene co-expression network in paired miRNA and mRNA expression profiling of endometriosis. By establishing the regulatory network in miRNA and mRNA expression profiling, our present study confirms and significantly extends the results of prior studies, thereby defining some crucial miRNAs, TFs and genes involved in the pathogenesis of endometriosis. The identified interactions could also have implications toward targeted therapeutic strategies for endometriosis. Further in-depth functional studies are encouraged to confirm our results.

Additional files

Additional file 1: Clinical characteristics of 30 enrolled patients with ovarian endometriosis. (DOCX 19 kb)

Additional file 2: Supplementary methods introduction for small RNA-seq and mRNA seq. (DOCX 21 kb)

Additional file 3: Primers had been used in qRT-PCR (DOCX 14 kb)

Additional file 4: Summary of the Small RNA sequencing data after filtering and mapping (DOCX 15 kb)

Additional file 5: List of 107 differentially expressed miRNAs in ectopic endometria compared with eutopic endometria (DOCX 17 kb)

Additional file 6: Summary of the mRNA sequencing data after filtering and mapping (DOCX 16 kb)

Additional file 7: Top 25 up-regulated and down-regulated mRNAs in ectopic endometria compared with paired eutopic endometria in ovarian endometriosis. (DOCX 15 kb)

Abbreviations

BP: Biological process; CC: GO cellular component; DEG: Differentially expressed gene; DEM: Differentially expressed miRNA; EC: Ectopic endometrium; EU: Eutopic endometrium; FBL: Feed-back loop; FC: Fold change; FDR: False discovery rate; FFL: Feed-forward loop; GO: Gene Ontology; KEGG: Kyoto Encyclopedia of Genes and Genomes; MF: Molecular function; miRNA: microRNA; mRNA: messenger RNA; PCC: Pearson correlation coefficient; qRT-PCR: Quantitative reverse transcription-polymerase chain reaction; r-AFS: Revised American fertility society; RPKM: Reads per kilobase of one gene per million reads; RPM: Reads per million total reads; small RNA-seq: Small RNA sequencing; TF: Transcription factors

Acknowledgements

The authors thank all patients for their participation.

Funding

This study was funded by the National Natural Science Foundation of China (grant number: 81571411).

Authors' contributions

WSF and YGM conceived and designed the experiments. LYZ, CLG, MXY and ZZ performed the experiments. LYZ, CLG and LLA analyzed the data. LYZ and CLG wrote the paper. WSF revised the manuscript for important intellectual content. YGM supervised the manuscript writing. All authors read and approved the final manuscript.

Competing interests

The authors declare that they have no competing interests.

Author details

[1]Department of Gynecology and Obstetrics, People's Liberation Army (PLA) Medical School, Chinese PLA General Hospital, Beijing 100853, China. [2]Department of Gynecology and Obstetrics, Peking University People's Hospital, Beijing, China. [3]Department of Gynecology and Obstetrics, the 309th Hospital of Chinese PLA, Beijing, China.

References

1. Kennedy S, Bergqvist A, Chapron C, D'Hooghe T, Dunselman G, Greb R, Hummelshoj L, Prentice A, Saridogan E. Endometriosis ESIGf, Endometrium guideline development G. ESHRE guideline for the diagnosis and treatment of endometriosis. Hum Reprod. 2005;20(10):2698–704.
2. Stern RC, Dash R, Bentley RC, Snyder MJ, Haney AF, Robboy SJ. Malignancy in endometriosis: frequency and comparison of ovarian and extraovarian types. Int J Gynecol Pathol. 2001;20(2):133–9.
3. Meuleman C, Vandenabeele B, Fieuws S, Spiessens C, Timmerman D, D'Hooghe T. High prevalence of endometriosis in infertile women with normal ovulation and normospermic partners. Fertil Steril. 2009;92(1):68–74.
4. Montgomery GW, Nyholt DR, Zhao ZZ, Treloar SA, Painter JN, Missmer SA, Kennedy SH, Zondervan KT. The search for genes contributing to endometriosis risk. Hum Reprod Update. 2008;14(5):447–57.
5. Bartel DP. MicroRNAs: genomics, biogenesis, mechanism, and function. Cell. 2004;116(2):281–97.
6. Eulalio A, Huntzinger E, Izaurralde E. Getting to the root of miRNA-mediated gene silencing. Cell. 2008;132(1):9–14.
7. Latchman DS. Transcription factors: an overview. Int J Biochem Cell Biol. 1997;29(12):1305–12.
8. Vaquerizas JM, Kummerfeld SK, Teichmann SA, Luscombe NM. A census of human transcription factors: function, expression and evolution. Nat Rev Genet. 2009;10(4):252–63.
9. Hobert O. Gene regulation by transcription factors and microRNAs. Science. 2008;319(5871):1785–6.
10. Arora S, Rana R, Chhabra A, Jaiswal A, Rani V. miRNA-transcription factor interactions: a combinatorial regulation of gene expression. Mol Gen Genomics. 2013;288(3–4):77–87.
11. Cui Q, Yu Z, Pan Y, Purisima EO, Wang E. MicroRNAs preferentially target the genes with high transcriptional regulation complexity. Biochem Biophys Res Commun. 2007;352(3):733–8.
12. Shalgi R, Lieber D, Oren M, Pilpel Y. Global and local architecture of the mammalian microRNA-transcription factor regulatory network. PLoS Comput Biol. 2007;3(7):e131.
13. Marson A, Levine SS, Cole MF, Frampton GM, Brambrink T, Johnstone S, Guenther MG, Johnston WK, Wernig M, Newman J, Calabrese JM, Dennis LM, Volkert TL, Gupta S, Love J, Hannett N, Sharp PA, Bartel DP, Jaenisch R, Young RA. Connecting microRNA genes to the core transcriptional regulatory circuitry of embryonic stem cells. Cell. 2008;134(3):521–33.
14. Sadeghi M, Ranjbar B, Ganjalikhany MR, MK F, Schmitz U, Wolkenhauer O, Gupta SK. MicroRNA and transcription factor gene regulatory network analysis reveals key regulatory elements associated with prostate cancer progression. PLoS One. 2016;11(12):e0168760.
15. Feng F, Wu J, Gao Z, Yu S, Cui Y. Screening the key microRNAs and transcription factors in prostate cancer based on microRNA functional synergistic relationships. Medicine (Baltimore). 2017;96(1):e5679.
16. Ohlsson Teague EM, Van der Hoek KH, Van der Hoek MB, Perry N, Wagaarachchi P, Robertson SA, Print CG, Hull LM. MicroRNA-regulated pathways associated with endometriosis. Mol Endocrinol. 2009;23(2):265–75.
17. Burney RO, Hamilton AE, Aghajanova L, Vo KC, Nezhat CN, Lessey BA, Giudice LC. MicroRNA expression profiling of eutopic secretory endometrium in women with versus without endometriosis. Mol Hum Reprod. 2009;15(10):625–31.
18. Filigheddu N, Gregnanin I, Porporato PE, Surico D, Perego B, Galli L, Patrignani C, Graziani A, Surico N. Differential expression of microRNAs between eutopic and ectopic endometrium in ovarian endometriosis. J Biomed Biotechnol. 2010;2010:369549.
19. Hawkins SM, Creighton CJ, Han DY, Zariff A, Anderson ML, Gunaratne PH, Matzuk MM. Functional microRNA involved in endometriosis. Mol Endocrinol. 2011;25(5):821–32.
20. Laudanski P, Charkiewicz R, Kuzmicki M, Szamatowicz J, Charkiewicz A, Niklinski J. MicroRNAs expression profiling of eutopic proliferative endometrium in women with ovarian endometriosis. Reprod Biol Endocrinol. 2013;11:78.
21. Abe W, Nasu K, Nakada C, Kawano Y, Moriyama M, Narahara H. miR-196b targets c-myc and Bcl-2 expression, inhibits proliferation and induces apoptosis in endometriotic stromal cells. Hum Reprod. 2013;28(3):750–61.

22. Braza-Boils A, Mari-Alexandre J, Gilabert J, Sanchez-Izquierdo D, Espana F, Estelles A, Gilabert-Estelles J. MicroRNA expression profile in endometriosis: its relation to angiogenesis and fibrinolytic factors. Hum Reprod. 2014;29(5):978–88.
23. Saare M, Rekker K, Laisk-Podar T, Soritsa D, Roost AM, Simm J, Velthut-Meikas A, Samuel K, Metsalu T, Karro H, Soritsa A, Salumets A, Peters M. High-throughput sequencing approach uncovers the miRNome of peritoneal endometriotic lesions and adjacent healthy tissues. PLoS One. 2014;9(11):e112630.
24. Laudanski P, Charkiewicz R, Tolwinska A, Szamatowicz J, Charkiewicz A, Niklinski J. Profiling of selected MicroRNAs in proliferative Eutopic Endometrium of women with ovarian endometriosis. Biomed Res Int. 2015; 2015:760698.
25. Yotova I, Hsu E, Do C, Gaba A, Sczabolcs M, Dekan S, Kenner L, Wenzl R, Tycko B. Epigenetic alterations affecting transcription factors and signaling pathways in Stromal cells of endometriosis. PLoS One. 2017;12(1):e0170859.
26. Canis M, Donnez JG, Guzick, DS, Halme JK, Rock JA, Schenken RS, Vernon MW. Revised American Society for Reproductive Medicine classification of endometriosis: 1996. Fertil Steril. 1997;67(5):817–21.
27. Noyes RW, Hertig AT, Rock J. Dating the endometrial biopsy. Am J Obstet Gynecol. 1975;122(2):262–3.
28. Chomczynski P, Sacchi N. The single-step method of RNA isolation by acid guanidinium thiocyanate-phenol-chloroform extraction: twenty-something years on. Nat Protoc. 2006;1(2):581–5.
29. Li H, Wu B, Geng J, Zhou J, Zheng R, Chai J, Li F, Peng J, Jiang S. Integrated analysis of miRNA/mRNA network in placenta identifies key factors associated with labor onset of large white and Qingping sows. Sci Rep. 2015;5:13074.
30. Aken BL, Ayling S, Barrell D, Clarke L, Curwen V, Fairley S, Fernandez Banet J, Billis K, Garcia Giron C, Hourlier T, Howe K, Kahari A, Kokocinski F, Martin FJ, Murphy DN, Nag R, Ruffier M, Schuster M, Tang YA, Vogel JH, White S, Zadissa A, Flicek P, Searle SM. The Ensembl gene annotation system. Database (Oxford). 2016;2016
31. Langmead B, Trapnell C, Pop M, Salzberg SL. Ultrafast and memory-efficient alignment of short DNA sequences to the human genome. Genome Biol. 2009;10(3):R25.
32. Kozomara A, Griffiths-Jones S. miRBase: annotating high confidence microRNAs using deep sequencing data. Nucleic Acids Res. 2014; 42(Database issue):D68–73.
33. Wang L, Feng Z, Wang X, Wang X, Zhang X. DEGseq: an R package for identifying differentially expressed genes from RNA-seq data. Bioinformatics. 2010;26(1):136–8.
34. Langmead B, Salzberg SL. Fast gapped-read alignment with bowtie 2. Nat Methods. 2012;9(4):357–9.
35. Trapnell C, Pachter L, Salzberg SL. TopHat: discovering splice junctions with RNA-Seq. Bioinformatics. 2009;25(9):1105–11.
36. Anders S, Pyl PT, Huber W. HTSeq–a python framework to work with high-throughput sequencing data. Bioinformatics. 2015;31(2):166–9.
37. Bisognin A, Sales G, Coppe A, Bortoluzzi S, Romualdi C. MAGIA(2): from miRNA and genes expression data integrative analysis to microRNA-transcription factor mixed regulatory circuits (2012 update). Nucleic Acids Res. 2012;40(Web Server issue):W13–21.
38. Grimson A, Farh KK, Johnston WK, Garrett-Engele P, Lim LP, Bartel DP. MicroRNA targeting specificity in mammals: determinants beyond seed pairing. Mol Cell. 2007;27(1):91–105.
39. Friard O, Re A, Taverna D, De Bortoli M, Cora D. CircuitsDB: a database of mixed microRNA/transcription factor feed-forward regulatory circuits in human and mouse. BMC Bioinformatics. 2010;11:435.
40. Wang J, Lu M, Qiu C, Cui Q. TransmiR: a transcription factor-microRNA regulation database. Nucleic Acids Res. 2010;38(Database issue):D119–22.
41. Shannon P, Markiel A, Ozier O, Baliga NS, Wang JT, Ramage D, Amin N, Schwikowski B, Ideker T. Cytoscape: a software environment for integrated models of biomolecular interaction networks. Genome Res. 2003;13(11):2498–504.
42. Huang DW, Sherman BT, Lempicki RA. Systematic and integrative analysis of large gene lists using DAVID bioinformatics resources. Nat Protoc. 2009;4(1):44–57.
43. Livak KJ, Schmittgen TD. Analysis of relative gene expression data using real-time quantitative PCR and the 2(–Delta Delta C(T)) method. Methods. 2001;25(4):402–8.
44. Nunez YO, Truitt JM, Gorini G, Ponomareva ON, Blednov YA, Harris RA, Mayfield RD. Positively correlated miRNA-mRNA regulatory networks in mouse frontal cortex during early stages of alcohol dependence. BMC Genomics. 2013;14:725.
45. Barabasi AL, Oltvai ZN. Network biology: understanding the cell's functional organization. Nat Rev Genet. 2004;5(2):101–13.
46. Teague EM, Print CG, Hull ML. The role of microRNAs in endometriosis and associated reproductive conditions. Hum Reprod Update. 2010;16(2):142–65.
47. Shi XY, Gu L, Chen J, Guo XR, Shi YL. Downregulation of miR-183 inhibits apoptosis and enhances the invasive potential of endometrial stromal cells in endometriosis. Int J Mol Med. 2014;33(1):59–67.
48. Rajewsky N. microRNA target predictions in animals. Nat Genet. 2006; 38(Suppl):S8–13.
49. Bou Kheir T, Futoma-Kazmierczak E, Jacobsen A, Krogh A, Bardram L, Hother C, Gronbaek K, Federspiel B, Lund AH, Friis-Hansen L. miR-449 inhibits cell proliferation and is down-regulated in gastric cancer. Mol Cancer. 2011;10:29.
50. Sandbothe M, Buurman R, Reich N, Greiwe L, Vajen B, Gurlevik E, Schaffer V, Eilers M, Kuhnel F, Vaquero A, Longerich T, Roessler S, Schirmacher P, Manns MP, Illig T, Schlegelberger B, Skawran B. The microRNA-449 family inhibits TGF-beta-mediated liver cancer cell migration by targeting SOX4. J Hepatol. 2017;
51. Zhang Z, Wang J, Gao R, Yang X, Zhang Y, Li J, Zhang J, Zhao X, Xi C, Lu X. Downregulation of microRNA-449 promotes migration and invasion of breast cancer cells by targeting tumor protein D52 (TPD52). Oncol Res. 2016;
52. Luo W, Huang B, Li Z, Li H, Sun L, Zhang Q, Qiu X, Wang E. MicroRNA-449a is downregulated in non-small cell lung cancer and inhibits migration and invasion by targeting c-met. PLoS One. 2013;8(5):e64759.
53. Jang SG, Yoo CW, Park SY, Kang S, Kim HK. Low expression of miR-449 in gynecologic clear cell carcinoma. Int J Gynecol Cancer. 2014;24(9):1558–63.
54. Wu J, Bao J, Kim M, Yuan S, Tang C, Zheng H, Mastick GS, Xu C, Yan W. Two miRNA clusters, miR-34b/c and miR-449, are essential for normal brain development, motile ciliogenesis, and spermatogenesis. Proc Natl Acad Sci U S A. 2014;111(28):E2851–7.
55. Hermeking H. The miR-34 family in cancer and apoptosis. Cell Death Differ. 2010;17(2):193–9.
56. Wang R, Ma J, Wu Q, Xia J, Miele L, Sarkar FH, Wang Z. Functional role of miR-34 family in human cancer. Curr Drug Targets. 2013;14(10):1185–91.
57. Misso G, Di Martino MT, De Rosa G, Farooqi AA, Lombardi A, Campani V, Zarone MR, Gulla A, Tagliaferri P, Tassone P, Caraglia M. Mir-34: a new weapon against cancer? Mol Ther Nucleic Acids. 2014;3:e194.
58. Rupaimoole R, Slack FJ. MicroRNA therapeutics: towards a new era for the management of cancer and other diseases. Nat Rev Drug Discov. 2017;
59. Feng X, Wang Z, Fillmore R, Xi Y. MiR-200, a new star miRNA in human cancer. Cancer Lett. 2014;344(2):166–73.
60. Matsuzaki S, Darcha C. Epithelial to mesenchymal transition-like and mesenchymal to epithelial transition-like processes might be involved in the pathogenesis of pelvic endometriosis. Hum Reprod. 2012;27(3):712–21.
61. Proestling K, Birner P, Gamperl S, Nirtl N, Marton E, Yerlikaya G, Wenzl R, Streubel B, Husslein H. Enhanced epithelial to mesenchymal transition (EMT) and upregulated MYC in ectopic lesions contribute independently to endometriosis. Reprod Biol Endocrinol. 2015;13:75.
62. Rekker K, Saare M, Roost AM, Kaart T, Soritsa D, Karro H, Soritsa A, Simon C, Salumets A, Peters M. Circulating miR-200-family micro-RNAs have altered plasma levels in patients with endometriosis and vary with blood collection time. Fertil Steril. 2015;104(4):938–46. e2
63. Li H, Wang J, Mor G, Sklar J. A neoplastic gene fusion mimics trans-splicing of RNAs in normal human cells. Science. 2008;321(5894):1357–61.
64. Vagnini LD, Renzi A, Oliveira-Pelegrin GR, Canas Mdo C, Petersen CG, Mauri AL, Oliveira JB, Baruffi RL, Cavagna M, Franco Junior JG. The TP73 gene polymorphism (rs4648551, a>G) is associated with diminished ovarian reserve. PLoS One. 2015;10(3):e0120048.
65. Mendell JT. miRiad roles for the miR-17-92 cluster in development and disease. Cell. 2008;133(2):217–22.
66. Han H, Sun D, Li W, Shen H, Zhu Y, Li C, Chen Y, Lu L, Li W, Zhang J, Tian Y, Li Y. A c-Myc-MicroRNA functional feedback loop affects hepatocarcinogenesis. Hepatology. 2013;57(6):2378–89.
67. Qiao J, Lee S, Paul P, Theiss L, Tiao J, Qiao L, Kong A, Chung DH. miR-335 and miR-363 regulation of neuroblastoma tumorigenesis and metastasis. Surgery. 2013;154(2):226–33.

68. Hsu KW, Wang AM, Ping YH, Huang KH, Huang TT, Lee HC, Lo SS, Chi CW, Yeh TS. Downregulation of tumor suppressor MBP-1 by microRNA-363 in gastric carcinogenesis. Carcinogenesis. 2014;35(1):208–17.
69. Li D, Ilnytskyy Y, Kovalchuk A, Khachigian LM, Bronson RT, Wang B, Kovalchuk O. Crucial role for early growth response-1 in the transcriptional regulation of miR-20b in breast cancer. Oncotarget. 2013;4(9):1373–87.
70. Hong S, Yu S, Li J, Yin Y, Liu Y, Zhang Q, Guan H, Li Y, Xiao H. MiR-20b displays tumor-suppressor functions in papillary thyroid carcinoma by regulating the MAPK/ERK signaling pathway. Thyroid. 2016;26(12):1733–43.
71. Li P, Xu Q, Zhang D, Li X, Han L, Lei J, Duan W, Ma Q, Wu Z, Wang Z. Upregulated miR-106a plays an oncogenic role in pancreatic cancer. FEBS Lett. 2014;588(5):705–12.
72. Zhi F, Zhou G, Shao N, Xia X, Shi Y, Wang Q, Zhang Y, Wang R, Xue L, Wang S, Wu S, Peng Y, Yang Y. miR-106a-5p inhibits the proliferation and migration of astrocytoma cells and promotes apoptosis by targeting FASTK. PLoS One. 2013;8(8):e72390.
73. Chen J, Gu L, Ni J, Hu P, Hu K, Shi YL. MiR-183 regulates ITGB1P expression and promotes invasion of endometrial Stromal cells. Biomed Res Int. 2015;2015:340218.
74. Zaret KS, Carroll JS. Pioneer transcription factors: establishing competence for gene expression. Genes Dev. 2011;25(21):2227–41.
75. Hannenhalli S, Kaestner KH. The evolution of fox genes and their role in development and disease. Nat Rev Genet. 2009;10(4):233–40.
76. Fu Z, Tindall DJ. FOXOs, cancer and regulation of apoptosis. Oncogene. 2008;27(16):2312–9.
77. Yin X, Pavone ME, Lu Z, Wei J, Kim JJ. Increased activation of the PI3K/AKT pathway compromises decidualization of stromal cells from endometriosis. J Clin Endocrinol Metab. 2012;97(1):E35–43.
78. Myatt SS, Wang J, Monteiro LJ, Christian M, Ho KK, Fusi L, Dina RE, Brosens JJ, Ghaem-Maghami S, Lam EW. Definition of microRNAs that repress expression of the tumor suppressor gene FOXO1 in endometrial cancer. Cancer Res. 2010;70(1):367–77.
79. Zhu X, Wei L, Bai Y, Wu S, Han S. FoxC1 promotes epithelial-mesenchymal transition through PBX1 dependent transactivation of ZEB2 in esophageal cancer. Am J Cancer Res. 2017;7(8):1642–53.
80. Xia L, Huang W, Tian D, Zhu H, Qi X, Chen Z, Zhang Y, Hu H, Fan D, Nie Y, Wu K. Overexpression of forkhead box C1 promotes tumor metastasis and indicates poor prognosis in hepatocellular carcinoma. Hepatology. 2013; 57(2):610–24.
81. Deng L, Liu T, Zhang B, Wu H, Zhao J, Chen J. Forkhead box C1 is targeted by microRNA-133b and promotes cell proliferation and migration in osteosarcoma. Exp Ther Med. 2017;14(4):2823–30.
82. Myatt SS, Lam EW. The emerging roles of forkhead box (fox) proteins in cancer. Nat Rev Cancer. 2007;7(11):847–59.
83. Tremblay JJ, Viger RS. GATA factors differentially activate multiple gonadal promoters through conserved GATA regulatory elements. Endocrinology. 2001;142(3):977–86.
84. Ren B, Cam H, Takahashi Y, Volkert T, Terragni J, Young RA, Dynlacht BD. E2F integrates cell cycle progression with DNA repair, replication, and G(2)/M checkpoints. Genes Dev. 2002;16(2):245–56.
85. Johnson DG. The paradox of E2F1: oncogene and tumor suppressor gene. Mol Carcinog. 2000;27(3):151–7.
86. Fujiwara K, Yuwanita I, Hollern DP, Andrechek ER. Prediction and genetic demonstration of a role for activator E2Fs in Myc-induced tumors. Cancer Res. 2011;71(5):1924–32.
87. Zhan L, Huang C, Meng XM, Song Y, XQ W, Miu CG, Zhan XS, Li J. Promising roles of mammalian E2Fs in hepatocellular carcinoma. Cell Signal. 2014;26(5):1075–81.
88. Dong Q, Meng P, Wang T, Qin W, Qin W, Wang F, Yuan J, Chen Z, Yang A, Wang H. MicroRNA let-7a inhibits proliferation of human prostate cancer cells in vitro and in vivo by targeting E2F2 and CCND2. PLoS One. 2010;5(4):e10147.
89. Zhang P, Iwasaki-Arai J, Iwasaki H, Fenyus ML, Dayaram T, Owens BM, Shigematsu H, Levantini E, Huettner CS, Lekstrom-Himes JA, Akashi K, Tenen DG. Enhancement of hematopoietic stem cell repopulating capacity and self-renewal in the absence of the transcription factor C/EBP alpha. Immunity. 2004;21(6):853–63.
90. Wang C, Ren R, Hu H, Tan C, Han M, Wang X, Zheng Y. MiR-182 is up-regulated and targeting Cebpa in hepatocellular carcinoma. Chin J Cancer Res. 2014;26(1):17–29.
91. Weltmeier F, Borlak J. A high resolution genome-wide scan of HNF4alpha recognition sites infers a regulatory gene network in colon cancer. PLoS One. 2011;6(7):e21667.
92. Cicchini C, Amicone L, Alonzi T, Marchetti A, Mancone C, Tripodi M. Molecular mechanisms controlling the phenotype and the EMT/MET dynamics of hepatocyte. Liver Int. 2015;35(2):302–10.
93. Goud PT, Goud AP, Joshi N, Puscheck E, Diamond MP, Abu-Soud HM. Dynamics of nitric oxide, altered follicular microenvironment, and oocyte quality in women with endometriosis. Fertil Steril. 2014;102(1):151–9. e5
94. Little AS, Smith PD, Cook SJ. Mechanisms of acquired resistance to ERK1/2 pathway inhibitors. Oncogene. 2013;32(10):1207–15.
95. McKinnon BD, Kocbek V, Nirgianakis K, Bersinger NA, Mueller MD. Kinase signalling pathways in endometriosis: potential targets for non-hormonal therapeutics. Hum Reprod Update. 2016;22(3)
96. Le TD, Zhang J, Liu L, Li J. Ensemble methods for MiRNA target prediction from expression data. PLoS One. 2015;10(6):e0131627.

6

Proteomic profile of human spermatozoa in healthy and asthenozoospermic individuals

Xiaodan Cao, Yun Cui, Xiaoxia Zhang, Jiangtao Lou, Jun Zhou, Huafeng Bei and Renxiong Wei*

Abstract

Asthenozoospermia is considered as a common cause of male infertility and characterized by reduced sperm motility. However, the molecular mechanism that impairs sperm motility remains unknown in most cases. In the present review, we briefly reviewed the proteome of spermatozoa and seminal plasma in asthenozoospermia and considered post-translational modifications in spermatozoa of asthenozoospermia. The reduction of sperm motility in asthenozoospermic patients had been attributed to factors, for instance, energy metabolism dysfunction or structural defects in the sperm-tail protein components and the differential proteins potentially involved in sperm motility such as COX6B, ODF, TUBB2B were described. Comparative proteomic analysis open a window to discover the potential pathogenic mechanisms of asthenozoospermia and the biomarkers with clinical significance.

Keywords: Proteome, Spermatozoa, Sperm motility, Asthenozoospermia, Infertility

Background

Infertility is defined as the lack of ability to achieve a clinical pregnancy after one year or more of unprotected and well-timed intercourse with the same partner [1]. It is estimated that around 15% of couples of reproductive age present with infertility, and about half of the infertility is associated with male partner [2, 3]. With the continuing world-wide increase in male infertility, it has become a major health problem attracting more clinical attention. Asthenozoospermia(AS) is a common cause of human male infertility characterized by reduced sperm motility with sperm motility< 50% or progressive motility< 25% [4]. The proteins involved in the normal physiology of the sperm motility is rather scarce and the molecular basis of asthenozoospermia is not yet fully understood [5–7]. The causes of poor sperm motility include abnormal metabolism in the testicular tissue or epididymis, structural deficiency in the sperm tail, and functional deficiency of the epididymis or other accessory sex glands [8–10]. Routine semen analysis on sperm motility is only a clinical indicator of male fertility and does not account for the underlying cause of defects associated with sperm movement. It is possible that individual protein defects in spermatozoa might cause fertilization failure [4] and it has become clear that identifying the precise proteins and the pathways involved in sperm motility is needed [5].

Application of proteomic techniques in male infertility

Proteomic approaches, such as two-dimensional (2D) polyacrylamide gel electrophoresis, mass spectrometry (MS), matrix-assisted laser desorption ionization time of flight (MALDI-TOF) and isobaric tags for relative and absolute quantitation (iTRAQ) could be useful in identifying a wide range of the proteins responsible for diagnosis of sperm dysfunctions and the regulatory mechanism of male fertility [11–17] (Fig. 1). A number of studies have utilized high-throughput techniques to study protein alterations in fertile versus infertile groups, for example, normal versus malformed, capacitated versus incapacitated and low versus high sperm motility [11, 18–20]. These techniques offers the comprehensive understanding of sperm proteins with their particular structure and also provides a new view to study different functional states of sperm [21, 22]. For example, Chan et al. performed MADLI-TOF to address altered protein phosphorylation and

* Correspondence: cxd0319@163.com
Department of Clinical Laboratory, Ningbo Municipal Hospital of Traditional Chinese Medicine, Ningbo 315000, China

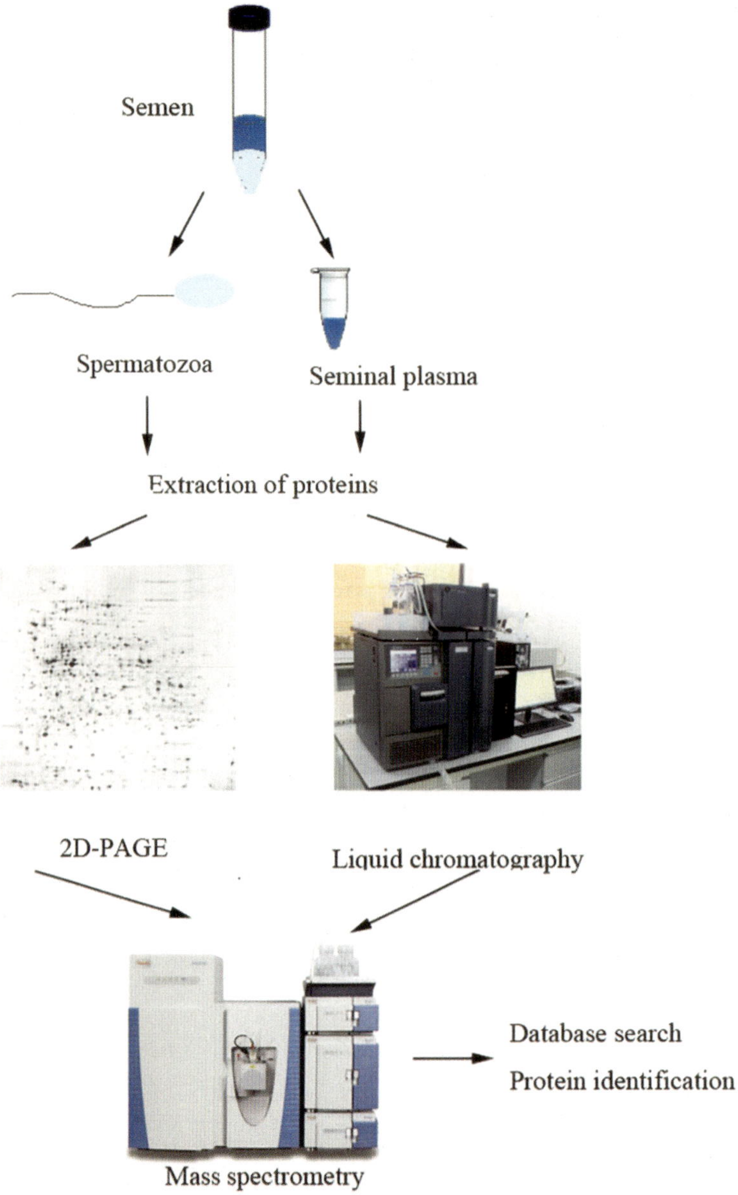

Fig. 1 Schematic diagram showing the proteomic analysis of the sperm cells and seminal plasma. After collection and liquefaction of ejaculated semen, the desired target components are purified through density gradients centrifugation. Proteins are extracted and separated by two-dimensional polyacrylamide gel electrophoresis (2D–PAGE) or liquid chromatography(LC), and then followed by identification using mass spectrometry and database search

aberrant sperm motility and 12 proteins were identified [18]. Secciani et al. employed MS/MS approach to analyze the protein profiles of capacitated versus ejaculated spermatozoa [23]. Sperm protein expression in asthenozoospermic patients and normozoospermic controls were compared, and several quantitative and qualitative significant variations were found [15]. Some of these differential proteins may be potential target proteins that could benefit further research on sperm function-related infertility and also shedding light on the key proteins involved in fertilization.

Spermatozoal proteome in asthenozoospermia

Sperm motility is an important prerequisite for successful fertilization. The proteomic studies on asthenozoospermic individuals are increasing and more and more proteins and pathways involved in sperm motility are identified (Table 1, Table 2). Hashemitabar et al. [24] investigated the protein expression profiles of human sperm tail from asthenozoospermic and normozoospermic individuals using the MALDI-TOF-TOF approach. Among the fourteen differentially expressed proteins, eleven proteins [(A-kinase anchor protein 4 (AKAP4),

Table 1 Sperm proteins with a significantly higher or lower expression in asthenozoospermia in different proteomic studies

Study	Method	Identified proteins	
		up-regulated in astheno	down-regulated in astheno
Hashemitabar et al.	2D electrophoresis MALDI-TOF-TOF analysis	CLU, KRT1, ASRGL1	AKAP4, ODF2, TUBB2B, COX6B, GSTMu3, PHGPx, GAPD-S, VDAC2, HSPA2, HSPA9 and SPANXB
Siva et al.	2D PAGE MALDI MS/MS analysis	TRIS, GPK2, SCOT1, unidentified	TUBB2C, tektin 1, PSMA3, HSPA2
Martı'nez-Heredia et al.	2D electrophoresis MS analysis	CLUpre, DLDpre, FHpre, HSPA2, IMPA1, PSMB3, SEMG1pre, TEX12, MPST/ECH1pre	ACTB, ANXA5, COX6B, histone H2A, PIP, PIPpre, calcium binding protein-S100A9
Shen et al.	2D electrophoresis MALDI-TOF analysis	PIPpre, flagellin, GPX4, GAPDH	TEKT4, Lacto, ODF2, SPANXB, PGK2, GRP78, Hsp70, DJ-1, CAB2, Actin, Heat shock protein 70 testis variant
Zhao et al.	2D electrophoresis MALDI-TOF analysis	PGM2, TPI, GOT-1, ODF, GS, semenogelin I precursor	IDH-α, CA-II, GDI-1, MSS1

outer dense fiber 2 (ODF2), tubulin beta 2B (TUBB2B), cytochrome c oxidase subunit 6B (COX6B), glutathione S-transferase Mu 3 (GSTMu3), phospholipid hydroperoxide glutathione peroxidase (PHGPx), glyceraldehyde-3-phosphate dehydrogenase, testis-specific (GAPD-S), voltage-dependent anion-selective channel protein 2 (VDAC2), heat shock-related 70 kDa protein 2 (HSPA2), stress-70 protein, mitochondrial (HSPA9), Sperm protein associated with the nucleus on the X chromosome B (SPANXB)] had increased amounts in normal controls, and three proteins [clusterin (CLU), keratin, type II cytoskeletal 1 (KRT1), isoaspartyl peptidase/L-asparaginase (ASRGL1)] had higher expression levels in asthenozoospermic samples. In the functional categorization, the majority fall into five groups: energy and metabolism (COX6B, GAPDS, PHGPx), movement and structural organization (TUBB2B, ODF2, AKAP4, KRT1, CLU), stress response and turn over (HSPA2, HSPA9), signaling and transport (VDAC2), and antioxidant activity (GSTMu3).

Proteins responsible for energy and metabolism (COX6B, GAPDS and PHGPx), associated with the production of ATP in distal regions of the flagellum [25, 26], had a decreased expression in asthenozoospermic sperm samples. The decreased level might affect the structure of fibrous sheath and ATP production, which might impair sperm motility. VDAC family proteins with an ATP binding site regulates mitochondrial outer membrane permeabilization to ions and ATP molecules [27, 28] and knockout of the VDAC2 and VDAC3 gene resulted in significantly reduced sperm motility and embryo development[29], suggesting that

Table 2 Summary of Gene Ontology(GO) analysis of differential sperm proteins in asthenozoospermia in different proteomic studies

Study	GO term	Protein names
Hashemitabar et al.	energy and metabolism	COX6B, GAPDS, PHGPx
	movement and structural organization	TUBB2B, ODF2, AKAP4, KRT1, CLU
	stress response and turn over	HSPA2, HSPA9
	signaling and transport	VDAC2
	antioxidant activity	GSTMu3
Siva et al.	energy and metabolism	TRIS, GPK2, SCOT1, unidentified
	movement and organization	TUBB2C, tektin 1
	protein turnover, folding and stress response	PSMA3, HSPA2
Martı'nez-Heredia et al.	energy production	COX6B, DLDpre, Fhpre, ECH1pre
	structure and movement	ACTB, H2A, PIP, PIPpre, SEMG1
	cell signalling and regulation	ANXA5, S100A9, IMPA1
Zhao et al.	metabolic enzymes	IDH-α, PGM2, TPI, GOT-1, CA-II
	structure	GDI-1,ODF
	other	14-kDa fragment and 17-kDa fragments of semenogelin I

VDACs are indispensable for sperm energy metabolism and successful fertilization.

Sperm is a highly polarized cell and its motility is fully dependent on flagellum. The ability of sperm to move forward is crucial for the successful fertilization of an egg [30]. The reduction of sperm motility in asthenozoospermic men has been attributed to factors such as structural defects in the sperm-tail protein components [8]. Sperm flagellum consists of an axoneme surrounded in distinct regions by accessory structures such as the fibrous sheath and ODF. AKAP3 and AKAP4 are the most abundant structural proteins in the fibrous sheath and have anchoring sites for cyclic-AMP-(cAMP)-dependent protein kinase that increases tyrosine phosphorylation of sperm proteins and regulating flagellar function [31]. Deleting AKAP4 gene in male mice caused dysplasia of the fibrous sheath (DFS) which lead to defective sperm motility [32]. Absence of AKAP4 resulted in loss of effective sperm motility because cAMP-dependent signaling processes fail to be associated with the fibrous sheath [33]. The fibrous sheath is involved in regulating sperm maturation, motility and capacitation and AKAP4 could influence the sperm locomotion and might be a biomarker of understanding prefertilization events. Numerous polypeptides such as ODF1 and ODF2 constitute the ODF sheath which help to preserve the elastic rigidity of sperm flagellum [34, 35]. An ultra structural study of asthenozoospermia individuals with DFS showed the abnormal extension of ODF to the principal piece[36]. Reduction of one or more ODF proteins might result in decreased elasticity of sperm flagellum and cause nonfunctional tails [37]. There is a possibility for a screening regarding the distribution of sperm tail proteins related to motility disorder.

Tubulin is known to play a key role in the formation of microtubules of flagellum. TUBB2C is a major cytoskeletal protein present in the head and flagellum of spermatozoa and existed actual influences on sperm motility [38, 39]. TUBB2B, expressed in post-mitotic cells in male germ cells, are essential for the the formation of meiotic spindles and cytoplasmic microtubules and also share in the organization of 9 + 2 of the axonemal microtubule in sperm tail [40]. Sperm in asthenozoospermic patients were defective in motility might due to the lower expression of tubulin with structural defects in sperm flagellum like dysplasia of the fibrous sheath (DFS) with missing axonemal central pairs and complete distortion of 9 + 2 axonemal structure [36].

HSP family proteins are stress response proteins which protect the cell against oxidative stress and pathological changes [41]. HSPA9 is predominant in the mitochondrial matrix and required during protein translocation into mitochondria and the refolding of mitochondria proteins [42]. GSTMu3 is a kind of antioxidant proteins and participates in the detoxification of toxins, drugs and oxidative stress products [43]. The down-regulated of HSPA9 and GSTMu3 in asthenozoospermia could lead to the accumulation of oxidative stress products and impair sperm motility.

Siva et al. [44] employed 2D PAGE MALDI MS/MS analysis to compare the sperm proteome of asthenozoospermic and normozoospermic patients. Eight proteins showing changes in levels between two groups were revealed and the differential proteins belonged to three functional groups: energy and metabolism [triose-phosphate isomerase(TRIS), glycerol kinase, testis specific 2 (GPK2) and succinyl-CoA:3-ketoacid CoA transferase 1 (SCOT1), unidentified], movement and organization [tubulin beta-2C chain(TUBB2C) and tektin 1] and protein turnover, folding and stress response [proteasome subunit alpha type 3 (PSMA3) and HSPA2]. It was interesting to note that proteins falling in the 'energy and metabolism' group are higher in asthenozoospermic individuals and the high expression may be because of the redundant cytoplasm (droplets) contained in immaturation spermatozoa, while proteins with altered intensity in other two functional groups are higher in normozoospermic donors. TUBB2C, TPIS, HSPA2 and PSMA3 have been reported to get S-nitrosylated in human sperm during capacitation [17], indicating an involvement of these proteins in various sperm functions associated with capacitation, including sperm motility. HSPA2 has been shown to be a marker for sperm maturity [45] with lower amounts in oligoteratozoospermic men [46].

Proteasomes have been detected in sperm from various species and the major function of proteasome is to degrade nuclear and cytosolic ubiquitinated proteins [47–49]. Its low expression in asthenozoospermia might lead to the accumulation of higher ubiquitinated molecules and was related to sperm motility [48]. Studies on the sperm proteome from asthenozoospermic samples have revealed that the relative expression of some component of the proteasome complex is different. Zhao et al. [15] reported that the 26S protease regulatory subunit 7 (MSS1) is decreased in asthenozoospermic patient, in contrast to the study by Martı'nez-Heredia et al. [50] which showed that PSMB3 is increased in asthenozoospermia. The different trend for proteasome subunit is not clear and may be attributed to ethnic differences (studies by Siva and Zhao group worked on Asian population and Martı'nez-Heredia et al., worked on European population). Further study on a larger sample size would be required to confirm these findings.

Martı'nez-Heredia et al. [50] compared the expression of asthenozoospermic samples to that of semen donor controls using two-dimensional proteomic analysis and seventeen protein spots have been identified at different amounts. Of these proteins identified,

COX6B, dihydrolipoamide dehydrogenase precursor (DLDpre), fumarate hydratase precursor (FHpre) and 3-mercapto-pyruvate sulfurtransferase/dienoyl-CoA isomerase precursor (MPST/ECH1pre) constitute the 'energy production' group; cytoskeletal actin-B (ACTB), histone H2A, prolactin-inducible protein (PIP), prolactin-inducible protein precursor (PIPpre), and semenogelin 1 precursor (SEMG1pre) constitute 'structure and movement' group; and the 'cell signalling and regulation' group is constituted by annexin-A5 (ANXA5), calcium binding protein-S100A9, and inositol-1 monophosphatase (IMPA1). It is interesting to note that six of these identified proteins are precursor forms [(DLDpre, FHpre, ECH1pre, PIPpre, SEMG1pre and clusterin precursor (CLUpre)] of mature proteins, which could suggest the presence of a generalized post-translation processing problem of these proteins. The accumulation of precursors in asthenozoospermic patients also might lead to the deregulation of some downstream proteins. DLDpre and Fhpre, associated with the major sources of ATP production in sperm, were upregulated in asthenozoospermic patients, which could be involved with a potential decrease in the mature protein and the failure of tail movement of sperm in asthenozoospermia [51, 52]. The results together with those of Zhao et al. [15] demonstrate the existence of a general deregulation in the pathways involved in energy and metabolism in asthenozoospermic patients.

PIP is a 17-kDa glycoprotein present in human seminal plasma. Its aspartyl-proteinase nature suggests its specificity to fibronectin that is one of the major protein constituents of the seminal coagulum [53–55], which indicates that PIP could contribute to the specifical degradation of fibronectin during liquefaction. Lower expression of PIP in asthenozoospermia might result in an incomplete liquefaction of the ejaculate and make a restriction for the movement of spermatozoa.

2D electrophoresis MALDI-TOF analysis was performed to compare sperm protein composition in asthenozoospermic patients with that of normozoospermic samples [15, 56]. Sixteen differentially expressed protein were identified by Shen et al. and tektin 4 (TEKT4) and ODF2 appeared only in normozoospermic samples [56]. Tektins and ODFs form the main components of the cytoskeleton in sperm flagella, and the reduction of sperm motility in asthenozoospermic men has been attributed to factors such as abnormal expression of the structural constituents of cytoskeleton [8]. 78 kDa glucose-regulated protein (GRP78), belonging to HSP protein located on endoplasmic reticulum(ER), is down-regulated in asthenozoospermic samples. GRP78 was able to bind to the acrosomal region of capacitated human spermatozoa and to modulate the binding interaction between sperm and the zona pellucida, which might affect intracellular signaling transduction and the capacitation of sperm [57, 58].

Ten differentially expressed proteins involved in the regulation of sperm motility were identified by Zhao et al. and these proteins were distributed into three categories: metabolic enzymes, tructure-associated proteins and other functional proteins [15]. Contrary to the previous studies, ODF protein showed higher expression in asthenozoospermia in this study and the disturbance of ODF protein may be associated with sperm motility defect. Half of the identified proteins are related with ATP metabolism to support sperm movement. The overexpression of phosphoglycerate mutase 2 (PGM2), triosephosphate isomerase(TPI) and glutamate oxaloacetate transaminase-1(GOT-1) in asthenozoospermic patients may be a compensatory reaction to the reduced motility sperm and weakened TCA cycle associated with low isocitrate dehydrogenase subunit α (IDH-α) expression [15].

Post-translational modifications in spermatozoa of asthenozoospermia

Post-translational modifications especially phosphorylation play an important role in sperm motility and protein phosphorylation is reported to be a prerequisite for spermatozoa to fertilize an egg. Chan et al. [23] performed 2D electrophoresis MALDI-TOF MS approach to analyze motility and protein phosphorylation in healthy and low-motility-sperm and identified twelve spots as having differential phosphorylation. Among these 12 proteins, 10 proteins were hypophosphorylated in asthenozoospermic sperm, while 2 proteins exhibited a relatively lower phosphorylation level in normal sperm. Parte et al. [59] investigated the expression of phosphoproteins in normal- and asthenozoo-sperm by Nano UPLC–MSE and Ingenuity Pathways Analysis to identify the differential phosphoproteins and the key pathways regulating sperm motility. 66 phosphoproteins were significantly different of which 27 proteins were decreased and 39 proteins were increased in asthenozoosperm compared with those in normal samples. The differentially regulated proteins contained the family of HSPs, cytoskeletal proteins and proteins involved in the fibrous sheath and energy metabolism. Pathway analysis indicated that carbohydrate and energy metabolism, cyclic AMP signaling, PI3K/AKT signaling and pathway regulating actin based motility by Rho were significantly altered. The data identified demonstrated that the signature molecules of metabolic enzymes, fibrous sheath associated proteins and cytoskeletal proteins have the potential as biomarkers for diagnosing axonemal defects, a defective fibrous sheath, and abnormal mitochondria in asthenozoospermia.

Proteome in the seminal plasma of asthenozoospermia

Seminal plasma is a mixture of secretions from the testis, epididymis and several male accessory glands and a growing number of seminal plasma proteins have been shown to be related with sperm motility. To further explore the impact of post-testicular processes on sperm motility, seminal plasma proteins from asthenozoospermia individuals and healthy men were collected and analyzed by LC-MS/MS. 101 differentially expressed proteins were identifed and Chain A, Human Dj-1 with sulfinic acid (DJ-1) was the most downregulated protein in the seminal plasma of asthenozoospermic patients. Most of these proteins enriched in the hydrolase activity, catalytic activity and enzyme regulator activity. In addition, the levels of reactive oxygen species (ROS) were higher in asthenozoospermia men and these data suggest that downregulation of the DJ-1 protein could lead to increased oxidative stress for spermatozoa which would influence the quality of the semen and sperm motility [60]. Saraswat et al. [61] have performed a differential proteomic analysis of the sperm and seminal plasma in normozoospermia and asthenozoospermia samples and identified 667 proteins for label-free analysis in sperm and 429 proteins in seminal plasma. Statistical and mathematical analysis including principal component analysis, OPLS-DA (S-Plot), ROC Curve analysis and self-organizing maps analysis were performed on the dataset. Various pathways were enriched in the proteomic datasets and some of these pathways were gluconeogenesis, glycolysis, stress response, nucleosome assembly, axoneme activation and focal adhesion assembly. The studies elucidated the pathways underlying the sperm motility which can lead to identification of novel treatment avenues.

Conclusion

In this review, we have compared data of proteome studies from asthenozoospermic men and normal individuals that evaluated the protein profile that controls infertility. Studies compiled in this work would contribute appreciably to the presently limited information available about molecular mechanism underlying sperm motility. There is a need to extend these studies to get a consistent view on the specific proteins involved in asthenozoospermia and their characterization could merit further investigation on sperm motility-related infertility. Ultimately, these findings will contribute towards the development of novel diagnostic markers of male infertility.

Abbreviations

AKAP4: A-kinase anchor protein 4; ANXA5: annexin-A5; ASRGL1: Isoaspartyl peptidase/L-asparaginase; CAB2: XPA binding protein 2, isoform CRA_b; CA-II: Carbonic anhydrase II; CLU: Clusterin; CLUpre: Clusterin precursor; COX6B: Cytochrome c oxidase subunit 6B; DFS: Dysplasia of the fibrous sheath; DJ-1: Chain A, Human Dj-1 with sulfinic acid; DLDpre: Dihydrolipoamide dehydrogenase precursor; Fhpre: Fumarate hydratase precursor; GAPDH: Glyceraldehyde-3-phosphate dehydrogenase; GAPD-S: Glyceraldehyde-3-phosphate dehydrogenase, testis-specific; GDI-1: Rho GDP-dissociation inhibitor 1; GKP2: Glycerol kinase, testis specific 2; GOT-1: Glutamate oxaloacetate transaminase-1; GPX4: Phospholipid hydroperoxide glutathione peroxidase; GRP78: 78 kDa glucose-regulated protein; GS: Glutamine synthetase; GSTMu3: Glutathione S-transferase Mu 3; HSP: Heat shock protein; HSPA2: Heat shock-related 70 kDa protein 2; HSPA9: Stress-70 protein, mitochondrial; IDH-α: Isocitrate dehydrogenase subunitα; IMPA1: Inositol-1 monophosphatase; iTRAQ: Isobaric tags for relative and absolute quantitation; KRT1: Keratin, type II cytoskeletal 1; Lacto: Lactoferrin; MALDI-TOF: Matrix-assisted laser desorption ionization time of flight; MPST/ECH1pre: 3-mercapto-pyruvate sulfurtransferase/dienoyl-CoA isomerase precursor; MS: Mass spectrometry; MSS1: 26S protease regulatory subunit 7; ODF: Outer dense fiber; PGK2: Phosphoglycerate kinase 2; PGM2: Phosphoglycerate mutase 2; PIP: Prolactin-inducible protein; PIPpre: Prolactin-inducible protein precursor; PSMA: Proteasome subunit alpha; PSMB3: Proteosome subunit beta 3; ROS: Reactive oxygen species; SCOT: Succinyl-CoA:3-ketoacid CoA transferase; SEMG1pre: Semenogelin 1 precursor; SPANXB: Sperm protein associated with the nucleus on the X chromosome B; TEKT4: Tektin 4; TEX12: Testis expressed sequence 12; TPI: Triosephosphate isomerase; TUBB2B: Tubulin beta 2B; TUBB2C: Tubulin beta 2C; VDAC2: Voltage-dependent anion-selective channel protein 2

Acknowledgments

Not applicable

Funding

This work was supported by the Natural Science Foundation of Ningbo (No. 2016A610200).

Authors' contributions

XDC, XXZ, JTL, JZ and HFB were involved in data acquisition, analysis and manuscript drifting. XDC was the major contributor in writing the manuscript. YC and RXW approved the final manuscript. All authors read and approved the final manuscript.

Competing interests

The authors declare that they have no competing interests.

References

1. Brugh VM 3rd, Lipshultz LI. Male factor infertility: evaluation and management. Med Clin North Am. 2004;88(2):367–85.
2. Luk BH, Loke AY. A review of supportive interventions targeting individuals or couples undergoing infertility treatment: directions for the development of interventions. J Sex Marital Ther. 2016;42(6):515–33.
3. Esteves SC, Chan P. A systematic review of recent clinical practice guidelines and best practice statements for the evaluation of the infertile male. Int Urol Nephrol. 2015;47(9):1441–56.
4. World Health Organization. Laboratory manual of the WHO for the examination of human semen and sperm-cervical mucus interaction. Ann Ist Super Sanita. 2001; 37(1):I-XII, 1–123.
5. Luconi M, Forti G, Baldi E. Pathophysiology of sperm motility. Front Biosci. 2006;11:1433–47.
6. Baccetti B, Collodel G, Estenoz M, Manca D, Moretti E, Piomboni P. Gene deletions in an infertile man with sperm fibrous sheath dysplasia. Hum Reprod. 2005;20(10):2790–4.
7. Rousseaux S, Caron C, Govin J, Lestrat C, Faure AK, Khochbin S. Establishment of male-specific epigenetic information. Gene. 2005;345(2):139–53.

8. Ryder TA, Mobberley MA, Hughes L, Hendry WF. A survey of the ultrastructural defects associated with absent or impaired human sperm motility. Fertil Steril. 1990;53(3):556–60.
9. Comhaire FH, Mahmoud AM, Depuydt CE, Zalata AA, Christophe AB. Mechanisms and effects of male genital tract infection on sperm quality and fertilizing potential: the andrologist's viewpoint. Hum Reprod Update. 1999;5(5):393–8.
10. Infante JP, Huszagh VA. Synthesis of highly unsaturated phosphatidylcholines in the development of sperm motility: a role for epididymal glycerol-3-phosphorylcholine. Mol Cell Biochem. 1985;69(1):3–6.
11. Pixton KL, Deeks ED, Flesch FM, Moseley FL, Bjorndahl L, Ashton PR, et al. Sperm proteome mapping of a patient who experienced failed fertilization at IVF reveals altered expression of at least 20 proteins compared with fertile donors: case report. Hum Reprod. 2004;19(6):1438–47.
12. Baker MA, Witherdin R, Hetherington L, Cunningham-Smith K, Aitken RJ. Identification of post-translational modifications that occur during sperm maturation using difference in two-dimensional gel electrophoresis. Proteomics. 2005;5(4):1003–12.
13. Johnston DS, Wooters J, Kopf GS, Qiu Y, Roberts KP. Analysis of the human sperm proteome. Ann N Y Acad Sci. 2005;1061:190–202.
14. Capkova J, Elzeinova F, Novak P. Increased expression of secretory actin-binding protein on human spermatozoa is associated with poor semen quality. Hum Reprod. 2007;22(5):1396–404.
15. Zhao C, Huo R, Wang FQ, Lin M, Zhou ZM, Sha JH. Identification of several proteins involved in regulation of sperm motility by proteomic analysis. Fertil Steril. 2007;87(2):436–8.
16. Baker MA, Reeves G, Hetherington L, Muller J, Baur I, Aitken RJ. Identification of gene products present in triton X-100 soluble and insoluble fractions of human spermatozoa lysates using LC-MS/MS analysis. Proteomics Clin Appl. 2007;1(5):524–32.
17. Lefievre L, Chen Y, Conner SJ, Scott JL, Publicover SJ, Ford WC, et al. Human spermatozoa contain multiple targets for protein S-nitrosylation: an alternative mechanism of the modulation of sperm function by nitric oxide? Proteomics. 2007;7(17):3066–84.
18. Secciani F, Bianchi L, Ermini L, Cianti R, Armini A, La Sala GB, et al. Protein profile of capacitated versus ejaculated human sperm. J Proteome Res. 2009;8(7):3377–89.
19. Bohring C, Krause W. The characterization of human spermatozoa membrane proteins–surface antigens and immunological infertility. Electrophoresis. 1999;20(4–5):971–6.
20. Bohring C, Krause W. Immune infertility: towards a better understanding of sperm (auto)-immunity. The value of proteomic analysis. Hum Reprod. 2003;18(5):915–24.
21. Anderson NL, Anderson NG. Proteome and proteomics: new technologies, new concepts, and new words. Electrophoresis. 1998;19(11):1853–61.
22. Wu TF, Chu DS. Sperm chromatin: fertile grounds for proteomic discovery of clinical tools. Mol Cell Proteomics. 2008;7(10):1876–86.
23. Chan CC, Shui HA, Wu CH, Wang CY, Sun GH, Chen HM, et al. Motility and protein phosphorylation in healthy and asthenozoospermic sperm. J Proteome Res. 2009;8(11):5382–6.
24. Hashemitabar M, Sabbagh S, Orazizadeh M, Ghadiri A, Bahmanzadeh M. A proteomic analysis on human sperm tail: comparison between normozoospermia and asthenozoospermia. J Assist Reprod Genet. 2015;32(6):853–63.
25. Miki K, Qu W, Goulding EH, Willis WD, Bunch DO, Strader LF, et al. Glyceraldehyde 3-phosphate dehydrogenase-S, a sperm-specific glycolytic enzyme, is required for sperm motility and male fertility. Proc Natl Acad Sci U S A. 2004;101(47):16501–6.
26. Ursini F, Heim S, Kiess M, Maiorino M, Roveri A, Wissing J, et al. Dual function of the selenoprotein PHGPx during sperm maturation. Science. 1999;285(5432):1393–6.
27. Pavlov E, Grigoriev SM, Dejean LM, Zweihorn CL, Mannella CA, Kinnally KW. The mitochondrial channel VDAC has a cation-selective open state. Biochim Biophys Acta. 2005;1710(2–3):96–102.
28. Choudhary OP, Ujwal R, Kowallis W, Coalson R, Abramson J, Grabe M. The electrostatics of VDAC: implications for selectivity and gating. J Mol Biol. 2010;396(3):580–92.
29. Kwon WS, Park YJ, Mohamed el SA, Pang MG. Voltage-dependent anion channels are a key factor of male fertility. Fertil Steril. 2013;99(2):354–61.
30. Turner RM. Moving to the beat: a review of mammalian sperm motility regulation. Reprod Fertil Dev. 2006;18(1–2):25–38.
31. Eddy EM, Toshimori K, O'Brien DA. Fibrous sheath of mammalian spermatozoa. Microsc Res Tech. 2003;61(1):103–15.
32. Miki K, Willis WD, Brown PR, Goulding EH, Fulcher KD, Eddy EM. Targeted disruption of the Akap4 gene causes defects in sperm flagellum and motility. Dev Biol. 2002;248(2):331–42.
33. Moretti E, Scapigliati G, Pascarelli NA, Baccetti B, Collodel G. Localization of AKAP4 and tubulin proteins in sperm with reduced motility. Asian J Androl. 2007;9(5):641–9.
34. Cao W, Gerton GL, Moss SB. Proteomic profiling of accessory structures from the mouse sperm flagellum. Mol Cell Proteomics. 2006;5(5):801–10.
35. Brohmann H, Pinnecke S, Hoyer-Fender S. Identification and characterization of new cDNAs encoding outer dense fiber proteins of rat sperm. J Biol Chem. 1997;272(15):10327–32.
36. Chemes HE, Olmedo SB, Carrere C, Oses R, Carizza C, Leisner M, et al. Ultrastructural pathology of the sperm flagellum: association between flagellar pathology and fertility prognosis in severely asthenozoospermic men. Hum Reprod. 1998;13(9):2521–6.
37. Petersen C, Fuzesi L, Hoyer-Fender S. Outer dense fibre proteins from human sperm tail: molecular cloning and expression analyses of two cDNA transcripts encoding proteins of approximately 70 kDa. Mol Hum Reprod. 1999;5(7):627–35.
38. Fujinoki M, Kawamura T, Toda T, Ohtake H, Shimizu N, Yamaoka S, et al. Identification of the 58-kDa phosphoprotein associated with motility initiation of hamster spermatozoa. J Biochem. 2003;134(4):559–65.
39. Cosson J, White D, Huitorel P, Edde B, Cibert C, Audebert S, et al. Inhibition of flagellar beat frequency by a new anti-beta-tubulin antibody. Cell Motil Cytoskeleton. 1996;35(2):100–12.
40. Fackenthal JD, Turner FR, Raff EC. Tissue-specific microtubule functions in drosophila spermatogenesis require the beta 2-tubulin isotype-specific carboxy terminus. Dev Biol. 1993;158(1):213–27.
41. Neuer A, Spandorfer SD, Giraldo P, Dieterle S, Rosenwaks Z, Witkin SS. The role of heat shock proteins in reproduction. Hum Reprod Update. 2000;6(2):149–59.
42. Schneider HC, Berthold J, Bauer MF, Dietmeier K, Guiard B, Brunner M, et al. Mitochondrial Hsp70/MIM44 complex facilitates protein import. Nature. 1994;371(6500):768–74.
43. Aitken J, Krausz C, Buckingham D. Relationships between biochemical markers for residual sperm cytoplasm, reactive oxygen species generation, and the presence of leukocytes and precursor germ cells in human sperm suspensions. Mol Reprod Dev. 1994;39(3):268–79.
44. Siva AB, Kameshwari DB, Singh V, Pavani K, Sundaram CS, Rangaraj N, et al. Proteomics-based study on asthenozoospermia: differential expression of proteasome alpha complex. Mol Hum Reprod. 2010;16(7):452–62.
45. Ergur AR, Dokras A, Giraldo JL, Habana A, Kovanci E, Huszar G. Sperm maturity and treatment choice of in vitro fertilization (IVF) or intracytoplasmic sperm injection: diminished sperm HspA2 chaperone levels predict IVF failure. Fertil Steril. 2002;77(5):910–8.
46. Cedenho AP, Lima SB, Cenedeze MA, Spaine DM, Ortiz V, Oehninger S. Oligozoospermia and heat-shock protein expression in ejaculated spermatozoa. Hum Reprod. 2006;21(7):1791–4.
47. Pizarro E, Pasten C, Kong M, Morales P. Proteasomal activity in mammalian spermatozoa. Mol Reprod Dev. 2004;69(1):87–93.
48. Sutovsky P, Hauser R, Sutovsky M. Increased levels of sperm ubiquitin correlate with semen quality in men from an andrology laboratory clinic population. Hum Reprod. 2004;19(3):628–38.
49. Sutovsky P, Turner RM, Hameed S, Sutovsky M. Differential ubiquitination of stallion sperm proteins: possible implications for infertility and reproductive seasonality. Biol Reprod. 2003;68(2):688–98.
50. Martinez-Heredia J, de Mateo S, Vidal-Taboada JM, Ballesca JL, Oliva R. Identification of proteomic differences in asthenozoospermic sperm samples. Hum Reprod. 2008;23(4):783–91.
51. Cardullo RA, Baltz JM. Metabolic regulation in mammalian sperm: mitochondrial volume determines sperm length and flagellar beat frequency. Cell Motil Cytoskeleton. 1991;19(3):180–8.
52. Coughlin EM, Christensen E, Kunz PL, Krishnamoorthy KS, Walker V, Dennis NR, et al. Molecular analysis and prenatal diagnosis of human fumarase deficiency. Mol Genet Metab. 1998;63(4):254–62.
53. Caputo E, Manco G, Mandrich L, Guardiola J. A novel aspartyl proteinase from apocrine epithelia and breast tumors. J Biol Chem. 2000;275(11):7935–41.

54. Lilja H, Abrahamsson PA, Lundwall A. Semenogelin, the predominant protein in human semen. Primary structure and identification of closely related proteins in the male accessory sex glands and on the spermatozoa. J Biol Chem. 1989;264(3):1894–900.
55. Autiero M, Abrescia P, Guardiola J. Interaction of seminal plasma proteins with cell surface antigens: presence of a CD4-binding glycoprotein in human seminal plasma. Exp Cell Res. 1991;197(2):268–71.
56. Shen S, Wang J, Liang J, He D. Comparative proteomic study between human normal motility sperm and idiopathic asthenozoospermia. World J Urol. 2013;31(6):1395–401.
57. Lachance C, Bailey JL, Leclerc P. Expression of Hsp60 and Grp78 in the human endometrium and oviduct, and their effect on sperm functions. Hum Reprod. 2007;22(10):2606–14.
58. Marin-Briggiler CI, Gonzalez-Echeverria MF, Munuce MJ, Ghersevich S, Caille AM, Hellman U, et al. Glucose-regulated protein 78 (Grp78/BiP) is secreted by human oviduct epithelial cells and the recombinant protein modulates sperm-zona pellucida binding. Fertil Steril. 2010;93(5):1574–84.
59. Parte PP, Rao P, Redij S, Lobo V, D'Souza SJ, Gajbhiye R, et al. Sperm phosphoproteome profiling by ultra performance liquid chromatography followed by data independent analysis (LC-MS(E)) reveals altered proteomic signatures in asthenozoospermia. J Proteome. 2012;75(18):5861–71.
60. Wang J, Wang J, Zhang HR, Shi HJ, Ma D, Zhao HX, et al. Proteomic analysis of seminal plasma from asthenozoospermia patients reveals proteins that affect oxidative stress responses and semen quality. Asian J Androl. 2009; 11(4):484–91.
61. Saraswat M, Joenvaara S, Jain T, Tomar AK, Sinha A, Singh S, et al. Human spermatozoa quantitative proteomic signature classifies Normo- and Asthenozoospermia. Mol Cell Proteomics. 2017;16(1):57–72.

7

Genetics of the human Y chromosome and its association with male infertility

Stacy Colaco and Deepak Modi[*]

Abstract

The human Y chromosome harbors genes that are responsible for testis development and also for initiation and maintenance of spermatogenesis in adulthood. The long arm of the Y chromosome (Yq) contains many ampliconic and palindromic sequences making it predisposed to self-recombination during spermatogenesis and hence susceptible to intra-chromosomal deletions. Such deletions lead to copy number variation in genes of the Y chromosome resulting in male infertility. Three common Yq deletions that recur in infertile males are termed as AZF (Azoospermia Factor) microdeletions viz. AZFa, AZFb and AZFc. As estimated from data of nearly 40,000 Y chromosomes, the global prevalence of Yq microdeletions is 7.5% in infertile males; however the European infertile men are less susceptible to Yq microdeletions, the highest prevalence is in Americans and East Asian infertile men. In addition, partial deletions of the AZFc locus have been associated with infertility but the effect seems to be ethnicity dependent. Analysis of > 17,000 Y chromosomes from fertile and infertile men has revealed an association of gr/gr deletion with male infertility in Caucasians and Mongolian men, while the b2/b3 deletion is associated with male infertility in African and Dravidian men. Clinically, the screening for Yq microdeletions would aid the clinician in determining the cause of male infertility and decide a rational management strategy for the patient. As these deletions are transmitted to 100% of male offspring born through assisted reproduction, testing of Yq deletions will allow the couples to make an informed choice regarding the perpetuation of male infertility in future generations. With the emerging data on association of Yq deletions with testicular cancers and neuropsychiatric conditions long term follow-up data is urgently needed for infertile men harboring Yq deletions. If found so, the information will change the current the perspective of androgenetics from infertility and might have broad implication in men health.

Keywords: Infertility, Y chromosome, Microdeletions, AZF, AZFc, gr/gr deletions, Prevalence, Spermatogenesis

Background

Human spermatogenesis is an intricate biological process that begins with the mitotic division of spermatogonia to give rise to primary spermatocytes which in turn undergo the first meiotic division to form secondary spermatocytes. After a second meiosis cycle, these secondary spermatocytes produce haploid cells called round spermatids, which subsequently form elongated spermatids which finally differentiate into mature spermatozoa. The spermatogenic process relies on the concerted actions of various hormones, local secretory factors and testis-specific genes. Defects at any of these levels can lead to accumulation of errors resulting in impaired spermatogenesis leading to male infertility. According to the World Health Organization [1], male infertility refers to the inability of the male partner to cause pregnancy in a clinically normal female. Almost 30 million males worldwide are infertile with the largest niches of male infertility occurring in central and Eastern Europe [8–12%] and Australia [8–9%] [2]. As per WHO 2010 male infertility can be classified based on seminogram under following categories:

- Azoospermia- Absence of sperm in the ejaculate, it can be classified as obstructive azoospermia [OA] where absence of sperm in the ejaculate is observed as a result of problems in sperm delivery or non-obstructive azoospermia [NOA] where there is absence of sperm in the semen due to abnormal sperm production. NOA constitutes 60% of all cases of azoospermia

* Correspondence: deepaknmodi@yahoo.com; modid@nirrh.res.in
Department of Molecular and Cellular Biology, ICMR-National Institute for Research in Reproductive Health, JM Street, Parel, Mumbai, Maharashtra 400012, India

- Oligozoospermia- Less than 15–20 × 10^6 spermatozoa in the ejaculate
- Severe oligozoospermia- Less than 5 × 10^6 spermatozoa in the ejaculate
- Normozoospermia- Normal values of sperms in the ejaculate
- Asthenozoospermia- Low levels of motility observed in less than 50% of sperms
- Teratozoospermia- Less than 30% of sperms have normal morphology
- Aspermia- Failure in ejaculating semen

Causes of male infertility

Male infertility can be attributed to several factors such as cryptorchidism [absence of one or both testes in the scrotum], varicocele [abnormal enlargement of the pampiniform venous plexus in the scrotum], endocrinological disorders, obstruction/absence of seminal pathways, infections, alcohol consumption or chemotherapy [3, 4]. However, genetic alterations have also emerged as one of the leading cause of male infertility. Genetic defects commonly observed in infertile males include karyotypic abnormalities, gene copy number variations [CNVs], single gene mutations/polymorphisms and deletions on the long arm of the Y chromosome [Yq microdeletions]. These genetic defects impede the development of the male gonads or urogenital tract during development, cause arrest of germ cell production and/or maturation or produce non-functional spermatozoa. Amongst the various factors, karyotypic abnormalities and Yq microdeletions are the leading genetic causes of male infertility. In this review, we present the current knowledge of the human Y chromosome, its genes and how the defects in these genes lead to male infertility.

The human Y chromosome

Mammalian sex chromosomes evolved from autosomes at least 180 million years ago. The first step in differentiation of the Y chromosome involved the acquisition of the testis-determining gene followed by large-scale inversions and sequential suppression of recombination between the X and Y chromosomes in a stepwise fashion [5–7]. A detailed overview on the evolution of the human Y chromosome and its present day status has been a subject of recent reviews [5]. Cytogenetically, the human Y is an acrocentric chromosome composed of two pseudoautosomal regions (PARs), a short arm (Yp) and the long arm (Yq) that are separated by a centromere (Fig. 1). While the PARs and the short arm are euchromatic, a large portion of the long arm is heterochromatic with the exception of the proximal portion juxtaposed to the centromere which is euchromatic in nature.

The pseudo autosomal regions (PARs)

The PAR1 and PAR2 of the Y chromosome are short regions of homology between the mammalian X and Y chromosomes; the PAR1 is located on the tip of the p arm and the PAR2 on the tip of the q arm (Fig. 1). Due

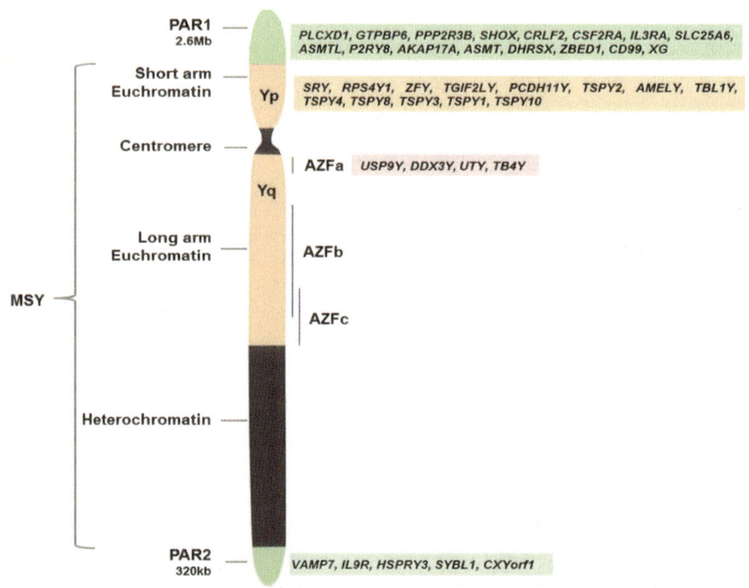

Fig. 1 Structure of the human Y chromosome. The Pseudo Autosomal Regions [PAR1 and PAR2] are located at the terminal ends of the Y chromosome. The green boxes show the genes encoded in these regions. Yp is the short arm of the Y chromosome and the genes within it are show in the peach box. The long arm, Yq, is composed of both euchromatin and the genetically inactive heterochromatin regions. This region contains the Azoospermia factors AZFa, AZFb and AZFc. The pink box shows the genes in the AZFa region. The heterochromatin is not known to harbor any known genes. The region beyond the PAR is termed as Male Specific Region on Y (MSY)

to the diversity in the genetic sequences of the X and Y chromosomes, they do not undergo pairing during meiosis, except for the regions in PAR which pair and recombine with the PARs in the X chromosome during meiosis. However, the recombination and pairing of PARs is temporally and genetically distinct from that of the rest of the genome [8]. The PARs have a delayed double stranded break (DSBs) formation and pairing as compared to autosomes due to the fact that the PARs initiate DSB formation only after all the autosomal DSBs have been repaired.

Despite this delayed recombination, the cross over rate in PAR1 occurs more rapidly than it does on the autosomes [9]. In mice, on average, one meiotic DSB forms every 10 mega base pairs [Mb] while in the PARs it spans a mere 0.7 Mb [10]. It is proposed that in the PARs, deoxyribonucleic acid [DNA] is packaged into several small loops as compared to fewer but larger loops in the autosomes, thus allowing greater DSB formation in the PARs. Indeed, reports indicate that PAR1 contains several recombination hotspots, which have activities that differ significantly among human populations [11]. The genetic control of DSB formation in PARs is also distinct from that of autosomes. Autosomal pairing is dependent on SPO11βm while the X-Y paring is SPO11α dependent. It has been observed that PAR DSBs are not formed in mice that lack SPO11α leading to X-Y mis-segregation and male infertility, the autosomal DSBs are somehow not majorly affected [8]. Interestingly, studies have also associated deletion of human PAR1 with total male sterility [12, 13], reduced recombination in PAR1 has been associated with increased frequency of sex chromosome aneuploidy in sperm, leading to X-chromosome monosomy (Turner syndrome) or XXY (Kleinfelter syndrome) in the offspring [14, 15]. These observations suggest that although the Y chromosome PARs behave like autosomes, the mechanisms by which they do so is different and also has a distinct genetic control.

Genes in PAR1 and PAR2

While the PARs have distinct genetic control as compared to autosomes, wide differences also exist between the two PARs in terms of their genetic content and their functions. Together the PARs contain at least 29 genes, with diverse roles in cell signalling, transcriptional regulation and mitochondrial function [16]. PAR1 contains genes, all of which are known to escape X inactivation (Fig. 1). Interestingly, defects in genes of the PAR1 are associated with mental and stature disorders. Loss of short stature homeobox [*SHOX*] gene in the PAR1 is related to short stature of Turner syndrome [17]; mutation in *SHOX* are reported in patients with idiopathic growth retardation [18]. PAR1 loci are also reported to be associated with schizophrenia and bipolar disorder [19, 20].

PAR2 on the other hand is a much shorter region, spanning only 320 kilobase pairs [kb]. Unlike in the PAR1, crossovers in PAR2 occur at a rate similar to the genome average, in both sexes, suggesting behaviour similar to many autosomal regions. PAR is not necessary for fertility [21]. Unlike PAR1 which is gene rich, the PAR2 region contains only five genes of which two, *HSPRY3* and *SYBL1*, are inactivated on Y chromosome and subjected to X inactivation in females [22]. Additional file 1: Table S2. lists the different 226 genes on the Y chromosome, their cellular expression 227 in testis, putative function and role in spermatogenesis.

Beyond the PAR1 and PAR2, reports also suggest the existence of a 3.5 Mb region termed as PAR3. This region is said to have originated at Xq21.3 when a 3.5 Mb region of the X chromosome underwent duplication and transposition on the Y chromosome at Yp11.2 approximately 5–6 million years ago [23]. It is reported that Yp11.2 and Xq21.3 have 98.78% identity and a high concentration of tandem repeats. Interestingly, allelic unequal recombination also occurs between the two X transposed regions [24]. This PAR3 region is however found only in 2% of the general population and the functional significance (if any) of this PAR is unknown.

The non-recombining region of Y (NRY)

NRY is defined as the locus beyond the PARs which does not undergo recombination during meiosis due to lack of homology with the X chromosome. Cytogenetically this region is divided into two regions viz. the heterochromatic and the euchromatic regions. The heterochromatic region of the Y chromosome comprises distal Yq that contains two highly repetitive sequences families, DYZ1 and DYZ2 [25]. Variation in the size of the Y chromosome long arm heterochromatin within an individual have been reported [26] however its clinical significance remains unknown.

The euchromatic region encompasses the para-centromeric region and the short and long arm of the Y. This region is also referred to as male specific region on Y (MSY) and was for a long time thought to be a functional wasteland. However research in the last two decades have revealed important roles of the euchromatic region ranging from sex determination to regulation of brain functions. Discussed below is our current understanding of the human MSY and alterations in this region that affect human health.

Euchromatic region of Y

The euchromatic region of the Y lies distal to the PAR1 and consists of the short arm para-centromeric region, the centromere and the long arm para-centromeric region (Fig. 1). This region contains sequences that are subdivided into three discrete classes: X-transposed, X-degenerate and ampliconic [27]. The X-transposed sequences are so named, because of a massive X to Y transposition that occurred about 3–4 million years ago. Most of these sequences are composed of repeat elements such as Alu, retroviral and Long interspersed nuclear elements [LINE1]. Some of the genes belonging to this region have ubiquitous tissue expression; the ampliconic sequences contain genes and transcription units that are expressed solely in the testes [28]. The protein products of the MSY genes, contribute to gonad formation, regulation of spermatogenesis, brain, heart, and kidney development [29, 30] suggesting its critical functions in tissue development and its adult functions. Approximately 70 genes have been identified on the Y chromosome and described below are some of these genes. Additional file 1: Table S2 enlists the different genes on the Y chromosome along with their expression, function and role in spermatogenesis.

Genes on the short arm of the Y chromosome [Yp]

Sex determining region on Y [*SRY*]

In the year 1959 two scientific reports on the Klinefelter syndrome and on the Turner syndrome [31, 32], described for the very first time that the human Y chromosome contained at least one sex-determining gene that was responsible for the maleness of the embryo. A large numbers of sex reversed patients were subsequently identified to have deletions in portions of the Yp (XY sex reversal) or had additional portions of the Yp (XX males). These patients immensely contributed to the discovery of the SRY gene which was responsible for testis determination during embryogenesis. In 1990, the gene responsible for testicular determination, *SRY* (Sex-determining Region on the Y chromosome), was identified [33, 34] and was found to be located on the short arm of the Y chromosome close to the pseudoautosomal boundary. This gene is thought to have been evolved by a mutation in the *SOX3* gene. The human *SRY* is a single exon that encodes a protein of 204 amino acids which contains a conserved DNA-binding domain. *SRY* is essential for initiating testis development and differentiation of the bi-potential gonad into Sertoli cells, which then support differentiation and development of the male germline. Hence this gene has been proposed to be the master gene regulating the cascade of testis determination [35]. Mutations in the SRY gene are identified in approximately 15% 46, XY females (Swyer syndrome); translocation of the *SRY* gene to the X chromosome is reported in a subset of 46, XX males [36]. Beyond its expression in developing testis, *SRY* is reportedly expressed in adult testis and even ejaculated spermatozoa [37] the functional significance of which is yet unclear. In addition *SRY* is also expressed in other somatic tissues such as adipose, oesophagus, thymus, adrenal glands, brain kidneys and also in some cancer cell lines [28, 29] suggesting its functions beyond sex determination.

Zinc Finger protein, Y linked [*ZFY*]

Another gene on the p arm of the Y chromosome is *ZFY* which encodes a zinc finger-containing protein and functions as a transcription factor. Expressed in almost all somatic tissues [28, 29], it is proposed to play a role in spermatogenesis, particularly in promoting meiotic division and sperm formation [38–41] Refer Additional file 1: Table S2. While mice knockout for Zfy genes are infertile [42], despite its expression in multiple tissues, a rare deletion of *ZFY* and *SRY* in a woman was not associated with Turner syndrome stigmata. So far, no mutations of *ZFY* have been reported, indicating that *ZFY* may not have any critical somatic functions [43].

Amelogenin, Y linked [*AMELY*]

The *AMELY*, encodes a member of the amelogenin family of extracellular matrix proteins which are involved in biomineralization during tooth enamel development. This gene has a paralogoue on the X chromosome, *AMELX* and a mutation in this gene leads to amelogenesis imperfecta. *AMELY* is expressed at only 10% of the level of *AMELX* and the amelogenin paralogoues, there exist men with deletion of *AMELY*, but have no apparent phenotype [44], suggesting that absence of *AMELY* has no major deleterious effects.

Transducin Beta-like 1Y [*TBL1Y*]

The Transducin Beta-like 1Y (*TBL1Y*), is a Y-linked homologue of *TBL1X* that is related with X-linked late-onset sensorineural deafness. *TBLR1*, a homologue of *TBL1Y*, and *TBL1X* act as a co-repressor/co-activator for several nuclear receptors and transcription factors. A recent study [45] has demonstrated differential expression of the *TBL1Y* during cardiac differentiation of human embryonic stem cells. Interestingly it was noted that the *TBL1Y* protein showed a significant increase during differentiation while the expression level of *TBL1X* simultaneously decreased. When the cellular levels of *TBL1Y* decreased, the authors observed reduced rates of cardiac differentiation as well as an increase in the probability of impaired contractions suggesting that *TBL1Y* knockdown may have negatively impacted cardiogenesis. Another study [46] has reported that the *TBL1Y(A)-USP9Y(A)* haplotype of the Y chromosome, present only in black people of African origin, contributed to a favourable lipoprotein pattern that most likely contributed to their reduced susceptibility to coronary heart disease. The role of *TBL1Y* in testis [if any] remains unknown.

Protocadherin 11, Y linked [*PCDH11Y*]

Another gene of the p arm of the human Y chromosome is, *PCDH11Y*. This gene has an homologue on the *PCDH11X*; is a protocadherin and expressed in multiple tissues including the testis and brain [28, 29, 47]. It is proposed to play a role in cell-cell recognition during brain development and establishment of cerebral asymmetries in humans [48]. Deletions of both the X and Y *PCDH11* are associated with language delay [49].

Testis-specific protein Y-linked [*TSPY*]

The Yp has an array of genes encoding the testis-specific protein Y linked (*TSPY*) which also has an X-homologue, *TSPX*. These proteins function as a proto-oncogene and a tumour suppressor respectively and are also cell cycle regulators [50]. Expressed in a variety of tissue including cancers, *TSPY* is a candidate gene for gonadoblastoma and variations in *TSPY* genes are associated with compromised spermatogenesis [51, 52] although a recent study has refuted this view [53]. For more information on the genes on the p arm of the Y chromosome refer to Additional file 1: Table S2.

Genes on the long arm of the Y chromosome [Yq]

While the short arm of the Y chromosome was yet assumed to have some transcribing genes, the long arm of the Y chromosome was believed to be genetically inert. This myth was disproved in 1997 when 12 novel genes or gene families with ten full-length complementary DNA sequence were identified in the human testis that were localized to the Yq [54]. Since this discovery, the Y chromosome has been well annotated in different species and several functional genes identified [7]. Based on the expression pattern, these genes fall in two categories viz., the housekeeping genes which have X homologoues that escape X inactivation; the second group, consisting of the gene families expressed specifically in testes. The genes perform an array of regulatory functions and belong to diverse clasess such as histone lysine demethylases (*KDM5D* and *UTY*); the transcription factor (*ZFY*), spliceosomal component (*RBMY*); translation initiation factors (*DDX3Y* and *EIF1AY*); and the deubiquitinase (*USP9Y*) suggesting that the genes can govern expression of targets throughout the genome (Fig. 1).

Genes and genetics of human Yq

Although the first demonstration of the functional capacity of the NRY of the human Y chromosome was in 1997, the involvement of this locus with male infertility was first made almost four decades ago. In 1976 Italian researchers, identified microscopically detectable deletions at the distal end of band q11 of the Y chromosome in six out of 1170 infertile males [55]. Analysis indicated that the fathers of two of the same six males had undeleted Y chromosomes, indicating that the deletions arose de novo and could be the underlying aetiology of their azoospermia. Based on these findings, the authors proposed the existence of a spermatogenesis factor, called the "azoospermia factor" [AZF] in the Yq locus. With the advent of the physical and molecular map of the human Y chromosome [56, 57] the studies in the AZF locus and male infertility were extensively propelled. Using a panel of molecular markers, a series of subfertile men who had deletions in the Yq were identified [58–60]. Based on the deletion analysis of these men three recurrently deleted non-overlapping sub-regions in proximal, middle, and distal Yq11 were defined and designated "AZFa," "AZFb," and "AZFc," respectively [61]. While the *DAZ* (Deleted in Azoospermia) gene was considered as a strong candidate for male infertility [60] little was known about the existence of other genes within this locus. With the availability of the first complete sequence of AZFc locus [62] and later the detailed structure of the MSY including the AZFa, b and c regions [27] a large number of genes were identified.

Our understanding of the roles of these genes have mainly stemmed from the genetic analysis of oligozoospermic and azoospermic men where the presence and absence of these genes within the AZF a, b and c loci has been studied. Many of these studies are heterogeneous in nature and would have included men with compromised or absent spermatogenesis (mainly non obstructive oligozoospermia and its forms and azoospermia). For the sake of simplicity we have often used the term "infertile men" to describe these men which essentially mean that these studies would have been done in either azoospermic or oligozoospermic subjects or both.

AZFa locus, its genes and its deletions

The AZFa encodes only single copy genes and is exclusively constituted by single-copy, ubiquitously expressed genes with X homologues that escape inactivation. Four genes have been mapped to AZFa.

Ubiquitin specific peptidase 9, Y linked [*USP9Y*]

Earlier known as known as *DFFRY* or Drosophila fat facets related Y, *USP9Y* was the first gene identified in the AZFa sub-region with a length of 170 k base pairs [kb], consisting of 46 exons [63]. This gene encodes a large polypeptide of 2555 amino acids that is approximately 300 kilo Dalton [kDa] in size and belongs to the C19 cysteine peptidase family with protease activity specific to ubiquitin. *USP9Y* regulates the protein turnover by preventing degradation of proteins by the proteasome through the removal of ubiquitin from protein–ubiquitin conjugates [64] and also stabilizes the de-ubiquitinated target proteins, thus playing an important role in the development of germ cells in males [65]. *USP9Y* is ubiquitously expressed in adult and embryonic tissues and shares 91% identity with its X-homologue, *USP9X*, which escapes X-inactivation and is also expressed in many tissues. Deletion of Usp9x in the mouse causes sterility due to block in spermatogenesis during meiosis [66].

The *USPY* is one of the candidate genes of the AZFa as there exist infertile men with deletion or mutation in *USPY* [64, 67]. However, refuting this view, evidences are also available describing deletions of *USP9Y* in men with normal sperm count [63, 68] suggesting that *USP9Y* is not essential for normal sperm production and fertility in males.

Besides its role in spermatogenesis, studies have discovered that a nine-residue peptide derived from *USP9Y* represents a minor histocompatibility antigen [H-Y antigen] involved in graft rejection [69]. Recently, an association of gene fusion involving *USP9Y* (*TTTY15-USP9Y*) with prostate cancer has also been reported [70] suggesting its functions beyond regulation of sperm production.

DEAD [asp-glu-ala-asp] box RNA helicases, Box 3, Y-linked [*DBY*]

DBY, also known as *DDX3Y*, was first identified by Lahn and Page [54] at the 5C region of the long arm of the Y chromosome at cytogenetic location Yq11.21 [53, 71]. *DBY*, which extends for 15.5 kb, consists of 17 exons and encodes a conserved ATP-dependent DEAD-box RNA helicase that is expressed only in germ cells with an alleged function at G1–S phase of the cell cycle [72]. *DBY* has a homologue on the X chromosome, *DBX* [53] and both of these genes have been reported to have > 95% sequence similarity while being expressed in two different stages of male germ cell line. While *DBY* protein expression is limited to only pre-meiotic male germ cells, the *DBX* protein is expressed in post-meiotic spermatids and in multiple somatic tissues [71].

Deletion analysis for the AZFa region in infertile males has revealed that males lacking *DBY* exhibit either Sertoli Cell Only syndrome [SCOS] or severe hypospermatogenesis suggesting that *DBY* plays a key role in the spermatogenic process [73, 74]. *DBY* protein has been reported to control the translation initiation of cyclin E1, which is essential for cell cycle progression from the G1 to S phase [75]. In drosophila, the *DBY* homologue, *Belle*, is essential for mitotic progression and survival of germline stem cells and spermatogonia [76]. Developmentally, *DBY* expression is initiated in the germ cells of human testis by 17 weeks of gestation implying that this protein may play a role in early spermatogonial proliferation [72]. This also suggests that, in males with AZFa deletion; germ cell depletion may begin prenatally. Indeed, complementation with *DBY* on the AZFa background, improved the formation of germ cell like cells from induced pluoripotent stem cells with AZFa deletion [77] suggesting that *DBY* functions in the earliest stages of human germ cell development.

Ubiquitously transcribed tetratricopeptide repeat containing, Y linked [*UTY*]

UTY and Ubiquitously transcribed tetratricopeptidete repeat, X [*UTX*] genes are members of the tetratricopeptide repeat [TPR] protein family which occur in proteins that control mitosis. The *UTY* gene is located at the 5C band of AZFa contains 50 exons and a 3'UTR region with several polyadenylation signals [78]. Two *UTY* transcripts are detected in various human tissues such as spleen, thymus, prostate, testis, intestine, colon, and in cells such as leukocytes, but is not transcribed in ovary [53].

The *UTY* encodes a male-specific histone demethylase that catalyzes trimethylated 'Lys-27' [H3K27me3] demethylation in histone H3 of DNA. *UTY* is also involved in protein-protein interactions and may act as a chaperone [79]. Reports also suggest that the *UTY* protein is a minor histocompatibility antigen that may induce graft rejection of stem cell grafts of males [80]. A recent study [81] has suggested that the *UTY* is involved in a transcriptional regulatory network that is essential for prostate differentiation and that disruption of this network predisposes males to prostate cancer. Another study [82] reported the occurrence of *UTY* copy number variation in males afflicted with urothelial bladder cancer. The role of *UTY* in testis is not clear. Several missense mutations in *UTY* are reported in dbSNP database and computational analysis of some of these, have been shown to be deleterious [80]. However the fertility status of these men is unknown.

Thymosin beta 4 Y linked, [*TB4Y*]

TB4Y, has been mapped to region 5D on the long arm of the human Y chromosome. *TB4Y* is expressed in various tissues, exists in a single copy and showing about 93% sequence similarity to its X chromosome homolog *TB4X* [53]. *TB4Y* encodes a novel human leukocyte antigen [HLA]-A*3303-restricted, minor histocompatibility antigen [83] and is a key activator of natural killer cell cytotoxicity [84]. The involvement of *TBY4* in testicular functions is unknown.

AZFb locus, its genes and its deletions

The AZFb locus is located in the central region of Yq11 [intervals 5M-6B] and spans 3.2 Mb of which 1.5 Mb overlaps with AZFc (Figs. 1 and 2). The AZFb region has a complex genomic structure and contains three single-copy regions, a Y chromosome specific repeated DNA family [DYZ] 19 satellite repeat array and 14 multi-copy sequence units called amplicons (Fig. 2). These amplicons are organized into six sequence families, with intra-family homology levels > 99%. Amplicon families are defined by a specific colour code [yellow, blue, turquoise, green, red or grey] and each family member is identified by a numeral (Fig. 2). Of the 14 amplicon units, seven [yel3, yel4, b5, b6, b1, t1, t2] are restricted to AZFb, while the

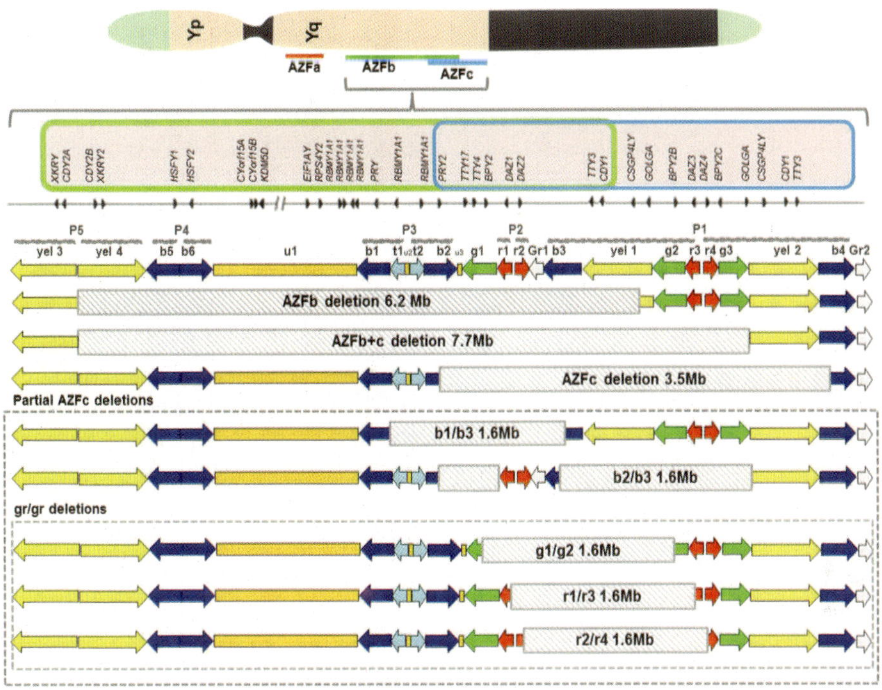

Fig. 2 Schematic organization of the AZFb and c loci depicting how the various microdeletions arise. The AZFb and c regions are located in the euchromatic region on the Yq. Both regions share a number of genes [pink box], the genes present in the AZFb region are shown in the green box while the genes present in the AZFc region are present in the blue box. The grey arrows depict the orientation of the genes and the grey bars depict the organisation of the amplicons into palindromes [P1 to P5]. The AZFb and AZFc loci are composed of numerous stretches of ampliconic sequences [block arrows] which are annotated as six colour-coded sequence families (yellow, blue, turquoise, green, red and grey) called amplicons. The size and orientation of the coloured arrows represents the length and orientation of the arrows. AZFb is defined by the P5/proximal P1 deletion (yel3/yel1) which removes 6.23 Mb of DNA and AZFc by the b2/b4 deletion which removes 3.5 Mb of DNA. The partial AZFc deletions b1/b3, b2/b3 and the three variations of the gr/gr deletions [g1/g2], [r1/r3] and [r2/r4] [in dotted box] remove almost half of the AZFc gene content. The shaded block depicts the exact location of the deletion. The information of the map is adapted from published data ([6, 27], and [62])

remaining are shared with AZFc. Amplicons are also categorized by a higher-order structural organization based on symmetrical arrays of contiguous repeat units called palindromes. AZFb contains palindromes P2 to P5 and the proximal part of P1 (Fig. 2). The presence of extensive ampliconic domains in AZFb allows for very complex rearrangements [62]. The critical AZFb interval necessary for spermatocyte maturation stretches from the center of palindrome P5 to the proximal edge of P3 within the *RBMY1* cluster, an interval of over 4 Mb containing 13 coding genes [85].

The AZFb is prone to NAHR [non-allelic homologous recombination] with AZFc, resulting in two frequent deletions of, 6.23 and 7.7 Mb. The 6.23 Mb, complete or classic AZFb deletion [P5/proximal P1] corresponds to the interval encompassed between amplicons yel3 and yel1 (Fig. 2) and occurs mainly due to unequal crossing over between homologous segments at their extremities [86]. This classical deletion overlaps within 1.5 Mb of the proximal portion of AZFc and leads to the loss of at least 32 coding genes and transcripts [87, 88]. Deletions of both AZFb and AZFc together occur in two breakpoints between P4/distal P1 (7.0 Mb, 38 gene copies removed) or between P5/distal P1 (7.7 Mb and 42 gene copies removed) [89]. The AZFb gene contains a total of five different single-copy transcription units as detailed in Fig. 2. However, not much is known about the biological functions of many of these genes.

Chromosome Y open reading frame 15 [*CYorf15*]

*CYorf15A*and *CYorf15B* are single copy genes in AZFb which have an X homologue, *CXorf15*, thought to be involved with the taxilin family of proteins which are implicated in intracellular vesicle traffic [6].

Ribosomal protein S4, Y linked [*RPS4Y2*]

Eukaryotic ribosomal protein S4 (S4e) is X-linked in mammals [90] and a Y linked homologue (*RPS4Y1*) is present in all primate lineages [91]. In humans, a second copy of the Y-linked gene (*RPS4Y2*) was described [27] which originated by duplication before the radiation of Old World Monkeys, approximately 35 million years ago [91]. The *RPS4Y1* is expressed in the testis and prostrate and is more highly expressed during spermatogenesis. It encodes a structurally conserved ribosomal protein subunit required for mRNA binding to the ribosome [92] and plays a role in the post-transcriptional regulation of the spermatogenic process.

Eukaryotic Translation Initiation Factor 1A, Y linked [*EIF1AY*]

This gene is ubiquitously expressed and is a Y-linked member of the EIF-1A family—a family involved in translation initiation. The EIF-1A proteins enhance ribosome dissociation into subunits and stabilize the binding of the 43S complex to the end of capped RNA during protein biosynthesis. Studies implicate this gene with ischemic stroke [93, 94]. Widely expressed in multiple tissues, the biological roles of this gene are unknown. However, a close homologue of this gene in the mouse (*Eif2s3y*) along with SRY is sufficient to induce testicular differentiation and initiate spermatogenesis until the round spermatid stage in XX mice [95] suggesting its role in spermatogenesis.

Lysine Demethylase 5D [KDM5D] / Selected Mouse cDNA, Y [*SMCY*]

This gene has several alternative names such as Jumonji At-Rich Interactive Domain 1D [*JARID1D*], Histocompatibility Y Antigen [*HY*] and H-Y Antigen [*HYA*]. It is thought that *KDM5D* plays a crucial role in chromosome condensation during meiosis by demethylating di- and tri-methylated H3K4 thus explaining the maturation arrest observed at the spermatocyte stage associated to AZFb deletions. The *KDM5D* enzyme is also known to form a protein complex with the MutS protein homolog 5 [MSH5] DNA repair factor during spermatogenesis which can be found on condensed DNA during the leptotene/zygotene stage, suggesting an involvement in male germ cell chromatin remodelling. Despite the apparently male germline-specific functions, this gene is ubiquitously expressed and is homologous to *KDM5C*, an X-borne gene. *KDM5D* has also been reported to have a tumour suppressor function in prostate cancer [96]. This gene regulates invasion-associated genes and the loss of *KDM5D* causes the cell to acquire invasiveness leading to the development of metastasis. A recent study [97] provides evidence that *KDM5D* plays an important role in determining docetaxel sensitivity, which is used in treating prostate cancer, by interacting with androgen receptor signalling and that its expression level is associated with clinical outcomes.

X linked Kell Blood group precursor, Y linked [*XKRY*]

The *XKRY* exists in two copies in the yellow amplicon of AZFb (Fig. 2) that encodes a protein which is similar to XK, a putative membrane transport protein. By analysis of a panel of partial Y chromosomes this gene was mapped to region 5 L on the long arm of the human Y chromosome [53]. The functions of this protein is unknown, no role for it has been ascribed in spermatogenesis.

Heat Shock transcription factor, Y linked [*HSFY*]

This gene maps to the blue amplicons with the two active copies located in b5 and b6 in the AZFb locus (Fig. 2). In the AZFb locus *HSFY* exists as two coding copies *HSFY1* and *HSFY2*. Although *HSFY* shows homology to the heat shock transcription factor-type (HSF) DNA-binding domain, it does not bind to heat shock elements and no HSFY-targeted promoters have been identified during spermatogenesis [98, 99]. *HSFY* has homologues at Xq28, *HSFX1* and *HSFX2* [27] but *HSFY* is expressed exclusively in the testis and principal cells of the epididymis.

That *HSFY* is functional and required for spermatogenesis is evident from the observations in four infertile males with a large 768 kb deletion around the P4 palindrome at the proximal end of the AZFb interval that resulted in loss of both *HSFY1* and *HSFY2*, and six non-coding transcription units *FAM41AY2*, *NCRNA00230B*, *TTTY9A*, *TTTY9B*, *NCRNA00185* and *TTTY14* [98]. Another study [99] also reported a partial AZFb deletion that removed the *HSFY* genes and three other genes [*KDM5D*, *CYorf15A and CYorf15B*] ostensibly only affecting the functional copies of *HSFY* in an azoospermic man.

The observations in genetic deletions are also backed by functional studies. *HSFY* is expressed in nuclei of germ cells with predominant expression in round spermatids. *HSFY* protein levels are decreased in testis of men with maturation arrest, associating this gene to the regulation of spermatogenesis [100–104].

PTPN13-like Y linked, [*PTPBL*]-Related gene on Y [*PRY*]

PRY is a testis specific gene that encodes a protein similar to protein tyrosine phosphatase, non-receptor type 13 [105]. Two nearly identical copies of this gene, *PRY* and *PRY2*, map to the blue amplicons of the AZFb region (Fig. 2), with the two functional units being restricted to b1 and b2 [106].

The expression of *PRY* in germ cells is heterogeneous, with the protein being detected only in a few sperm and spermatids. Furthermore, *PRY* levels are increased in ejaculated sperm obtained from males with abnormal semen parameters, suggesting a link between its expression and defective spermatogenesis [107]. The *PRY* genes are thought to be involved in the regulation of apoptosis implicated in the removal of abnormal sperm [107]. Deletions that include the *PRY1* and *PRY2* genes have also been reported to cause meiotic arrest [108]. Studies reveal that in cases where all the genes in the AZFb region, excluding *RBMY* and *PRY* are deleted, there is hypospermatogenesis however if both *RBMY* and *PRY* are deleted, spermatogenesis is arrested completely [109]. This indicates that these two genes are the major genes involved in fertility [108, 110].

Ribonucleic Acid [RNA]-Binding Motif, Y linked [*RBMY*]

The *RBMY* is one of the most important genes of the AZFb region with approximately six copies of this gene being dispersed within the Y chromosome [111]. The *RBMY1A1* gene family was identified [112] as a multicopy gene family designated *YRRM* (Y chromosome RNA recognition motif) and the first candidate azoospermia facto (Fig. 2). The proteins of the *RBM* gene family are characterised by the presence of an N-terminal RNA recognition motif [RRM] responsible for its interaction with target RNA molecules. Contrasting with the other RBM genes, *RBMY1A1* contains a C-terminal protein interaction repeat domain enriched in serine, arginine, glycine, and tyrosine [SRGY]. This serves as a probable regulatory region for the modulation of *RBMY1A1* function [113].

RBMY1A1 is involved in several aspects of meiotic and pre-meiotic regulation via the establishment of multiple protein-protein and protein-RNA complexes. *RBMY1* encodes a testis-specific RNA binding protein that is expressed in the nuclei of spermatogonia, spermatocytes and round spermatids [114–118] and the expression of the protein is reduced in testis of men with AZFb deletions [117]. Interestingly, the subcellular distribution of *RBMY* differs in spermatogenic cells as they progress through meiosis [115], Fig. 3. In the spermatogonia, *RBMY* is localized as two foci, with one in the nucleolus and the other in the sub nuclear region. However in the spermatocytes, *RBMY* is distributed in a punctuate manner in the nucleus but the subnuclear foci is retained. In the pachytene cells, *RBMY* is spread along the length of the condensing chromosomes. Interestingly, in the round and elongating spermatids *RBMY* is excluded from the nucleus and restricted to the cytoplasm while it is retained in the mid-piece of ejaculated sperm (Fig. 3). These observations suggest that *RBMY* must have diverse functional roles during different stages of spermatogenesis. Indeed analysis of the human testicular *RBMY* bound transcriptome have led to identification of 20 target genes some of which are testis specific and have diverse cellular functions and is proposed to regulate alternate splicing during the course of spermatogenesis [119].

Molecular analysis of infertile men have has indicated a positive correlation between number of *RBMY1* copies and sperm count and motility [120]. Deletion of *RBMY1* copies leads to decrease in sperm count; however the persistence of the two proximal *RMBY1* copies is sufficient to avoid spermatogenic failure despite the total absence of the *PRY* gene [121]. These reports emphasized that the presence of *RMBY1* was sufficient for spermatogenesis to remain qualitatively complete although quantitatively reduced. Interestingly, unlike the humans, mice knockout of Rbmy undergo normal spermatogenesis but have abnormal spermatozoa [122] indicating that atleast in rodents Rbmy is dispensable for spermatogenesis but might be required in spermiogenesis. Indeed, even in humans, *RBMY* protein is detected in elongating spermatids and also in ejaculated sperm [115], Fig. 3. Sperm with high motility carry more *RBMY1* protein than those with relatively low motility [120]; inhibition of *RBMY* using a functionally neutralizing antibody inhibits sperm motility in vitro [115].

Beyond the testis, *RBMY* has been shown to play a role in liver cancers where *RBMY* was expressed exclusively in the testis of 36% of cases with hepatocellular carcinoma (HCCs), in 67% cases with hepatoblastoma and also in a liver cancer cell line [123, 124]. Gain of functions of *RBMY* in mouse fibroblast or in vivo in the liver results in vivo tumor formation [123, 124] down-regulating *RBMY* in liver cancer cells reduces their tumorigenic potential [124]. *RBMY* is reportedly increased mainly in the hepatic stem cells of patients with HCC where it aberrantly signals GSK3β-WNT-β catenin signaling complex resulting in cell proliferation [124]. These observations imply that beyond the testis *RBMY*

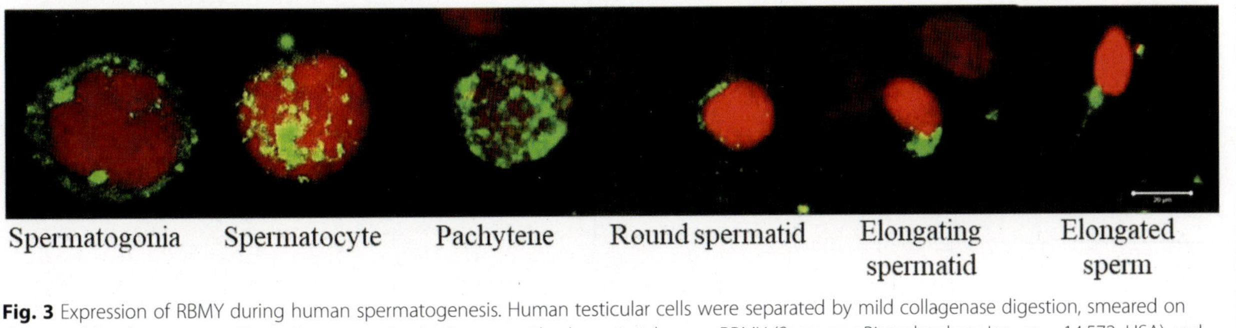

Fig. 3 Expression of RBMY during human spermatogenesis. Human testicular cells were separated by mild collagenase digestion, smeared on slides and fixed in acetone. The cells were probed using an antibody against human RBMY (Santacruz Biotechnology Inc., sc – 14,572, USA) and detected using a FITC labeled secondary antibody. The cells were imaged under a fluorescent microscope and different stages were identified based on the cell and nuclear size. Green staining represents RBMY, red is nuclei. Bar represents 20 μm. For details of the methods see Abid et al. [115]

may act as an oncogene and this might explain the male predominance of various cancers including HCC.

AZFc locus, its genes and its deletions

The AZFc is located at the distal part of deletion interval 6 (subintervals 6C–6E) on the Y chromosome (Figs. 1, 2). While the AZFa and AZFb regions are essential in initiating spermatogenesis, the AZFc region is essential to complete the process of spermatogenesis. The AZFc is the most commonly deleted region of the AZF locus in infertile men [27, 125].

The AZFc region spans 4.5 Mb and codes for 21 candidate genes and 11 families of transcription units (Fig. 2) that are exclusively expressed in the testis [100, 126]. This region contains six distinct families of amplicons; turquoise, grey and yellow, which occur twice in the AZFc locus, the green amplicon which occurs thrice and the blue and red amplicons which occur four times in the locus (Fig. 2). The members of each amplicon family are nearly identical and are arranged to form six large inverted repeats and three large direct repeats (Fig. 2). Three of the six inverted repeats are palindromes, or near palindromes, with large, inverted duplications containing much shorter intervening sequences. In the AZFc region, six distinct inverted repeat amplicon families are arranged in a complex repetitive pattern forming three palindromes that are believed to have formed as a result of the duplications and tandem inversions during evolution [62]. Together, palindromes P1, P2 and P3 encompass 4.0 of the 4.5 Mb of sequence (Fig. 2). Palindrome P1 is 1.5 Mb long with a span of 3 Mb and arm-to-arm identity of 99.97%. Within the arms of P1 lie two smaller palindromes, P1.1 and P1.2, each spanning 24 kb. The three uncoloured segments u1, u2 and u3 occur once each in this region (Fig. 2). u1 shows 70–85% identity to a locus on Yp, u2 shows 70–90% identity to an interspersed Y-specific repeated locus and u3 falls within a 65-kb block of 99.7% identity to Yp. The uncoloured 2 kb segments at the centres of the P1 and P2 palindromes are identical to each other (Fig. 2). The repetitive and palindromic nature of this locus and the fact that it is bordered with a highly repetitive heterochromatic region of Yq12 make this region highly susceptible to intra-chromosomal rearrangements during meiotic recombination thus making the AZFc locus prone to deletions, duplications and copy number variations of the eight gene families that are harboured within it [62].

There are no single-copy sequences in the AZFc (Fig. 2). The AZFc region includes 12 genes and transcription units, each present in a variable number of copies making a total of 32 copies. Amongst the various transcriptional units, only active copies of four protein-coding gene families map to the AZFc interval. These include the *PRY2, BPY2, DAZ* and *CDY1*. These genes locate to the blue, green, red and yellow-coded amplicons, respectively, with one transcription unit per amplicon copy (Fig. 2).

Deleted in Azoospermia [*DAZ*]

DAZ originated on the Y chromosome as a transposition of a DNA segment containing the autosomal germ-cell specific gene *DAZL* almost 35 million years ago [87, 127]. Two autosomal *DAZ* homologs, *BOULE* and *DAZL*, have also been identified in humans with *BOULE* being considered a founding member of the *DAZ* gene family due to its conservation across the metazoan lineages [128, 129]. A loss of function mutation of the *Drosophila* homologue *boule* results in azoospermia thus emphasizing the role of *DAZ* in spermatogenesis [129].

DAZ was the first candidate gene to be isolated from the AZFc locus and was originally identified as a frequently deleted gene on the Y chromosome of infertile males [60, 130]. It was later found that the AZFc region contained palindromic duplications of *DAZ* as two clusters of four genes, *DAZ 1* and *2* and *DAZ 3* and *4* [131–133]. The four *DAZ* copies are expressed in spermatogonia, encoding an RNA-binding protein important for spermatogenesis [106] and these genes are expressed in all stages of germ cell development. Using human embryonic stem cells, it is shown that *DAZ* family genes function in germ cell formation and meiotic progression [134]. Therefore, all *DAZ* family genes are regarded critical for germ cell development.

Like the *RMBY* genes, the *DAZ* genes too, are known to contain an RNA recognition motif [RRM], expressed in the cytoplasm of pre-meiotic testicular germ cells, making these genes candidates for the maintenance of germ stem cell populations. The *DAZ* proteins are characterized by the presence of one or more *DAZ* repeat [24 amino acids rich in Asn, Tyr, and Gln residues], while in some cases, the *DAZ* motif is thought to mediate interaction with other proteins [135]. The human *DAZ* proteins carry out transportation, translational activation of developmentally regulated transcripts and their storage [136].

Deletion of *DAZ* accounts for 10% of cases of males with spermatogenic defects [136, 137]. Infertile males showing a loss of copies of *DAZ* genes are highly predisposed to azoospermia or severe oligozoospermia [138–140]. However due to the presence of the functional homologue (*DAZLA*) on human chromosome 3, a direct association between deletions in *DAZ* and azoospermia is difficult to conclude. Studies have also identified a single nucleotide polymorphism of *DAZL* that confers susceptibility to defects in spermatogenesis [141] and the deletion of the *DAZ1/DAZ2* doublet has been considered responsible for severe oligozoospermia, incomplete maturation arrest and for the testicular phenotype of residual spermiogenesis [140, 142].

While *DAZ* gene copies are deleted in men with complete and partial AZFc deletions, we and others have reported that individual *DAZ* copies can get deleted or duplicated even in absence of complete deletions [138, 140, 143–145]. While *DAZ* gene copy deletions/duplications are reported even in fertile men, deletion of *DAZ* and *CDY1* copies results in reduced sperm count and motility [140, 143]. These observations underscore the importance of *DAZ* genes in spermatogenesis. Functionally, the mechanism by which *DAZ* would regulate spermatogenesis remains unexplored, it is suspected to do so by regulation of RNA translation [146]. The targets of human *DAZ* gene have not been identified; human *DAZ* is known to interact with several other proteins that not necessarily have a role in protein translation [146] suggesting possibility of alternate mechanisms.

Chromodomain Protein Y linked [*CDY*]

The human Y chromosome has two identical copies of this gene within the AZFc region [*CDY1A* and *CDY1B*] and a pair of closely related genes in the palindrome P5 [*CDY2A* and *CDY2B*, Fig. 2]. The *CDY1* gene encodes a protein containing an N-terminal chromatin-binding domain [chromo domain], which aids in regulation of gene expression, chromatin remodelling and encodes a histone acetyltransferase. This protein has been reported to concentrate in the round spermatid nucleus, where histone hyperacetylation occurs and causes the replacement of histones by the sperm-specific DNA packaging proteins, TNPs and PRMs [114, 147]. Although found only in primates, *CDY1* is believed to have been retroposed directly into MSY from a transcript of the autosomal gene *CDYL* more than 150 million years ago, making it one of the oldest genes on the Y chromosome [106].

The *CDY1* and *DAZ* families display autosomal homologues and hence some degree of functional redundancy between the Y-borne and the autosomal copies may partially account for the production of mature sperm in AZFc deleted males. One of the two copies of the *CDY1* gene is deleted in men with partial deletion of the AZFc locus [88, 105]. Based on analyses of gene copy deletions in the AZFc locus of infertile men, Machev et al. [148] discriminated four types of *DAZ-CDY1* partial deletions and found that only one deletion type, *DAZ3/4-CDY1a*, was associated with male infertility. In a similar study concomitant deletion of both *DAZ* and *CDY1* copies in males predisposes them to azoospermia or severe oligozoospermia [140, 149] deletion of *CDY1b* copy alone is also reported to be associated with oligo/azoospermia [150]. However, the fact that some men with *CDY1* deletions (alone or in combination with *DAZ*) are fertile/normozoopermic suggest that these genes are not indispensible for spermatogenesis [140, 151]. Beyond its function as a histone acetyltransferase, little is known about the molecular functions of *CDY1*.

Basic Protein Y linked, 2 [*BPY2*]

The *BPY2* gene is expressed specifically in testis and its protein product is involved in male germ cell development. Three nearly identical copies of this gene exist on Y chromosome, *BPY2A*, *BPY2B* and *BPY2C*, of which two copies of are located at the boundaries of the gr/gr deletion, flanking the *DAZ* gene clusters (Fig. 2). *BPY2* is localized in the nuclei of spermatocytes, round spermatids and spermatogonia [152]. The *BPY2* gene encodes for a small positively charged protein which is thought to be involved in cytoskeletal regulation in spermatogenesis. Due to its small size and high charge, it is thought that *BPY* proteins may functionally interact with DNA in a manner that resembles chromatin-associated proteins such as histones and high mobility group proteins which are known to play a role in the regulation of processes such as transcription, replication, recombination and DNA repair [153]. The frequency of *BPY2* copy number alterations in infertile males is reported to be significantly high in the Chinese population [138] and also in Indian population (Modi et al. unpublished data). Some genetic variants in *BPY2* gene are associated with SCOs [154].

Golgi autoantigen, golgi subfamily a, 2-like, Y-linked [*GOLGA2LY*]

GOLGA exists as two copies viz. *GOLGA2P2Y* and *GOLGA2P3Y* on the AZFc locus, arranged in opposite orientation in palindrome P1 (Fig. 2). This gene is reported to be transcribed and expressed only in the testis where it encodes a 108 amino acid protein [27, 106, 155]. However we have failed to amplify specific *GOLGA2LY* transcripts in the human testis, sequence analysis of some residual bands in RT-PCR experiments have been shown to arise out of non-specific amplifications from its homologs (Modi et al. unpublished data). *GOLGA2LY* protein has not been reported in any of the testicular proteomes [156]. Thus it is yet unclear if *GOLGA2LY* is a pseudogene or is transcriptionally active.

Partial AZFc deletion involves deletion of one of the two copies of the *GOLGA2LY* gene (Fig. 2). Although no function has been attributed to *GOLGA2LY*, it is interesting to note that males harbouring *GOLGA2P3Y* deletion have low sperm concentration and motility compared with males without deletion or with deletion of *GOLGA2P2Y*, suggesting the differential roles of the two copies spermatogenesis [138, 143]. The frequency of *GOLGA2P3Y* deletion is significantly higher in oligozoospermic men compared with normozoospermic men (odds ratio of 9), whereas the frequency of *GOLGA2P2Y* deletion was comparable between oligozoospermic and normozoospermic men [157]. Furthermore, men with *GOLGA2P3Y* deletion have reduced sperm concentration and motility compared with men without deletion or with deletion of *GOLGA2P2Y* [157] suggesting that loss of *GOLGA2P3Y* is an independent risk factor for oligozoospermia. However, assuming that the *GOLGA2LY* is a pseudogene and does not transcribe/translate in the testis, how these deletion result in infertility is difficult to ascertain. Positional shifts in the AZFc locus due to such deletions might offer a possible explanation.

Chondroitin Sulfate Proteoglycan 4 Pseudogene 1, Y-linked [*CSPG4P1Y*]

Like the *GOLGA*, *CSPG4P1Y* the family of transcription units exist in two copies (Fig. 2) and is regarded as a pseudogene [32]. One of the two copies of the *CSPG4LY* gene is deleted in the b2/b3 deletion within the AZFc region [105]. Not much is known about the functions of this gene or its copies in maintenance of spermatogenesis.

Testis-Specific Transcript, Y-Linked 4 [*TTY4*]

The *TTY4* gene has three copies (Fig. 2), *TTY4A*, *TTY4B* and *TTY4C*. This gene has not been studied in detail and is considered to be an RNA that does not encode any protein [88, 105]. *TTY4* copy deletions are rare in Indian population but, loss of one or more copies of *TTY4C* have been found to be associated with male infertility (Modi et al. unpublished data). In summary, it appears that the Y chromosome harbours genes that not only play integral roles in spermatogenesis but also in several aspects of human health. Several Y encoded genes are expressed not only in the testis but also in tissues involved in immune functions. [Refer Additional file 1: Table S2] However the putative functions of several Y borne genes still remains unknown and future studies may provide answers towards this end.

Y chromosome microdeletions and male infertility

The human Y chromosome is genetically dynamic and is also prone to significant variation owing to the high proportion of segmental duplications which form the basis of the wide variety of deletions and duplications seen in various loci of this chromosome. Since the Yq locus contains large numbers of genes that are transcribed in the testis and have well defined role in spermatogenesis loss of these regions would cause infertility. Clinically, the Y chromosome alterations can be classified as (1) AZF deletions (complete loss of one or more of the AZF loci), (2) partial AZFc deletions and duplications and, (3) the gene copy number variations (CNVs). Described below are the prevalence and association of these deletions with male infertility.

Yq microdeletions

Y chromosome microdeletions are small submicroscopic segmental deletions in the proximal Yq that remove the entire or parts of AZF region (complete deletions). Based on extensive deletion mapping studies in infertile men, five different deletions patterns on Yq have been reported [88]. However, in clinical practice, these are clubbed and termed as AZFa, AZFb, and AZFc deletions (Fig. 2). These deletions are one of the leading causes of spermatogenic failure and hence the screening for AZF deletions has become part of the routine diagnostic work-up of infertile men [158–160]. With the availability of the specific markers, simple PCR strategies to study the AZF locus are now available from various parts of the world that have shown the prevalence of Yq microdeletions. With a few exceptions of early reports, with refinements in the technologies, Yq microdeletions are detected exclusively in men with abnormal spermiograms and not been observed in large series of fertile men [158–160] suggesting that these deletions are the cause of failure of spermatogenesis and hence infertility. However, there are case reports where fathers of infertile men have been shown to carry these Yq deletions [161, 162] and this casts doubt on the whether these deletions themselves are sufficient to cause infertility or additional defects in the genome would be required to manifest the phenotype.

Based on global data, Yq microdeletions are estimated to occur in about 1: 4000 men in the general population, but its frequency in infertile men is about 1:12. Of the > 30,000 Y chromosomes analysed for AZF microdeletions (by STS-PCR method), the global prevalence of AZF microdeletions in infertile men is estimated to be **7% (95% CL 6.74–6.79)**, (Fig. 4). As evident there is a wide variation in the frequency of Yq microdeletions in different parts of the world (Fig. 4), this could reflect underlying differences in sample size, methodology used and the population screened. The country wise published data of Yq deletion in infertile men is provided in Additional file 1: Table S1. However; pooled estimates based on geographic locations suggest that the lowest prevalence of Yq microdeletions is in Europe **(3% 95% CL 2.9–3.0)** and Australia **(5.3% 95% CL 5.9–7.8)**; while the rest of the world has an average of 8–9% (Fig. 5). What makes the Europeans and Australian infertile men less susceptible to Yq microdeletions warrants investigation. Amongst the Asians we observed that the highest prevalence of Yq microdeletions is amongst the East and South East Asians and lowest amongst South Asians (Fig. 5). This indicates that the susceptibility of the Yq to undergo microdeletions is perhaps race or ethnicity dependent. An influence of the Y chromosome genetic background (e.g. haplogroups) has been suggested to influence the susceptibility of partial AZFc deletions (see below). Whether these haplogroups also contribute to the

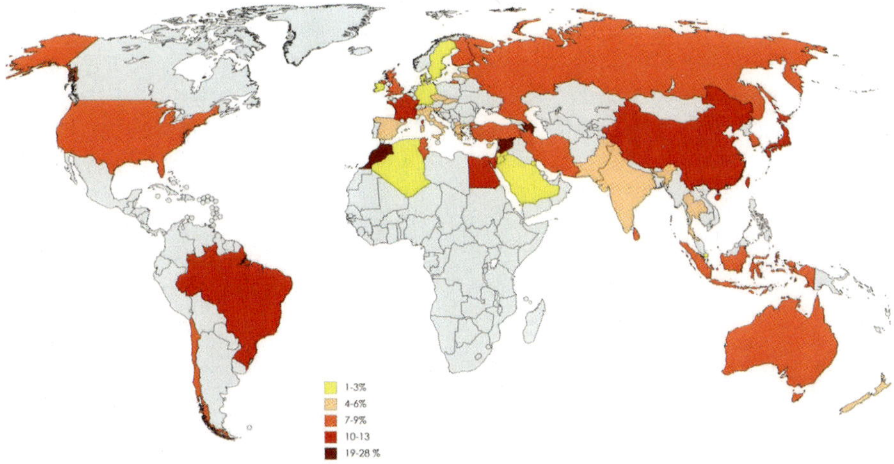

Fig. 4 World map depicting the prevalence of Yq microdeletions in infertile males in different countries. The prevalence of Yq microdeletions in different countries of the world was estimated from published data of 40,127 Y chromosomes from infertile men. (oligozoospermic or azoospermic men). Only those articles published in English were considered and total number of infertile men studied and those having deletions were recorded along with the country. For each country data from different studies were pooled and the average estimated

occurrence of Yq microdeletions needs to be investigated. Since the global data is collated from diverse groups and not all studies have reported the ethnicity of the population investigated we are unable to determine the influence of different genetic background on prevalence of Yq microdeletions.

Irrespective of the population under study, the AZFc is most frequently deleted locus in infertile men [60–70%] followed by AZFa [0.5–4%], AZFb [1–5%] and AZFb+c [1–3%] deletion [11]. While these are global estimates, it is intriguing that the frequencies of the various AZF loci that are deleted in infertile men differ amongst various populations. While the frequency of AZFc deletion is lower in Indian population as compared to western counterparts (45% versus 60%), the frequency of AZFa deletion is almost double (11 versus 5%). Further, the frequency of double deletions (AZF a + b, b + c) is also higher in the Indian population as opposed to world literature [159]. A similar difference in the frequency of deletion of different AZF loci has been observed in Iranian population [163]. Also there are unusual combinations of deletions like the AZFa+c deletion observed

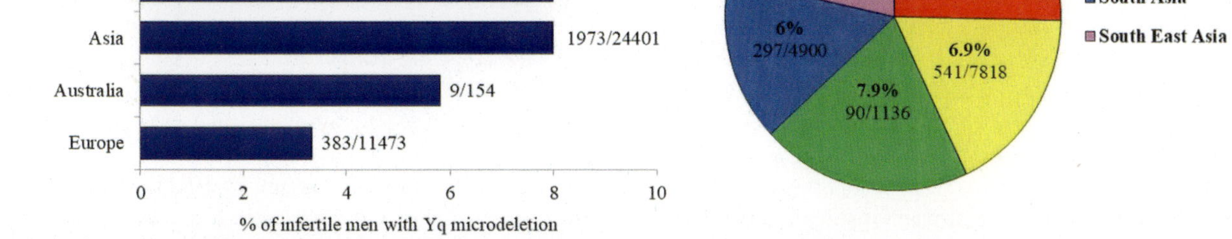

Fig. 5 Prevalence of Yq microdeletions in infertile men. The average prevalence of the Yq microdeletions in different continents of the world was estimated from published data of 40,127 Y chromosomes from infertile men. Infertile men could be oligozoospermic or azoospermic men. Pie chart gives distribution of Yq microdeletions in the Asian region. The numbers were estimated from the data of Asian men based on geographical. In both the cases, only those articles published in English were considered and total number of infertile men studied and those having deletions were recorded along with the country. Data from different studies from same continent were pooled and the average estimated (for details see Additional file 1: Table S1)

in some populations but not the others [159, 164–166]. It is suggested that since the unusual combination of deletions are detected only by isolated markers and not confirmed by additional analyses these are perhaps methodological artefacts [158]. Nevertheless, it is important to note here that these deletions recurred in various populations and were detected using a variety of STS markers exclusively in infertile men; hence these deletion patterns should not be disregarded. Additional data will be needed to understand the molecular basis of such deletions.

Phenotypic manifestations of Yq microdeletions

AZF deletions are specific to infertile men and hence it is appropriate to consider Y deletions as a cause of oligo/azoospermia rather than a cause of 'infertility'. Overall, 25–55% of males with extreme testicular pathologies such as hypospermatogenesis, sperm maturation arrest and SCOS and 5–25% males with severe oligozoospermia or azoospermia harbour Y chromosome microdeletions [167]. However, depending on the AZF locus deleted the phenotypic manifestations reportedly vary.

AZFa deletions

In general, deletions of the entire AZFa region invariably result in Sertoli cell only syndrome (SCOS) and azoospermia [58, 168–172]. Since genes within the AZFa locus are expressed in the germ cells prenatally, it is possible that the loss of these genes could lead to germ cell death developmentally leading to SCOS [72]. The partial AZFa deletions are however associated with phenotypes ranging from azoospermia to normozoospermia [173] indicating that the amount of genetic content lost is a critical determinant of azoospermia due to AZFa deletions. Hence the diagnosis of a complete deletion of the AZFa region implies the virtual impossibility to retrieve testicular spermatozoa for intracytoplasmic sperm injection (ICSI).

AZFb deletions

The genes in the AZFb locus support the growth and maturity of sperm and are considered critical for efficient progression of sperm through meiosis into spermiogenesis. Not unexpectedly, patients with deletions of the AZFb region have a testicular phonotype of maturation arrest, frequently at the spermatocyte stage with an absence of post-meiotic germ cells in the majority of the tubules [6, 86, 174]. A clear correlation between the extent of the AZFb deletion and testicular histological findings is observed. Hypospermatogenesis is frequently observed among partial AZFb/b + c deleted specimens, but more severe findings are observed in complete AZFb and AZFb+c deleted specimens indicating that the AZFb deletions do not confer a severe phenotype but cause a block in spermatogenesis. The maturation arrest phenotype associated to AZFb deletions most probably stems from a combination of genetic disruption with structural defects in the chromosome [175].

It is generally accepted that the chance to retrieve mature sperm cells either from the ejaculate or via testicular sperm extraction is negligible in cases with AZFb deletion [175–177] although sperm have been retrieved from testis of men harbouring AZFb deletions [178–182]. While these differences could reflect the heterogeneity in extent of deletion in different patients; the likelihood of finding sperm cells in males with complete versus partial AZFb deletions is significantly lower [175].

AZFc deletions

Men with AZFc deletions by far have the most variable phenotype ranging from complete azoospermia to mild oligozoospermia [126]. In general, the testis of men with AZFc deletions will have elongating spermatids and sperm can be retrieved in a reasonable numbers of AZFc deleted infertile males [166, 170]. In most men with AZFc deletion, spermatogenesis is completed, but on a reduced scale resulting in oligozoospermia [171].

By semen analysis, complete AZFc deletions are associated with drastic reduction in sperm count and most AZFc deleted males are severely oligozoospermic [158, 159, 171] however some may even be azoospermic [158, 159]. There also exist rare AZFc deleted males who have conceived multiple children naturally but all of the sons of these males have been found to be infertile [151, 161, 162].

While the AZFc deletions by themselves are less pathogenic, in prospective follow up case studies, it is observed that that in a subset of men with AZFc microdeletions there is progressive decline in sperm count and the patient progresses from oligozoospermia to its severe form or even become azoospermia [183–185]. This implies a temporally deteriorating effect of AZFc deletions on spermatogenesis leading to worsening in sperm numbers and quality. Thus although men with AZFc deletion may have sperm in the ejaculate, they must be offered semen cryopreservation to prevent invasive techniques like TESA in later stages of life for sperm retrieval.

Partial AZFc deletions

The AZFc region is comprised of repeated sequences and palindromes hence making it most vulnerable to deletions. A complete deletion of AZFc involves the b2/b4 region which contains 12 genes and transcriptional units in multiple copy numbers (Fig. 2). In addition to b2/b4, the AZFc locus has many partial deletions that include b1/b3 (1.6 Mb), b2/b3 (1.8 Mb) and gr/gr (1.6 Mb) [186]. These deletions remove unique portions of the AZFc; however the genes removed are almost similar (Fig. 2). Three types of gr/gr deletions are reported that are caused by homologous recombination flanking the g1/g2, r1/r3 and r2/r4 amplicons in P1 and P2 palindromes in the AZFc (Fig. 2). However all the three are referred to as gr/gr and not classified further during analysis.

None of the partial deletions completely eliminate any gene family, but reduces the copy number of gene families with the exception of b1/b3 deletion that results in the loss of the six copies of *RBMY1* and both functional copies of PRY (Fig. 2). The gr/gr deletion results in loss of two of the four *DAZ* gene copies, one of the two *CDY1* and *BPY2* gene copies along with one of three copies of *BPY2* and two of the four *DAZ* genes. The b2/b3 deletion is derived from a gr/gr or b2/b3 inversion and removes almost the same gene content as gr/gr (Fig. 2).

Prevalence of partial AZFc deletions and male infertility

The AZFc is of particular interest to both geneticist and a reproductive biologist as it harbours multicopy genes and provides an opportunity to study gene dosage effects in regulation of spermatogenesis. It is believed that the partial deletions lead to extensive copy number variations in the AZFc which might compromise the amounts of the protein produced thereby affecting spermatogenesis. This has formed the basis for analysis of the partial AZFc deletions in clinical evaluation of an infertile male. The ease of a well-designed PCR strategy has further fuelled this practice in various clinics and laboratories globally.

Since their first description, a wealth of information regarding partial AZFc deletions has accumulated in the past 15 years and it is clear that the association of partial AZFc deletions and male infertility is not as lucid as in the case of complete AZF deletions. This is because 1) there is wide heterogeneity in the types of partial AZFc deletions and 2) fertile and normozoospermic men harbour the AZFc partial deletions. Thus doubts have been cast on the involvement of AZFc partial deletions and male infertility. Three well designed meta-analysis and one study of > 20,000 Y chromosomes are published in recent times that have analysed the association of partial AZFc deletions and male infertility [126, 167, 187, 188]. Described below is the picture that has emerged out of these studies with large sample sizes.

Several controversies exist about the association of gr/gr deletion with male infertility. Early on it was reported that the gr/gr deletion was present in 3.8% of infertile males and 2.2% of fertile males (of unknown sperm counts) but absent in normozoospermic males [186] suggesting that the gr/gr deletion was associated with decreased sperm production resulting from the reduced dose of AZFc genes. However subsequent studies in many populations have yielded controversial findings where gr/gr deletions have been identified even in fertile males with normal sperm counts (see [167, 187]). While some studies have suggested that frequency of gr/gr deletion is significantly higher in infertile men as compared to fertile/normozoospermic controls; others have reported no such association. In two meta-analysis studies [167, 187] a significant association of gr/gr deletions and male infertility has however been observed. We analysed the available data [167] and observed that of the of the 10,978 Y chromosomes analysed from infertile men and 6704 from fertile/normozoospermic controls, twice the number of infertile men had gr/gr deletions as compared to controls (Fig. 6); with an OR of 1.8. Interestingly, the gr/gr deletions are common in African and Asian men (10–15%), they occur at a frequency of less than 5% in other population (Fig. 6). Furthermore, the association of gr/gr deletion with male infertility is observed in Australian, Asian and European and Australian men; the association is weak or negligible in American men and African men. The association of gr/gr deletion and male infertility is also ethnicity dependent [167, 187]. Amongst the different races, the association of gr/gr deletions and male infertility is strongest in Caucasian men and weaker in Mongolian men, but no association is observed in Dravidian and Nigro-Caucasian lineages (Fig. 6). Why the prevalence of gr/gr deletions and it association to male infertility differ with populations (geographically and ethnicity) is a matter of debate. It is suggested that such differences in susceptibility gr/gr deletions to male infertility is dependent on the Y chromosome background mainly the haplogroups [6]. A second school of thought is the high heterogeneity in the gene copy deletions in men with gr/gr deletions. It is shown that not all men with gr/gr deletions have identical amounts of DNA lost. Based on copy number estimates of *DAZ* and *CDY1* genes, it is observed that only those men with two *DAZ* and one *CDY1* copy deleted will have azoospermia or oligozoospermia, retention of any one of these genes will be almost always be associated with normozoospermia [139, 140, 143, 145, 149]. Along with *DAZ* and *CDY1*, studies have also identified *GOLGA2LY* and *BPY2* copy numbers have a protective effect on fertility of men with gr/gr deletions [138, 143, 157]. Thus it appears that the gene content and the gene dosage effect in the AZFc locus is a determinant of fertility in men harbouring gr/gr deletions.

Nevertheless, irrespective of the population, in individual studies as well as pooled estimates men with gr/gr deletions have significantly lower sperm counts and motility as compared to non-deleted controls [126, 167, 187] indicating that the gr/gr deletion might not be a direct cause of infertility, but does compromise process of spermatogenesis leading to lower sperm counts.

b2/b3 deletion

As compared to the gr/gr, the b2/b3 is a slightly a larger deletion (1.6 Mb versus 1.8 Mb) and derived as an inversion (Fig. 2). Unlike the gr/gr, the correlation of b2/b3

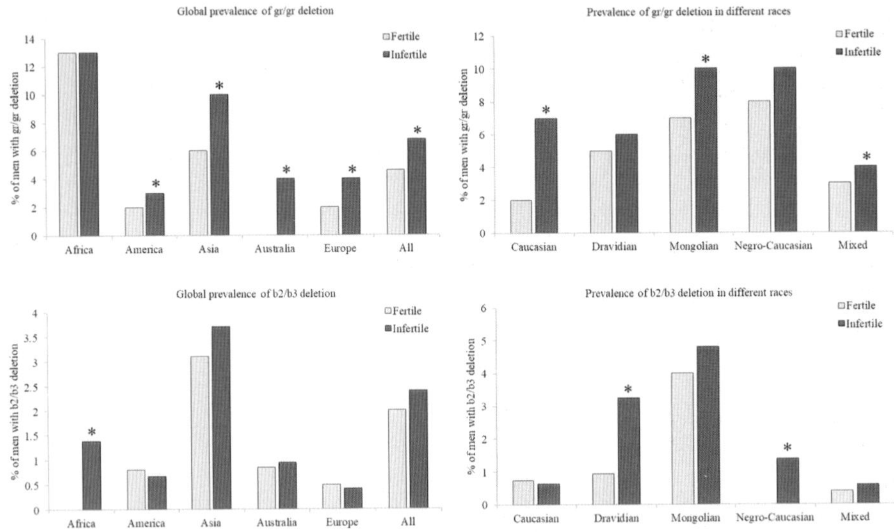

Fig. 6 Association of gr/gr and b2/b3 deletions with male infertility. Data was obtained from previous studies [105, 126, 167, 188]. Data for gr/gr is derived out of 10,978 and 6704 Y chromosomes from infertile and fertile men respectively. For b2/b3 the data is derived out of 9981 and 5990 Y chromosomes from fertile and infertile men respectively. Infertile men could be oligozoospermic or azoospermic men. Fertile men would be normozoospermic/proven fertile men with unknown sperm counts. Data was divided based on continents or by race. * indicates value significantly different form fertile counterpart

partial deletions with spermatogenic failure is uncertain. Analysis of 17,784 Y chromosomes from infertile men and 11,684 Y chromosomes from fertile/normozoospermic men [188], showed a poor (but statistically significant) correlation of b2/b3 deletion and male infertility (Fig. 6). Like in case of gr/gr, the prevalence and association of male infertility and b2/b3 deletion differs geographically and is based on the ethnicity of the study population. Irrespective of the fertility status, the prevalence of b2/b3 deletion is highest amongst Asians (~ 3%) and lowest in Europeans (~ 0.5%) and in both these cases there is no significant difference in its frequency in fertile and infertile men; no association of b2/b3 deletions with male infertility has been noted in Australian men (Fig. 6). Intriguingly, while gr/gr deletions is not significantly associated with male infertility in African men, the prevalence of b2/b3 deletion is higher in infertile men of African origin as compared to its normozoospermic/fertile counter parts (1.17 vs. 0.25) and this difference is significant (Fig. 6). A similar association is observed in Chilean men where b2/b3 deletions are exclusively reported in infertile men. However, the b2/b3 deletion does not seem to be associated with male infertility in American men [126].

Like, the gr/gr, the association of b2/b3 deletions and male infertility also seems to be ethnicity dependent. The b2/b3 deletion is strongly association with male infertility in Dravidian and Negro-Caucasian men, weekly in Mongolian men but not in Caucasian men (Fig. 6). This pattern seems to be complementary to gr/gr deletions. The gr/gr but not b2/b3 deletion is strongly associated with male infertility in Caucasian men, the b2/b3 but not gr/gr is associated with male infertility in Dravidian and Negro-Caucasian men. In the Mongolian population both deletion carry a risk of infertility albeit weakly (Fig. 6). These observations are interesting and suggest that irrespective of the type of deletion and the population, the loss of gene copies in AZFc increases the susceptibility of an individual to reduction in sperm count. However, why one kind of deletion is pathogenic in one population but not the other needs further investigation.

b1/b3 deletion

The b1/b3 deletion differs from the gr/gr and b2/b3 deletions because this deletion encompasses the part of AZFb and results in loss of the six copies of RBMY1 and both the copies of PRY (Fig. 6). Very few studies have reported association of b1/b3 deletion and male infertility. In an analysis of 20,000 Y chromosomes [126], the b1/b3 deletion is estimated to occur in one of every 994 men but this deletion increases the risk of spermatogenetic failure (OR 2.5). However, this deletion is very infrequent in most population and hence its association with male infertility is not known in most populations.

Copy Number Variation in Y chromosome and male infertility

A Copy Number Variation [CNV] is defined as a DNA segment longer than 1 kb with a variable copy number of genes in comparison with a reference genome [189]. CNVs produce phenotype via diverse mechanisms, including gene dosage, presence of an interrupting gene, creating a fusion gene, unmasking of recessive coding region, mutation or other functional SNPs and position effect. All the different AZF microdeletions can be considered as large CNVs because they modify the copy number of genes on the Y chromosome. Further, the unstable AZFc region is predisposed to undergo several types of rearrangements resulting in changes in the cumulative copy number of the gene families contained within it. These complete or partial AZF deletions leading to CNVs of genes within it compromise spermatogenesis [138, 140, 143, 157, 190]. In addition to these AZF loci, CNVs across the entire length of the Y chromosome have been investigated in male infertility [125, 191–193]. In a CNV analysis of the MSY in healthy males, large duplications encompassing the *AMELY* and *TBL1Y* genes, partial deletions of the *TSPY* cluster, a variation in the number of *RBMY* genes and duplication of two segments overlapping the AZFa region have been reported [194] indicating that the Y chromosome is highly polymorphic in terms of its genetic content in general population. To understand the association of gene CNVs and male infertility, 68 well-defined histopathologically confirmed cases of males with idiopathic testicular maturation arrest were analysed by SNP arrays [103]. The results revealed PAR 1 and PAR 2 CNVs in 5 cases, PAR 3 CNVs in 19 cases and *TSPY2* gene gain in 16 cases. Men with normal spermatogenesis have not been investigated in this study; it is difficult to ascertain the significance of these CNVs. However, the discovery of PAR CNVs is biologically significant as X and Y chromosome pairing is made possible by the PARs and aberrations in chromosome structure at the PARs due to these CNVs would logically disrupt meiotic synapsis resulting in gametogenic failure and can be one of the aetiological factors underlying maturation arrest. In addition, the PAR regions are rich in genes that escape X inactivation to maintain dosage compensation (Fig. 1) it is plausible that these CNVs (deletions or duplications) of PARs may result in under- or over-expression of these genes resulting in a pathological phenotype. However, with the exception of genes in AZFc, no direct studies have been done comparing the CNVs with gene expression and spermatogenesis arrest.

Clinical significance of genetic testing of Y chromosome and male infertility

Although there is universal agreement on the need for chromosome analysis by karyotyping in the workup of male infertility, there is still a lack of consensus regarding the clinical utility of testing for Y chromosome microdeletions in azoospermic and oligozoospermic males. While the American Society of Reproductive Medicine recommends the use of both, karyotyping and Y chromosome microdeletion studies, in males preparing to undergo Intracytoplasmic Sperm Injection [ICSI], the National Institute for Health and Care Excellence recommends only karyotyping for this group of patients [4]. In which patients molecular screening of the Y chromosome should be performed remains a dilemma. Based on data of several thousands of patients, Yq microdeletions are found in a high proportion of patients with azoospermia or severe oligozoospermia; the occurrence of deletion in infertile patients with sperm concentration $> 5 \times 10^6$/mL is usually less [195]. However there are population specific differences [159] and in this scenario country specific guidelines are necessary. While analysis of Yq microdeletions is not indicated in patients with chromosomal abnormalities, obstructive azoospermia or hypogonadotropic hypogonadism, there are a number of examples of deletion carriers among non-idiopathic infertile men including Klinefelter syndrome and varicocele [159]. Therefore, the presence of any diagnosis accompanied by azoo- or severe oligozoospermia should be an indication for AZF testing. We recommend Yq microdeletion testing in routine clinical practice for the following reasons

1. Identifying the cause of infertility: The Y chromosome contains several genes required for spermatogenesis and loss of one or more of such genes can cause impairment of this process. By investigating the presence of Y chromosome microdeletions it is possible to determine the underlying genetic aetiology of male factor infertility and implement appropriate screening strategies for abnormal phenotypes. Knowledge regarding these deletions will also help clinicians to provide more effective solutions to problems faced by infertile couples. For example, low sperm count and motility can be treated with hormones, anti-oxidants and lifestyle changes to improve the seminogram. However, these strategies of treatment will fail if the cause of infertility is genetic. Also AZF screening is important before varicocoelectomy because deletion carriers will most likely not benefit from the surgical procedure. Therefore, if the male partner is detected with a deletion the couple can directly be offered assisted reproductive techniques [ART] and not subjected to medical treatments to improve sperm count and motility.
2. Predicting the prognosis of infertile males: While there exist numerous cases reports of AZFc deleted men can father a child, it is clinically observed that individuals harbouring Y chromosome microdeletions have progressive decline in sperm counts and can progress to azoospermia over time (discussed above). Thus males with mild or moderate oligozoospermia and Yq microdeletions would require a multiple followed-up for their possible progression to azoospermia. Thus the

knowledge of the Yq status would aid in counselling these men and provide them an option of sperm cryopreservation for biological parenthood in future.

3. Predicting outcome of testicular sperm aspiration [TESA]: Most males with Y chromosome microdeletions would be infertile and have absence of or very few sperms in ejaculate. To achieve pregnancy, sperm can be retrieved directly from the testes using techniques like testicular sperm extraction [TESE] or testicular sperm aspiration [TESA]. The occurrence and type of Yq microdeletion has been found to correlate with testicular phenotype and chance of sperm retrieval. Hence, screening for Y chromosome microdeletions can aid to predict the success of obtaining biological parenthood before undertaking invasive procedures.
4. Predicting the success of ART: Most men with Yq microdeletions would require ART for biological parenthood. Although yet controversial, Studies have reported slower fertilization rate, poor embryo quality, impaired blastocyst rate and lower overall success of ART in men with AZF deletions [140, 157, 166, 195]. Hence, Yq microdeletion screening would also help in counselling couples regarding the probability of success rates after taking up ART to aid the couple in a rational decision making.
5. Prevention of vertical transmission of the genetic defects: With the advent of ICSI, several live births are reported in couples where the male partner has a Yq microdeletion. However, in all these cases, the Yq microdeletion is passed down to the male offspring who are also infertile, thus resulting in a 100% transmission of the genetic defect and infertility from the fathers. In some instances the partial AZFc deletion in the father has resulted in full deletion in the offspring [196] which is a definite case of spermatogenic failure. Thus Y chromosome microdeletion testing is highly recommended for all infertile males who opt for ICSI so that the couple can make an informed choice of having biological parenthood at the risk of perpetuating infertility in the family.
6. Risk of testicular cancers: The Y chromosome has long been a suspect candidate for gonadal cancers. In individuals with gonadal dysgenesis that bear a full or even partial fragments of Y chromosome (even in a few of the cells) have a high risk of developing gonadal tumours specifically gonadoblastoma [197–200]. In addition the Yq microdeletions and/or its CNVs are suggested to be a risk factor for the development of testicular cancer [201]. While these are limited observational studies, results of large case control studies are yet awaited. It is becoming increasingly apparent that beyond infertility, the knowledge of Yq microdeletions should also aid in predicting occurrence of cancers in men.
7. Neuropsychiatric disorders and Yq microdeletions: While Yq microdeletions are strongly associated with infertility, reports are now emerging that atleast a subset of men with Y chromosome defects have higher prevalence of mental disorders. In a recent analysis of 42 Chilean patients diagnosed with Yq microdeletions a significantly higher proportion of abnormal height was seen amongst patients with terminal AZFb+c deletions compared with infertile cases without microdeletions. Intriguingly, 5/42 men (11%) had some forms of neuropsychiatric disorders including two with bipolar disorder and three with severe clinical depression. Clinical histories also documented language delay, attention-deficit hyperactivity disorder (ADHD) and emotional and behavioural problems including anxiety and social disabilities in this cohort [202]. However none of the infertile patients with non-terminal Yq microdeletions had any medical history of neuropsychiatric abnormalities [202]. While further long term clinical follow-up data of men with Yq microdeletions is required; these preliminary observations do indicate the occurrence of other health risks beyond infertility in such men and this warrants testing of Y chromosome genetics in a clinical situation.

Conclusion and future directions

Male infertility is a complex multifactorial condition that presents with highly heterogeneous phenotypes. The Y chromosome plays a central role in regulation of spermatogenesis as it harbours Y-linked genes that are expressed in the testis and involved in various processes during spermatogenesis. The importance of these genes is evident from the observations that the removal of these genes causes distinct pathological testis phenotypes. After 20 years from the first molecular definition of the AZF, Yq deletion screening has now become a routine test for infertile males in many countries to identify the cause of male infertility. With clear-cut cause–effect relationship with severely impaired spermatogenesis, this test is now of help in even determining the success rates of sperm retrieval and prediction of success of assisted reproduction. Further as the deletion has 100% transmission rate to male offspring's, the couple needs to be aware that the males in the future generation will also be infertile. Further as the gr/gr deletions are known to undergo expansion leading to full deletions [138, 196] the couple should be aware that besides the obligatory transmission of a genetic risk factor for impaired sperm production (gr/gr deletion) to the male offspring, there is a higher risk for the transmission of a complete AZFc deletion, which is a causative factor for spermatogenic failure.

Beyond these immediate applications, there are some clinically relevant issues associated with Yq deletions that need urgent attention. Presently, there is no long term follow-up data of men harbouring Yq microdeletions and there is an urgent need for data on the health status of children born from AZF deletion carriers. It is especially relevant in two conditions 1) Increased risk of testicular cancers 2) Possible occurrence of neurological dysfunctions. Due to the instable nature of the deleted Y chromosome, there is an increased risk of the expansion of deletions which might be a viewed as a "genomic instability". Such progressive loss of genetic material during spermatogenesis might lead to sex chromosome mosaicism in germ cells which might predispose them to testicular/germ cell tumours. However, little data exist on the incidence of testicular tumours in men with Yq microdeletions especially in second generation males born to fathers carrying the deletion. Secondly, recent reports have demonstrated a significantly higher deletion load not only on the sex chromosome but also on autosomes of infertile men ([203, 204]) indicate more widespread effects of such deletions on genomic stability. Coupled with the fact that many Y linked genes are also expressed in multiple tissues; how genomic instability and disturbances in gene expression owing to Yq deletions affect general physiological functions has not been investigated the long term implications of such effects are obscure. With the recent data on higher prevalence of neurological problems in infertile men with Yq deletions it is imperative that we carry out detailed analysis of men with Yq deletions with an outlook beyond infertility. We hope that careful clinical observations coupled with detailed genetic information will provide important insights into these unanswered basic questions and give a different perspective to the field of androgenetics.

Abbreviations

ADHD: Attention-deficit hyperactivity disorder; Alu: *Arthrobacter luteus*; *AMELX*: Amelogenin, X-Linked; *AMELY*: Amelogenin, Y-Linked; AZF: Azoospermia factor; *BPY2*: Basic Charge, Y-Linked, 2; *CDY*: Chromodomain Protein, Y linked; CNV: Copy number variations; *CSPG4P1Y*: Chondroitin Sulfate Proteoglycan 4 Pseudogene 1, Y-Linked; *CXorf15*: Chromosome X Open Reading Frame 15; *CYorf15*: Chromosome Y Open Reading Frame 15; *DAZ*: Deleted in Azoospermia; *DAZL*: Deleted in Azoospermia like; dbSNP: The Single Nucleotide Polymorphism database; *DBY*: DEAD [asp-glu-ala-asp] box RNA helicases, Box 3, Y-linked; *DDX3Y*:-DEAD-Box Helicase 3, Y-Linked; *DFFRY*: Drosophila fat facets related Y; DNA: Deoxyribonucleic acid; DSB: Double stranded break; DYZ1: DNA Y chromosome Z [number of repetitive segments at one site] 1; *EIF1AY*: Eukaryotic Translation Initiation Factor 1A, Y linked; *FAM41AY2*: Family With Sequence Similarity 41 Member A, Y-Linked 2; *GOLGA2P2Y*: Golgi autoantigen, golgi subfamily a, 2-like, Y-linked; GSK3β -WNT: Glycogen synthase kinase 3 – wingless integrated pathway; HCC: Hepatocellular carcinoma; HLA: Human leukocyte antigen; HSFY: Heat Shock transcription factor, Y linked; *HSPRY3*: *Homo Sapiens* Sprouty homolog 3; *HY*: Histocompatibility Y Antigen; *HYA*: Histocompatibility Y Antigen; ICSI: Intracytoplasmic sperm injection; *JARID1D*: Jumonji At-Rich Interactive Domain 1D; KDa: kiloDalton; *KDM5D*: Lysine Demethylase 5D; Mb: Mega base pairs; MSH5: MutS protein homolog 5; MSY: Male specific region; NAHR: Non-allelic homologous recombination; *NCRNA00185*: Non-protein coding RNA 185; *NCRNA00230B*: Non-Protein Coding RNA 230B; NOA: Non obstructive azoospermia; NRY: Non-recombining region; OA: Obstructive azoospermia; PAR 2: Pseudoautosomal regions 2; PAR: Pseudoautosomal regions; PAR1: Pseudoautosomal regions 1; *PCDH11Y*: Protocadherin 11, Y linked; PRM: Protamine; *PRY*: PTPN13-like Y linked, [PTPBL]-Related gene on Y; *RBMY*: Ribonucleic Acid -Binding Motif, Y linked; *RPS4Y1*: Ribosomal protein S4, Y linked; RRM: RNA recognition motif; SCOS: Sertoli Cell Only syndrome; *SHOX*: Stature homeobox; *SMCY*: Selected cDNA on Y, Mouse, homolog of; *SOX3*: *Sry Box 3*; SPO11α: Sporulation 11; *SRY*: Sex determining region on Y; *SYBL1*: *Synaptobrevin like 1*; *TB4Y*: Thymosin beta 4 Y linked; *TBL1Y*: Transducin Beta-like 1Y; *TBLR1*: Transducin Beta-like 1 K linked receptor; TESA: Testicular sperm aspiration; TESE: Testicular sperm extraction; TNP: Transition Nuclear Protein; TPR: Tetratricopeptide repeat; *TSPY*: Testis-specific protein Y-linked; *TTTY*: Testis-Specific Transcript, Y-Linked; *USP9Y*: Ubiquitin specific peptidase 9, Y linked; UTR: Untranslated region; *UTY*: Ubiquitously transcribed tetratricopeptide repeat containing, Y linked; WHO: World Health Organisation; *XKRY*: X linked Kell Blood group precursor, Y linked; *ZFY*: Zinc Finger protein, Y linked

Acknowledgements

We thank Mr. Anshul Bhide (project JRF, NIRRH) for help in preparing the figures. The manuscript bears the NIRRH ID: IR/569/11-2017. DM lab is supported by grants from the Indian Council of Medical Research, Department of Science and Technology, Department of Biotechnology, Government of India. SC is a recipient of the ICMR postdoctoral grant.

Funding

Indian Council of Medical Research [ICMR] and the ICMR-Post Doctoral Program.

Authors' contributions

DM contributed towards the design and structure of the manuscript, performed the analysis and designed the figures. SC collected and analyzed the data. Both authors wrote the manuscript and approve the final manuscript.

Authors' information

DM is scientist E and Head of Molecular Biology, Indian Council of Medical Research, National Institute for Research in Reproductive Health, Mumbai, India. SC is a post-doctoral fellow, Indian Council of Medical Research, National Institute for Research in Reproductive Health, Mumbai, India.

Competing interests

The authors declare that they have no competing interests.

References

1. WHO. Laboratory manual for the examination and processing of human semen. 5th ed. Geneva: World Health Organization; 2010.
2. Agarwal A, Mulgund A, Hamada A, Chyatte MR. A unique view on male infertility around the globe. Reprod Biol Endocrinol. 2015;13:37–46.
3. Hotaling J, Carrell DT. Clinical genetic testing for male factor infertility: current applications and future directions. Andrology. 2014;2:339–50.
4. Colaco S, Lakdawala A, Modi D. Role of Y chromosome microdeletions in the clinical evaluation of infertile males. MGM J Med Sci. 2017;4:79–88.
5. Hughes JF, Page DC. The biology and evolution of mammalian Y chromosomes. Annu Rev Genet. 2015;49:507–27.
6. Navarro-Costa P, Gonçalves J, Plancha CE. The AZFc region of the Y chromosome: at the crossroads between genetic diversity and male infertility. Hum Reprod Update. 2010;18:525–42.
7. Bellott DW, Hughes JF, Skaletsky H, Brown LG, Pyntikova T, Cho TJ, Koutseva N, Zaghlul S, Graves T, Rock S, Kremitzki C. Mammalian Y chromosomes retain widely expressed dosage-sensitive regulators. Nature. 2014;508:494–9.
8. Kauppi L, Barchi M, Baudat F, Romanienko PJ, Keeney S, Jasin M. Distinct properties of the XY pseudoautosomal region crucial for male meiosis. Science. 2011;331:916–20.
9. Page DC, Mosher R, Simpson EM, Fisher EM, Mardon G, Pollack J, McGillivray B, de la Chapelle A, Brown LG. The sex-determining region of the human Y chromosome encodes a finger protein. Cell. 1987;51:1091–104.
10. Barchi M, Roig I, Di Giacomo M, de Rooij DG, Keeney S, Jasin M. ATM promotes the obligate XY crossover and both crossover control and chromosome axis integrity on autosomes. PLoS Genet. 2008;4:e1000076.
11. Hinch AG, Altemose N, Noor N, Donnelly P, Myers SR. Recombination in the human pseudoautosomal region PAR1. PLoS Genet. 2014;10:e1004503.
12. Mohandas TK, Speed RM, Passage MB, Yen PH, Chandley AC, et al. Role of the pseudoautosomal region in sex-chromosome pairing during male meiosis: meiotic studies in a man with a deletion of distal Xp. Am J Hum Genet. 1992;51:526–33.
13. Gabriel-Robez O, Rumpler Y, Ratomponirina C, Petit C, Levilliers J, Croquette MF, Couturier J. Deletion of the pseudoautosomal region and lack of sex-chromosome pairing at pachytene in two infertile men carrying an X; Y translocation. Cytogenet Cell Genet. 1990;54:38–42.
14. Shi Q, Martin RH. Aneuploidy in human spermatozoa: FISH analysis in men with constitutional chromosomal abnormalities, and in infertile men. Reproduction. 2001;121:655–66.
15. Hassold TJ, Sherman SL, Pettay D, Page DC, Jacobs PA. XY chromosome nondisjunction in man is associated with diminished recombination in the pseudoautosomal region. Am J Hum Genet. 1991;49:253–60.
16. Ross MT, Grafham DV, Coffey AJ, Scherer S, McLay K, et al. The DNA sequence of the human X chromosome. Nature. 2005;434:325–37.
17. Ellison JW, Wardak Z, Young MF, GehronRobey P, Laig-Webster M, Chiong W. PHOG, a candidate gene for involvement in the short stature of turner syndrome. Hum Mol Genet. 1997;6:1341–7.
18. Rao E, Weiss B, Fukami M, Rump A, Niesler B, Mertz A, Muroya K, Binder G, Kirsch S, Winkelmann M, Nordsiek G, Heinrich U, Breuning MH, Ranke MB, Rosenthal A, Ogata T, Rappold GA. Pseudoautosomal deletions encompassing a novel homeobox gene cause growth failure in idiopathic short stature and turner syndrome. Nat Genet. 1997;16:54–63.
19. Lencz T, Morgan TV, Athanasiou M, Dain B, Reed CR, et al. Converging evidence for a pseudoautosomal cytokine receptor gene locus in schizophrenia. Mol Psychiatry. 2007;12:572–80.
20. Flaquer A, Jamra RA, Etterer K, Di'az GO, Rivas F, et al. A new susceptibility locus for bipolar affective disorder in PAR1 on Xp22.3/Yp11.3. Am J Med Genet. 2010;153B:1110–4.
21. Mangs Helena A, Morris BJ. The human pseudoautosomal region (PAR): origin, function and future. Curr Genomics. 2007;8:129–36.
22. Charchar FJ, Svartman M, El-Mogharbel N, Ventura M, Kirby P, Matarazzo MR, Ciccodicola A, Rocchi M, D'Esposito M, Graves JA. Complex events in the evolution of the human pseudoautosomal region 2 (PAR2). Genome Res. 2003;13:281–6.
23. Lopes AM, Ross N, Close J, Dagnall A, Amorim A, Crow TJ. Inactivation status of PCDH11X: sexual dimorphisms in gene expression levels in brain. Hum Genet. 2006;119:267–75.
24. Veerappa AM, Padakannaya P, Ramachandra NB. Copy number variation-based polymorphism in a new pseudoautosomal region 3 (PAR3) of a human X-chromosome-transposed region (XTR) in the Y chromosome. Funct Integr Genomics. 2013;13:285–93.
25. Manz E, Alkan M, Bühler E, Schmidtke J. Arrangement of DYZ1 and DYZ2 repeats on the human Y-chromosome: a case with presence of DYZ1 and absence of DYZ2. Mol Cell Probes. 1992;6:257–9.
26. Cotter PD, Norton ME. Y chromosome heterochromatin variation detected at prenatal diagnosis. Prenat Diagn. 2005;25:1062–3.
27. Skaletsky H, Kuroda-Kawaguchi T, Minx PJ, Cordum HS, Hillier L, Brown LG, Repping S, Pyntikova T, Ali J, Bieri T, et al. The male-specific region of the human Y chromosome is a mosaic of discrete sequence classes. Nature. 2003;423:825–37.
28. Maan AA, Eales J, Akbarov A, Rowland J, Xu X, Jobling MA, Charchar FJ, Tomaszewski M. The Y chromosome: a blueprint for men's health? Eur J Hum Genet. 2017;25:1181–8.
29. Meyfour A, Pooyan P, Pahlavan S, Rezaei-Tavirani M, Gourabi H, Baharvand H, Salekdeh GH. Chromosome-centric human proteome project allies with developmental biology: a case study of the role of Y chromosome genes in organ development. J Prot Res. 2017; https://doi.org/10.1021/acs.jproteome.7b00446.
30. Rengaraj D, Kwon WS, Pang MG. Bioinformatics annotation of human Y chromosome-encoded protein pathways and interactions. J Prot Res. 2015; 14:3503–18.
31. Jacobs PA, Strongs JA. A case of human intersexuality having a possible XXY sex determining mechanism. Nature. 1959;183:302–3.
32. Ford CE, Jones KW, Polani PE, De Almeida JC, Briggs JH. A sex-chromosome anomaly in a case of gonadal dysgenesis (Turner's syndrome). Lancet. 1959; 1:711–3.
33. Koopman P, Sinclair A, Lovell-Badge R. Of sex and determination: marking 25 years of Randy, the sex-reversed mouse. Development. 2016;143:1633–7.
34. Sinclair AH, Berta P, Palmer MS, Hawkins JR, Griffiths BL, Smith MJ, Foster JW, Frischauf AM, Lovell-Badge R, Goodfellow PN. A gene from the human sex-determining region encodes a protein with homology to a conserved DNA-binding motif. Nature. 1990;346:240–4.
35. She ZY, Yang WX. Sry and SoxE genes: how they participate in mammalian sex determination and gonadal development? Semin Cell Dev Biol. 2017;63:13–22.
36. Quinn A, Koopman P. The molecular genetics of sex determination and sex reversal in mammals. Semin Reprod Med. 2012;30:351–63.
37. Modi D, Shah C, Sachdeva G, Gadkar S, Bhartiya D, Puri C. Ontogeny and cellular localization of SRY transcripts in the human testes and its detection in spermatozoa. Reproduction. 2005;130:603–13.
38. Decarpentrie F, Vernet N, Mahadevaiah SK, Longepied G, Streichemberger E, Aknin-Seifer I, Ojarikre OA, Burgoyne PS, Metzler-Guillemain C, Mitchell MJ. Human and mouse ZFY genes produce a conserved testis-specific transcript encoding a zinc finger protein with a short acidic domain and modified transactivation potential. Hum Mol Genet. 2012;21:2631–45.
39. Yamauchi Y, Riel JM, Ruthig V, Ward MA. Mouse Y-encoded transcription factor Zfy2 is essential for sperm formation and function in assisted fertilization. PLoS Genet. 2015;11:e1005476.
40. Vernet N, Mahadevaiah SK, Yamauchi Y, Decarpentrie F, Mitchell MJ, et al. Mouse Y-linked Zfy1 and Zfy2 are expressed during the male-specific interphase between meiosis I and meiosis II and promote the 2nd meiotic division. PLoS Genet. 2014;10:e1004444.
41. Vernet N, Mahadevaiah SK, Decarpentrie F, Longepied G, de Rooij DG, et al. Mouse Y-encoded transcription factor Zfy2 is essential for sperm head Remodelling and sperm tail development. PLoS One. 2016;11:e0145398.
42. Nakasuji T, Ogonuki N, Chiba T, Kato T, Shiozawa K, Yamatoya K, Tanaka H, Kondo T, Miyado K, Miyasaka N, Kubota T, Ogura A, Asahara H. Complementary critical functions of Zfy1 and Zfy2 in mouse spermatogenesis and reproduction. PLoS Genet. 2017;13:e1006578.

43. Müller U, Kirkels VG, Scheres JM. Absence of turner stigmata in a 46, XYp-female. Hum Genet. 1992;90:239–42.
44. Jobling MA, Lo IC, Turner DJ, Bowden GR, Lee AC, Xue Y, Carvalho-Silva D, Hurles ME, Adams SM, Chang YM, Kraaijenbrink T. Structural variation on the short arm of the human Y chromosome: recurrent multigene deletions encompassing Amelogenin Y. Hum Mol Genet. 2006;16:307–16.
45. Meyfour A, Ansari H, Pahlavan S, Mirshahvaladi S, Rezaei-Tavirani M, Gourabi H, Baharvand H, Salekdeh GH. Y chromosome missing protein, TBL1Y, may play an important role in cardiac differentiation. J Proteome Res. 2017; https://doi.org/10.1021/acs.jproteome.7b00391.
46. Russo P, Siani A, Miller MA, Karanam S, Esposito T, Gianfrancesco F, Barba G, Lauria F, Strazzullo P, Cappuccio FP. Genetic variants of Y chromosome are associated with a protective lipid profile in black men. Arterioscler Thromb Vasc Biol. 2008;28:1569–74.
47. Johansson MM, Lundin E, Qian X, Mirzazadeh M, Halvardson J, Darj E, Feuk L, Nilsson M, Jazin E. Spatial sexual dimorphism of X and Y homolog gene expression in the human central nervous system during early male development. Biol Sex Differ. 2016; https://doi.org/10.1186/s13293-015-0056-4.
48. Priddle TH, Crow TJ. The protocadherin 11X/Y (PCDH11X/Y) gene pair as determinant of cerebral asymmetry in modern Homo Sapiens. Ann N Y Acad Sci. 2013;1288:36–47.
49. Speevak MD, Farrell SA. Non-syndromic language delay in a child with disruption in the Protocadherin11X/Y gene pair. Am J Med Genet B Neuropsychiatr Genet. 2011;156:484–9.
50. Li Y, Zhang DJ, Qiu Y, Kido T, Lau YF. The Y-located proto-oncogene TSPY exacerbates and its X-homologue TSPX inhibits transactivation functions of androgen receptor and its constitutively active variants. Hum Mol Genet. 2017;26:901–12.
51. Delbridge ML, Longepied G, Depetris D, Mattei MG, Disteche CM, Graves JA, Mitchell MJ. TSPY, the candidate gonadoblastoma gene on the human Y chromosome, has a widely expressed homologue on the X-implications for Y chromosome evolution. Chromosome Res. 2004;12: 345–56.
52. Krausz C, Giachini C, Forti G. TSPY and male fertility. Genes. 2010;1:308–16.
53. Yang X, Leng X, Tu W, Liu Y, Xu J, Pei X, Ma Y, Yang D, Yang Y. Spermatogenic phenotype of testis-specific protein, Y-encoded, 1 (TSPY1) dosage deficiency is independent of variations in TSPY-like 1 (TSPYL1) and TSPY-like 5 (TSPYL5): a case-control study in a Han Chinese population. Reprod Fertil Dev. 2017; https://doi.org/10.1071/RD17146.
54. Lahn BT, Page DC. Functional coherence of the human Y chromosome. Science. 1997;278:675–80.
55. Tiepolo L, Zuffardi O. Localization of factors controlling spermatogenesis in the nonfluorescent portion of the human Y chromosome long arm. Hum Genet. 1976;34(2):119–24.
56. Vergnaud G, Page DC, Simmler MC, Brown L, Rouyer F, Noel B, Botstein D, De La Chapelle A, Weissenbach J. A deletion map of the human Y chromosome based on DNA hybridization. Am J Hum Genet. 1986;38:109–24.
57. Vollrath D, Foote S, Hilton A, Brown LG, Beer-Romero P, Bogan JS, Page DC. The human Y chromosome: a 43-interval map based on naturally occurring deletions. Science. 1992;258:52–60.
58. Vogt PH. Human Y chromosome function in male germ cell development. Adv Dev Biol 1992. 1996;4:191–257.
59. Reijo R, Alagappan RK, Page DC, Patrizio P. Severe oligozoospermia resulting from deletions of azoospermia factor gene on Y chromosome. Lancet. 1996; 347:1290–3.
60. Reijo R, Lee TY, Salo P, Alagappan R, Brown LG, Rosenberg M, Rozen S, Jaffe T, Straus D, Hovatta O, de la Chapelle A. Diverse spermatogenic defects in humans caused by Y chromosome deletions encompassing a novel RNA–binding protein gene. Nat Genet. 1995;10:3383–93.
61. Vog PH, Edelmann A, Kirsch S, Henegariu O, Hirschmann P, Kiesewetter F, Köhn FM, Schill WB, Farah S, Ramos C, Hartmann M. Human Y chromosome azoospermia factors (AZF) mapped to different subregions in Yq11. Hum Mol Genet. 1996;5:933–43.
62. Kuroda-Kawaguchi T, Skaletsky H, Brown LG, Minx PJ, Cordum HS, Waterston RH, Wilson RK, Silber S, Oates R, Rozen S, Page DC. The AZFc region of the Y chromosome features massive palindromes and uniform recurrent deletions in infertile men. Nat Genet. 2001;29:279–86.
63. Luddi A, Margollicci M, Gambera L, Serafini F, Cioni M, De Leo V, Balestri P, Piomboni P. Spermatogenesis in a man with complete deletion of USP9Y. N Engl J Med. 2009;360:881–5.
64. Brown GM, Furlong RA, Sargent CA, Erickson RP, Longepied G, Mitchell M, Jones MH, Hargreave TB, Cooke HJ, Affara NA. Characterisation of the coding sequence and fine mapping of the human DFFRY gene and comparative expression analysis and mapping to the Sxr-b interval of the mouse Y chromosome of the Dffry gene. Hum Mol Genet. 1998;7:97–107.
65. Ho LK, Jee SG, Soo KI, Woong KS, Jae-Seung P, Ha CC, Kunsoo R. Ubiquitin-specific protease activity of USP9Y, a male infertility gene on the Y chromosome. Reprod Fertil Dev. 2003;15:129–33.
66. Kishi K, Uchida A, Takase HM, Suzuki H, Kurohmaru M, Tsunekawa N, Kanai-Azuma M, Wood SA, Kanai Y. Spermatogonial deubiquitinase USP9X is essential for proper spermatogenesis in mice. Reproduction. 2017; https://doi.org/10.1530/REP-17-0184.
67. Sun C, Skaletsky H, Birren B, Devon K, Tang Z, Silber S, Oates R, Page DC. An azoospermic man with a de novo point mutation in the Y-chromosomal gene USP9Y. Nat Genet. 1999;23:429–32.
68. Tyler-Smith C, Krausz C. The will-o'-the-wisp of genetics—hunting for the azoospermia factor gene. N Engl J Med. 2009;360:925–7.
69. Vogt MHJ, de Paus RA, Voogt PJ, Willemze R, Falkenburg JHF. DFFRY codes for a new human male-specific minor transplantation antigen involved in bone marrow graft rejection. Blood. 2000;95:1100–5.
70. Zhu Y, Ren S, Jing T, Cai X, Liu Y, Wang F, Zhang W, Shi X, Chen R, Shen J, Lu J. Clinical utility of a novel urine-based gene fusion TTTY15-USP9Y in predicting prostate biopsy outcome. Urol Oncol. 2015;33:384.e9–20.
71. Ditton HJ, Zimmer J, Kamp C, Rajpert-De Meyts E, Vogt PH. The AZFa gene DBY (DDX3Y) is widely transcribed but the protein is limited to the male germ cells by translation control. Hum Mol Genet. 2004;13:2333–41.
72. Gueler B, Sonne SB, Zimmer J, Hilscher B, Hilscher W, Græm N, Rajpert-De Meyts E, Vogt PH. AZFa protein DDX3Y is differentially expressed in human male germ cells during development and in testicular tumours: new evidence for phenotypic plasticity of germ cells. Hum Reprod. 2012;27: 1547–55.
73. Foresta C, Ferlin A, Moro E. Deletion and expression analysis of AZFa genes on the human Y chromosome revealed a major role for DBY in male infertility. Hum Mol Genet. 2000;9:1161–9.
74. Lardone MC, Parodi DA, Valdevenito R, Ebensperger M, Piottante A, Madariaga M, Smith R, Pommer R, Zambrano N, Castro A. Quantification of DDX3Y, RBMY1, DAZ and TSPY mRNAs in testes of patients with severe impairment of spermatogenesis. Mol Hum Reprod. 2007;13:705–12.
75. Lai MC, Chang WC, Shieh SY, Tarn WY. DDX3 regulates cell growth through translational control of cyclin E1. Mol Cell Biol. 2010;30:5444–53.
76. Kotov AA, Olenkina OM, Godneeva BK, Adashev VE, Olenina LV. Progress in understanding the molecular functions of DDX3Y (DBY) in male germ cell development and maintenance. Biosci Trends. 2017;11:46–53.
77. Ramathal C, Angulo B, Sukhwani M, Cui J, Durruthy-Durruthy J, Fang F, Schanes P, Turek PJ, Orwig KE, Pera RR. DDX3Y gene rescue of a Y chromosome AZFa deletion restores germ cell formation and transcriptional programs. Sci Rep. 2015;5:15041.
78. Laaser I, Theis FJ, de Angelis MH, Kolb H-J, Adamski J. Huge splicing frequency in human Y chromosomal UTY gene. OMICS. 2011;15:141–54.
79. Walport LJ, Hopkinson RJ, Vollmar M, Madden SK, Gileadi C, Oppermann U, Schofield CJ, Johansson C. Human UTY(KDM6C) is a male-specific N -methyl lysyl demethylase. J Biol Chem. 2014;289:18302–13.
80. Nailwal M, Chauhan JB. Computational analysis of high risk missense variant in human UTY gene: a candidate gene of AZFa sub-region. J Reprod Infertil. 2017;18:298–306.
81. Dutta A, Le Magnen C, Mitrofanova A, Ouyang X, Califano A, Abate-Shen C. Identification of an NKX3. 1-G9a-UTY transcriptional regulatory network that controls prostate differentiation. Science. 2016;352:1576–80.
82. Ahn J, Kim KH, Park S, Ahn YH, Kim HY, Yoon H, Lee JH, Bang D, Lee DH. Target sequencing and CRISPR/Cas editing reveal simultaneous loss of UTX and UTY in urothelial bladder cancer. Oncotarget. 2016;7:63252.
83. Torikai H, Akatsuka Y, Miyazaki M, Warren EH 3rd, Oba T, Tsujimura K, Motoyoshi K, Morishima Y, Kodera Y, Kuzushima K, Takahashi T. A novel HLA-A*3303-restricted minor histocompatibility antigen encoded by an unconventional open reading frame of human TMSB4Y gene. J Immunol. 2004;173:7046–54.
84. Lee HR, Yoon SY, Kang HB, Park S, Kim KE, Cho YH, Kim S, Kim CW, Cho BJ, Lee WJ, Bang SI, Park H, Cho D. Thymosin beta 4 enhances NK cell cytotoxicity mediated by ICAM-1. Immunol Lett. 2009;123:72–6.
85. Kichine E, Rozé V, Di Cristofaro J, Taulier D, Navarro A, Streichemberger E, Decarpentrie F, Metzler-Guillemain C, Lévy N, Chiaroni J, Paquis-Flucklinger

V. HSFY genes and the P4 palindrome in the AZFb interval of the human Y chromosome are not required for spermatocyte maturation. Hum Reprod. 2011;27:615–24.
86. Soares AR, Costa P, Silva J, Sousa M, Barros A, Fernandes S. AZFb microdeletions and oligozoospermia—which mechanisms? Fertil Steril. 2012;97:858–63.
87. Ravel C, Chantot-Bastaraud S, El Houate B, Rouba H, Legendre M, Lorenço D, Mandelbaum J, Siffroi JP, McElreavey K. Y-chromosome AZFc structural architecture and relationship to male fertility. Fertil Steril. 2009;92:1924–33.
88. Repping S, Skaletsky H, Lange J, Silber S, van der Veen F, Oates RD, Page DC, Rozen S. Recombination between palindromes P5 and P1 on the human Y chromosome causes massive deletions and spermatogenic failure. Am J Hum Genet. 2002;71:906–22.
89. Zorrilla M, Yatsenko AN. The genetics of infertility: current status of the field. Curr Genet Med Rep. 2013;1:247–60.
90. Fisher E, Beer-Romero P, Brown L, Ridley A, McNeil J, Lawrence J, Willard H, Bieber F, Page DC. Homologous ribosomal protein genes on the human X and Y chromosomes: escape from X inactivation and possible implications for turner syndrome. Cell. 1990;63:1205–18.
91. Andrés O, Kellermann T, López-Giráldez F, Rozas J, Domingo-Roura X, Bosch M. RPS4Y gene family evolution in primates. BMC Evol Biol. 2008;8:142.
92. Lopes AM, Miguel RN, Sargent CA, Ellis PJ, Amorim A, Affara NA. The human RPS4 paralogue on Yq11. 223 encodes a structurally conserved ribosomal protein and is preferentially expressed during spermatogenesis. BMC Mol Biol. 2010;11:33. https://doi.org/10.1186/1471-2199-11-33.
93. Tian Y, Stamova B, Jickling GC, Xu H, Liu D, Ander BP, Bushnell C, Zhan X, Turner RJ, Davis RR, Verro P. Y chromosome gene expression in the blood of male patients with ischemic stroke compared with male controls. Gend Med. 2012;9:68–75.
94. Yu A, Zhang J, Liu H, Liu B, Meng L. Identification of nondiabetic heart failure-associated genes by bioinformatics approaches in patients with dilated ischemic cardiomyopathy. Exp Ther Med. 2016;11:2602–8.
95. Yamauchi Y, Riel JM, Stoytcheva Z, Ward MA. Two Y genes can replace the entire Y chromosome for assisted reproduction in the mouse. Science. 2013; 3:1242544.
96. Li N, Dhar SS, Chen TY, Kan PY, Wei Y, Kim JH, Chan CH, Lin HK, Hung MC, Lee MG. JARID1D is a suppressor and prognostic marker of prostate cancer invasion and metastasis. Cancer Res. 2016;76:831–4.
97. Komura K, Jeong SH, Hinohara K, Qu F, Wang X, Hiraki M, Azuma H, Lee GS, Kantoff PW, Sweeney CJ. Resistance to docetaxel in prostate cancer is associated with androgen receptor activation and loss of KDM5D expression. Proc Natl Acad Sci U S A. 2016;113:6259–64.
98. Zhang W, Shao Y, Qin Y, Wu Y. Expression pattern of HSFY in the mouse testis and epididymis with and without heat stress. Cell Tissue Res. 2016;366:763–70.
99. Vinci G, Raicu F, Popa L, Popa O, Cocos R, McElreavey K. A deletion of a novel heat shock gene on the Y chromosome associated with azoospermia. Mol Hum Reprod. 2005;11:295–8.
100. Yu XW, Wei ZT, Jiang YT, Zhang SL. Y chromosome azoospermia factor region microdeletions and transmission characteristics in azoospermic and severe oligozoospermic patients. Int J Clin Exp Med. 2015;8:14634.
101. Shinka T, Sato Y, Chen G, Naroda T, Kinoshita K, Unemi Y, Tsuji K, Toida K, Iwamoto T, Nakahori Y. Molecular characterization of heat shock-like factor encoded on the human Y chromosome, and implications for male infertility. Biol Reprod. 2004;71:297–306.
102. Stahl PJ, Mielnik AN, Barbieri CE, Schlegel PN, Paduch DA. Deletion or underexpression of the Y-chromosome genes CDY2 and HSFY is associated with maturation arrest in American men with nonobstructive azoospermia. Asian J Androl. 2012;14:676682.
103. Halder A, Kumar P, Jain M, Iyer VK. Copy number variations in testicular maturation arrest. Andrology. 2017;5:460–72.
104. Tessari A, Salata E, Ferlin A, Bartoloni L, Slongo ML, Foresta C. Characterization of HSFY, a novel AZFb gene on the Y chromosome with a possible role in human spermatogenesis. Mol Hum Reprod. 2004;10(4): 253—8.
105. Repping S, van Daalen SK, Korver CM, Brown LG, Marszalek JD, Gianotten J, Oates RD, Silber S, van der Veen F, Page DC, Rozen S. A family of human Y chromosomes has dispersed throughout northern Eurasia despite a 1.8-Mb deletion in the azoospermia factor c region. Genomics. 2004;83:1046–52.
106. Alechine E, Corach D. High-throughput screening for spermatogenesis candidate genes in the AZFc region of the Y chromosome by multiplex real time PCR followed by high resolution melting analysis. PLoS One. 2014;9: e97227.
107. Stouffs K, Lissens W, Verheyen G, Van Landuyt L, Goossens A, Tournaye H, Van Steirteghem A, Liebaers I. Expression pattern of the Y-linked PRY gene suggests a function in apoptosis but not in spermatogenesis. Mol Hum Reprod. 2004;10:15–21.
108. Vogt PH. Human chromosome deletions in Yq11, AZF candidate gene and male infertility: history and update. Mol Hum Reprod. 1998;4:739–44.
109. Ferlin A, Raicu F, Gatta V, Zuccarello D, Palka G, Foresta C. Male infertility: role of genetic background. Reprod BioMed Online. 2007;14:734–45.
110. O'Flynn O'Brien KL, Varghese AC, Agarwal A. The genetic causes of male infertility: a review. Fertil Steril. 2010;93:1–12.
111. Tahmasbpour E, Balasubramanian D, Agarwal A. A multi-faceted approach to understanding male infertility: gene mutations, molecular defects and assisted reproductive techniques (ART). J Assist Reprod Genet. 2014;31:1115–37.
112. Ma K, Inglis JD, Sharkey A, Bickmore WA, Hill RE, Prosser EJ, Speed RM, Thomson EJ, Jobling M, Taylor K, et al. A Y chromosome gene family with RNA-binding protein homology: candidates for the azoospermia factor AZF controlling human spermatogenesis. Cell. 1993;75:1287–95.
113. Elliott DJ. The role of potential splicing factors including RBMY, RBMX, hnRNPG-T and STAR proteins in spermatogenesis. Int J Androl. 2004;27:328–34.
114. Vogt PH. AZF deletions and Y chromosomal haplogroups: history and update based on sequence. Hum Reprod Update. 2005;11:309–36.
115. Abid S, Sagare-Patil V, Gokral J, Modi D. Cellular ontogeny of RBMY during human spermatogenesis and its role in sperm motility. J Biosci. 2013;38:85–92.
116. Elliott DJ, Oghene K, Makarov G, Makarova O, Hargreave TB, Chandley AC, Eperon IC, Cooke HJ. Dynamic changes in the subnuclear organisation of pre-mRNA splicing proteins and RBM during human germ cell development. J Cell Sci. 1998;111:1255–65.
117. Elliott DJ, Millar MR, Oghene K, Ross A, Kiesewetter F, Pryor J, McIntyre M, Hargreave TB, Saunders PT, Vogt PH, Chandley AC. Expression of RBM in the nuclei of human germ cells is dependent on a critical region of the Y chromosome long arm. Proc Natl Acad Sci U S A. 1997;94:3848–53.
118. Alikhani M, Tabar MS, Mirshahvaladi S, Kheimeh A, Gilani MA, Sabbaghian M. Expression analysis of RNA-binding motif gene on Y chromosome (RBMY) protein isoforms in testis tissue and a testicular germ cell cancer-derived cell line (NT2). Iran Biomed J. 2013;17:54–61.
119. Zeng M, Liang S, Zhao S, Liu Y, Sun H, Zhang S. Identifying mRNAs bound by human RBMY protein in the testis. J Reprod Dev. 2011;57:107–12.
120. Yan Y, Yang X, Liu Y, Shen Y, Tu W, Dong Q, Yang D, Ma Y, Yang Y. Copy number variation of functional RBMY1 is associated with sperm motility: an azoospermia factor-linked candidate for asthenozoospermia. Hum Reprod. 2017;32:1521–31.
121. Plotton I, Ducros C, Pugeat M, Morel Y, Lejeune H. Transmissible microdeletion of the Y-chromosome encompassing two DAZ copies, four RBMY1 copies, and both PRY copies. Fertil Steril. 2010;94:2770.e11–6. https://doi.org/10.1016/j.fertnstert.2010.04.038.
122. Mahadevaiah SK, Odorisio T, Elliott DJ, Rattigan Á, Szot M, Laval SH, Washburn LL, McCarrey JR, Cattanach BM, Lovell-Badge R, Burgoyne PS. Mouse homologues of the human AZF candidate gene RBM are expressed in spermatogonia and spermatids, and map to a Y chromosome deletion interval associated with a high incidence of sperm abnormalities. Hum Mol Genet. 1998;7:715–27.
123. Tsuei DJ, Hsu HC, Lee PH, Jeng YM, Pu YS, Chen CN, Lee YC, Chou WC, Chang CJ, Ni YH, Chang MH. RBMY, a male germ cell-specific RNA-binding protein, activated in human liver cancers and transforms rodent fibroblasts. Oncogene. 2004;23:5815–22.
124. Tsuei DJ, Lee PH, Peng HY, Lu SL, Su DS, Jeng YM, Hsu HC, Hsu SH, Wu JF, Ni YH, Chang MH. Male germ cell-specific RNA binding protein RBMY: a new oncogene explaining male predominance in liver cancer. PLoS One. 2011;6:e26948.
125. Song SH, Chiba K, Ramasamy R, Lamb DJ. Recent advances in the genetics of testicular failure. Asian J Androl. 2016;18:350–5.
126. Rozen SG, Marszalek JD, Irenze K, Skaletsky H, Brown LG, Oates RD, Silber SJ, Ardlie K, Page DC. AZFc deletions and spermatogenic failure: a population-based survey of 20,000 Y chromosomes. Am J Hum Genet. 2012;91:890–6.
127. Seboun E, Barbaux S, Bourgeron T, Nishi S, Algonik A, Egashira M, Nikkawa N, Bishop C, Fellous M, McElreavey K, Kasahara M. Gene sequence, localization, and evolutionary conservation of DAZLA, a candidate male sterility gene. Genomics. 1997;41:227–35.
128. Xu EY, Moore FL, Pera RA. A gene family required for human germ cell development evolved from an ancient meiotic gene conserved in metazoans. Proc Natl Acad Sci U S A. 2001;98:7414–9.

129. Eberhart CG, Maines JZ, Wasserman SA. Meiotic cell cycle requirement for a fly homologue of human deleted in Azoospermia. Nature. 1996;381:783–5.
130. Foresta C, Moro E, Garolla A, Onisto M, Ferlin A. Y chromosome microdeletions in cryptorchidism and idiopathic infertility. J Clin Endocrinol Metab. 1999;84:3660—5.
131. Saxena R, de Vries JW, Repping S, Alagappan RK, Skaletsky H, Brown LG, et al. Four *DAZ* genes in two clusters found in the *AZFc* region of the human Y chromosome. Genomics. 2000;67:256–67.
132. Vogt PH, Fernandes S. Polymorphic DAZ gene family in polymorphic structure of *AZFc* locus: art work for functional for human spermatogenesis? APMIS. 2003;111:115–26.
133. Kim B, Lee Y, Kim Y, Lee KH, Chun S, Rhee K, et al. Polymorphic expression of DAZ proteins in the human testis. Hum Reprod. 2009;24:1507–15.
134. Kee K, Angeles VT, Flores M, Nguyen HN, Reijo RA. Human DAZL, *DAZ* and *BOULE* genes modulate primordial germ-cell and haploid gamete formation. Nature. 2009;462:222–5.
135. Fu XF, Cheng SF, Wang LQ, Yin S, De Felici M, Shen W. DAZ family proteins, key players for germ cell development. Int J Biol Sci. 2015;11:1226–135.
136. Ferlin A, Moro E, Garolla A, Foresta C. Human male infertility and Y chromosome deletions: role of the AZF-candidate genes DAZ, RBM and DFFRY. Hum Reprod. 1999;4:1710–6.
137. Kuo PL, Wang ST, Lin YM, Lin YH, Teng YN, Hsu CC. Expression profiles of the DAZ gene family in human testis with and without spermatogenic failure. Fertil Steril. 2004;81:1034–40.
138. Lu C, Jiang J, Zhang R, Wang Y, Xu M, Qin Y, Lin Y, Guo X, Ni B, Zhao Y, Diao N. Gene copy number alterations in the azoospermia-associated AZFc region and their effect on spermatogenic impairment. Mol Hum Reprod. 2014;20:836–43.
139. Shahid M, Dhillon VS, Khalil HS, Sexana A, Husain SA. Associations of Y-chromosome subdeletion gr/gr with the prevalence of Y-chromosome haplogroups in infertile patients. Eur J Hum Genet. 2011;19:23–9.
140. Sen S, Ambulkar P, Hinduja I, Zaveri K, Gokral J, Pal A, Modi D. Susceptibility of gr/gr rearrangements to azoospermia or oligozoospermia is dependent on DAZ and CDY1 gene copy deletions. J Assist Reprod Genet. 2015;32:1333–41.
141. Teng YN, Lin YM, Lin YH, Tsao SY, Hsu CC, Lin SJ, Tsai WC, Kuo PL. Association of a single-nucleotide polymorphism of the deleted-in-azoospermia-like gene with susceptibility to spermatogenic failure. J Clin Endocrinol Metab. 2002;87:5258–64.
142. Fernandes S, Huellen K, Goncalves J, Dukal H, Zeisler J, Rajpert De Meyts E, Skakkebaek NE, Habermann B, Krause W, Sousa M, Barros A, Vogt PH. High frequency of DAZ1/DAZ2 gene deletions in patients with severe oligozoospermia. Mol Hum Reprod. 2002;8:286–98.
143. Noordam MJ, Westerveld GH, Hovingh SE, van Daalen SK, Korver CM, van der Veen F, van Pelt AM, Repping S. Gene copy number reduction in the azoospermia factor c (AZFc) region and its effect on total motile sperm count. Hum Mol Genet. 2011;20:2457–63.
144. Mozdarani H, Ghoraeian P, Mozdarani S, Fallahi P, Mohseni-Meybodi A. High frequency of de novo DAZ microdeletion in sperm nuclei of subfertile men: possible involvement of genome instability in idiopathic male infertility. Hum Fertil. 2017;19:1–9.
145. Alimardanian L, Saliminejad K, Razi S, Ahani A. Analysis of partial azoospermia factor c deletion and DAZ copy number in azoospermia and severe oligozoospermia. Andrologia. 2016;48:978–82.
146. Van Gompel MJ, Xu EY. The roles of the DAZ family in spermatogenesis: more than just translation? Spermatogenesis. 2011;1:36–46.
147. Lahn BT, Tang ZL, Zhou J, Barndt RJ, Parvinen M, Allis CD, Page DC. Previously uncharacterized histone acetyltransferases implicated in mammalian spermatogenesis. Proc Natl Acad Sci U S A. 2002;99:8707–12.
148. Machev N, Saut N, Longepied G, Terriou P, Navarro A, Levy N, Guichaoua M, Metzler-Guillemain C, Collignon P, Frances AM, Belougne J. Sequence family variant loss from the AZFc interval of the human Y chromosome, but not gene copy loss, is strongly associated with male infertility. J Med Genet. 2004;41:814–25.
149. Ghorbel M, Baklouti-Gargouri S, Keskes R, Chakroun N, Sellami A, Fakhfakh F, Ammar-Keskes L. Gr/gr-DAZ2-DAZ4-CDY1b deletion is a high-risk factor for male infertility in Tunisian population. Gene. 2016;592:29–35.
150. Ghorbel M, Baklouti-Gargouri S, Keskes R, Chakroun N, Sellami A, Fakhfakh F, Ammar-Keskes L. Deletion of CDY1b copy of Y chromosome CDY1 gene is a risk factor of male infertility in Tunisian men. Gene. 2014;548:251–5.
151. Saut N, Terriou P, Navarro A, Lévy N, Mitchell MJ. The human Y chromosome genes BPY2, CDY1 and DAZ are not essential for sustained fertility. Mol Hum Reprod. 2000;6:789–93.
152. Tse JY, Wong EY, Cheung AN, O WS, Tam PC, Yeung WS. Specific expression of VCY2 in human male germ cells and its involvement in the pathogenesis of male infertility. Biol Reprod. 2003;69:746–51.
153. Singh I, Ozturk N, Cordero J, Mehta A, Hasan D, Cosentino C, Sebastian C, Krüger M, Looso M, Carraro G, Bellusci S. High mobility group protein-mediated transcription requires DNA damage marker γ-H2AX. Cell Res. 2015; 25:837–50.
154. Choi J, Koh E, Suzuki H, Maeda Y, Yoshida A, Namiki M. Alu sequence variants of the BPY2 gene in proven fertile and infertile men with Sertoli cell-only phenotype. Int J Urol. 2007;14:431–5.
155. Jangravi Z, Alikhani M, Arefnezhad B, Sharifi Tabar M, Taleahmad S, Karamzadeh R, Jadaliha M, Mousavi SA, Ahmadi Rastegar D, Parsamatin P, Vakilian H. A fresh look at the male-specific region of the human Y chromosome. J Prot Res. 2012;12:6–22.
156. Ahmadi Rastegar D, Sharifi Tabar M, Alikhani M, Parsamatin P, Sahraneshin Samani F, Sabbaghian M, Sadighi Gilani MA, Mohammad Ahadi A, Mohseni Meybodi A, Piryaei A, Ansari-Pour N. Isoform-level gene expression profiles of human Y chromosome azoospermia factor genes and their X chromosome paralogs in the testicular tissue of non-obstructive azoospermia patients. J Prot Res. 2015;14:3595–605.
157. Sen S, Agarwal R, Ambulkar P, Hinduja I, Zaveri K, Gokral J, Pal A, Modi D. Deletion of GOLGA2P3Y but not GOLGA2P2Y is a risk factor for oligozoospermia. Reprod BioMed Online. 2016;32:218–24.
158. Krausz C, Hoefsloot L, Simoni M, Tuttelmann F, European Academy of Andrology, European Molecular Genetics Quality Network. EAA/EMQN best practice guidelines for molecular diagnosis of Y-chromosomal microdeletions: state-of-the-art 2013. Andrology. 2014;2:5–19.
159. Sen S, Pasi AR, Dada R, Shamsi MB, Modi D. Y chromosome microdeletions in infertile men: prevalence, phenotypes and screening markers for the Indian population. J Assist Reprod Genet. 2013;30:413–22.
160. Simoni M, Bakker E, Krausz C. EAA/EMQN best practice guidelines for molecular diagnosis of y-chromosomal microdeletions. State of the art 2004. Int J Androl. 2004;27:240–9.
161. Chang PL, Sauer MV, Brown S. Y chromosome microdeletion in a father and his four infertile sons. Hum Reprod. 1999;14:2689–94.
162. Gatta V, Stuppia L, Calabrese G, Morizio E, Guanciali-Franchi P, Palka G. A new case of Yq microdeletion transmitted from a normal father to two infertile sons. J Med Genet. 2002;39:e27.
163. Yousefi-Razin E, Nasiri MJ, Omrani MD. Frequency of Y chromosome microdeletions among Iranian infertile men with azoospermia and severe oligozoospermia: a meta-analysis. J Reprod Infertil. 2016;17:208–12.
164. Foresta C, Moro E, Ferlin A. Y chromosome microdeletions and alterations of spermatogenesis. Endocr Rev. 2001;22:226–39.
165. Massart A, Lissens W, Tournaye H, Stouffs K. Genetic causes of spermatogenic failure. Asian J Androl. 2012;14:40–8.
166. Simoni M, Tuttelman F, Gromoll J, Nieschalg E. Clinical consequences of microdeletions of the Y chromosome: the extended Munster experience. Reprod BioMed Online. 2008;16:289–303.
167. Bansal SK, Jaiswal D, Gupta N, Singh K, Dada R, Sankhwar SN, Gupta G, Rajender S. Gr/gr deletions on Y-chromosome correlate with male infertility: an original study, meta-analyses, and trial sequential analyses. Sci Rep. 2016; 6:19798.
168. Kamp C, Huellen K, Fernandes S, Sousa M, Schlegel PN, Mielnik A, Kleiman S, Yavetz H, Krause W, Küpker W, Johannisson R. High deletion frequency of the complete AZFa sequence in men with Sertoli-cell-only syndrome. Mol Hum Reprod. 2001;7:987–94.
169. Krausz C, Quintana-Murci L, McElreavey K. Prognostic value of Y deletion analysis: what is the clinical prognostic value of Y chromosome microdeletion analysis? Hum Reprod. 2000;15:1431–4.
170. Hopps CV, Mielnik A, Goldstein M, Palermo GD, Rosenwaks Z, Schlegel PN. Detection of sperm in men with Y chromosome microdeletions of the AZFa, AZFb and AZFc regions. Hum Reprod. 2003;18:1660–5.
171. Abid S, Maitra A, Meherji P, Patel Z, Kadam S, Shah J, Shah R, Kulkarni V, Baburao V, Gokral J. Clinical and laboratory evaluation of idiopathic male infertility in a secondary referral center in India. J Clin Lab Anal. 2008;22:29–38.
172. Kleiman SE, Almog R, Yogev L, Hauser R, Lehavi O, et al. Screening for partial AZFa microdeletions in the Y chromosome of infertile men: is it of clinical relevance? Fertil Steril. 2012;98:43–7.

173. Wei W, Fitzgerald T, Ayub Q, Massaia A, Smith BB, Dominiczak AA, Morris AA, Porteous DD, Hurles ME, Tyler-Smith C, Xue Y. Copy number variation in the human Y chromosome in the UK population. Hum Genet. 2015;134:789–800.
174. Costa P, Gonçalves R, Ferrás C, Fernandes S, Fernandes AT, Sousa M, Barros A. Identification of new breakpoints in AZFb and AZFc. Mol Hum Reprod. 2008;14:251–8.
175. Kleiman SE, Yogev L, Lehavi O, Hauser R, Botchan A, Paz G, Yavetz H, Gamzu R. The likelihood of finding mature sperm cells in men with AZFb or AZFb-c deletions: six new cases and a review of the literature (1994–2010). Fertil Steril. 2011;95:2005–12.
176. Jungwirth A, Giwercman A, Tournaye H, Diemer T, Kopa Z, Dohle G, Krausz C, EAU Working Group on Male Infertility. European Association of Urology guidelines on male infertility: the 2012 update. Eur Urol. 2012;62:324–32.
177. Sadeghi-Nejad H, Farrokhi F. Genetics of azoospermia: current knowledge, clinical implications, and future directions. Part II: Y chromosome microdeletions. Urol J. 2007;4:192–206.
178. Liu XY, Wang RX, Fu Y, Luo LL, Guo W, Liu RZ. Outcomes of intracytoplasmic sperm injection in oligozoospermic men with Y chromosome AZFb or AZFc microdeletions. Andrologia. 2017;49:e12602.
179. Zhang YS, Li LL, Xue LT, Zhang H, Zhu YY, Liu RZ. Complete AZFb deletion of Y chromosome in an infertile male with severe oligoasthenozoospermia: case report and literature review. Urology. 2016;1:26–33.
180. Shi YC, Cui YX, Zhou YC, Wei L, Jiang HT, Xia XY, Lu HY, Wang HY, Shang XJ, Zhu WM, Li XJ, Huang YF. A rare Y chromosome constitutional rearrangement: a partial AZFb deletion and duplication within chromosome Yp in an infertile man with severe oligoasthenoteratozoospermia. Int J Androl. 2011;34:461–9.
181. Stouffs K, Vloeberghs V, Gheldof A, Tournaye H, Seneca S. Are AZFb deletions always incompatible with sperm production? Andrology. 2017;5:691–4.
182. Choi JM, Chung P, Veeck L, Mielnik A, Palermo GD, Schlegel PN. AZF microdeletions of the Y chromosome and in vitro fertilization outcome. Fertil Steril. 2004;81:337–41.
183. Simoni M, Gromoll J, Dworniczak B, Rolf C, Abshagen K, Kamischke A, et al. Screening for deletions of the Y chromosome involving the DAZ (deleted in Azoospermia) gene in azoospermia and severe oligozoospermia. Fertil Steril. 1997;67:542–7.
184. Krausz C, Forti G. Sperm cryopreservation in male infertility due to genetic disorders. Cell Tissue Bank. 2006;7:105–12.
185. Fu L, Xiong DK, Ding XP, Li C, Zhang LY, et al. Genetic screening for chromosomal abnormalities and Y chromosome microdeletions in Chinese infertile men. J Assist Reprod Genet. 2012;29:521–7.
186. Repping S, Skaletsky H, Brown L, van Daalen SK, Korver CM, Pyntikova T, Kuroda-Kawaguchi T, de Vries JW, Oates RD, Silber S, van der Veen F, Page DC, Rozen S. Polymorphism for a 1.6-Mb deletion of the human Y chromosome persists through balance between recurrent mutation and haploid selection. Nat Genet. 2003;35:247–51.
187. Stouffs K, Lissens W, Tournaye H, Haentjens P. What about gr/gr deletions and male infertility? Systematic review and meta-analysis. Hum Reprod Update. 2011;17:197–209.
188. Bansal SK, Gupta G, Rajender S. Y chromosome b2/b3 deletions and male infertility: a comprehensive meta-analysis, trial sequential analysis and systematic review. Mutat Res Rev Mutat Res. 2016;768:78–90.
189. Krausz C, Chianese C, Giachini C, Guarducci E, Laface I, Forti G. The Y chromosome-linked copy number variations and male fertility. J Endocrinol Investig. 2011;34:376–82.
190. Vodicka R, Vrtel R, Dusek L, Singh AR, Krizova K, Svacinova V, Horinova V, Dostal J, Oborna I, Brezinova J, Sobek A. TSPY gene copy number as a potential new risk factor for male infertility. Reprod BioMed Online. 2007;14:579–87.
191. Lee C, Iafrate AJ, Brothman AR. Copy number variations and clinical cytogenetic diagnosis of constitutional disorders. Nat Genet. 2007;39:S48–54.
192. Tüttelmann F, Simoni M, Kliesch S, Ledig S, Dworniczak B, Wieacker P, Röpke A. Copy number variants in patients with severe oligozoospermia and Sertoli-cell-only syndrome. PLoS One. 2011;6:e19426.
193. Dong Y, Pan Y, Wang R, Zhang Z, Xi Q, Liu RZ. Copy number variations in spermatogenic failure patients with chromosomal abnormalities and unexplained azoospermia. Genet Mol Res. 2015;14:16041–9.
194. Krausz C, Casamonti E. Spermatogenic failure and the Y chromosome. Hum Genet. 2017;136:637–55.
195. Mateu E, Rodrigo L, Martínez MC, Peinado V, Milán M, Gil-Salom M, Martínez-Jabaloyas JM, Remohí J, Pellicer A, Rubio C. Aneuploidies in embryos and spermatozoa from patients with Y chromosome microdeletions. Fertil Steril. 2010;94:2874–7.
196. Zhang F, Lu C, Li Z, Xie P, Xia Y, Zhu X, Wu B, Cai X, Wang X, Qian J, Wang X. Partial deletions are associated with an increased risk of complete deletion in AZFc: a new insight into the role of partial AZFc deletions in male infertility. J Med Genet. 2007;44:437–44.
197. Modi D, Bhartiya D. Y chromosome mosaicism and occurrence of gonadoblastoma in cases of turner syndrome and amenorrhoea. Reprod BioMed Online. 2007;15:547–53.
198. Jørgensen A, Johansen ML, Juul A, Skakkebaek NE, Main KM, Rajpert-De Meyts E. Pathogenesis of germ cell neoplasia in testicular dysgenesis and disorders of sex development. Semin Cell Dev Biol. 2015;45:124–37.
199. Kido T, Lau YF. Roles of the Y chromosome genes in human cancers. Asian J Androl. 2015;17:373–80.
200. Huang H, Wang C, Tian Q. Gonadal tumour risk in 292 phenotypic female patients with disorders of sex development containing Y chromosome or Y-derived sequence. Clin Endocrinol. 2017;86:621–7.
201. Nathanson KL, Kanetsky PA, Hawes R, Vaughn DJ, Letrero R, Tucker K, Friedlander M, Phillips KA, Hogg D, Jewett MA, Lohynska R. The Y deletion gr/gr and susceptibility to testicular germ cell tumor. Am J Hum Genet. 2005;77:1034–43.
202. Castro A, Rodríguez F, Flórez M, López P, Curotto B, Martínez D, Maturana A, Lardone MC, Palma C, Mericq V, Ebensperger M. Pseudoautosomal abnormalities in terminal AZFb+ c deletions are associated with isochromosomes Yp and may lead to abnormal growth and neuropsychiatric function. Hum Reprod. 2017;32:465–75.
203. Krausz C, Escamilla AR, Chianese C. Genetics of male infertility: from research to clinic. Reproduction. 2015;150:R159–74.
204. Lopes AM, Aston KI, Thompson E, Carvalho F, Gonçalves J, Huang N, Matthiesen R, Noordam MJ, Quintela I, Ramu A, Seabra C. Human spermatogenic failure purges deleterious mutation load from the autosomes and both sex chromosomes, including the gene DMRT1. PLoS Genet. 2013;9:e1003349.

8

Obesity as disruptor of the female fertility

Erica Silvestris[1*], Giovanni de Pergola[2], Raffaele Rosania[1] and Giuseppe Loverro[1]

Abstract

Both obesity and overweight are increasing worldwide and have detrimental influences on several human body functions including the reproductive health. In particular, obese women undergo perturbations of the 'hypothalamic pituitary ovarian axis', and frequently suffer of menstrual dysfunction leading to anovulation and infertility. Besides the hormone disorders and subfertility that are common in the polycystic ovary syndrome (PCOS), in obesity the adipocytes act as endocrine organ. The adipose tissue indeed, releases a number of bioactive molecules, namely adipokines, that variably interact with multiple molecular pathways of insulin resistance, inflammation, hypertension, cardiovascular risk, coagulation, and oocyte differentiation and maturation. Moreover, endometrial implantation and other reproductive functions are affected in obese women with complications including delayed conceptions, increased miscarriage rate, reduced outcomes in assisted conception treatments.
On the contrary, weight loss programs through lifestyle modification in obese women, have been proven to restore menstrual cyclicity and ovulation and improve the likelihood of conception.

Keywords: Obesity, Infertility, Adipokines, Anovulation, Oocytes

Background

Major functions of the female gonads include the production of gametes, the oocytes, and sex hormones that control the development of the female secondary sexual characters and support the pregnancy. In physiology, these functions are cyclically exerted between puberty and menopause, and are regulated by endocrine and paracrine factors that interact with several cell types located in ovaries [1]. Thus, besides other pathological outcomes, dysfunctional or altered regulation of these mechanisms can either directly or indirectly result in infertility.

According to the American Society of Reproductive Medicine Practice Committee [2], infertility is a disease generally defined as *failure to conceive after twelve or more months of attempts of natural fertilization* and is a rising problem in our society today. The WHO worldwide estimation suggests that this pathology currently affects up to 50–80 millions of women, with a variable incidence that in several instances may raise up to about 50% of all women [3].

A number of factors appear to concur to provoke infertility in women mainly including ovulatory dysfunction, tubal, cervical and/or uterine factors, as well as endometriosis although 20–30% of cases remain unexplained [4]. Recently, the effects of lifestyle on female reproductive health have received great attention as well as the body mass index (BMI), foods and nutrients, sport and physical activity, stressing jobs and other conditions, are currently widely claimed as having a negative impact on the female fertility [5].

Here, we critically review the potential influence of the altered metabolic state on the reproductive health of women, focusing the effects of obesity on fertility, and the management of infertility in obese and overweight women.

Pathophysiology of the woman infertility

A number of differential conditions concur to affect the woman fertility. Several of them are strictly related to the pathophysiology of reproductive organs whereas others are mainly dependent on occupational aspects including the lifestyle factors as the hypercaloric nutrition usually resulting in metabolic derangements and increase in the body weight promoting obesity.

* Correspondence: ericasilvestris85@gmail.com
[1]Interdisciplinary Department of Medicine, Section of Obstetrics and Gynecology, University of Bari Aldo Moro, P.za G.Cesare, 11-70124 Bari, Italy
Full list of author information is available at the end of the article

Below are listed the major causes of infertility belonging to both of these pathogenic conditions as next detailed.

Dysfunction of reproductive organs

- ***Deregulated ovarian function*** – Since the ovulation is the result of a complex balance and interaction of hormones, any alteration of these mechanisms may influence its physiology. The most common cause of ovulation failure includes the polycystic ovary syndrome (PCOS) [6]. This condition is related to the arrest of the follicle maturation resulting in formation of small follicles, defective ovulation and dysmenorrhea. Other causes include malfunctions of the hypothalamus or pituitary gland leading to the production of immature eggs, or the result of invasive surgery for repeated ovarian cysts as well as ovulatory disorders dependent on extraovarian pathologies including either hypothyroidism or hyperthyroidism.
- ***Tubal infections*** – The factors responsible for tubal disease are different and derive from post-infection damage, obstruction, pelvic adhesion even after surgery, and probably undefined others. In this contest, the pelvic inflammatory disease is a major etiologic event of anatomic and functional disorders of tubae and is predominantly associated to infections by *Chlamydia Trachomatis* and *Neisseria Gonorrhoea* which can ultimately lead to tubal related infertility [7].
- ***Endometriosis*** – It is a chronic condition characterized by the growth of endometrial tissue in areas other than the uterine cavity, most commonly in the pelvic cavity, including the ovaries. Tubal damage can occur as a result of the chronic inflammation associated to the growing endometrioid tissue and approximately 20–30% of women with endometriosis suffer of subfertility [8].
- ***Cervical factor*** – The cervix plays an important role in the reproduction activity. It provides the passage way for sperms, allowing them to access into the uterine cavity and ultimately into the fallopian tubes. The ability of the sperm to gain access to the upper tract is influenced by the cervical mucus within the cervical canal. Therefore, all conditions modifying the mucosal film of the cervix may concur to prevent the progression of sperms toward the tubae.
- ***Uterine factors*** – Dysfunction in uterus such as defect of adhesion molecules, polyps, submucous fibroids, asymptomatic tumors, recurrent miscarriages as well as other endometrial pathologies and infections, may dramatically affect the blastocyst engraftment. Exploration of the uterine cavity by hysteroscopy is thus mandatory in the presence of unexplained bleeding.
- ***Unknown causes of infertility*** – In addition to the described major reproductive pathologies, other causes including hormone alterations, constitutive defects of inflammatory soluble factors and/or chronic alterations of metabolic pathways of reproductive organs, are related to infertility and remain to be assessed in clinical investigative studies [9].

Lifestyle and infertility

Recently, great interest has been focused on several lifestyle factors including the emotional state, typical of stress or anxiety condition, modifiable habits and ways of life that can greatly influence overall health and well being. Below are listed several of those factors for which there is a defined evidence of a negative impact on fertility.

- ***Psychological stress for social life and work*** – Particularly in western countries there is a larger incidence of depression and anxiety, which is partially related to the lifestyle and to a number of stressing jobs. Thus, the symptoms related to both depression and anxiety have been reported as more prominent in infertile than in fertile women. In a series of studies it has been indeed described that infertile women are more likely to experience higher levels of psychological distress [10], as well as high levels of reactive depression [11], and increased likelihood of anxiety [12]. A probability based study also suggested that the general distress levels are lower in the presence of higher socioeconomic status, or conversely, higher in the presence of highly stressing jobs, poor economic conditions or missing work. These aspects concur to generate a persistent condition of psychological stress in addition to the detrimental well being feeling, may alter the physiologic maturation of oocytes [13].
- ***Smoking*** – Although in the absence of defined molecular mechanisms, there is an apparently negative influence of smoking resulting in reduced fertility in female smokers. Several effects on negative reproductive consequences of chronic smoking include rapid depletion of ovarian follicles, conception delay, increased risk of spontaneous miscarriage in both natural and assisted conception cycles as well as increased risk of birth defects [14].
- ***Drugs, caffeine and alcohol*** – There are a number of daily or occasionally assumed drugs that are known to impact fertility. Non-steroidal anti-inflammatory drugs, commonly used to treat pain or

inflammation are defined ovulation inhibitors whereas cytotoxic chemotherapy drugs used in anti-cancer treatments are primarily responsible of the ovarian failure in women [15]. On the other hand, higher introduction of caffeine has been associated with an increased risk of pregnancy loss whereas in alcohol abusers the liver metabolic alterations and/or psyconeurologic damages concur with stress factors to restrain the oocyte maturation.

- ***Diet and variations of body weight*** – Inadequate diets as those with poor calories and protein content or, vice versa, based on habitual hypercaloric food assumption, leading to severe thinness or overweight, definitely affect the ovarian function and increase the risk of women infertility. To this regard, it has been reported that the time to conceive is longer in women with BMI over 25 kg/m^2 or, vice versa, less than 19 kg/m^2, and that obesity and overweight are significantly associated with decreased pregnancy rates, increased requirements for gonadotrophins and higher miscarriage events. High BMI is also associated with adverse pregnancy outcomes such as gestational diabetes, hypertension and premature lebor.

Evidence on the effect of diet composition in fertility is scarce. Several studies investigating the effect of various dietary factors on fertility have been completed on data from extended studies including 116,678 women in the Nurses' Health Study II. In these reports, it has been described a reduced risk of fertility due to ovulatory disorder in women whose diet included prevalently foods with low glycaemic content and limited intake of nutrients. This dietary restriction, indeed, may increase insulin resistance, such as lower trans fatty acid intake [16] thus supporting the pivotal role exerted by the glucose homeostasis and insulin sensitivity in the normal ovulatory function and fertility as occurs in women with normal weight.

- ***Physical activity*** – The excess in physical activity could be closely linked to considerable negative effects on the whole body including skeletal pathologies or functional derangements in endocrine, cardiovascular, reproductive and central nervous systems. In contrast with the vantages of sport activities in decreasing the abdominal fat, blood glucose, lipids and insulin resistance as well as in regulating the menstrual cyclicity, ovulation and fertility due to the lowered testosterone levels and increase of sex hormone binding globulin (SHBG), the intensively exerted agonistic sports may typically produce the *'female athlete triad'*, a syndrome characterized by amenorrhea, osteoporosis and eating disorder as defined by the American College of Sports Medicine [17].
- ***Environmental pollutants*** – Based on several investigative studies, the OSHA (Occupational Safety and Health Administration, USA) provided evidence that chronic exposure to specific chemicals as organic solvents, aromatic amines, heavy metals, phytodrugs, vegetal toxins and others is associated with reduced fertility as well as to increased tendency to either occasional or recurrent abortions [18]. The pathogenic mechanisms leading to unsuccessful fertility by these conditions are unclear and further studies are required to clarify the effect of environmental pollutants on female fertility.

The growing interest and the amount of research in this field emphasize the role of lifestyle factors in affecting the woman fertility and particularly obesity may represent a major condition in which both alteration of metabolic pathways and inflammatory factors concur to reduce the oocyte viability leading to subfertility or infertility.

Molecular and endocrinological influence of obesity on woman fertility

In female mammals, a number of evolutionary mechanisms are enrolled to integrate environmental, nutritional and hormonal cues in order to guarantee reproduction in normal energetic conditions and, vice versa, to inhibit it in case of food scarcity. This metabolic strategy could be an advantage in nutritionally poor environments, but nowadays is affecting women's health since the energy states may influence the female reproductive health in conditions of under or overweight.

Obesity and strenuous physical activity are conditions that alter the profiles of specific hormones such as insulin and adipokines and, thus, definitely impair the women fertility. Furthermore, there is undoubtedly a tight interconnection between energy metabolism and fertility, above all in females.

Obesity is a common problem among women of reproductive age. Obesity and overweight involves an abnormal and excessive fat accumulation that negatively affects the health status. According to the World Health Organization (WHO), if BMI is equal or greater than 25 kg/m^2, it is considered overweight, whereas the BMI higher than 30 kg/m^2 defines obesity [19]. The WHO reports that 60% of women are overweight in the United States and in most European countries while 30% of the female population are obese. Moreover, 6% of all women are morbidly obese (BMI $\geq$ 35 kg/m^2) [20]. The negative effects of obesity on the reproductive physiology are known, since obese women frequently undergo menstrual irregularity with ovulatory disorders, endometrial pathology, and infertility.

The impact of obesity on reproductive function, especially ovulatory disorders, are mainly attributable to endocrine mechanisms [21], which interfere with neuroendocrine and ovarian functions, and reduce the ovulation omeostatic [22]. In obese women, gonadotropin secretion is affected as effect of the increased peripheral aromatization of androgens to estrogens while the insulin resistance and hyperinsulinemia lead to hyperandrogenemia. Furthermore, the sex hormone-binding globulin (SHBG), growth hormone (GH), and insulin-like growth factor binding proteins (IGFBP) are decreased and leptin levels are increased. Thus, the neuroregulation of the hypothalamic-pituitary-ovarian (HPO) axis may be severely deranged while the obese condition also increases the risk of miscarriage, poor pregnancy outcomes, and impaired fetal well being [23].

The risk of infertility has been shown to be threefold higher in obese than in non-obese women, and several studies have demonstrated that the obese females need longer time to pregnancy. In particular, two studies performed in large cohorts of Danish women planning pregnancies showed an inverse relation of fecundity with respect to the BMI increase [24]. It is noteworthy that obese women remain subfertile even in the absence of ovulatory dysfunction and Gesink and coworkers showed reduced fecundity in eumenorrheic obese women by examining a large American cohort of more than 7000 women in whom the probability of spontaneous conception linearly declined with each BMI point > 29 kg/m^2 as in a parallel study completed in a Dutch cohort of more than 3000 women with normal cycles [25].

Moreover, fertility in obese women seems to be impaired also in assisted conception programs. In fact, overweight and obesity are also associated with negative outcomes for patients undergoing in vitro fertilization (IVF) due to the poor oocyte quality, as well as the lower preimplantation rate and uterine receptivity. Therefore, in these women it is strongly recommend the weight loss in order to improve the fertility functions [26].

The molecular and endocrinological aspects of obesity, its effects and consequences on the reproductive system as well as benefits from modifying lifestyles improving the reproductive outcomes, are next reviewed.

Adipokines as major fat tissue soluble products

The adipose tissue is considered an endocrine organ that plays important roles in the regulation of many physiological events, such as reproduction, immune response, glucose and lipid metabolism, through the secretion of a variety of bioactive cytokines, named adipokines, commonly involved in metabolic regulation and inflammatory processes.

During the last years, the dysfunction of the adipose tissue has been implicated in the pathophysiology of infertility based on recently discovered effects of adipokines. Their normal levels are critical to maintain the integrity of hypothalamus-pituitary-gonadal axis as well as to regulate ovulatory processes, successful embryo implantation, and in general the physiologic pregnancy.

The family of adipokines includes the adipose-specific cytokines, namely secreted by adipocytes, such as leptin, adiponectin (APN), resistin, visfatin and omentin, and the non adipose specific cytokines such as retinol binding protein-4 (RBP4), lipocalin-2 (LCN2), chemerin, interleukin 6 (IL6), interleukin 1β (IL1β), and tumor necrosis factor α (TNFα). The panel of adipokines is depicted in Table 1.

Abnormal levels of these factors have been shown to be strongly associated with both insulin resistance (IR) and type 2 diabetes mellitus (T2DM) and in patients with the PCOS, a severe dysfunction of adipose tissue has been observed leading to over-production of pro-inflammatory adipokines such as TNFα and, concurrently, reduction of a few "beneficial adipokines" such as APN. Peculiarities of each bioactive cytokine are next summarized.

- ***Leptin*** - Leptin is a 167-amino acid protein encoded by the *"ob"* gene. It is an important hormone involved in the regulation of food intake, energy balance, and body weight. Leptin is the first discovered adipokine to realize the endocrine functions of adipose tissue Fig. 1. It's predominantly secreted by adipose tissue and largely available in many organs as stomach, placenta, hypothalamus, pituitary, and mammary gland. The leptin receptor (LEPR) is a single transmembrane domain receptor that is highly expressed in the choroid plexus. There are six isoforms of the LEPR (Ob-Ra, b, c, d, e, and f) due to the alternative RNA splicing. Leptin is constitutively secreted by adipocytes in relation to the extent of the adipose mass and is abundant in subjects with extensive abdominal fat. It suppresses the food intake and promotes energy expenditure mainly via its direct effects on hypothalamic neurons, and is thus considered an anti-obesity hormone. Its levels decrease with fasting and increase after food intake [27].

Higher circulating levels of leptin may lead to chronic down-regulation of LEPR in the brain of obese women, and higher leptin-BMI ratios may well explain lower rates of pregnancy with IVF. Jain et al., found that the amplitude of LH pulsatility was significantly lower in

Table 1 Major effects of adipokines in fertility of the obese woman

Adipokines	Serum Levels	Effects
Leptin	↑	Inhibits insulin induced ovarian steroidogenesis Inibiths LH stimulated E2 production by the granulosa cells
Adiponectin	↓	Plasma insulin levels increase
Resistin	↑	Causes insulin resistance
Visfatin	↑	Increased insulin sensitivity
Omentin	↓	Increased insulin sensitivity
Chemerin	↑	Negatively regulates FSH_induced follicular steroidogenesis

LH Luteinizing hormone, *FSH* Follicle stimulating Hormone, *E2* Estradiol

eumenorrheic obese women, thus suggesting a central defect. Moreover, higher serum levels of leptin in obese women correlate with higher levels of leptin in the follicular fluid. In vitro studies have shown that leptin affects steroidogenic pathways in granulosa cells and decreases both estrogen and progesterone production in a dose-dependent manner [28]. This negative effect of obesity on the oocyte physiology could have downstream effects on endometrial receptivity and embryo implantation.

- ***Adiponectin*** - Adiponectin (APN) is the most abundant secreted protein expressed exclusively in adipose tissue. There are three forms of APN: at *low molecular weight* (APN-LMW); at *medium molecular weight* (APN-MMW); and at *high molecular weight* (APN-HMW). Three receptors have been thus identified for APN: AdipoR1, AdipoR2, and T-cadherin.

AdipoR1 and AdipoR2 receptors are ubiquitously expressed and largely on female reproductive tissues, including ovary, placenta, endometrium, and oviduct [29]. It has been shown that APN inhibits LH and GNRH release, indicating its possible role in modulating the central reproductive endocrine axis [30].

Circulating APN levels decrease with obesity and increase with weight loss and major effects of APN are devoted to increase the insulin sensitivity by stimulating glucose uptake in liver and muscles, while decreasing hepatic gluconeogenesis, and promoting the fatty acid β-oxidation in the skeletal muscle. Consequently, APN reduces triglyceride (TG) accumulation and enhances the insulin sensitivity [31].

Reduced expression of AdipoR1 and AdipoR2 has been also observed in endometria of women with recurrent implantation failure compared with fertile women, suggesting an important role of APN signaling in uterine receptivity and its possible contribution to implantation failures and pregnancy loss in women with maternal metabolic conditions such as obesity and PCOS [32].

- ***Resistin*** - Resistin is a small cysteine-rich 94-amino acid polypeptide. This adipokine is considered a potential link between obesity and T2DM as result of its inhibitory effect on adipocyte differentiation and its association with IR. Resistin is mainly secreted by peripheral blood mononuclear cells including macrophages and by stromal cells in adipose tissue, but its mRNA has been also found in hypothalamus-pituitary axis [33].

The resistin gene polymorphism is associated with BMI in women with PCOS, suggesting that it might be related to adiposity in PCOS. A randomized placebo-controlled study recently showed that treatment with

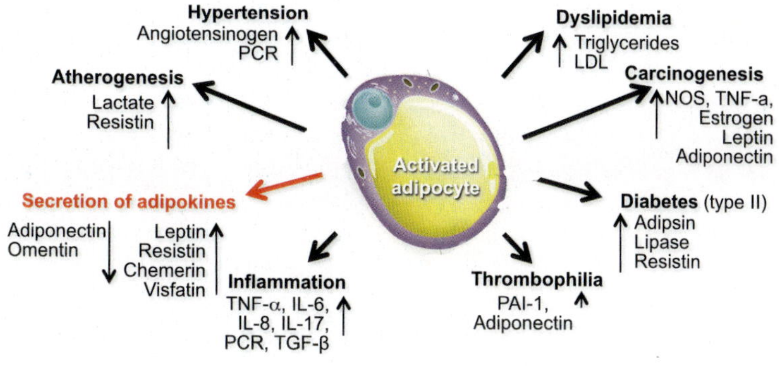

Fig. 1 Functional properties of adipocites

the insulin sensitizer rosiglitazone significantly reduces the serum resistin levels in overweight women with PCOS, thus implying the contribution of this adipokine to the insulin sensitivity improvement during treatment [34]. In summary, resistin seems to be an important adipokine that is involved in obesity, IR, PCOS and endocrine dysfunction.

- ***Visfatin*** - Visfatin is a protein expressed by a variety of tissues and cell types, including adipocytes, lymphocytes, bone marrow, liver, muscle, trophoblast, and fetal membranes.

In vitro studies have demonstrated that visfatin stimulates the glucose uptake in both adipocytes and muscle cells while suppressing the release of glucose by hepatocytes. A recent meta-analysis revealed that plasma visfatin is significantly increased in both overweight and obese subjects, or in patients with T2DM and metabolic syndrome [35]. It has been also reported that the gene expression and the circulating levels of visfatin are increased in women with PCOS as compared with age and BMI matched controls. A positive correlation, however, has been found between plasma visfatin concentration and fasting insulin in a homeostasis model assessment (HOMA)-IR [36].

- ***Omentin*** - Omentin-1, also named intelectin-1, a 313-amino acid peptide, is an anti-inflammatory adipokine preferentially expressed in stromal vascular cells of visceral adipose tissue. It is suggested that this substance makes an important contribution to the physiological difference between visceral and subcutaneous adipose tissue. It is also abundant in vasculature, small intestine, colon, thymus and heart.

Omentin-1 is the major circulating form but other homologues are known. Genes of both omentin-1 and omentin-2 are located as adjacent to each other at 1q22-q23, exactly in the region linked to type 2 diabetes mellitus. Both omentin homologues as circulating forms correlate with expression in visceral fat tissue [37]. Omentin-1 increases the insulin signal transduction as well as the insulin-stimulated glucose transport in human adipocytes though with no effect on basal glucose uptake, and contributes to the regulation of lipid metabolism. Its role, however, in the reproduction's physiology is unclear.

Dysendocrine effects of obesity: hyper- and hypo-androgenism

- ***Obesity, hyperandrogenism and anovulation*** - Obesity, body fat location as upper versus lower body disposition, and muscle mass have important effects on the reproductive function and fertility. The majority of obese women have normal ovulatory menstrual cycles, remain fertile and have no apparent hyperandrogenism thus suggesting that obesity per se is not the only factor involved in the genesis of hyperandrogenism and ovulatory dysfunction. However, elevated androgen levels in obese women appear to be a common finding in the presence of amenorrhea. The mechanism by which the excess adipose tissue can be associated with hyperandrogenism remains controversial although the hyperinsulinemia plays a primary role in influencing obesity in hyperandrogenism.

Hyperinsulinemia and insulin resistance are the underlying causes that lead to obesity, accompanied by hyperandrogenism and alterations in steroidogenesis, in those patients with stromal hyperplasia of the ovaries. Both hyperinsulinemia and hyperandrogenism affect the ovarian function in both obese and non-obese women although the mechanism by which how hyperandrogenism and/or hyperinsulinemia inhibit the regular ovulation has not been fully understood. It has been experimentally shown that insulin has specific actions on steroidogenesis through its own receptor since it stimulates the theca cells to produce androgens and exert a growth stimulatory effect on stromal cells, thus priming the production of extradiol [38] Fig. 2. Another proposed mechanism of hyperandrogenism induced by hyperinsulinemia, which can be found in the PCOS patient obese or not, occurs through the insulin-like growth factor-I (IGF-I) which is secreted by human ovarian tissue while its receptors are also located in ovaries.

Insulin can bind IGF-I receptors (IGF-IR) as well as its own receptors and activates the tyrosine kinase of the β-subunit resulting in triggering the intracellular events that potentiate those normally mediated by IGF-I. Therefore, the insulin-like growth factor binding proteins (IGFBP) include a group of secreted proteins which bind to IGF-I and IGF-II with high affinity and modulate the biological actions of IGF [38]. When the IGFBPs bind and activate the IGF-IR, the hepatic synthesis of IGFBP-I is decreased thus making IGF-I more biologically available with the final effect of enhancing the androgen production by theca interstitial and stromal cells Fig. 3.

Willis et al., showed that insulin also reinforces the activity of the LH on granulosa cells by exerting two distinct effects on the preovulatory follicle, namely the steroidogenesis activation and the inhibition of mitosis thus restraining the terminal differentiation of those cells [39]. As a result of the enhanced steroidogenesis due to insulin and its interaction with LH, the unfavorable

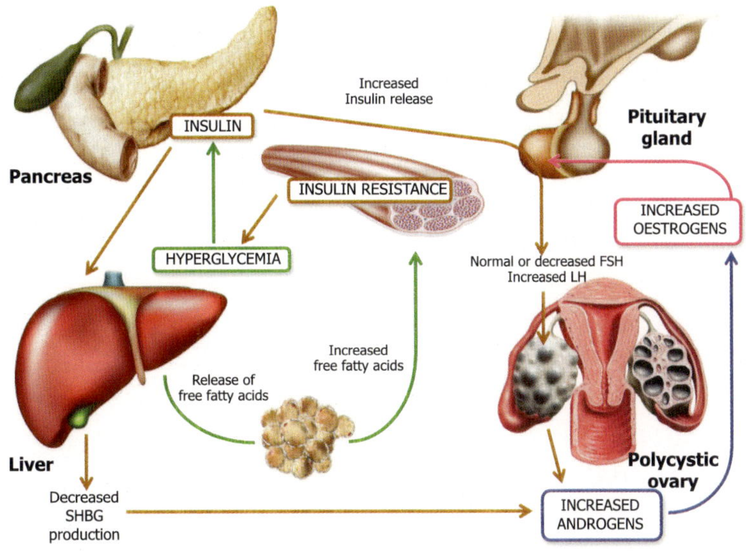

Fig. 2 Pathophysioly of insuline resistance. This figure illustrates the complex interactions underlying the pathophysiology of PCOS. Insulin resistance and the resulting hyperinsulinemia are responsible for the majority of the changes found in PCOS. Insulin resistance in PCOS does not occur in all tissues, but rather appears to be tissue-specific. Skeletal-muscle and adipose tissue become insulin resistance resulting in decrease glucose uptake and increased lipolysis, respectively, whereas the ovary, adrenal and liver remain insulin sensitive. In PCOS, hyperinsulinemia occurs as a compensatory response to insulin resistance. This resulting hyperinsulinemia has a stimulatory effect on the ovaries and adrenal glands that leads to enhanced androgen production by these organs. More specifically, excess insulin enhances androgen production in ovarian theca cells in response to luteinizing hormone (LH) stimulation, resulting in follicular arrest and anovulation. In contrast hyperinsulinemia acts to suppress hepatic production of sex hormone-binding globulin (SHBG), the primary binding protein for testosterone in the serum. Therefore, insuline resistance whith compensatory hyperinsulinemia results in hyperandrogenemia

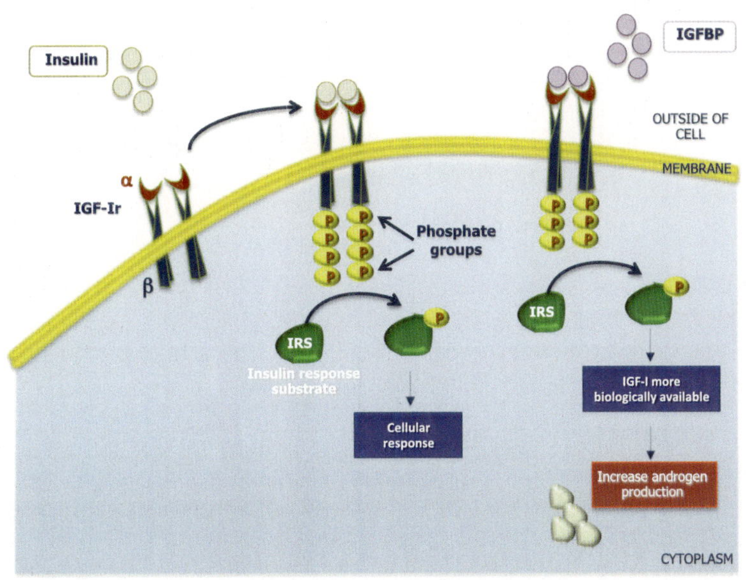

Fig. 3 Insulin receptor tyrosine kinases. The α subunit binds insulin and the β transmits a signal from bound insulin to the cytoplasm. The insulin signal activates the receptor's protein kinases domain in the cytoplasm. Proteine kinases from the receptor phosphorylate insuline-response substrates triggering other chemical responses inside the cell. When IGFBPs binds and therefore activates the IGF-Ir, the hepatic synthesis of IGFBP-I is decreased, making IGF-I more biologically available, thus enhancing androgen production by theca interstitial and stromal cells

milieu produces the blockage of the follicle growth. Thus, the premature luteinization and the consequent follicular arrest result in menstrual cycle disorders and oligo-anovulation which appears strictly related to the obesity [40]. The increased estrogen production, due to peripheral conversion, impairs the function of HPG axis and renders both estrogen excess and hyperandrogenism as major causes of anovulation in these patients.

A nature-experiment of the association obesity/infertility is related to the Laron syndrome (LS), a rare autosomal recessively inherited disease described in consanguineous families originating from Mediterranean, middle-east or south Asian regions [41]. This syndrome is characterized by a primary GH insensitivity or resistance caused by deletions or mutations in the GH receptor gene, which leads to absence of GH activity and congenital IGF-I deficiency [42]. However, one of the intriguing characteristics of LS, in addition to dwarfism, is the chronic obesity which occurs in early childhood and does not decrease with long-term IGF-I treatment. In parallel with a remarkable increase of both subcutaneous and visceral fat, the majority of patients with LS progressively develop signs of metabolic syndrome as hyperlipidemia and non-alcoholic fatty liver disease. Based on this deeply altered metabolism of lipids, the women with LS are usually subfertile and require a treatment to induce ovulation for the chronic defects in their reproductive function [43]. Therefore, given the tight interconnection between energy metabolism and reproduction, the impact that obesity induces on fertility in these women can be considered an aggravating factor in this clinical condition.

- ***Obesity, menstrual cycle and fertility in hypoandrogenic women*** - Whether most of the studies on menstrual cycle and fertility in obesity have been completed in hyperandrogenic women, very few studies examined women without hyperandrogenism and/or with normal menstrual cycle.

One cross-sectional study performed in more than 250 overweight and obese non-hyper-androgenic women partially claiming problems of infertility, showed that 64% of these women were eumenorrheic with normal menstrual cycles, whereas in the original population 21% of them had oligomenorrhea and only 14% were hyper or polimenorrheic, thus proving that oligomenorrhea is the most frequent alteration of menstrual cycle in apparently fertile obese women [44].

The same study showed that abdominal fat accumulation measured by waist circumference, is the most predictive parameter of oligomenorrhea in apparently fertile women, independently from hyperinsulinemia, insulin resistance or other parameters. However, obese non-hyperandrogenic women, even with normal menstrual cycles and apparent normal fertility, have lower circulating levels of gonadotropins, estradiol and inhibin during the follicular phase, thus suggesting an inhibitory effect of obesity per se on the production of these hormones [45]. By contrast, the number of ovary follicles does not seem to be influenced by insulin and body mass in these patients 46].

Lastly, free testosterone (FT) levels are usually higher in obese premenopausal women without hyrsutism and normal/lower circulating levels of other androgens including dehidro-epiandrosterone (DHEA), DHEA-sulphate, androstenedione and 17-OH-progesterone [46], raising the possibility that increased concentrations of FT may have a negative effect on fertility. DHEA is a hormone intermediary in the testosterone- and estrogen-pathway. Its plasma levels are significantly lower in morbid obesity [47], and are inversely correlated with total body fat. These relationships might be the expression of a lower production of DHEA by adrenal glands and/or of higher DHEA uptake in adipose tissue, as well as of a lipomobilizing effect of DHEA. On the other hand, this hormone stimulates resting metabolic rate (RMR) and lipid oxidation at the level of visceral adipose tissue in particular, and enhances the glucose disposal by increasing the expression of GLUT-1 and GLUT-4 on fat cell plasma membrane [48]. For these reasons several IVF units administer DHEA to improve the endocrine environment and the influences on the oocytes.

Therefore, on the basis of these information, it is evident that the decrease of DHEA levels may furtherly enhance the fat accumulation, thus generating a vicious circle in obesity and contributing to higher insulin concentrations and lower fertility in obese women.

Obesity effects on reproduction apparatus

Obesity may affect the woman fertility by a number of events as impairment of ovarian follicles development, qualitative and quantitative defects of oocyte maturation, altered fertilization, disrupted meiosis and mitochondrial dynamics derangements leading to abnormal embryo preimplantation [49]. The excess of free fatty acids may exert a toxic effect in reproductive tissues producing a persistent cell damage and a chronic low-grade inflammatory state. To this regard, several mechanisms have been postulated to explain why obesity and/or the overweight affect the quality of female gametes and several hypotheses are related to plasmatic levels of reproductive hormones and their metabolism.

In this contest, Machtinger et al., explored the oocytes failed to be fertilized in IVF cycles of morbidly obese women, and described disarrayed meiotic spindles with misaligned metaphase chromosomes [50]. Independently from aneuploidy, obesity also appears to alter the mitochondrial function in the oocyte. One potential mechanism for oocyte organelle damage in obesity is the lipotoxicity. In fact, the excess fatty acids obtained from the diet can be stored as triglycerides in adipocytes although they are apparently unable to induce the cellular damage in this storage compartment. However, when this capacity is overwhelmed with continued dietary excess, fatty acids accumulate in other tissues and exert their toxic effects known as lipotoxicity [51].

Furthermore, obese women have higher levels of circulating free fatty acids, which damage non adipose cells by increasing reactive oxygen species (ROS) that, in turn, induce mitochondrial and ER stress resulting in apoptosis of multiple cell types including oocytes [52]. This effect is related to the chronic low grade inflammatory state related to obesity which is proven by the increased circulating levels of C-reactive protein (CRP), as well as lactate and triglyceride concentrations in follicular fluid, and by the enhanced expression of pro-inflammatory (CXCL2) and oxidative stress related (DUSP) genes [53].

The preimplantation embryo is also affected by the endometrial obese environment. Comparison of human IVF cycles with autologous oocytes show that obese women are more likely to create poor quality embryos [54] as effect of the lipotoxicity of embryonic cells in a similar fashion as described for the oocyte. However, there are conflicting data as to whether obesity has a significant effect on the endometrium. Although many factors contribute to restrain reproductive outcomes in obese women, Rhee JS et al., in their study emphasize the importance of decidualization defects in obese women which would alter the endometrial receptivity resulting in poor implantation [55].

The 'at risk' fertility in obese women

Although in a high percentage of obese women the pregnancy occurs with normal accomplishment, several risks in their conception plans need to be considered and are briefly discussed.

Impact on egg viability and quality

The constitutive ovarian reserve in fertile women is not unlimited and the number of maturing oocytes usually declines with aging. For this reason, the impact of maternal environment and obesity on the differentiation of these cells is particularly consequential and negative environmental exposures may affect the developmental competence of the oocyte, defined as the ability of mature oocytes to be fertilized and support the embryo development [56]. Thus, based on the systemic inflammatory state associated to the obesity, the oocyte maturation is variably affected by the altered balance of driver hormones as SHBG with other soluble factors including insulin, glucose, lactate, triglycerides, and C reactive protein [53].

High BMI values also alter the concentration of certain adipokines. In rodent models, high concentrations of leptin impair the follicle development, ovulation, and oocyte maturation [57], whereas leptin deficient mice (ob/ob) are the animal experimental model to investigate the effects of obesity, and female ob/ob mice develop low numbers of antral follicules resulting in impaired folliculogenesis, reduced ovulation rate, and accelerated apoptosis of granulosa cells [58].

Furthermore, elevated levels of leptin associated with high BMI also impairs the steroidogenesis. The mechanisms by which leptin regulates the steroidogenesis in human granulosa cells have been investigated by Lin Q. et al., in experimental studies completed in 40 granulosa cell lines obtained from explanted human granulosa samples during in vitro fertilization program [59]. They show that human granulosa cells after exposure to high dosage of recombinant human leptin, inhibit 8-bromo cAMP-stimulated progesterone production in a dose-dependent manner with downregulation of StAR mRNA levels, a steroidogenic regulatory protein, produced for the progesterone synthesis. Therefore, they suggest that leptin interferes with the secretion of gonadotropin-stimulated proge-sterone in these cells and with induction of StAR protein by cAMP which, thus, is significantly reduced. They also proved that both cAMP-regulated steroidogenic enzymes and progesterone production could be inhibited by leptin via the MAPK pathway. These results confirm that leptin acts through its receptor to initiate the MAPK pathway and downregulates the cAMP-induced steroidogenesis in human granulosa cells [59].

Leptin receptors are structurally similar to the class I cytokine receptor family [53]. In humans, the leptin receptor (OB-R) is produced in several alternatively spliced forms, designated OB-Ra, OB-Rb, OB-Rc, OB-Re [60]. Each of these isoforms shows an extracellular domain and a transmembrane domain in common, with a variable intracellular domain typical for each isoform. Based on the variable intracellular domain, these isoforms are classified as short (OB-Ra), long (OB-Rb) and secreted (OB-Re) leptin receptor. Other than the classical JAK/STAT signalling pathways, leptin may act through OB-Ra or OB-Rb to trigger the MAPK cascade in two different ways, namely via tyrosine phosphorylation of JAK2 receptor-associated activation, or independently from the receptor phosphorylation [61]. Thus, the stimulation of granulosa cells by leptin was used to investigate the activation of MAPK pathway suggesting that MAPK cascades are involved in leptin mediated inhibition of steroidogenesis in granulosa cells by the phosphorylation of ERK, p38 and JNK.

Adiponectin is primarily secreted by adipocytes, but its serum levels drop down in obesity and in insulin resistance while increasing with weight loss [62]. It has been demonstrated that in obese women where circulating levels are lower, there would just reflect the insulin sensitivity and that this effect may negatively influence the control of ovulation since adiponectin is variably detectable in ovaries, follicular fluid, oocyte, corpus luteum, theca cells, while is weakly expressed by granulosa cells [63]. However, the direct effect of adiponectin in ovarian function remains unclear. In animal models, the protein has been described to influence both folliculogenesis and the follicular remodelling as well as to modulate the sex steroid secretion via activation of its own receptors R1 and R2, and by modulating the insulin/IGF system [64].

Ledoux and co-workers examined the effects of recombinant porcine adiponectin on porcine ovarian granulosa cells in vitro and demonstrated that the protein at physiologically levels equal to 10–25 μg/ml, provokes expression of genes committed to the periovulatory remodelling of the ovarian follicle over a time frame of 6-24 h. These include cyclooxygenase-2, prostaglandin E synthase, and vascular endothelial growth factor. Therefore, adiponectin modulates steroid synthetic protein gene expression by increasing the steroidogenic acute regulatory protein transcript and, concurrently, by reducing the cytochrome P450 aromatase. Finally, these studies demonstrated that the MAPK pathway, via phosphorylation of ERK1/2, is involved in mediation of the adiponectin signal in ovarian granulosa cells, rather than the protein kinase A, or the classic adiponectin transducer AMP-activated protein kinase. These results suggested that since adiponectin synthesis is reduced in obesity, this defect may play a substantial role in obesity-related ovarian dysfunction [64].

Other adipokines such as interluekin-6 (IL6), plasminogen activator inhibitor (PAI) type-1, or TNF family members may affect oocyte competence or maturation through alterations in steroidogenesis and interaction with other metabolic hormones [65]. While the mechanisms by which adipokines impact the oocyte quality have not been elucidated yet, their altered concentrations due to obesity represent the major potential factor by which obesity may negatively impact on the oocyte health thus affecting the fertility in women.

Obesity and miscarriage rate

The association between obesity and miscarriage has been assessed in a number of studies in both natural and assisted conceptions in which the miscarriage risk was as high as up to approximately 40% in obese women with respect to less than 15% in females with a normal BMI. However, despite these findings, there is no consensus about the causative mechanisms in obese women [66].

A major pathogenic factor could be related to the impaired stromal decidualization in obese women which is responsible of placental abnormalities, stillbirth and preeclampsia [67], although the most frequent cause of first trimester miscarriages usually related to embryo chromosomal pathologies, does not seem to be increased in overweight women [68].

AMH in obese patients

Anti-Mullerian hormone (AMH) is a product of the granulosa cells of small antral and pre-antral follicles, and clinically, it may be reflective of the prediction of ovarian reserve in women undergoing fertility evaluation and treatment [69]. For this reason, is important to evaluate the change in the levels of AMH, as a fertility parameter in obese women with or without PCOS, submitted to aerobic exercise with the aim of losing weight. The slimming via exercise or diet is considered one of the most important targets in lifestyle modification programmes capable to induce an improvement in reproductive function among obese women with PCOS [70]. Exercise interventions of moderate activity are one of the most important lifestyle modifications that positively influence on fertility and assisted reproductive technology outcomes [71].

Einas AE and coworkers, have studied the possible correlation with adiposity, clinical and hormonal parameters in PCOS and normo-ovulatory women, conducting a one-year study among obese women with or without polycystic ovary syndrome. All patients were classified into three age-matched groups; group A: controls, group B: PCOS patients and group C: obese women. The AMH, was measured at baseline and following 12 weeks of supervised aerobic exercise. They conclude that the change in AMH levels correlated significantly with physical activity, therefore the authors claim that a moderate aerobic training for 12 weeks had a positive significant effect on reproductive functions via modulating adiposity, AMH and fertility in obese women with or without PCOS [72].

Influence of obesity on fertility treatments

Overweight and obese women have lower outcomes following fertility treatments than normal population. They poorly respond to induction of ovulation, require higher doses of gonadotropins and longer treatment courses for follicular development and ovulatory cycles. In addition, the oocyte yield is lower in obese women resulting in a higher rate of cycle cancellation [73]. Ovarian stimulation for assisted reproduction produces fewer follicles leading to the harvest of fewer oocytes. Thus, the fertilization rates are scarce and the embryo quality is impaired in younger obese undergoing fertility treatments who definitely show low pregnancy rate with increased risk of early pregnancy loss.

Glueck CJ et al., report in their study that insulin sensitising-lowering agents ameliorate the reproductive, and metabolic disorders, typical of the obese patient [74]. The action of metformin is widely discussed in the literature, which is considered as the first-line medication for the treatment of type 2 diabetes. Women with PCOS receiving metformin improved pregnancy outcomes, and this has been attributed to its ability to reduce the insulin resistance as well as hyperinsulinaemia and the inhibitor of the hypofibrinolytic plasminogen activator resulting in improvement of oocyte quality and folliculogenesis for amelioration of PCOS.

The major effects of metformin include its property to decrease the liver glucose production by suppressing hepatic gluconeogenesis as well as the increase of insulin sensitivity and peripheral glucose uptake [75]. The molecular mechanism of metformin is incompletely understood. Multiple potential mechanisms of action have been proposed, including; inhibition of the mitochondrial respiratory chain (complex I), activation of AMP-activated protein kinase (AMPK), inhibition of glucagon induced elevation of cyclic adenosine monophosphate (cAMP) with reduced activation of protein kinase A (PKA), inhibition of mitochondrial glycerophosphate dehydrogenase, and an effect on gut microbiota [76]. All these activities may have contributed to improve the oocyte maturation in PCOS and may exert a definitive favorable effect on infertility associated to inefficient oocyte differentiation and maturation.

Benefits from weight loss

Weight loss has been shown to improve reproductive outcomes by ameliorating fertility, as well as by regularizing menstrual cycles and increasing the chance of spontaneous ovulation and conception in anovulatory overweight and obese women.

Available data suggest that the weight loss equal to 5%–10% of the body weight may definitely improve the fertility rate [77], whereas other studies prove that 5% of weight loss results in significant improvement of endocrine parameters, such as decrease of free testosterone, and LH and insulin levels, with the improvement of ovulation frequency [78].

Sim and collaborators investigated the effects of weight loss in overweight and/or obese women undergoing assisted reproductive procedures on their subsequent pregnancy outcome. In their observation, the weight loss achieved by diet and lifestyle change resulted in significantly increased pregnancy rates and/or live birth in overweight and/or obese women undergoing assisted reproductive technology (ART) in 8 of the 11 studies reviewed. In addition, regularization of the menstrual pattern, decrease in cancellation rates, increase in number of embryos available for transfer, reduction in the number of ART cycles required to achieve pregnancy, and a significant decrease in miscarriage rates were reported. Interestingly, an increase of the number of natural conceptions in five of the six studies was also reported [79].

However, the decision to postpone the treatment of fertility to allow weight loss often results in a further increase in maternal age in women who are not very young. A recent study demonstrated that the effect of BMI on IVF success was strongly influenced by age. In fact, the effect of BMI reduction alone is apparently reduced with increasing age, and in women aged 36 yrs. or older, the weight loss may sometimes result not functional in favouring the woman fertility [80].

Conclusions

Overweight and obese women need longer time to conceive and undoubtedly are at higher risk of infertility. Higher BMI is also associated with adverse pregnancy outcomes, such as gestational diabetes and hypertension and women undergoing undergoing in vitro fertilization may experience negative outcomes at higher rate than normal weight females. However, as early symptoms of dysfunctional oocyte maturation and hormone derangements, oligomenorrhea and alterations of menstrual cycles should primarily alert overweight and obese women on their potentially defective fertility. The impact of obesity on reproductive function, especially associated with ovulatory disorders, is mainly due to neuroendocrine mechanisms, which interfere with ovarian functions, and are able to affect the ovulation rate and the endometrial receptivity. Obese women, even with normal menstrual cycles and apparently normal fertility, have lower circulating levels of gonadotropins, estradiol and inhibin in the follicular phase, suggesting an inhibitory effect of the obesity condition per se on the production of these hormones.

Since the obesity is pathogenically associated to inflammation, all mechanisms enrolled in oocyte differentiation and maturation including hormones, proteins and soluble factors released by adipocytes are deregulated and affected in their physiology. The direct effect of adipose tissue in lowering the fertility potential in women is thus based on the derangement of major molecular mechanisms that regulate the normal biological activity of cell components of the woman reproductive organs also controlled through the hypothalamus hypophysis ovaries axis.

In conclusion, in terms of human and social impact of obesity in women during the reproductive phase, this disease does not affect only the cardiovascular system and the skeleton health for higher incidence of osteoporosis and dramatically restrains the physical activity in addition to the unfavourable aesthetic impact in women, but also provides suffering in relation to the lower probabilities to conceive and normal pregnancies as in non-obese females.

Abbreviations

IL1β: Interleukin 1β; TNFα: Tumor necrosis factor α; AMH: Anti-Mullerian hormone; AMPK: AMP-activated preotein kinas; APN: Adiponectin; APN-LMW: Adiponectin at low molecular weight; APN-MMW: at medium molecular weight; APN-HMW: at high molecular weight; ART: Assisted reproductive technology; BMI: Body mass index; cAMP: Cyclic adenosine monophosphate; DHEA: Dehidro-epiandrosterone; FT: Free testosterone; GH: Growth hormone; HOMA: Homeostasis model assessment; HPO: Hypothalamic-pituitary-ovarian; IGFBP: Insulin-like growth factor binding proteins; IGF-I: Insulin-like growth factor-I; IGF-IR: IGF-I receptors; IL6: Interleukin 6; IL6: Interluekin-6; IR: Insulin resistance; LCN2: Lipocalin-2 (LCN2); LEPR: Leptin receptor; LS: Laron syndrome; OSHA: Occupational Safety and Health Administration; PAI: Plasminogen activator inhibitor; PCOS: Polycystic ovary syndrome; PKA: Protein kinase A; RBP4: Protein-4; RMR: Resting metabolic rate; ROS: Reactive oxygen species; SHBG: Sex hormone binding globulin; SHBG: Sex hormone-binding globulin; T2DM: Type 2 diabetes mellitus; TG: Triglyceride

Acknowledgements

None.

Funding

No funding was requested for this review.

Authors' contributions

ES and GL conceived the idea. GDP and RR were involved in literature collection. All authors independently and critically reviewed the selected manuscripts. ES and GDP were involved in drafting the early manuscript and equally contributed to the first draft, which was then expanded and improved by all authors. All authors read and approved the final manuscript.

Competing interests

The authors declare they have no competing interests.

Author details

[1]Interdisciplinary Department of Medicine, Section of Obstetrics and Gynecology, University of Bari Aldo Moro, P.za G.Cesare, 11-70124 Bari, Italy. [2]Departmentof Biomedical Sciences and Human Oncology, Section of Internal Medicine and Clinical Oncology, University of Bari Aldo Moro, P.za G.Cesare, 11-70124 Bari, Italy.

References

1. McGee EA, Hsueh AJ. Initial and cyclic recruitment of ovarian follicles. Endocr Rev. 2000;21:200–14.
2. Habbema JD, Collins J, Leridon H, et al. Towards less confusing terminology in reproductive medicine: a proposal. Hum Reprod. 2004;19:1497–501.
3. Willem Ombelet, Ian Cooke, Sylke Dyer, Gamal Serour and Paul Devroey. Infertility and the provision of infertility medical services in developing countries . Human Reproud Hupdate. 2008;14(6):605-21.
4. Templeton A. Infertility and the establishment of pregnancy-overview. Br Med Bull. 2000;56:577–87.
5. Chavarro JE, Rich-Edwards JW, Rosner BA, Willett WC. Diet and lifestyle in the prevention of ovulatory disorder infertility. Obstet Gynecol. 2007;110: 1050–8.
6. Balen AH, Rutherford AJ. Managing anovulatory infertility and polycystic ovary syndrome. BMJ. 2007;335(7621):663–6.
7. Khalaf Y. Tubal subfertility. BMJ. 2003;327(7415):610–3.
8. Johnson N, Farquhar C. Endometriosis. BJM Clin Evid. 2007;2007:0802.
9. Quaas A, Dokras A. Diagnosis and treatment of unexplained infertility. Rev Obstet Gynecol. 2008;1(2):69–76.
10. Greil AL, Slauson-Blevins K, McQuillan J. The experience of infertility: a review of recent literature. Sociol Health Illn. 2010;32(1):140–62.
11. Cousineau TM, Domar AD. Psychological impact of infertility. Best Pract Res Cl Ob. 2007;21(2):293–308.
12. King RB. Subfecundity and anxiety in a nationally representative sample. Soc Sci Med. 2003;56(4):739–51.
13. Klonoff-Cohen H, Natarajan L. The concerns during assisted reproductive technologies (CART) scale and pregnancy outcomes. Fertil Steril. 2004;81(4):982–8.
14. Dorfman SF. Tobacco and fertility: our responsabilities. Fertil Steril. 2008; 89(3):502–4.
15. Curtis KM, Savitz DA, Arbuckle TE. Effect of cigarette smoking, caffeine consumption, and alcohol intake on fecundability. Am J Epidemiol. 1997; 146:32–41.
16. Janet W, et al. Adolescent body mass index and infertility caused by ovulatory disorder. AJOG. 1994;171(1):171–7.
17. Orio F, et al. Effects of physical exercise on the female reproductive system. Minerva Endocrinol. 2013 Sep;38(3):305–19.
18. Lawson C, et al. Occupational exposures among nurses and risk of spontaneous abortion. Am J Obstet Gynecol. 2012;206(4):327.e1–327.8.
19. World Health Organization. Preventing and managing the global epidemic. In: Report of the World Health Organization on obesity. Geneva: World Health Organization; 1997. http://www.who.int/nutrition/publications/obesity/WHO_TRS_894/en/.
20. Haslam DW, James WP. Obesity. Lancet. 2005;366:1197–209.
21. ASRM-American Society for Reproductive Medicine. Practice Committee of American Society for reproductive medicine. De nitions of infertility and recurrent pregnancy loss. Fertil Steril. 2008;90:S60.
22. Pasquali R, Pelusi C, Genghini S, Cacciari M, Gambineri A. Obesity and Reproductive disorders in women. Hum Reprod Update. 2003;9:359–72.
23. Talmor A, Dunphy B. Female obesity and infertility. Best Pract Res Clin Obstet Gynaecol. 2015;29:498–506.
24. Wise LA, Rothman KJ, Mikkelsen EM, Sorensen HT, Riis A, Hatch EE. An internet-based prospective study of body size and time-to-pregnancy. Hum Reprod. 2010;25:253–64.
25. Gesink Law DC, Maclehose RF, Longnecker MP. Obesity and time to pregnancy. Hum Reprod. 2007, 22:414–20.
26. Bellver J, Ayllon Y, Ferrando M, Melo M, Goyri E, Pellicer A, Remohi J, Meseguer M. Female obesity impairs in vitro fertilization outcome without affecting embryo quality. Fertil Steril. 2010;93:447–54.
27. Budak E, Fernandezsanchez M, Bellver J, Cervero A, Simon C, Pellicer A. Interactions of the hormones leptin, ghrelin, adiponectin, resistin, and PYY3-36 with the reproductive system. Fertil Steril. 2006;85:1563–81.
28. Brannian JD, Zhao Y, McElroy M. Leptin inhibits gonadotrophin-stimulated granulosa cell progesterone production by antagonizing insulin action. Hum Reprod. 1999;14:1445–8.
29. Hug C, Wang J, Ahmad NS, Bogan JS, Tsao TS, Lodish HF. T-cadherin is a receptor for hexameric and high-molecular-weight forms of Acrp30/adiponectin. PNAS. 2004;101:10308–13.
30. Psilopanagioti A, Papadaki H, Kranioti EF, Alexandrides TK, Varakis JN. Expression of adiponectin and adiponectin receptors in human pituitary gland and brain. Neuroendocrinology. 2009;89:38–47.
31. Michalakis KG, Segars JH. The role of adiponectin in reproduction: from polycystic ovary syndrome to assisted reproduction. Fertil Steril. 2010;94: 1949–57.
32. Kim KH, Lee K, Moon YS, Sul HS. A cysteine-rich adipose tissue specific secretory factor inhibits adipocyte differentiation. J Biol Chem. 2001;276: 11252–6.

33. Schwartz DR, Lazar MA. Human resistin: found in translation from mouse to man. Trends Endocrinol Metab. 2011;22:259–65.
34. Spicer LJ, Schreiber NB, Lagaly DV, Aad PY, Douthit LB, Grado-Ahuir JA. Effect of resistin on granulosa and theca cell function in cattle. Anim Reprod Sci. 2011; 124:19–27.
35. Fukuhara A, Matsuda M, Nishizawa M, Segawa K, Tanaka M, Kishimoto K, Matsuki Y, Murakami M, Ichisaka T, Murakami H, et al. Visfatin: a protein secreted by visceral fat that mimics the effects of insulin. Science. 2005;307:426–30.
36. Tan BK, Chen J, Digby JE, Keay SD, Kennedy CR, Randeva HS. Increased visfatin messenger ribonucleic acid and protein levels in adipose tissue and adipocytes in women with polycystic ovary syndrome: parallel increase in plasma visfatin. J Clin Endocrinol Metab. 2006a;91:5022–8.
37. De Souza Batista CM, Yang RZ, Lee MJ, Glynn NM, Yu DZ, Pray J, et al. Omentin plasma levels and gene expression are decreased in obesity. Diabetes. 2007;56:1655–61.
38. Poretsky L, Grigorescu F, Seibel M, Moses AC, Flier JS. Distribution and characterization of insulin and insulin-like growth factor 1 receptors in normal human ovary. J Clin Endocrinol Metab. 1985;61:728–34.
39. Hillier SG. Current concepts of the roles of follicle stimulating hormone and luteinizing hormone in folliculogenesis. Hum Reprod. 1994;9:188–91.
40. Franks S, Robinson S, Willis D. Nutrition, Insulin and polycistic ovary syndrome. Rev Reprod. 1996;1:47–53.
41. Laron Z, Pertzelan A, Mannheimer S. Genetic pituitary dwarfism with high serum concentation of growth hormone – a new inborn error of metabolism? Isr J Med Sci. 1966;2:152–5.
42. Laron Z. Laron syndrome (primary growth hormone resistance or insensitivity): the personal experience 1958–2003. J Clin Endocrinol Metab. 2004;89:1031–44.
43. Hull KL, Harvey S. Growth hormone: roles in female reproduction. J Endocrinol. 2001;168:1–23.
44. De Pergola G, Tartagni M, d'Angelo F, Centoducati C, Guida P, Giorgino R. Abdominal fat accumulation, and not insulin resistance, is associated to oligomenorrhea in non-hyperandrogenic overweight/obese women. J Endocrinol Investig. 2009;32:98–101.
45. De Pergola G, Maldera S, Tartagni M, Pannacciulli N, Loverro G, Giorgino R. Inhibitory effect of obesity on gonadotropin, estradiol, and inhibin B levels in fertile women. Obesity 2006;14:1954–1960.
46. Giagulli VA, De Pergola G, Giorgino F, Cignarelli M, Abbaticchio GF, Vermeulen A, Giorgino R. Increased free testosterone but normal 5α-reduced testosterone metabolites in obese premenopausal women. Clin Endocrinol. 1992;36:553–8.
47. De Pergola G, Giagulli VA, Garruti G, Cospite MR, Giorgino F, Cignarelli M, Giorgino R. Low dehydrooepiandrosterone circulating levels in premenopausal obese women with very high body mass index. Metabolism. 1991;40:187–90.
48. De Pergola G. The adipose tissue metabolism: role of testosterome and dehydroepiandro-sterone. Int J Obes. 2000;24(suppl. 2):S59–63.
49. Jungheim ES, Travieso JL, Hopeman MM. Weighing the impact of obesity on female reproductive function and fertility. Nutr Rev. 2013;71:3–8.
50. Machtinger R, Combelles CM, Missmer SA, Correia KF, Fox JH, Racowsky C. The association between severe obesity and characteristics of failed fertilized oocytes. Hum Reprod. 2012;27:3198–207.
51. Sorensen TI, Virtue S, Vidal-Puig A. Obesity as a clinical and public health problrm: is there a need for a new definition based on lipotoxicity effects? Biochim Biophys Acta. 2010;1801:400–4.
52. Broughton DE, Jungheim ES. A focused look at obesity and the preimplantation trophoblast. Semin Reprod Med. 2016;34:5–10.
53. Robker RL, Akison LK, Bennet BD, Thrupp PN, Chura LR, Russell DL, et al. Obese women exhibit differences in ovarian metabolites, hormones, and gene expression compared with moderate-weight women. J Clin Endocrinol Metab. 2009;94:1533–40.
54. Carrell DT, Jones KP, Peterson CM, Aoki V, Emery BR, Campbell BR. Body mass index is inversely related to intrafollicular hCG concentrations, embryo quality and IVF outcome. Reprod BioMed Online. 2001;3:109–11.
55. Rhee JS, Saben JL, Mayer AL, Schulte MB, Asghar Z, Stephens C, et al. Diet induced obesity impairs endometrial stromal cell decidualization: a potential role for impaired autophagy. Hum Reprod. 2016;31:1315–26.
56. Purcell SH, Moley KH. The impact of obesity on egg quality. J Assist Reprod Genet. 2011;28:517–24.
57. Duggal PS, Van Der Hoek KH, Milner CR, Ryan NK, Armstrong DT, Magoffin DA, et al. The in vivo and in vitro effects of exogenous leptin on ovulation in the rat. Endocrinology. 2000;141(6):1971.
58. Pallares P, Garcia-Fernandez RA, Criado LM, Letelier CA, Fernandez-Toro JM, Esteban D, et al. Substantiation of ovarian effects of leptin by challenging a mouse model of obesity/type 2 diabetes. Theriogenology. 2010;73:1088–95.
59. Lin Q, Poon SL, Chen J, Cheng L, HoYuen B, Leung PC. Leptin interferes with 3',5'-cyclic adenosine monophosphate (cAMP) signaling to inhibit steroidogenesis in human granulosa cells. Reprod Biol Endocrinol. 2009;7:115.
60. Poretsky L, Cataldo NA, Rosenwaks Z, Giudice LC. The insulin- related ovarian regulatory system in health and disease. Endocr Rev. 1999;20:535–82.
61. Diamond MP, Moley KH, Pellicer A, Vaughn WK, DeCherney AH. Effects of streptozotocin and alloxan-induced diabetes mellitus on mouse follicular and early embryo development. J Reprod Fertil. 1989;86:1–10.
62. Gosman GG, Katcher HI, Legro RS. Obesity and the role of gut and adipose hormones in female reproduction. Hum Reprod Update. 2006;12:585–601.
63. Pierre P, Froment P, Negre D, Rame C, Barateau V, Chabrolle C, Lecomte P, Dupont J. Role of adiponectin receptors, AdipoR1 and AdipoR2, in the steroidogenesis of the human granulosa tumor cell line, KGN. Hum Reprod. 2009;24:2890–901.
64. Ledoux S, Campos DB, Lopes FL, Dobias-Goff M, Palin MF, Murphy BD. Adiponectin induces periovulatory changes in ovarian follicular cells. Endocrinology. 2006;147:5178–86.
65. Brewer CJ, Balen AH. The adverse effects of obesity on conception and implantation. Reproduction. 2010;140:347–64.
66. Metwally M, Tuckerman EM, Laird SM, Ledger WL, Li TC. Impact of high body mass index on endometrial morphology and function in the peri-implantation period in women with recurrent miscarriage. Reprod BioMed Online. 2007;14:328–34.
67. Ruebel ML, Cotter M, Sims CR, Moutos DM, Badger TM, Cleves MA, Shankar K, Andres A. Obesity modulates inflammation and lipid metabolism oocyte gene expression: a single cell transcriptome perspective. J Clin Endocrinol Metab. 2017; https://doi.org/10.1210/jc.2016-3524.
68. Bellver J, Cruz F, Martínez MC, Ferro J, Ramírez JF, Pellicer A, Garrido N. Female overweight is not associated with a higher embryo euploidy rate in first trimester miscarriages karyotyped by hysteroembryoscopy. Fertil Steril. 2011;96:931–3.
69. Anderson RA, Nelson SM, Wallace WH. Measuring anti-Müllerian hormone for the assessment of ovarian reserve: when and for whom is it indicated? Maturitas. 2012;71(1):28–33.
70. Crosignani PG, Colombo M, Vegetti W, Somigliana E, Gessati A, Ragni G. Overweight and obese anovulatory patients with polycystic ovaries: parallel improvements in anthropometric indices, ovarian physiology and fertility rate induced by diet. Hum Reprod. 2003;18:1928–32.
71. Rich-Edwards JW, Spiegelman D, Garland M, Hertzmark E, Hunter DJ, Colditz GA, et al. Physical activity, body mass index, and ovulatory disorder infertility. Epidemiology. 2002;13:184–90.
72. Einas AE, Sami AG, Ahmad HA. Effects of supervised aerobic training on the levels of anti-Mullerian hormone and adiposity measures in women with normo-ovulatory and polycystic ovary syndrome. J Pak Med Assoc. 2017;67:4.
73. Fedorcsak P, Dale PO, Storeng R, Ertzeid G, Bjercke S, Oldereid N, et al. Impact of overweight and underweight on assisted reproduction treatment. Hum Reprod. 2004;19:2523–8.
74. Glueck CJ, Streicher P, Wang P. Treatment of polycystic ovary syndrome with insulin-lowering agents. Expert Opin Pharmacother. 2002 Aug;3(8):1177–89.
75. Collier CA, Bruce CR, Smith AC, Lopaschuk G, Dyck DJ. Metformin counters the insulin-induced suppression of fatty acid oxidation and stimulation of triacylglycerol storage in rodent skeletal muscle. Am J Physiol Endocrinol Metab. 2006;291(1):E182–9.
76. Rena G, Pearson ER, Sakamoto K. Molecular mechanism of action of metformin: old or new insights? Diabetologia. 2013;56(9):1898–906.
77. Clark AM, Ledger W, Galletly C, Tomlinson L, Blaney F, Wang X, et al. Weight loss results in significant improvement in pregnancy and ovulation rates in anovulatory obese women. Hum Reprod. 1995;10:2705–12.
78. Kiddy DS, Hamilton-Fairley D, Bush A, Short F, Anyaoku V, Reed MJ, et al. Improvement in endocrine and ovarian function during dietary treatment of obese women with polycystic ovary syndrome. Clin Endocrinol. 1992;36: 105–11.
79. Sim KA, Partridge SR, Sainsbury A. Does weight loss in overweight or obese women improve fertility treatment outcomes? A systematic review. Obes Comorbidity. 2014;15:839–50.
80. Sneed ML, Uhler ML, Grotjan HE, Rapisarda JJ, Lederer KJ, Beltsos AN. Body mass index: impact on IVF success appears age-related. Hum Reprod. 2008; 23:1835–9.

9

Suppressive regulatory T cells and latent transforming growth factor-β-expressing macrophages are altered in the peritoneal fluid of patients with endometriosis

Tetsuro Hanada[1], Shunichiro Tsuji[1*], Misako Nakayama[2], Shiro Wakinoue[1], Kyoko Kasahara[1], Fuminori Kimura[1], Takahide Mori[3], Kazumasa Ogasawara[2] and Takashi Murakami[1]

Abstract

Background: Endometriosis is a known cause of infertility. Differences in immune tolerance caused by regulatory T cells (Tregs) and transforming growth factor-β (TGF-β) are thought to be involved in the pathology of endometriosis. Evidence has indicated that Tregs can be separated into three functionally and phenotypically distinct subpopulations and that activated TGF-β is released from latency-associated peptide (LAP) on the surfaces of specific cells. The aim of this study was to examine differences in Treg subpopulations and LAP in the peripheral blood (PB) and peritoneal fluid (PF) of patients with and without endometriosis.

Methods: PB and PF were collected from 28 women with laparoscopically and histopathologically diagnosed endometriosis and 20 disease-free women who were subjected to laparoscopic surgery. Three subpopulations of $CD4^+$ T lymphocytes ($CD45RA^+FoxP3^{low}$ resting Tregs, $CD45RA^-FoxP3^{high}$ effector Tregs, and $CD45RA^-FoxP3^{low}$ non-Tregs) and $CD11b^+$ mononuclear cells expressing LAP were analyzed by flow cytometry using specific monoclonal antibodies.

Results: Proportions of suppressive Tregs (resting and effector Tregs) were significantly higher in the PF samples of patients with endometriosis than in those of control women ($P = 0.02$ and $P < 0.01$, respectively) but did not differ between the PB samples of patients and controls. The percentage of $CD11b^+LAP^+$ macrophages was significantly lower in PF samples of patients with endometriosis than in those of controls ($P < 0.01$) but was not altered in the PB samples.

Conclusion: Proportions of suppressive Tregs and LAP^+ macrophages are altered locally in the PF of endometriosis patients.

Keywords: Regulatory T cell, TGF-β, Latency-associated peptide, Endometriosis

Background

Endometriosis, defined by the presence of endometrial glands and stroma outside the uterus, is a common, chronic, estrogen-dependent disease contributing to dysmenorrhea and infertility. One leading theory hypothesizes that peritoneal lesions are derived from steroid hormone-sensitive endometrial cells and tissues that are implanted on the peritoneal surface during retrograde menstruation, eliciting an inflammatory response. Although most women exhibit retrograde menstruation, affected women may suffer from immune dysfunction that interferes with the clearing of such lesions [1].

FoxP3-expressing $CD4^+$ regulatory T cells (Tregs) play an indispensable role in the maintenance of self-tolerance and immune homeostasis [2] and are involved in various human diseases, such as autoimmune diseases, allergies, and cancer [3–5]. $FoxP3^+$ cells, however, are heterogeneous in function and phenotype. Miyara et al. suggested that human FoxP3-expressing $CD4^+$ Tregs can be separated into three functionally and phenotypically distinct subpopulations: 1) $CD45RA^+FoxP3^{low}$ resting Tregs (rTregs), 2) $CD45RA^-FoxP3^{high}$ effector Tregs (eTregs), and 3)

* Correspondence: tsuji002@belle.shiga-med.ac.jp
[1]Department of Obstetrics and Gynecology, Shiga University of Medical Science, Seta Tsukionowa-cho, Otsu, Shiga 520-2192, Japan
Full list of author information is available at the end of the article

cytokine-secreting CD45RA$^-$FoxP3^{low} non-Tregs (non-Tregs) [6, 7]. rTregs and eTregs have been shown to be suppressive Tregs, whereas non-Tregs are non-suppressive. Although rTregs do not exhibit proliferative potential in vitro, upon antigenic stimulation, they acquire an eTreg phenotype, i.e., FoxP3 is upregulated, followed by proliferation and eventual differentiation into eTregs. In humans, conflicting results have been obtained regarding whether populations of Tregs in the peritoneal fluid (PF) or peripheral blood (PB) differ significantly between patients with endometriosis and controls [8–10]. Moreover, the association between endometriosis and Treg subpopulations has not been well studied. Thus, in this study, we focused on assessing the association of each Treg subpopulation with endometriosis.

Transforming growth factor-β (TGF-β) induces FoxP3$^+$ Tregs and inhibits the proliferation of immune cells and cytokine production via FoxP3-dependent and -independent mechanisms [11]. TGF-β is secreted as an inactive form that is trapped by latency-associated peptide (LAP) to form the small latent complex. The addition of the latent TGF-β-binding protein forms the large latent complex, which is deposited onto the extracellular matrix. After being released from LAP, activated TGF-β plays important roles in the control of cell proliferation, differentiation, and apoptosis [12]. According to several studies, a strong association between TGF-β levels in PF and endometriosis has been observed [13]. PF mainly comprises macrophages, with smaller numbers of lymphocytes, natural killer cells, and mesothelial cells [14, 15]. However, the contribution of activated TGF-β released from macrophages remains unclear, as the surface expression of LAP on the macrophages of endometriosis patients has not yet been determined.

Therefore, in the present study, we assessed the immunotolerance of patients with endometriosis by analyzing Treg subpopulations and LAP expression in macrophages and monocytes derived from the PF and PB, respectively, of patients with endometriosis and controls.

Methods

Patients

This single-center study was approved by the Ethics Committee of Shiga University of Medical Science (approval number: 26–217) prior to patient recruitment. Patients were recruited the day before surgery when they were hospitalized in the University Hospital. All participants were Japanese, and only women who still exhibited a menstrual cycle were recruited; patients who were menstruating at the time of admission were not recruited. All patients accepted the recruitment, and they were distributed into endometriosis group or control group based on the findings of laparoscopic surgery and post-surgical histopathology. Five patients were excluded (4 due to insufficient volume of the PF and 1 due to an acute inflammatory finding during surgery and a diagnosis of chlamydia peritonitis after surgery), and a total of 28 women diagnosed with endometriosis (mean age: 34.3 years, range: 23–46 years) were enrolled. All patients with endometriosis were classified as stage I–IV according to the revised American Society for Reproductive Medicine classification [16]. In the endometriosis group, 12 patients were in the proliferative phase, and 16 were in the secretory phase. Patients without visible endometriotic foci and pelvic inflammation who underwent laparoscopic excision of benign ovarian tumors and uterine myomas or diagnostic laparoscopy for infertility were assigned to the control group. A total of 20 women were enrolled in the control group (mean age: 36.1 years, range: 19–46 years). In the control group, 10 were in the proliferative phase, and 10 were in the secretory phase. Samples in the proliferative phase were collected on days 5–10 of the menstrual cycle, and samples in the secretory phase were collected on days 3–10 after ovulation. None of the patients were being treated with pharmacological medications, such as gonadotropin-releasing hormone agonists, low-dose estrogen and progestin, or dienogest, and all patients were free from other acute or chronic inflammatory diseases. Table 1 shows a summary of patient characteristics, including phase of the menstrual cycle and stage of endometriosis.

Sample collection

PB samples were obtained from patients and controls and were added to heparin-containing tubes within 24 h of surgery. PB mononuclear cells (PBMCs) were isolated from residual blood cells by density gradient centrifugation using Ficoll-Paque PLUS (GE Healthcare, Little Chalfont, UK). Cells were washed twice with phosphate-buffered saline by centrifugation at 400×*g* for 10 min. PF was aspirated by a laparoscopic procedure and added to heparin-containing tubes. The supernatant from the ascites was collected by centrifugation at 400×*g* for 5 min. Mononuclear cells (MNCs) were isolated following the same method used for PBMCs. All samples were transferred to our laboratory within 30 min of collection, and the aforementioned procedure was started immediately.

Monoclonal antibodies

Monoclonal antibodies against CD4-FITC (RPA-T4), CD11b-APC (ICRF44), CD45RA-APC (5H9), and FoxP3-PE (259D/C7) were purchased from Becton Dickinson (Franklin Lakes, NJ, USA). LAP-PE (clone 27,232) was purchased from R&D Systems (Minneapolis, MN, USA). Mouse IgG1-FITC, mouse IgG1-PE, and mouse IgG1-APC were purchased from eBioscience (San Diego, CA, USA) and were used as isotype-matched negative controls. Human Fc receptor blocker was purchased from Becton

Table 1 Summary of patient characteristics

		Endometriosis ($n = 28$)		Control ($n = 20$)	*P value*
Age in years, mean (range)		34.3 (23–46)		36.1 (19–36)	0.13
BMI, mean (range)		20.3 (17.3–24.0)		21.0 (18.5–25.7)	0.45
Gravida, mean (range)		0.68 (0–2)		1.0 (0–4)	0.67
Para, mean (range)		0.39 (0–2)		0.75 (0–3)	0.46
Smokers		none		1	Not applicable
Stage of Menstrual Cycle	Proliferative	12		10	Not applicable
	Secretory	16		10	Not applicable
Stage of Endometriosis		I	7	Not applicable	
		II	6		
		III	11		
		IV	4		

Differences between groups were analyzed by Mann-Whitney *U*-tests

Dickinson. Ethidium monoazide bromide was purchased from Molecular Probes, Inc. (Eugene, OR, USA).

Flow cytometry analysis

For Treg assays, PBMCs and MNCs were blocked with human Fc receptor blocker for 10 min on ice and stained for 20 min on ice in the dark using antibodies against CD4 and CD45RA. After washing, the cells were stained with ethidium monoazide bromide for 20 min on ice and permeabilized using a FoxP3 Staining Kit (Becton Dickinson), according to the manufacturer's protocol. Cells were analyzed using a FACS Aria flow cytometer (BD Biosciences, CA, USA), and 20,000 $CD4^+$ cells were obtained (Fig. 1a and b). For monocyte and macrophage LAP staining assays, PBMCs and MNCs were stained to detect CD11b and LAP. Cells were analyzed using a FACS Aria flow cytometer, and 20,000 $CD11b^+$ cells were obtained (Fig. 1c and d).

Evaluation of TGF-β concentration in the PF

The frozen plasma samples of the PF were preserved at −80 °C until analysis. Subsequently, the samples were sent to SRL Inc. (Tokyo, Japan) for evaluation of the concentration of TGF-β1 by enzyme-linked immunosorbent assay (ELISA) using a Quantikine human TGF-β1 immunoassay (R&D Systems; Minneapolis, MN, USA), which was performed according to the manufacture's recommendation.

Statistical analysis

Statistical analyses were performed using GraphPad Prism version 6 (GraphPad Software, Inc., La Jolla, CA, USA). Continuous variables were analyzed using Mann-Whitney *U*-tests. Fisher's exact tests were performed for comparisons between two groups. Differences with $P < 0.05$ were considered statistically significant.

Results

Treg subpopulations in the PF and PB of patients with endometriosis and controls

We gated $CD4^+$ T lymphocytes and determined the proportions of three subpopulations of cells in the PB and PF: $CD45RA^+FoxP3^{low}$ rTregs, $CD45RA^-FoxP3^{high}$ eTregs, and $CD45RA^-FoxP3^{low}$ non-Tregs (Fig. 1a and b). We did not detect cyclical changes in these subpopulations in patients with endometriosis or controls (Table 2). FACS analysis revealed that the frequencies of rTregs and eTregs in the PF were significantly higher in the endometriosis group (medians: 0.60% and 3.4%, respectively) than in the control group [medians: 0.25% ($P = 0.02$) and 1.7% ($P < 0.01$), respectively]; however, these did not differ between the two groups in the PB [median rTregs: 1.4% (endometriosis) and 1.9% (control), $P = 0.31$; median eTregs: 0.70% (endometriosis) and 0.90% (control), $P = 0.29$] (Fig. 2a and b). There were no significant differences in non-Tregs between patients and controls in either the PB or PF (Fig. 2c). Significant differences were also observed in comparisons based on the menstrual cycle stage (Table 3). Comparison of rTregs and eTregs in the PF with severity of endometriosis (rASRM stage I and II vs. III and IV) showed no significant difference between the two groups [median rTregs: 0.75% (stage I and II) and 0.65% (stage III and IV), $P = 0.59$; median eTregs: 2.8% (stage I and II) and 3.6% (stage III and IV), $P = 0.28$].

$CD11b^+LAP^+$ MNCs in the PF and PB of patients with endometriosis

PBMCs and MNCs were examined using side light scattering and analysis of CD11b expression to detect monocytes and macrophages by flow cytometry (Fig. 1c and d). We then determined the frequencies of LAP^+ cells among $CD11b^+$ monocytes and macrophages in the PB and PF (Fig. 1e). We did not detect cyclical changes in the

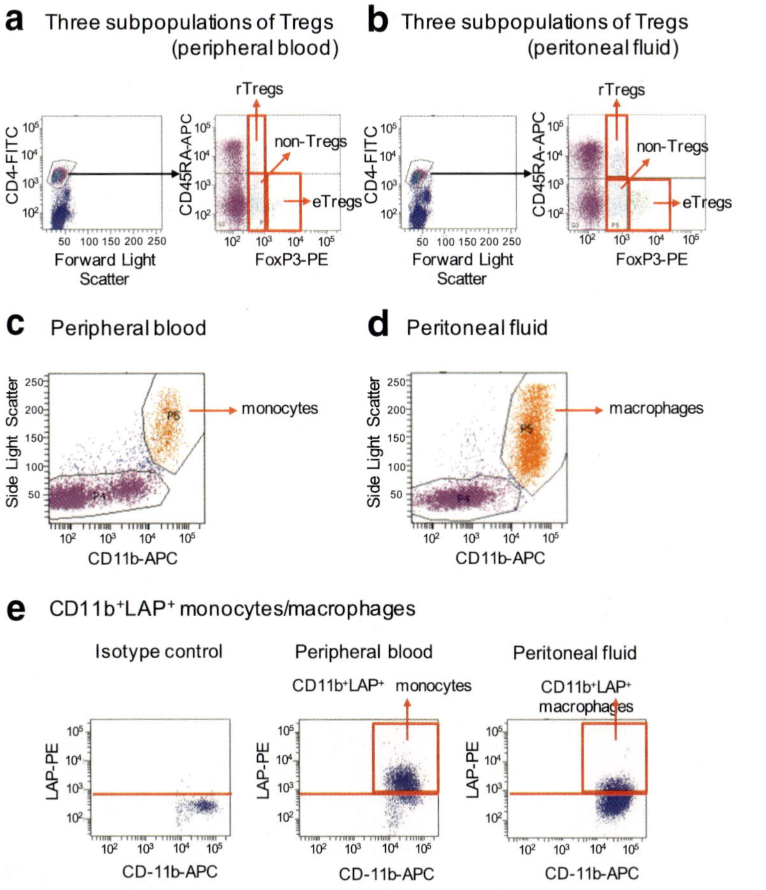

Fig. 1 Determination of frequencies of Tregs and LAP$^+$ macrophages and monocytes. **a**, **b** Gating of CD4$^+$ T lymphocytes and determination of the proportions of three subpopulations in the peripheral blood (**a**) and peritoneal fluid (**b**): CD45RA$^+$FoxP3^{low} resting Tregs (rTregs), CD45RA$^-$FoxP3^{high} effector Tregs (eTregs), and CD45RA$^-$FoxP3^{low} non-Tregs (non-Tregs). **c**, **d** Side light scattering and staining with CD11b gating to detect CD11b$^+$ monocytes and macrophages from the peripheral blood (**c**) and peritoneal fluid (**d**). **e** Staining with isotype control, CD11b$^+$LAP$^+$ monocytes from the peripheral blood, and CD11b$^+$LAP$^+$ macrophages from the peritoneal fluid

Table 2 Comparison of Treg subpopulations, LAP$^+$CD11b$^+$ monocytes, and TGF-β between proliferative and secretory phases in each group (mean ± SD)

Peritoneal fluid											
	Phase	rTregs (%)	*P*	eTregs (%)	*P*	nonTregs (%)	*P*	LAP+CD11b + Macrophages	*P*	TGF-β	*P*
Endometriosis	Proliferative (*n* = 12)	0.73 ± 0.56	ns	3.9 ± 1.7	ns	7.7 ± 2.7	ns	13.0 ± 14.4	ns	1.12 ± 0.57	ns
	Secretory (*n* = 16)	0.82 ± 0.75		3.1 ± 2.8		6.0 ± 3.0		12.1 ± 16.4		1.09 ± 0.32	
Control	Proliferative (*n* = 10)	0.47 ± 0.60	ns	2.2 ± 1.5	ns	5.8 ± 2.1	ns	80.0 ± 19.7	ns	0.85 ± 0.26	ns
	Secretory (*n* = 10)	0.30 ± 0.24		1.8 ± 1.3		8.6 ± 1.6		81.3 ± 17.3		0.79 ± 0.26	
Peripheral blood											
	Phase	rTregs (%)	*P*	eTregs (%)	*P*	nonTregs (%)	*P*	LAP+CD11b + Monocytes	*P*		
Endometriosis	Proliferative (*n* = 12)	1.3 ± 0.61	ns	1.2 ± 2.2	ns	2.4 ± 1.9	ns	83.5 ± 16.7	ns		
	Secretory (*n* = 16)	2.1 ± 1.6		0.9 ± 1.0		3.0 ± 1.8		80.3 ± 19.7			
Control	Proliferative (*n* = 10)	1.3 ± 2.6	ns	1.2 ± 0.8	ns	4.4 ± 2.6	ns	79.2 ± 19.1	ns		
	Secretory (*n* = 10)	0.8 ± 2.8		0.8 ± 0.4		3.9 ± 2.2		85.9 ± 11.5			

Differences between groups were analyzed by Mann-Whitney *U*-tests. ns, not significant

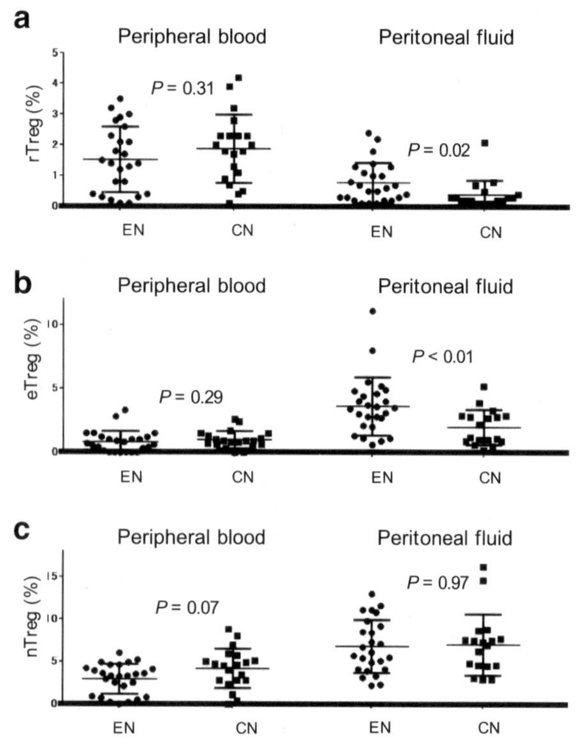

Fig. 2 Proportion of Tregs in peripheral blood and peritoneal fluid of patients with endometriosis and controls. Proportions of $CD45RA^{+}FoxP3^{low}$ (rTregs) (**a**), $CD45RA^{-}FoxP3^{high}$ (eTregs) (**b**), and $CD45RA^{-}FoxP3^{low}$ (non-Tregs) cells (**c**) among the $CD4^{+}$ population in the peripheral blood and peritoneal fluid of patients with endometriosis (EN, $n = 28$) and controls (CN, $n = 10$). Horizontal bars represent medians. Differences between groups were analyzed by Mann-Whitney *U*-tests

proportions of LAP^{+} macrophages in patients with endometriosis or controls (Table 2). We found that the proportion of LAP^{+} macrophages in the PF was significantly lower in patients with endometriosis (median: 6.2%) than in controls (median: 21.2%, $P < 0.01$), as shown in Fig. 3. There were no significant differences in the proportion of LAP^{+} monocytes in the PB of patients with endometriosis and controls (median: 89.4% and 89.2%, respectively; $P = 0.86$). Significant differences were also observed in comparisons based on the menstrual cycle stage (Table 3). Comparison of LAP^{+} macrophages in the PF with severity of endometriosis (rASRM stage I and II vs. III and IV) showed no significant difference between the two groups [median 31.1% (stage I and II) and 13.7% (stage III and IV), $P = 0.23$].

Evaluation of TGF-β concentration in the PF

The concentration of TGF-β in the PF was significantly increased in patients with endometriosis (median 1.08 ng/mL) compared with that in the controls (median 0.75 ng/mL, $P < 0.01$, as shown in Additional file 1: Figure S1).

Discussion

In the present study, we demonstrated that frequencies of rTregs and eTregs in the PF were higher in patients with endometriosis than in controls, but this pattern was not observed in the PB. In *Papio anubis*, induction of endometriosis alters the peripheral and endometrial populations of Tregs [17], whereas in humans, several studies have shown that Tregs are present in eutopic and ectopic endometrial tissues [18, 19] and that *FOXP3* mRNA levels are elevated in human endometriotic lesions [20]. These findings and our results together

Table 3 Comparison of Treg subpopulations, $LAP^{+}CD11b^{+}$ monocytes, and TGF-β concentrations in proliferative and secretory phases (mean ± SD) between endometriosis and control groups

Peritoneal fluid										
Proliferative	rTregs (%)	P	eTregs (%)	P	nonTregs (%)	P	LAP+CD11b + Macrophages	P	TGF-β	P
Endometriosis ($n = 12$)	0.73 ± 0.56	< 0.05	3.9 ± 1.7	< 0.05	7.7 ± 2.7	ns	13.0 ± 14.4	< 0.05	1.12 ± 0.57	< 0.05
Control ($n = 10$)	0.47 ± 0.60		2.2 ± 1.5		5.8 ± 2.1		80.0 ± 19.7		0.85 ± 0.26	
Secretory	rTregs (%)	P	eTregs (%)	P	nonTregs (%)	P	LAP+CD11b + Macrophages	P	TGF-β	P
Endometriosis ($n = 16$)	0.82 ± 0.75	< 0.05	3.1 ± 2.8	< 0.05	6.0 ± 3.0	ns	12.1 ± 16.4	< 0.05	1.09 ± 0.32	< 0.05
Control ($n = 10$)	0.30 ± 0.24		1.8 ± 1.3		8.6 ± 1.6		81.3 ± 17.3		0.79 ± 0.26	
Peripheral blood										
Proliferative	rTregs (%)	P	eTregs (%)	P	nonTregs (%)	P	LAP+CD11b + Monocytes	P		
Endometriosis ($n = 12$)	1.3 ± 0.61	ns	1.2 ± 2.2	ns	2.4 ± 1.9	ns	83.5 ± 16.7	ns		
Control ($n = 10$)	1.3 ± 2.6		1.2 ± 0.8		4.4 ± 2.6		79.2 ± 19.1			
Secretory	rTregs (%)	P	eTregs (%)	P	nonTregs (%)	P	LAP+CD11b + Monocytes	P		
Endometriosis ($n = 12$)	2.1 ± 1.6	ns	0.9 ± 1.0	ns	3.0 ± 1.8	ns	80.3 ± 19.7	ns		
Control ($n = 10$)	0.8 ± 2.8		0.8 ± 0.4		3.9 ± 2.2		85.9 ± 11.5			

Differences between groups were analyzed by Mann-Whitney *U*-tests. ns, not significant

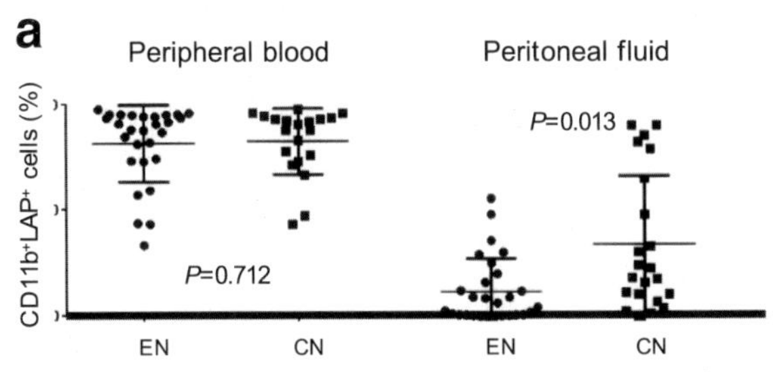

Fig. 3 CD11b^{+}LAP^{+} cells in peripheral blood and peritoneal fluid of patients with endometriosis and controls. Endometriosis, EN ($n = 28$); control, CN ($n = 20$). Horizontal bars represent medians. Columns and vertical bars indicate the 25th–75th percentiles and 10th–90th percentiles, respectively. Differences between groups were analyzed by Mann-Whitney *U*-tests

suggest that in humans, elevations in rTregs and eTregs in patients with endometriosis are not systemic but are locally induced in the peritoneal cavity. In contrast, in a recent report, there were no significant differences in Treg subpopulations in the PF of individuals with or without endometriosis [21]. The discrepancy in this result from ours may be caused by the different methods used to analyze Treg subpopulations: in this previous study, specimens were stored at − 80 °C before analysis by flow cytometry, and all specimens were obtained from patients with severe endometriosis. It has been reported that cryopreservation and thawing of specimens alter the phenotype and function of Tregs [22, 23].

Our results also demonstrated low LAP expression on the surfaces of macrophages in the PF of patients with endometriosis. Macrophage numbers are increased in the peritoneal cavities of women with endometriosis [24, 25]; therefore, the present study focused on macrophages in the PF. Disruption of the noncovalent interactions between LAP and TGF-β by either conformational changes or the complete dissociation of LAP can be induced under extreme conditions, e.g. extreme pH, heat, or the presence of serine protease plasmin, thrombospondin-1, reactive oxygen species, or integrin αγβ6 [26–28]. Active TGF-β can be released following this disruption, limiting tissue repair and promoting the development of tissue fibrosis [29–31]. Elevated concentrations of TGF-β in the PF of patients with endometriosis have been repeatedly reported [13, 32], and this result was further confirmed in our study (Additional file 1: Figure S1). Our results suggest that activated TGF-β released from the latent complex on macrophage surfaces may act to decrease LAP expression and increase the concentration of TGF-β in the PF of patients with endometriosis.

The overexpression of TGF-β has been implicated in fibrotic diseases of the kidney, liver, lung, skin, and other organs, and trapping TGF-β by increasing the expression of LAP in organ-specific cells leads to the suppression of fibrosis in the skin, hepatic tissue, and renal tissue [29, 33, 34]. Thus, higher levels of TGF-β may account for the peritoneal tissue fibrosis found in patients with endometriosis and are related to the severity of endometriosis [35]. In 2015, the results of a phase II clinical trial of fresolimumab, a neutralizing antibody against TGF-β1, β2, and β3, for skin sclerosis were reported. Fresolimumab treatment did not change the thickness of the dermis, but decreased the number of myofibroblasts [36]. Clinical studies using molecular targeted drugs for treatment of endometriosis have not yet been conducted, but monoclonal antibodies against TGF-β and LAP may be a promising approach for control of the disease.

As this is a cross-sectional study, it is difficult to determine whether the changes in TGF-β, LAP^{+} macrophages and suppressive Tregs are the cause or result of endometriosis; moreover, the trigger for LAP release also remains unknown. Though our data suggest a potential source of activated TGF-β, namely the reduced LAP expression on the surfaces of macrophages, TGF-β is produced by several types of cells including immune cells [37], and it has been reported that the peritoneum is a source of TGF-β in patients with endometriosis [38]. Additionally, as rASRM classification is based on macroscopic findings, potential endometriosis patients might be included in the control group, resulting in some data overlap between the groups. Regarding the limitation of the laboratory method, it is difficult to completely eliminate leucocytes from the PF derived from the PB due to contamination during operation. Furthermore, the participants of this study may include patients with dysmenorrhea symptoms such as pelvic pain and excessive menstruation, and infertility. There are some reports that endometriosis is related to infertility, pain, socioeconomic condition, stress, nickel allergy, vitamin D intake [39–42], and these potential confounding factors cannot be excluded completely with only the variabilities that we adjusted. However, owing to the small sample size of this study, it was difficult to adjust for all of these factors. We believe that such studies could clarify the pathophysiology of endometriosis and establish new treatment modalities.

Conclusions

Our results revealed increases in the proportions of rTregs and eTregs in the PF of women with endometriosis, as well as reduced expression of LAP on macrophages, resulting in the release of activated TGF-β. These observations may be associated with suppressed immune responses, which may initiate and promote endometriosis in the pelvic cavity. Further studies on the relevance of Tregs and LAP-TGF-β are needed, and elucidation of this cascade may lead to the establishment of effective approaches for the control of endometriosis.

Additional file

Additional file 1: Figure S1. Transforming growth factor-β (TGF-β) concentrations in peritoneal fluid of patients with endometriosis and controls. Concentrations determined by enzyme-linked immunosorbent assay. Endometriosis, EN ($n = 28$); control, CN ($n = 20$). Horizontal bars represent medians. Columns and vertical bars indicate the 25th–75th percentiles and 10th–90th percentiles, respectively. Differences between groups were analyzed by Mann-Whitney *U*-tests. (PDF 14 kb)

Abbreviations

eTregs: $CD45RA^{-}FoxP3^{high}$ effector Tregs; LAP: Latency-associated peptide; MNCs: Mononuclear cells; non-Tregs: $CD45RA^{-}FoxP3^{low}$ non-Tregs; PB: Peripheral blood; PBMCs: Peripheral blood mononuclear cells; PF: Peritoneal fluid; rTregs: $CD45RA^{+}FoxP3^{low}$ resting Tregs; TGF-β: Transforming growth factor-β; Tregs: Regulatory T cells

Acknowledgements

We would like to thank Mr. Mori and Mr. Yamamoto (Central Research Laboratory, Shiga University of Medical Science) for their technical support in the flow cytometry analysis.

Funding

None to declare.

Authors' contributions

TH and ST were involved in study design, clinical material collection, material preparation and flow cytometry measurements, data collection, analysis and interpretation, manuscript drafting, and critical discussion. MN was involved in analysis and interpretation. SW, KK, and FK were involved in data interpretation. TMo, KO, and TMu were involved in study conception and design, data analysis, drafting the article, and its final edition. All authors read and approved the final manuscript.

Competing interests

The authors declare that they have no competing interests.

Author details

[1]Department of Obstetrics and Gynecology, Shiga University of Medical Science, Seta Tsukionowa-cho, Otsu, Shiga 520-2192, Japan. [2]Department of Pathology, Division of Pathology and Disease Regulation, Shiga University of Medical Science, Seta Tsukionowa-cho, Otsu, Shiga 520-2192, Japan. [3]Academia for Repro-Regenerative Medicine, Nonprofit Organization, 394-1 Higashi-Hinodono-cho, Ichijo-Shinmachi-Higashiiru, Kamigyo-ku, Kyoto 602-0917, Japan.

References

1. Giudice LC. Clinical practice. Endometriosis. N Engl J Med. 2010;362:2389–98.
2. Sakaguchi S, Yamaguchi T, Nomura T, Ono M. Regulatory T cells and immune tolerance. Cell. 2008;133:775–87.
3. Curiel TJ, Coukos G, Zou L, Alvarez X, Cheng P, Mottram P, et al. Specific recruitment of regulatory T cells in ovarian carcinoma fosters immune privilege and predicts reduced survival. Nat Med. 2004;10:942–9.
4. Ehrenstein MR, Evans JG, Singh A, Moore S, Warnes G, Isenberg DA, et al. Compromised function of regulatory T cells in rheumatoid arthritis and reversal by anti-TNFalpha therapy. J Exp Med. 2004;200:277–85.
5. Miyara M, Amoura Z, Parizot C, Badoual C, Dorgham K, Trad S, et al. Global natural regulatory T cell depletion in active systemic lupus erythematosus. J Immunol. 2005;175:8392–400.
6. Miyara M, Sakaguchi S. Human FoxP3(+)CD4(+) regulatory T cells: their knowns and unknowns. Immunol Cell Biol. 2011;89:346–51.
7. Miyara M, Yoshioka Y, Kitoh A, Shima T, Wing K, Niwa A, et al. Functional delineation and differentiation dynamics of human CD4+ T cells expressing the FoxP3 transcription factor. Immunity. 2009;30:899–911.
8. Gogacz M, Winkler I, Bojarska-Junak A, Tabarkiewicz J, Semczuk A, Rechberger T, et al. T regulatory lymphocytes in patients with endometriosis. Mol Med Rep. 2014;10:1072–6.
9. Olkowska-Truchanowicz J, Bocian K, Maksym RB, Bialoszewska A, Wlodarczyk D, Baranowski W, et al. CD4(+) CD25(+) FOXP3(+) regulatory T cells in peripheral blood and peritoneal fluid of patients with endometriosis. Hum Reprod. 2013;28:119–24.
10. Takamura M, Koga K, Izumi G, Hirata T, Harada M, Hirota Y, et al. Simultaneous detection and evaluation of four subsets of CD4+ T lymphocyte in lesions and peripheral blood in endometriosis. Am J Reprod Immunol. 2015;74:480–6.
11. Yoshimura A, Wakabayashi Y, Mori T. Cellular and molecular basis for the regulation of inflammation by TGF-beta. J Biochem. 2010;147:781–92.
12. Annes JP, Munger JS, Rifkin DB. Making sense of latent TGFbeta activation. J Cell Sci. 2003;116:217–24.
13. Harada T, Iwabe T, Terakawa N. Role of cytokines in endometriosis. Fertil Steril. 2001;76:1–10.
14. Ho HN, Wu MY, Yang YS. Peritoneal cellular immunity and endometriosis. Am J Reprod Immunol. 1997;38:400–12.
15. Dmowski WP, Steele RW, Baker GF. Deficient cellular immunity in endometriosis. Am J Obstet Gynecol. 1981;141:377–83.
16. American Society for Reproductive Medicine. Revised American Society for Reproductive Medicine classification of endometriosis: 1996. Fertil Steril. 1997;67:817–21.
17. Braundmeier A, Jackson K, Hastings J, Koehler J, Nowak R, Fazleabas A. Induction of endometriosis alters the peripheral and endometrial regulatory T cell population in the non-human primate. Hum Reprod. 2012;27:1712–22.
18. Berbic M, Hey-Cunningham AJ, Ng C, Tokushige N, Ganewatta S, Markham R, et al. The role of Foxp3+ regulatory T-cells in endometriosis: a potential controlling mechanism for a complex, chronic immunological condition. Hum Reprod. 2010;25:900–7.
19. Wan YY, Flavell RA. TGF-beta and regulatory T cell in immunity and autoimmunity. J Clin Immunol. 2008;28:647–59.
20. Budiu RA, Diaconu I, Chrissluis R, Dricu A, Edwards RP, Vlad AM. A conditional mouse model for human MUC1-positive endometriosis shows the presence of anti-MUC1 antibodies and Foxp3+ regulatory T cells. Dis Model Mech. 2009;2:593–603.
21. Tanaka Y, Mori T, Ito F, Koshiba A, Takaoka O, Kataoka H, et al. Exacerbation of endometriosis due to regulatory T cell dysfunction. J Clin Endocrinol Metab. 2017;102:3206–17.
22. Florek M, Schneidawind D, Pierini A, Baker J, Armstrong R, Pan Y, et al. Freeze and thaw of CD4+CD25+Foxp3+ regulatory T cells results in loss of CD62L expression and a reduced capacity to protect against graft-versus-host disease. PLoS One. 2015;10:e0145763.
23. Weiner J, Duran-Struuck R, Zitsman J, Buhler L, Sondermeijer H, McMurchy AN, et al. Restimulation after cryopreservation and thawing preserves the phenotype and function of expanded baboon regulatory T cells. Transplant Direct. 2015;1:1–7.
24. Dmowski WP. Immunological aspects of endometriosis. Int J Gynaecol Obstet. 1995;50(Suppl 1):S3–S10.
25. Oral E, Arici A. Pathogenesis of endometriosis. Obstet Gynecol Clin N Am. 1997;24:219–33.
26. Oklu R, Hesketh R. The latent transforming growth factor beta binding protein (LTBP) family. Biochem J. 2000;352(Pt 3):601–10.
27. Munger JS, Harpel JG, Gleizes PE, Mazzieri R, Nunes I, Rifkin DB. Latent transforming growth factor-beta: structural features and mechanisms of activation. Kidney Int. 1997;51:1376–82.

28. Todorovic V, Jurukovski V, Chen Y, Fontana L, Dabovic B, Rifkin DB. Latent TGF-beta binding proteins. Int J Biochem Cell Biol. 2005;37:38–41.
29. Border WA, Noble NA. Transforming growth factor beta in tissue fibrosis. N Engl J Med. 1994;331:1286–92.
30. De Crescenzo G, Grothe S, Zwaagstra J, Tsang M, O'Connor-McCourt MD. Real-time monitoring of the interactions of transforming growth factor-beta (TGF-beta) isoforms with latency-associated protein and the ectodomains of the TGF-beta type II and III receptors reveals different kinetic models and stoichiometries of binding. J Biol Chem. 2001;276:29632–43.
31. Walton KL, Makanji Y, Chen J, Wilce MC, Chan KL, Robertson DM, et al. Two distinct regions of latency-associated peptide coordinate stability of the latent transforming growth factor-beta1 complex. J Biol Chem. 2010;285:17029–37.
32. Oosterlynck DJ, Meuleman C, Waer M, Koninckx PR. Transforming growth factor-beta activity is increased in peritoneal fluid from women with endometriosis. Obstet Gynecol. 1994;83:287–92.
33. Dooley S, Delvoux B, Lahme B, Mangasser-Stephan K, Gressner AM. Modulation of transforming growth factor beta response and signaling during transdifferentiation of rat hepatic stellate cells to myofibroblasts. Hepatology. 2000;31:1094–106.
34. Zhang Y, McCormick LL, Gilliam AC. Latency-associated peptide prevents skin fibrosis in murine sclerodermatous graft-versus-host disease, a model for human scleroderma. J Invest Dermatol. 2003;121:713–9.
35. Pizzo A, Salmeri FM, Ardita FV, Sofo V, Tripepi M, Marsico S. Behaviour of cytokine levels in serum and peritoneal fluid of women with endometriosis. Gynecol Obstet Investig. 2002;54:82–7.
36. Rice LM, Padilla CM, McLaughlin SR, Mathes A, Ziemek J, Goummih S, et al. Fresolimumab treatment decreases biomarkers and improves clinical symptoms in systemic sclerosis patients. J Clin Invest. 2015;125:2795–807.
37. Lawrence DA. Transforming Growth factor-beta: a general review. Eur Cytokine Netw. 1996;7:363–74.
38. Young VJ, Brown JK, Saunders PT, Duncan WC, Horne AW. The peritoneum is both a source and target of TGF-beta in women with endometriosis. PLoS One. 2014;9:e106773.
39. Mangtani P, Booth M. Epidemiology of endometriosis. J Epidemiol Community Health. 1993;47:84–8.
40. Syegh L, Fuleihan Gel-H, Nassar AH. Vitamine D in endometriosis: a causative or confounder factor? Metabolism. 2014;63:32–41.
41. Cuevas M, Cruz ML, Ramirez AE, Flores I, Thompson KJ, Bayona M, et al. Stress during development of experimental endometriosis influence nerve growth and disease progression. Reprod Sci. 2017;1933719117737846 (Epub).
42. Yuk JS, Shin JS, Shin JY, Oh E, Kim H, Park WI. Nickel allergy is a risk factor for endometriosis: an 11-year population-based nested case-control study. PLoS One. 2015;10:e0139388.

10

Functional role of AKT signaling in bovine early embryonic development: potential link to embryotrophic actions of follistatin

Mohamed Ashry[1,3,4], Sandeep K. Rajput[1,3], Joseph K. Folger[1,3], Jason G. Knott[2,3], Nabil A. Hemeida[4], Omaima M. Kandil[5], Refaat S. Ragab[4] and George W. Smith[1,3*]

Abstract

Background: TGF-β signaling pathways regulate several crucial processes in female reproduction. AKT is a non-SMAD signaling pathway regulated by TGF-β ligands essential for oocyte maturation and early embryonic development in the mouse, but its regulatory role in bovine early embryonic development is not well established. Previously, we demonstrated a stimulatory role for follistatin (a binding protein for specific members of TGF-β superfamily) in early bovine embryonic development. The objectives of the present studies were to determine the functional role of AKT signaling in bovine early embryonic development and embryotrophic actions of follistatin.

Methods: We used AKT inhibitors III and IV as pharmacological inhibitors of AKT signaling pathway during the first 72 h of in vitro embryo culture. Effects of AKT inhibition on early embryonic development and AKT phosphorylation were investigated in the presence or absence of exogenous follistatin.

Results: Pharmacological inhibition of AKT signaling resulted in a significant reduction in early embryo cleavage, and development to the 8- to 16-cell and blastocyst stages (d7). Treatment with exogenous follistatin increased AKT phosphorylation and rescued the inhibitory effect of AKT inhibitors III and IV on AKT phosphorylation and early embryonic development.

Conclusions: Collectively, results suggest a potential requirement of AKT for bovine early embryonic development, and suggest a potential role for follistatin in regulation of AKT signaling in early bovine embryos.

Keywords: AKT, Follistatin, TGF-β, AKT inhibitor, Bovine, Embryos

Background

Poor oocyte quality limits the efficiency of in vitro embryo production in cattle and women [1]. Our previous studies demonstrated a positive association between the transcript abundance of follistatin and oocyte developmental competence using the prepubertal calf and brilliant cresyl blue screening models [2, 3]. We also found that maternally derived follistatin is essential for bovine early embryonic development and exogenous supplementation of follistatin during first 72 h (h) of in vitro embryo culture has a stimulatory effect on early cleavage, embryonic development to 8- to 16-cell and blastocyst stages and blastocyst cell lineage allocation [4]. The functional requirement of follistatin in oocyte and early embryonic development has been described in bovine and other mono-ovulatory species [5].

Follistatin is a transforming growth factor β (TGF-β) superfamily binding protein that may exert its embryotrophic effects through modulation of one or more of the SMAD [6, 7] or non-SMAD [8–10] signaling pathways. We previously demonstrated that the embryotrophic actions of follistatin on development to 8- to 16-cell and blastocyst stages are linked to the SMAD signaling pathways [11, 12]. However, how follistatin promotes early embryonic development, particularly early cleavage, is still not fully understood.

* Correspondence: smithge7@msu.edu
[1]Laboratory of Mammalian Reproductive Biology and Genomics, Michigan State University, East Lansing, MI 48824, USA
[3]Department of Animal Science, Michigan State University, East Lansing, MI 48824, USA
Full list of author information is available at the end of the article

Follistatin was first identified as a high affinity Activin binding protein [13] and its binding affinity to select bone morphogenetic proteins (BMPs) has also been established [14, 15]. Both BMPs [16] and Activin [17] are major regulators of AKT signaling pathway that promotes cell cycle progression during G2/M transition. Studies have shown that AKT stimulates the transition from metaphase I (MI) to metaphase II (MII) in bovine [18], porcine [19], mouse [20, 21] and Xenopus [22] oocytes by activation of Phosphodiesterase 3A (PDE3A) and cyclin dependent kinase 1 (CDK1) required for resumption and regulation of meiosis. AKT was primarily identified as a serine/threonine specific protein kinase that functions downstream of Phosphatidylinositol 3-kinase (PI3K) [23]. Inhibition of AKT with a synthetic small molecule inhibitor (AKT inhibitor III) resulted in arrest of bovine oocytes at MI stage [18]. AKT plays an important role during entry of one cell mouse embryos into the first mitosis as inhibition of AKT resulted in arrest of cell cycle in G1 and G2 phases [24]. Moreover, inhibition of AKT activity compromised the development of mouse embryos to the blastocyst stage [25, 26]. Considering the role of AKT in cell cycle progression in oocytes and embryos, we hypothesized that AKT signaling is required for bovine early embryonic development and is linked to the embryotrophic actions of follistatin during in vitro embryo culture. To test this hypothesis, we determined the functional role of AKT in bovine early embryonic development and investigated the relationship between AKT signaling and the embryotrophic actions of follistatin. Effects of treatment with the AKT inhibitors III and IV on development of early bovine embryos and AKT phosphorylation were analyzed. Effects of exogenous follistatin supplementation on AKT phosphorylation and developmental potential of AKT inhibitor treated embryos were also investigated.

Methods

All chemicals and reagents used were purchased from Sigma- Aldrich (St. Louis, MO) unless stated otherwise.

Oocyte collection and in vitro embryo production

Bovine oocytes were retrieved from ovaries collected at local abattoir in the state of Michigan. Oocyte aspiration, in vitro maturation (IVM), in vitro fertilization (IVF), and in vitro embryo culture (IVC) were performed as previously described [3, 27]. Briefly, morphologically good quality cumulus oocyte complexes (COCs), which have three or more layers of compact cumulus cell and granular, homogenous cytoplasm, were matured in TCM-199 media [supplemented with 50 μg/ml gentamycin sulfate, 0.2 mM sodium pyruvate, 3.67 nM 17β-estradiol, 15.6 nM bovine FSH (Sioux Biochemical, Sioux Center, IA), 156 nM bovine LH (Sioux Biochemical), and 10% *v*/v defined fetal bovine serum (FBS) (Hyclone, Logan, UT)] at 38.5 °C in 5% CO_2 and humidified air for 24 h. IVF was conducted using motile spermatozoa separated by Percoll gradient technique from frozen thawed bovine semen. The matured COCs were co-incubated with motile spermatozoa (1×10^6 sperm/ml) for 18–20 h in fertilization media FIV (114 mM NaCl, 25 mM $NaHCO_3$, 3.2 mM KCl, 0.34 mM NaH_2PO_4, 0.183 mM penicillin-G, 16.6 mM sodium lactate, 0.5 mM $MgCl_26H_2O$, 2.7 mM $CaCl_22H_2O$, 0.2 mM sodium pyruvate, 6 mg/ml BSA, and 1.5 U of heparin) at 38.5 °C in 5% CO_2 and humidified air. After IVM and IVF, the cumulus cells were stripped off by vortexing for 6 min. Then, presumptive zygotes were washed and cultured in potassium simplex optimization medium (KSOM; EMD Millipore, Billerica, MA) supplemented with 0.3% fatty acid free bovine serum albumin (BSA) until 72 h post insemination (hpi). Then, 8- to 16-cell stage embryos were separated and cultured in fresh KSOM medium supplemented with 0.3% BSA and 10% FBS under same conditions until d 7.

Effect of AKT inhibitors III & IV on early embryonic development

AKT inhibitor III, known as SH6, is a cell permeable reversible substrate competitive phosphatidylinositol analog that prevents the generation of PIP3 by PIK3 which is required for AKT phosphorylation. AKT inhibitor IV is a cell permeable reversible benzimidazole compound that inhibits AKT phosphorylation/activation by targeting the ATP binding site of a kinase upstream of AKT, but downstream of PI3K [28]. The effects of AKT inhibitors III and IV treatment on early embryonic development were investigated as described in Fig. 1. Presumptive zygotes were cultured in KSOM medium supplemented with 0.3% BSA in the presence of 0, 25, 50 or 75 μM AKT inhibitor III (ALX-270-350 - Enzo Life Sciences, Farmingdale, NY), or 0, 1.5, 2.5 or 3.5 μM AKT inhibitor IV (Sigma, 124,011-1MG) until 72 hpi ($n = 25–30$ presumptive zygotes/group, $n = 4$ replicates/inhibitor). Embryos at 8- to 16-cell stage were separated, washed and cultured in fresh KSOM medium supplemented with 0.3% BSA and 10% FBS in the absence of inhibitor until d 7. The effects of AKT inhibition on indices of embryo developmental progression including early cleavage rate determined at 30 hpi, total cleavage rate determined at 48 hpi, percentage of embryos developing to the 8- to 16-cell stage at 72 hpi and percentage of embryos developing to the blastocyst stage at d 7 were recorded.

Effect of AKT inhibitors III & IV on AKT phosphorylation in early bovine embryos

To investigate the effect of AKT inhibitors III & IV treatment on AKT signaling activity in bovine embryo,

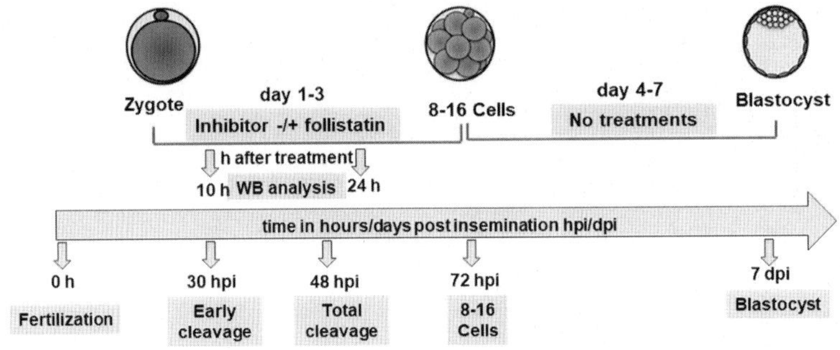

Fig. 1 Experimental design. To establish the role of AKT in early bovine embryonic development, bovine zygotes were cultured in the presence or absence of different doses of AKT inhibitors III or IV for 3 days. The optimized dose of each inhibitor was supplemented with or without 10 ng/ml follistatin to determine the effects on AKT phosphorylation at 10 h after treatment and development of AKT inhibitor treated embryos. On day 3 of development, embryos were washed and cultured in fresh media without any treatment for an additional 4 days. Indices of embryo development including early cleavage rate (30 hpi), total cleavage rate (48 hpi), percentage of embryos developing to the 8- to 16-cell stage (72 hpi), and percentage of embryos developing to the blastocyst stage (day 7) were recorded

AKT-Ser473 and AKT-Thr308 phosphorylation levels were analyzed. Presumptive zygotes were cultured in KSOM medium supplemented with 0.3% BSA in the presence of 0, 25, 50 or 75 μM AKT inhibitor III (Fig. 1) [18], or 0, 1.5, 2.5 or 3.5 μM AKT inhibitor IV for 10 h. Then, samples were collected for Western blot analysis of phosphorylated (p)-AKT-Ser473 or pAKT-Thr308, total (t)-AKT and actin ($n = 3$ replicates/inhibitor/phosphorylation site, $n = 20$ presumptive zygotes/group). All the doses of AKT inhibitors used in this study were selected based on previously published studies in bovine and mice [18, 19, 21].

Effects of follistatin supplementation on the developmental capacity of AKT inhibitor treated bovine embryos

Experiment was performed as described in Fig. 1. After IVM and IVF, presumptive zygotes were cultured with 0 or 10 ng/ml recombinant human follistatin (R&D Systems, Minneapolis, MN) [4] in the presence or absence of AKT inhibitor III (75 μM) or AKT inhibitor IV (3.5 μM) until 72 hpi ($n = 4$ replicates/inhibitor, $n = 20–30$ zygotes/group). Then, 8- to 16-cell stage embryos from each group were separated and cultured in fresh KSOM medium supplemented with 0.3% BSA and 10% FBS without any treatment until d 7. Effects of exogenous follistatin on early and total cleavage, development to 8–16-cell and d7 blastocyst rates were recorded.

Effect of follistatin supplementation on activity of AKT signaling pathway in AKT inhibitor treated early bovine embryos

Effects of follistatin supplementation on AKT signaling activity were investigated by analysis of AKT phosphorylation levels at 10 and 24 h after follistatin supplementation in the presence and absence of AKT inhibitor III or IV (Fig. 1). Presumptive zygotes were cultured with 0 or 10 ng/ml recombinant human follistatin in the presence or absence of AKT inhibitor III (75 μM) or AKT inhibitor IV (3.5 μM) during the initial 72 h of in vitro embryo culture. Samples were collected at 10 h after treatment administration ($n = 6$ replicates/inhibitor, $n = 20$ zygotes/group). For the second experiment, follistatin (0 or 10 ng/ml) was supplemented during the same time window and samples collected at 24 h after treatment administration ($n = 5$ replicates/inhibitor, $n = 20$ zygotes/group). Samples were subjected to Western blot analysis of pAKT-Ser473, pAKT-Thr308, tAKT and actin.

Western blot analysis

Western blot analysis was performed as described before [3]. Proteins (20 oocytes/embryos per sample) were separated by SDS-PAGE electrophoresis using 4–20% gradient pre-casted gel (Bio-Rad, Hercules, CA) and transferred to a polyvinylidene difluoride (PVDF, Millipore) membrane. After transfer, membranes were blocked with 5% BSA in Tris Buffered Saline with 0.5% Tween 20 (TBST) for 1 h at room temperature before overnight incubation with the appropriate primary antibody diluted in TBST with 5% BSA at 4 °C. The membrane was then washed and incubated with the appropriate HRP-conjugated secondary antibody diluted in TBST with 5% BSA for 1 h at room temperature. Protein signals were detected with SuperSignal West Dura Chemiluminescent Substrate (Thermo Scientific, Waltham, MA) and Images were captured using myECL Imager (Thermo Scientific). ImageJ software was used to measure the band intensities of the target proteins [29]. Relative abundance of each protein was normalized to the total–actin expression in corresponding lane, and phosphorylation level was expressed as phosphorylated (p) AKT/total (t) AKT. Membranes were probed sequentially with primary pAKT-Ser473 rabbit polyclonal antibody [1:1000 (Vol/Vol), Santa Cruz, sc-7985-R] or pAKT-Thr308 rabbit polyclonal antibody [1:1000 (Vol/Vol), Cell Signaling Technology, 9275]. After detection of pAKT membranes were striped with restore Western blot stripping buffer (Thermo Scientific) for 15 min at room temperature and re-probed with tAKT Rabbit polyclonal antibody [1:2000 (Vol/Vol), Santa Cruz, sc-8312]. After detection of tAKT, membranes were stripped and re-probed with actin monoclonal antibody (1:5000 (Vol/Vol) Millipore; MAB1501). HRP-conjugated Anti-Rabbit-IgG (Cell Signaling Technology, 7074), and Anti-Mouse-IgG (Thermo Scientific, A16011) were used as secondary antibodies at a 1:5000 (Vol/Vol) dilution.

Statistical analysis

Differences in phosphorylation levels obtained by Western-blot analysis were analyzed by ANOVA using the general linear models' procedure of SAS (SAS Institute Inc., Cary, NC). For experiments studying the effects of AKT inhibitors and follistatin supplementation on early embryonic development, data were arcsine transformed prior to analysis by mixed linear models' analysis procedures. Differences among treatment means were compared using Fisher's protected least significant difference test. In all cases data are presented as untransformed mean ± standard error ($P < 0.05$).

Results

AKT inhibition during the initial 72 h of in vitro culture reduced indices of embryonic developmental progression

To elucidate the potential role of AKT in bovine early embryogenesis, effects of AKT inhibitor III and AKT inhibitor IV supplementation (during the initial 72 h of in vitro embryo culture) on different developmental indices (early cleavage, total cleavage, 8- to 16-cell and blastocyst formation rates) were determined. The addition of 25, 50 and 75 μM AKT inhibitor III to the culture medium delayed early cleavage therefore no cleavage was observed at 30 hpi (Fig. 2a). Treatment with AKT inhibitor III significantly reduced the total cleavage rate, percentage of embryos that reached 8- to 16-cell stage at 72 hpi, and d 7 blastocyst rate relative to controls at 75 μM dose (Fig. 2b-d). However, no significant effects on total cleavage were observed in response to both 25 and 50 μM doses compared with control (Fig. 2b, c). Additionally, the 25-mM dose didn't impact the development to 8-to 16-cell or blastocyst stages (Fig. 2c-d). The addition of AKT inhibitor IV resulted in a dose dependent reduction in early cleavage, development to 8- to 16-cell and blastocyst stage with maximum response observed for 3.5 μM dose which delayed early cleavage and completely blocked development to blastocyst. Total cleavage wasn't impacted by lower doses of AKT inhibitor IV (1.5, 2.5 μM) whereas the higher dose (3.5 μM) significantly reduced the number of embryos

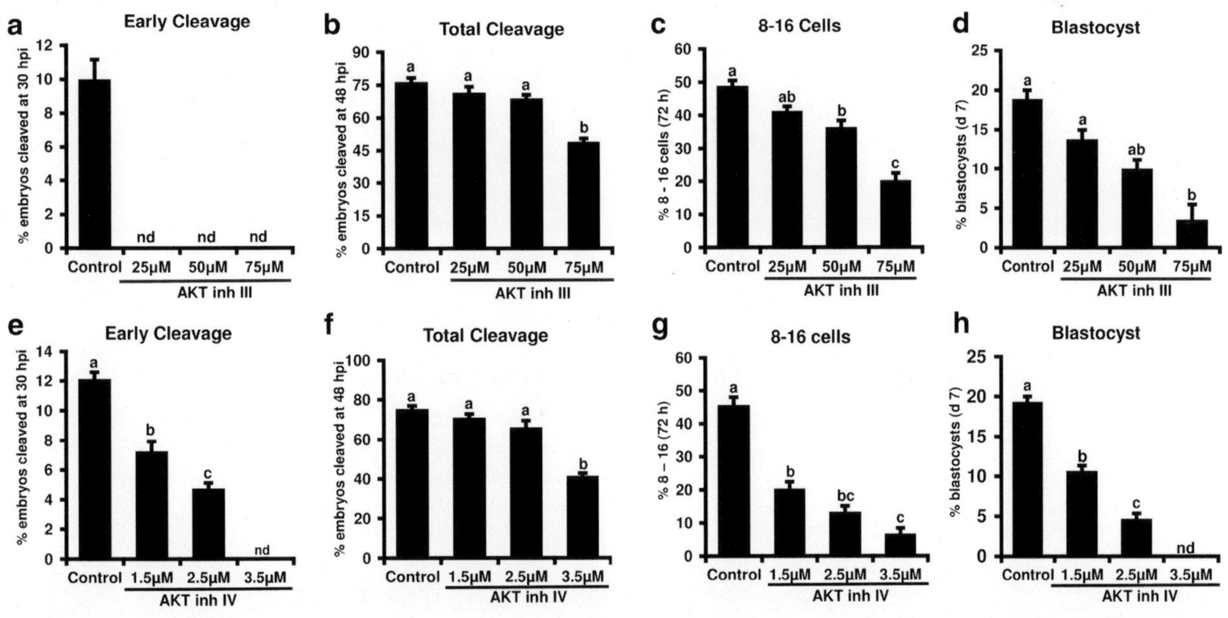

Fig. 2 Effects of AKT inhibitors III and IV treatment on bovine early embryonic development. Presumptive zygotes were cultured in the presence of 0, 25, 50 or 75 μM AKT inhibitor III or 0, 1.5, 2.5 or 3.5 μM AKT inhibitor IV until 72 hpi, then washed and cultured in fresh culture media lacking inhibitors until d 7 ($n = 4$ replicates/inhibitor, $n = 25–30$ embryos/treatment). Effects of each AKT inhibitor treatment on (**a**, **e**) early cleavage, (**b**, **f**) total cleavage, (**c**, **g**) development to 8- to 16-cell stage and (**d**, **h**) d7 blastocyst rates were determined. Data are expressed as mean ± SEM. Values with different superscripts among treatments indicate significant differences ($P < 0.05$)

reaching two cells at 48 hpi (Fig. 2e-h). Results demonstrate that inhibition of AKT delayed early embryonic cleavage at 30 hpi, and consequently reduced development to the later endpoints, suggesting a potential requirement of AKT for early embryonic development.

Effects of AKT inhibitors III & IV on AKT phosphorylation in early bovine embryos

Dose response studies were conducted to determine the effects of different concentrations of AKT inhibitor III (25, 50, and 75 μM) or AKT inhibitor IV (1.5, 2.5 and 3.5 μM) on AKT-Ser 473 and Thr308 phosphorylation levels in early embryos after 10 h of treatment. AKT-Thr308 phosphorylation level was significantly reduced in response to high doses of AKT inhibitor III (75 μM) and AKT inhibitor IV (3.5 μM) whereas slight non-significant reduction ($P < .09$) in phosphorylation level was also observed with lower doses of AKT inhibitor III (25 or 50 μM) or AKT inhibitor IV (1.5 and 2.5 μM) (Fig. 3a, b). On the other hand, AKT-Ser473 phosphorylation level was not impacted by treatment with the 25 μM AKT inhibitor III dose, whereas 50, and 75 μM doses, resulted in a significant reduction after 10 h of supplementation (Additional file 1: Figure S1a). Treatment with AKT inhibitor IV didn't show any effect on AKT-Ser437 phosphorylation at this time point (Additional file 1: Figure S1b).

Follistatin supplementation rescues the adverse effects of AKT inhibition on early embryo development

Our previous studies established a functional requirement of maternally derived follistatin for bovine early embryogenesis and embryotrophic effects of exogenous follistatin supplementation on early embryo development including enhanced early cleavage, and increased blastocyst formation rate and trophectoderm cell numbers. The AKT signaling pathway is regulated by members of TFG-β superfamily [8]. Hence, we investigated if follistatin supplementation can rescue the negative effects of AKT inhibition on early embryonic development. In the absence of the AKT inhibitors, follistatin supplementation (10 ng/ml) significantly increased the proportion of embryos reaching 2-cell stage at 30 hpi (early cleavage), the proportion of embryos reaching 8- to 16-cell stage at 72 h and d7 blastocyst rates compared with untreated controls. In addition, follistatin supplementation rescued the inhibitory effects of AKT inhibitors on early embryonic development (Fig. 4a-h). Follistatin supplementation was able to rescue the effects of AKT inhibitor III on early cleavage, total cleavage and development to 8- to 16-cell stage to levels similar to controls (Fig. 4a-c), and to partially rescue the effects of AKT inhibitor III on blastocyst development rate (Fig. 4d). Using AKT inhibitor IV with same experimental design, we observed that follistatin supplementation (10 ng/ml) partially rescued the negative effects of AKT inhibitor IV on total cleavage, early cleavage, 8- to 16-cell and blastocysts development rates (Fig. 4e-h). Collectively, results suggest a potential requirement of AKT for bovine early embryonic development, and a possible relationship between the embryotrophic actions of follistatin and the AKT signaling pathway.

Follistatin supplementation modulates the AKT signaling pathway in early bovine embryos

Our results revealed that exogenous follistatin could rescue the negative effects of AKT inhibition on various developmental endpoints in bovine embryos. Therefore, we analyzed the effect of exogenous follistatin supplementation

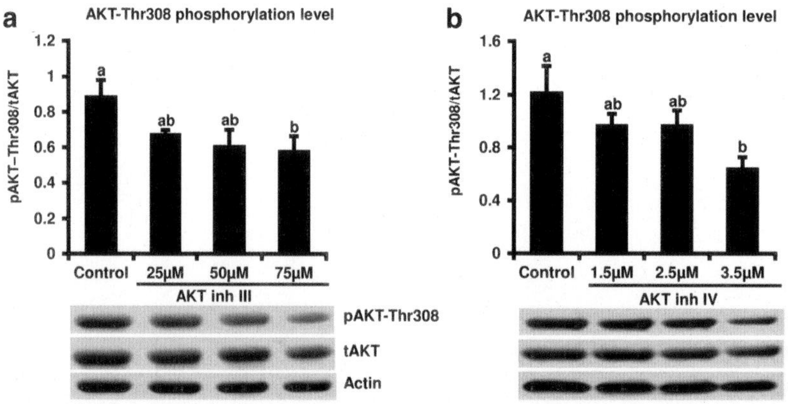

Fig. 3 Effect of AKT inhibitors III and IV treatments on AKT-Thr308 phosphorylation levels in early bovine embryos. Presumptive zygotes were cultured in presence of 0, 25, 50 or 75 μM AKT inhibitor III or 0, 1.5, 2.5 or 3.5 μM AKT inhibitor IV for 10 h, then subjected to Western blot for phosphorylated (p)AKt-Th308, total AKT (tAKT) and actin analysis ($n = 3$ replicates, $n = 20$ embryos/treatment). Data were normalized relative to abundance of actin and phosphorylation levels were expressed as pAKT/tAKT (**a**, **b**). Representative Western blot images are shown. Data are expressed as mean ± SEM. Values with different superscripts among treatments indicate significant differences ($P < 0.05$)

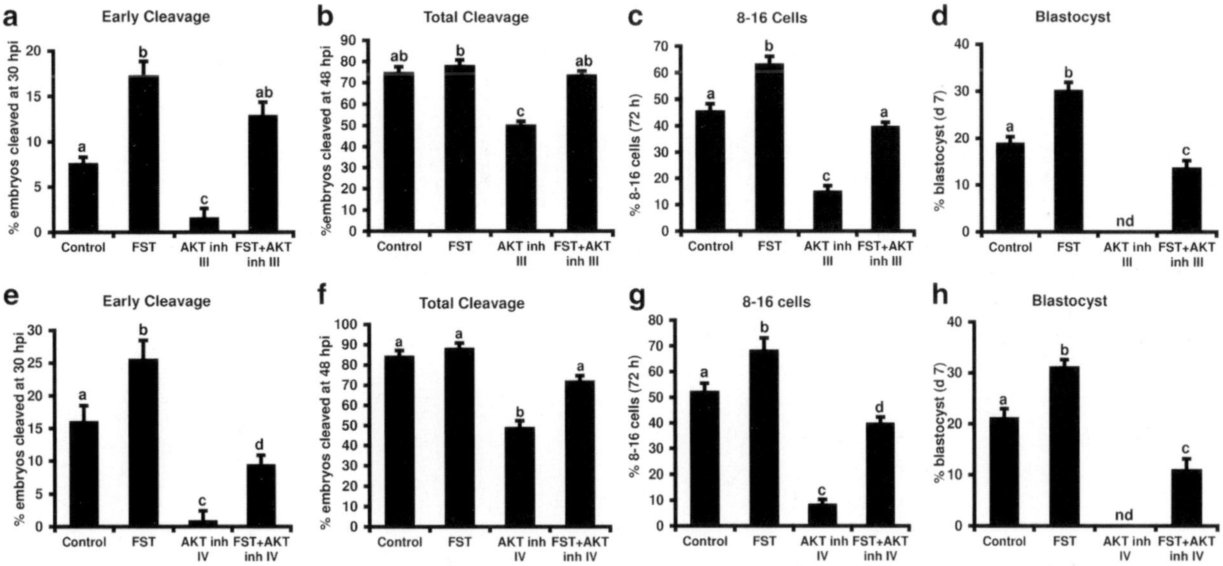

Fig. 4 Effect of follistatin supplementation on development of AKT inhibitors treated bovine embryos. Presumptive zygotes were cultured with 0 or 10 ng/ml recombinant human follistatin in the presence or absence of AKT inhibitor III (75 μM) or AKT inhibitor IV (3.5 μM) until 72 hpi then washed and cultured in fresh media lacking inhibitors and follistatin until d 7 ($n = 4$ replicates/inhibitor, $n = 25$–30 embryos/treatment). Effects of follistatin on multiple developmental endpoints for AKT inhibitor III or AKT inhibitor IV treated embryos were determined including; (**a**, **e**) early cleavage, (**b**, **f**) total cleavage, (**c**, **g**) development to 8- to 16-cell stage and (**d**, **h**) d7 blastocyst rates. Data are expressed as mean ± SEM. Values with different superscripts among treatments indicate significant differences ($P < 0.05$)

on AKT signaling activity in the presence or absence of AKT inhibitors to determine whether follistatin rescue the effects of AKT inhibition through modulation of AKT signaling. Western blot analysis showed that AKT inhibitor IV treatment resulted in a significant reduction in AKT-Thr308 phosphorylation level in zygotes 10 h post treatment that was rescued by supplementation with exogenous follistatin. However, no effect of follistatin treatment on basal levels of AKT phosphorylation was observed in the absence of inhibitor treatment (Fig. 5a). Similar pattern was observed in response to AKT inhibitor III treatment (Additional file 2: Figure S2a). We further investigated if follistatin supplementation has any effect on basal

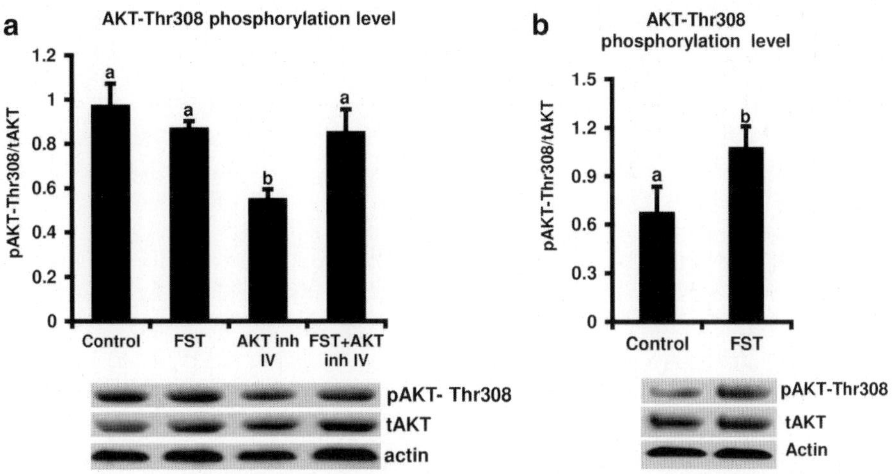

Fig. 5 Effect of follistatin treatment on AKT-Thr308 phosphorylation levels in early bovine embryos. Presumptive zygotes were cultured with 0 or 10 ng/ml recombinant human follistatin in the presence or absence of AKT inhibitor IV (3.5 μM) for 10 h ($n = 5$ replicates, $n = 20$ zygotes/group) (**a**), or Presumptive zygotes were cultured in the presence or absence of 10 ng/ml follistatin for 24 h ($n = 5$ replicates, $n = 20$ zygotes/group) (**b**). Samples were subjected to Western blot analysis for pAKT-Thr308, tAKT and Actin. Expression levels were normalized to the abundance of an endogenous control actin. Phosphorylation level was expressed as pAKT/tAKT. Data are expressed as mean ± standard error. Values with different superscripts among treatments indicate significant differences ($P < 0.05$). Representative Western blots are shown

AKT phosphorylation at a later time point. At 24 h post treatment administration, follistatin supplementation resulted in a significant increase in AKT phosphorylation relative to embryos cultured in the absence of follistatin (Fig. 5b, Additional file 2: Figure S2b).

Discussion

A growing body of evidence supports an important intrinsic role for follistatin in bovine oocyte quality and early embryo developmental progression in vitro [3, 4, 11, 12]. While follistatin is best known for its ability to bind and inhibit activity of select TGF-β superfamily ligands, the intrinsic ligands and signaling pathways linked to trophic actions of follistatin on early embryos are not known. Results of the present study demonstrated that pharmacological inhibition of AKT signaling pathway in early bovine embryos reduced their developmental capacity as assessed by early cleavage, total cleavage and rates of development to 8–16-cell and blastocyst stages. Follistatin supplementation during the first 72 h of in vitro embryo culture rescued the adverse effects of AKT signaling inhibition on embryo development and increased the level of AKT phosphorylation, suggesting a potential role for follistatin in regulation of AKT signaling in early bovine embryos. Results demonstrate follistatin regulation of non-canonical TGF-beta superfamily signaling in bovine embryos and a functional link to developmental progression.

AKT is serine/threonine-specific protein kinase that regulates crucial cellular processes such as glucose metabolism, transcription, cellular growth and proliferation [30–32]. Full activation of AKT requires translocation to the plasma membrane and phosphorylation at Thr308 and Ser473 motifs [33]. Previous studies have established a functional role of AKT during oocyte maturation in various species including bovine [18] and in early embryogenesis in mouse and pigs [19, 20, 34]. In bovine embryo, activation of PI3K/AKT pathway by insulin like growth factor – 1 (IGF-1) has been shown to block heat shock induced apoptosis [35]. In addition, pharmacological inhibition of PI3K, upstream kinase of AKT, using LY294002 resulted in significant decrease in total cleavage, 8 cells and blastocyst development rates in bovine [36]. In the present study, we used two different pharmacological inhibitors of AKT activity to investigate its role in early bovine embryo development. Pharmacological inhibition was selected over siRNA mediated knockdown because inhibitors are membrane permeable and can function immediately by specifically targeting AKT activity without affecting its total protein abundance in embryo. As inhibitors can function in reversible manner, this allowed us to inhibit AKT signaling for define period (d1–3) of in vitro embryo culture in this study. Our does dependent study showed that AKT inhibitor III at 75 μm or AKT inhibitor IV at 3.5 μM doses exhibited about 50% reduction in AKT phosphorylation levels and therefore were selected as most effective dose to inhibit AKT signaling. These results were in accordance with the previously published studies in bovine and mice [18, 19, 21]. In addition, higher doses of AKT inhibitor III used in this study has been previously reported to have no nonspecific effect on other kinases downstream to PDK1 [18].

Our results showed that inhibition of AKT during first 3 days of in vitro embryo culture (before zygotic genome activation) resulted in pronounced reduction in multiple indices of early embryonic development. Early embryonic cleavage at 30 hpi was not detected for all tested doses of AKT inhibitor III. Total cleavage, rates of development to 8- to 16-cell and day 7 blastocyst rates were significantly reduced in embryos treated with the highest dose of AKT inhibitor III. We observed similar effects of AKT signaling inhibition on embryo development using AKT inhibitor IV. Data from other species [37, 38] suggest that AKT is implicated in regulation of mitotic cell cycle transition from G2 to M phase through activation of M-phase promoting factor (MPF). Therefore, upon inhibition of AKT, the MPF complex remains inactive and the cells are arrested in G1 or G2 stages of the cell cycle [24, 39]. Reduction of AKT phosphorylation/activity may delay cell cycle progression [40] or compromise the developmental capacity of treated embryos. Therefore, early cleavage at 30 hpi was not detected, and total cleavage, development to 8- to 16-cell and blastocyst stages were reduced compared with untreated embryos. Collectively, these results demonstrated that inhibition of AKT signaling using two different AKT inhibitors similarly reduced the development of early bovine embryos in vitro suggesting an important functional role of AKT signaling in early bovine embryogenesis. However, further mechanistic studies are required to conclusively elucidate how the AKT signaling pathway regulates early embryonic development in bovine.

We previously established a positive association between follistatin and oocyte developmental competence [2, 3]. Supplementation of exogenous follistatin during in vitro embryo culture has embryotropic effects in bovine and non-human primates [4, 41]. Although, follistatin was originally identified as an activin antagonist [13], the embryotropic actions of follistatin are presumably not mediated by inhibition of activin action as exogenous supplementation of activin mimicked the embryotrophic effects of follistatin [4]. As a TGF-β superfamily growth factor binding protein, follistatin may exert its embryotrophic actions by modulating SMAD dependent (SMAD1/5/8 or SMAD2/3) or non-SMAD dependent (AKT, ERK, P38 and JNK) pathways implicated in signaling by this growth factor family [8]. Previous studies in our laboratory demonstrated that, exogenous follistatin supplementation rescued the effects of SMAD2/3 and SMAD4 inhibition/knockdown on early cleavage but not the effects on development to 8- to 16-cell and blastocyst stages, suggesting that the embryotrophic effects of follistatin on early cleavage are SMAD independent [11, 12]. In the current study, the effects of follistatin supplementation on development of AKT inhibitor treated embryos were investigated. Treatment with 10 ng/ml follistatin during the initial 72 h of in vitro embryo culture reversed the inhibitory effects of AKT inhibitor III on early cleavage, total cleavage and development to the 8- to 16-cell stage and partially rescued development to the blastocyst stage. Results also demonstrated that AKT inhibitors significantly reduced the levels of AKT phosphorylation in the absence of follistatin. In addition, follistatin treatment not only reverse the AKT inhibitors effect on phosphorylation level but also increase the AKT phosphorylation when supplemented independently for 24 h. These results suggest that follistatin may be playing a role in returning the AKT phosphorylation to the levels required for rescuing the adverse effect of AKT inhibitors on early cleavage. Collectively, results suggest a potential functional link between follistatin action and AKT signaling linked to its embryotropic actions in bovine embryos. As the effects of other signaling pathways can't be disregarded, further studies may be required to elucidate the effects of inhibition of multiple signaling pathways on the development of early bovine embryos and to dissect the specific effects of each signaling pathway.

Effects of TGF-β superfamily stimulation on AKT signaling appear to be pleiotropic and cell type dependent. It has been demonstrated that members of TGF-β superfamily activate PI3K pathway through phosphorylation of its downstream effector AKT [42–44]. TGF-β can induce a physical interaction between the p85 regulatory subunit of PI3K and the TβRII and TβRI receptors converting phosphatidylinositol-4,5-bisphosphate (PIP_2) to phosphatidylinositol-3,4,5-triphosphate (PIP_3) and subsequently AKT phosphorylation [45–47]. Studies on somatic cell lines indicate that follistatin treatment activates PI3K/AKT signaling pathway [48, 49]. In the present studies, follistatin treatment reversed the inhibitory effects of AKT inhibitor treatment on AKT phosphorylation levels at 10 h post treatment, but a follistatin dependent increase in basal AKT phosphorylation was not observed in the absence of AKT inhibitor treatment. However, follistatin treatment did increase basal AKT phosphorylation levels 24 h post treatment administration. The exact reason for time dependent effects on AKT signaling observed in response to follistatin treatment are not known but may be reflecting time/treatment induced differences in endogenous growth factor milieu and bioaffinity for specific ligands. Results suggest that follistatin plays a role in regulation of AKT signaling in early bovine embryos. However, AKT seems to not be required for the embryotrophic actions of follistatin.

Conclusions

Results of the present study demonstrate that inhibition of AKT signaling reduce the developmental competence of early bovine embryos suggesting a potential requirement of AKT signaling for bovine early embryonic development. Follistatin supplementation rescued the developmental competence of AKT inhibitor treated embryos suggesting that the examined embryotrophic effects of follistatin do not require AKT signaling. However, follistatin supplementation increased the relative abundance of pAKT in AKT inhibitor treated embryos and increased the level of AKT phosphorylation when supplemented without AKT inhibitor, suggesting that follistatin plays a role in regulation of AKT signaling in early bovine embryos. Together, the results reported here, provide additional insights into understanding the regulation of early embryonic development and the mechanism of action of the embryotrophic agent, follistatin, in early bovine embryos.

Additional files

Additional file 1: Figure S1. Effect of AKT inhibitors III and IV treatments on AKT-Ser473 phosphorylation levels in early bovine embryos. IVF embryos were cultured in presence of 0, 25, 50 or 75 μM AKT inhibitor III or 0, 1.5, 2.5 or 3.5 μM AKT inhibitor IV for 10 h, then subjected to Western blot for pAKT-Ser473, tAKT and actin analysis ($n = 3$ replicates/antibody, $n = 20$ embryos/treatment). Data were normalized relative to abundance of actin and phosphorylation levels (**a, b**) were expressed as pAKT/tAKT. Representative Western blot images are shown. Data are expressed as mean ± SEM. Values with different superscripts among treatments indicate significant differences ($P < 0.05$). (TIFF 650 kb)

Additional file 2: Figure S2. Effect of follistatin treatment on AKT-Ser473 phosphorylation in early bovine embryos. Presumptive zygotes were cultured with 0 or 10 ng/ml recombinant human follistatin in the presence or absence of AKT inhibitor III (75 μM) for 10 h ($n = 5$ replicates, $n = 20$ zygotes/group) (**a**), or Presumptive zygotes were cultured in the presence or absence of 10 ng/ml follistatin for 24 h ($n = 5$ replicates, $n = 20$ zygotes/group) (**b**). Samples were subjected to Western blot analysis for pAKT-Ser473, tAKT and Actin. Expression levels were normalized to the abundance of an endogenous control actin. Phosphorylation level was expressed as pAKT/tAKT. Data are expressed as mean ± standard error. Values with different superscripts among treatments indicate significant differences ($P < 0.05$). Representative Western blots are shown. (TIFF 542 kb)

Abbreviations

AKT/PKB: Protein Kinase B; BMPs: Bone Morphogenetic Proteins; BSA: Bovine Serum Albumin; CDK1: Cyclin Dependent Kinase 1; COCs: Cumulus Oocyte Complexes; D: Day; Dpi: Days post insemination; FBS: Fetal Bovine Serum; FSH: Follicle Stimulating Hormone; H: Hour; Hpi: Hour Post Insemination; IGF-1: Insulin Like Growth Factor – 1; Inh: Inhibitor; IVC: In Vitro Culture; IVF: In Vitro Fertilization; IVM: In Vitro Maturation; KSOM: Potassium Simplex

Optimization Medium; LH: Luteinizing Hormone; MI: Metaphase I; MII: Metaphase II; pAKT: Phosphorylated AKT; PDE3A: Phosphodiesterase 3A; PVDF: Polyvinylidene Difluoride; Ser: Serine; tAKT: Total AKT; TBST: Tris Buffered Saline; TGF-β: Transforming growth factor β; Thr: Threonine; WB: Western blotting; μM: Micro molar

Acknowledgements
Not applicable.

Funding
This study was supported by the National Institute of Child Health and Human Development of the National Institutes of Health under award number R01HD072972 and by Michigan State University AgBioResearch. MA was supported by the Egyptian Government Joint supervision grant JS2687. The funding agencies had no role neither in study design, data collection, analysis, or interpretation nor in the writing of the report; or in the decision to submit the paper for publication.

Authors' contributions
This study was conceptualized and designed by MA, SKR, JKF and GWS. Investigations and data curation were done by MA with guidance of SKR. Fund acquisition was done by GWS, JGK and MA. Statistical analysis was done by MA and JKF. Original draft was prepared by MA, reviews and editing were completed by MA, SKR, JKF, JGK, NAH, OMK, RSR and GWS. All authors read and approved the final manuscript.

Competing interests
The authors declare that they have no competing interests.

Author details
[1]Laboratory of Mammalian Reproductive Biology and Genomics, Michigan State University, East Lansing, MI 48824, USA. [2]Developmental Epigenetics Laboratory, Michigan State University, East Lansing, MI 48824, USA. [3]Department of Animal Science, Michigan State University, East Lansing, MI 48824, USA. [4]Department of Theriogenology, Faculty of Veterinary Medicine, Cairo University, Giza, Egypt. [5]Department of Animal Reproduction and Artificial Insemination, Veterinary Research Division, National Research Center, Giza, Egypt.

References

1. Ashry M, Smith GW. Application of embryo transfer using in vitro produced embryos: intrinsic factors affecting efficiency. Cattle Practice. 2015;23:8.
2. Patel OV, Bettegowda A, Ireland JJ, Coussens PM, Lonergan P, Smith GW. Functional genomics studies of oocyte competence: evidence that reduced transcript abundance for follistatin is associated with poor developmental competence of bovine oocytes. Reproduction. 2007;133:95–106.
3. Ashry M, Lee K, Mondal M, Datta TK, Folger JK, Rajput SK, Zhang K, Hemeida NA, Smith GW. Expression of TGFbeta superfamily components and other markers of oocyte quality in oocytes selected by brilliant cresyl blue staining: relevance to early embryonic development. Mol Reprod Dev. 2015;82:251–64.
4. Lee KB, Bettegowda A, Wee G, Ireland JJ, Smith GW. Molecular determinants of oocyte competence: potential functional role for maternal (oocyte-derived) follistatin in promoting bovine early embryogenesis. Endocrinology. 2009;150:2463–71.
5. Rajput SK, Lee K, Zhenhua G, Di L, Folger JK, Smith GW. Embryotropic actions of follistatin: paracrine and autocrine mediators of oocyte competence and embryo developmental progression. Reprod Fertil Dev. 2013;26:37–47.
6. Moustakas A, Souchelnytskyi S, Heldin CH. Smad regulation in TGF-beta signal transduction. J Cell Sci. 2001;114:4359–69.
7. Attisano L, Wrana JL. Signal transduction by the TGF-beta superfamily. Science. 2002;296:1646–7.
8. Zhang YE. Non-Smad pathways in TGF-beta signaling. Cell Res. 2009;19:128–39.
9. Mu Y, Gudey S, Landström M. Non-Smad signaling pathways. Cell Tissue Res. 2012;347:11–20.
10. Ikushima H, Miyazono K. TGFbeta signalling: a complex web in cancer progression. Nat Rev Cancer. 2010;10:415–24.
11. Zhang K, Rajput SK, Lee KB, et al. Evidence supporting a role for SMAD2/3 in bovine early embryonic development: potential implications for Embryotropic actions of Follistatin. Biol Reprod. 2015;93(4):86.
12. Lee KB, Zhang K, Folger JK, Knott JG, Smith GW. Evidence supporting a functional requirement of SMAD4 for bovine preimplantation embryonic development: a potential link to embryotrophic actions of follistatin. Biol Reprod. 2014;91:62.
13. Nakamura T, Takio K, Eto Y, Shibai H, Titani K, Sugino H. Activin-binding protein from rat ovary is follistatin. Science. 1990;247:836–8.
14. Iemura S, Yamamoto TS, Takagi C, Uchiyama H, Natsume T, Shimasaki S, Sugino H, Ueno N. Direct binding of follistatin to a complex of bone-morphogenetic protein and its receptor inhibits ventral and epidermal cell fates in early Xenopus embryo. Proc Natl Acad Sci U S A. 1998;95:9337–42.
15. Lin SY, Morrison JR, Phillips DJ, de Kretser DM. Regulation of ovarian function by the TGF-beta superfamily and follistatin. Reproduction. 2003;126:133–48.
16. Ghosh-Choudhury N, Abboud SL, Nishimura R, Celeste A, Mahimainathan L, Choudhury GG. Requirement of BMP-2-induced phosphatidylinositol 3-kinase and Akt serine/threonine kinase in osteoblast differentiation and Smad-dependent BMP-2 gene transcription. J Biol Chem. 2002;277:33361–8.
17. Do TV, Kubba LA, Antenos M, Rademaker AW, Sturgis CD, Woodruff TK. The role of activin a and Akt/GSK signaling in ovarian tumor biology. Endocrinology. 2008;149:3809–16.
18. Tomek W, Smiljakovic T. Activation of Akt (protein kinase B) stimulates metaphase I to metaphase II transition in bovine oocytes. Reproduction. 2005;130:423–30.
19. Kalous J, Kubelka M, Solc P, Susor A, Motlik J. AKT (protein kinase B) is implicated in meiotic maturation of porcine oocytes. Reproduction. 2009; 138:645–54.
20. Kalous J, Solc P, Baran V, Kubelka M, Schultz RM, Motlik J. PKB/AKT is involved in resumption of meiosis in mouse oocytes. Biol Cell. 2006;98:111–23.
21. Hoshino Y, Sato E. Protein kinase B (PKB/Akt) is required for the completion of meiosis in mouse oocytes. Dev Biol. 2008;314:215–23.
22. Andersen CB, Roth RA, Conti M. Protein kinase B/Akt induces resumption of meiosis in Xenopus oocytes. J Biol Chem. 1998;273:18705–8.
23. Bellacosa A, Testa JR, Staal SP, Tsichlis PN. A retroviral oncogene, akt, encoding a serine-threonine kinase containing an SH2-like region. Science. 1991;254:274–7.
24. Baran V, Fabian D, Rehak P. Akt/PKB plays role of apoptosis relay on entry into first mitosis of mouse embryo. Zygote. 2013;21:406–16.
25. Li Y, Chandrakanthan V, Day ML, O'Neill C. Direct evidence for the action of phosphatidylinositol (3,4,5)-trisphosphate-mediated signal transduction in the 2-cell mouse embryo. Biol Reprod. 2007;77:813–21.
26. Riley JK, Carayannopoulos MO, Wyman AH, Chi M, Ratajczak CK, Moley KH. The PI3K/Akt pathway is present and functional in the preimplantation mouse embryo. Dev Biol. 2005;284:377–86.
27. Bettegowda A, Patel OV, Ireland JJ, Smith GW. Quantitative analysis of messenger RNA abundance for ribosomal protein L-15, cyclophilin-a, phosphoglycerokinase, beta-glucuronidase, glyceraldehyde 3-phosphate dehydrogenase, beta-actin, and histone H2A during bovine oocyte maturation and early embryogenesis in vitro. Mol Reprod Dev. 2006;73:267–78.
28. Bhutani J, Sheikh A, Niazi AK. Akt inhibitors: mechanism of action and implications for anticancer therapeutics. Infect Agent Cancer. 2013;8:49.
29. Schneider CA, Rasband WS, Eliceiri KW. NIH image to ImageJ: 25 years of image analysis. Nat Meth. 2012;9:671–5.
30. Kandel ES, Skeen J, Majewski N, Di Cristofano A, Pandolfi PP, Feliciano CS, Gartel A, Hay N. Activation of Akt/protein kinase B overcomes a G(2)/m cell cycle checkpoint induced by DNA damage. Mol Cell Biol. 2002;22: 7831–41.
31. Song G, Ouyang G, Bao S. The activation of Akt/PKB signaling pathway and cell survival. J Cell Mol Med. 2005;9:59–71.
32. Kandel ES, Hay N. The regulation and activities of the multifunctional serine/ Threonine Kinase Akt/PKB. Exp Cell Res. 1999;253:210–29.

33. Downward J. Mechanisms and consequences of activation of protein kinase B/Akt. Curr Opin Cell Biol. 1998;10:262–7.
34. Feng C, Yu A, Liu Y, Zhang J, Zong Z, Su W, Zhang Z, Yu D, Sun QY, Yu B. Involvement of protein kinase B/AKT in early development of mouse fertilized eggs. Biol Reprod. 2007;77:560–8.
35. Jousan FD, Oliveira LJ, Hansen PJ. Short-term culture of in vitro produced bovine preimplantation embryos with insulin-like growth factor-i prevents heat shock-induced apoptosis through activation of the Phosphatidylinositol 3-Kinase/Akt pathway. Mol Reprod Dev. 2008;75:681–8.
36. Aparicio IM, Garcia-Herreros M, Fair T, Lonergan P. Identification and regulation of glycogen synthase kinase-3 during bovine embryo development. Reproduction. 2010;140:83–92.
37. Katayama K, Fujita N, Tsuruo T. Akt/protein kinase B-dependent phosphorylation and inactivation of WEE1Hu promote cell cycle progression at G2/M transition. Mol Cell Biol. 2005;25:5725–37.
38. Okumura E, Fukuhara T, Yoshida H, Hanada Si S, Kozutsumi R, Mori M, Tachibana K, Kishimoto T. Akt inhibits Myt1 in the signalling pathway that leads to meiotic G2/M-phase transition. Nat Cell Biol. 2002;4:111–6.
39. Roberts EC, Shapiro PS, Nahreini TS, Pages G, Pouyssegur J, Ahn NG. Distinct cell cycle timing requirements for extracellular signal-regulated kinase and phosphoinositide 3-kinase signaling pathways in somatic cell mitosis. Mol Cell Biol. 2002;22:7226–41.
40. Ornelas IM, Silva TM, Fragel-Madeira L, Ventura ALM. Inhibition of PI3K/Akt pathway impairs G2/M transition of cell cycle in late developing progenitors of the avian embryo retina. PLoS One. 2013;8:e53517.
41. VandeVoort CA, Mtango NR, Lee YS, Smith GW, Latham KE. Differential effects of follistatin on nonhuman primate oocyte maturation and pre-implantation embryo development in vitro. Biol Reprod. 2009;81:1139–46.
42. Bakin AV, Tomlinson AK, Bhowmick NA, Moses HL, Arteaga CL. Phosphatidylinositol 3-kinase function is required for transforming growth factor beta-mediated epithelial to mesenchymal transition and cell migration. J Biol Chem. 2000;275:36803–10.
43. Lamouille S, Derynck R. Cell size and invasion in TGF-beta-induced epithelial to mesenchymal transition is regulated by activation of the mTOR pathway. J Cell Biol. 2007;178:437–51.
44. Lamouille S, Xu J, Derynck R. Molecular mechanisms of epithelial-mesenchymal transition. Nat Rev Mol Cell Biol. 2014;15:178–96.
45. Yi JY, Shin I, Arteaga CL. Type I transforming growth factor beta receptor binds to and activates phosphatidylinositol 3-kinase. J Biol Chem. 2005;280: 10870–6.
46. Moustakas A, Heldin C-H. Non-Smad TGF-β signals. J Cell Sci. 2005;118: 3573–84.
47. Guo X, Wang XF. Signaling cross-talk between TGF-beta/BMP and other pathways. Cell Res. 2009;19:71–88.
48. Winbanks CE, Weeks KL, Thomson RE, Sepulveda PV, Beyer C, Qian H, Chen JL, Allen JM, Lancaster GI, Febbraio MA, et al. Follistatin-mediated skeletal muscle hypertrophy is regulated by Smad3 and mTOR independently of myostatin. J Cell Biol. 2012;197:997–1008.
49. Li X, Liu H, Wang H, Sun L, Ding F, Sun W, Han C, Wang J. Follistatin could promote the proliferation of duck primary myoblasts by activating PI3K/Akt/ mTOR signalling. Biosci Rep. 2014;34:e00143.

11

Expression of cystatin C in the female reproductive tract and its effect on human sperm capacitation

Robert Kuo-Kuang Lee[1,2,3†], Huan-Chin Tseng[1†], Yuh-Ming Hwu[2,4,5], Chi-Chen Fan[6,7], Ming-Huei Lin[2,5], Jhih-Jie Yu[1], Ling-Yu Yeh[1] and Sheng-Hsiang Li[1,5*]

Abstract

Background: Cystatin C (CST3), a cysteine protease inhibitor in seminal plasma, is expressed in animal uteri. However, its expression in the human female reproductive tract and its effect on human sperm capacitation are unclear.

Methods: The cellular localization of CST3 was observed using immunohistochemistry. The binding of CST3 to sperm was examined using immunocytochemistry. Sperm motility parameters were analyzed using computer-assisted sperm analysis. Sperm capacitation was evaluated by analyzing cholesterol content, protein tyrosine phosphorylation levels, and the acrosome reaction.

Results: Immunohistochemical staining demonstrated that CST3 is prominently expressed in the female reproductive tract, including the epithelial lining and cervix and endometrium fluids, particularly at times near ovulation. It can bind to human sperm on the post-acrosomal head region and the mid and principal piece of the tail. CST3 enhances sperm motility and inhibits the signal initiating sperm capacitation, i.e., efflux of cholesterol from the sperm plasma membrane and a late sperm capacitation event, i.e., the increase in the sperm protein tyrosine phosphorylation. The suppressive trend on sperm acrosome reaction further supports CST3's ability to inhibit sperm capacitation.

Conclusions: These findings suggest that cervical CST3 may prevent precocious capacitation and acrosome reaction, thus preserving sperm fertilizing ability before it reaches the fallopian tube. Additionally, CST3 may help sperm enter the upper reproductive tract by enhancing sperm motility.

Background

Cystatin C (CST3), a small secretory protein encoded by the *CST3* gene, is extensively expressed in various tissues and body fluids and possesses potent inhibitory activity against cysteine proteases [1]. CST3 level is high in blood serum and is removed from the bloodstream via the kidney's glomerular filtration; thus, it is a simple, accurate, and rapid endogenous marker of glomerular filtration rate [2, 3].

CST3 is prominently expressed in the male reproductive tract with high levels in seminal plasma, approximately 37-fold higher than in serum [4, 5]. The prostasome, an exosome-like vesicle in seminal plasma secreted by the prostate epithelium [6], can inhibit sperm capacitation [7, 8]; CST3 was demonstrated to be associated with the prostasome [9]. Thus, CST3 may be important in sperm physiology too.

Ejaculated sperm must reside in the female reproductive tract to be able to fertilize an egg, known as capacitation first described and defined in the early 1950s [10, 11]. The sperm's surface is exposed to protein-rich secretions from the seminal plasma, cervix, uterus, or fallopian tubes during transit. Thus, proteins secreted by these tissues interact with and modify changes in sperm physiology to make fertilization possible [12, 13]. Capacitation is a physiologically complex change and may be initiated by cholesterol removal from the sperm plasma membrane, leading to changes in the membrane's structure and fluidity and increasing the sperm's calcium and bicarbonate ion permeability [14, 15]. This activates a cyclic AMP (cAMP)-

* Correspondence: lsh@mmh.org.tw
†Equal contributors
[1]Department of Medical Research, Mackay Memorial Hospital, Tamsui District, New Taipei City 251, Taiwan
[5]Mackay Junior College of Medicine, Nursing, and Management, Beitou District, Taipei City 112, Taiwan
Full list of author information is available at the end of the article

dependent protein kinase and induces tyrosine phosphorylation of a subset of sperm proteins [16, 17].

Seminal plasma, a mix of male accessory sexual gland secretions, has been demonstrated to reverse sperm capacitation [18]. The affecting factor, defined as decapacitation factor (DF), is removed from the sperm surface before or during capacitation [13]. Previous studies have reported that potential DFs are primarily present in human and rodent seminal plasma [19–29]. However, as human sperm enters the cervix, it must migrate through interstices formed by cervical mucus [30]. The interstices are smaller than the sperm head; thus, proteins derived from seminal plasma and bound to sperm surface are potentially stripped from sperm when it passes the cervix because seminal proteins are speculated to weakly associate with sperm membrane [31]. This seemingly suggests that seminal plasma DFs become effective before sperm enters the cervix. How sperm can preserve its fertility before reaching the fertilization site, i.e., the ampulla of the fallopian tube, warrants further studies. Previous studies have evaluated the importance of oviductal components like hyaluronic acid [32] and some oviductal proteins [33, 34] in the female reproductive tract that contribute to preserve sperm viability and motility until fertilization. Human sperm can prolong acrosomal integrity as it stays in the cervix for up to five days [35]. This indicates that secretory proteins in the cervix are important in preserving sperm fertility.

We believe that, except seminal DFs, some proteins secreted by the lower female reproductive tract, such as cervical mucus or uterine fluid, may protect sperm from premature capacitation and thus preserve the sperm's fertilization ability until it reaches the fallopian tube. Previous studies have reported CST3 expression in the endometrial luminal epithelium and glandular epithelium, secreted into the uterine cavity, and upregulated by progesterone in the ovine uterus [36]. In rat uterus, CST3 was expressed in the glandular epithelium, secreted into the uterine lumen, and downregulated by estrogen during the peri-implantation period [37]. In pigs, *CST3* mRNA levels increased in the endometrial epithelium during pregnancy, whereas progesterone decreased CST3 expression in the epithelium but increased it in the stromal compartment [38]. However, CST3 cellular distribution in the human female reproductive tract has not been explored. Here, we investigated the cellular localization of CST3 in the human female reproductive tract and its effect on human sperm capacitation.

Methods

Samples and ethics

Formalin-fixed and paraffin-embedded tissues, including the cervix, uterine endometrium, and fallopian tubes in the proliferative and secretory phases, were obtained from the Department of Pathology, Mackay Memorial Hospital (Taipei, Taiwan). Patients with the following features were excluded: > 40 or < 20 years old, menstruation irregular or regular with hormone treatment, a malignant disease requiring surgery, and systemic disease. Semen samples were collected via masturbation after 2–3 days of sexual abstinence. After liquefaction for at least 30 min, routine semen analysis was conducted according to the 2010 World Health Organization criteria [39]. Semen samples with > 40% motility and sperm counts > 15 million/ml were included. Clinical paraffin section and semen usage was reviewed and approved by the hospital's institutional review board (approval number 15MMHIS101).

Immunohistochemical staining

An automatic staining machine (BenchMark XT; Ventana Medical Systems, Tucson, AZ, USA) was used for immunohistochemical staining using the XT ultraView (UV) 3, 3′-diaminobenzidine (DAB) detection kit (Ventana Medical Systems). Tissue sections (4 µm) on slides were deparaffinized, hydrated, and heated to induce antigen retrieval according to a previously described method [40]. After inactivating endogenous peroxidase activity using a UV inhibitor, the sections were incubated with a rabbit monoclonal anti-CST3 antibody (ab109508; Abcam, Cambridge, MA, USA) or a control antibody (1:5000) in a blocking solution at 37 °C for 30 min. Sections were rinsed and then incubated with UV horseradish peroxidase (HRP) at 37 °C for 8 min. Staining signals were developed using UV DAB and hydrogen peroxide at 37 °C for 8 min. Slides were finally incubated with UV copper for 4 min to enhance signal intensity, counterstained with hematoxylin (Vector Laboratories, Burlingame, CA, USA), and photographed using TissueFaxs software on an automated acquisition system (TissueGnostics, Vienna, Austria).

Human sperm preparation

Sperms were prepared using the swim-up method. Briefly, 1.0 ml liquefied semen was mixed with 6 ml 1X diluted Earle's balanced salt (E-7510; Sigma-Aldrich, St. Louis, MO, USA) medium supplemented with 0.3 mM sodium pyruvate (hereafter abbreviated as EBSS). After centrifuging at 500 *g* for 10 min, approximately 0.2 ml of the lowest layer was collected, resuspended, and transferred to an Eppendorf tube containing 1 ml EBSS medium. The tube was set at a 45° angle to make sperm swim-up in a 5% (*v*/v) CO_2 atmosphere in humidified air for 30 min. Sperm with progressive motility were collected from the upper layer.

Highly motile sperm was purified using two-layer PureSperm (Nidacon International AB, Mölndal, Sweden) discontinuous density gradient centrifugation. Briefly, 1.0 ml liquefied semen was layered above the upper layer of the PureSperm gradient solution prepared by layering 1.0 ml

PureSperm40 on 1.0 ml PureSperm80 solution. After centrifuging at 300 *g* for 20 min, the upper supernatant was removed except the lowest 0.5 ml and resuspended in 5 ml EBSS medium. After washing with EBSS by centrifugation again, the lowest 0.1 ml was collected. The sperm's working concentration could be arranged by centrifugation and then be resuspended in a suitable volume of medium.

Immunolocalization of CST3 on human sperm

To evaluate whether CST3 is a sperm-binding protein, sperm isolated using the swim-up method was smeared on slides, fixed in 4% (*w*/*v*) paraformaldehyde, allowed to air-dry, and washed twice with phosphate-buffered saline (PBS). The slides were incubated in a blocking solution, PBS containing 10% (*v*/*v*) normal goat serum, for 1 h at room temperature and then incubated with the anti-CST3 antibody (1:250; ab109508; Abcam) or control antiserum (1:100 in blocking solution) for 1 h. After repeatedly washing thrice with PBS for 5 min each to remove excess antibodies, the slides were incubated with fluorescein isothiocyanate (FITC)-conjugated goat anti-rabbit IgG (Vector Laboratories, 1:500 in blocking solution) for 40 min. The slides were then washed using previously described procedure, counterstained with 5 μg/ml Hoechst 33,258, and mounted in Prolong Gold antifade medium (Invitrogen Molecular Probes, Eugene, OR, USA) after briefly rinsing with PBS. The staining signal was visualized using an epifluorescence microscope equipped with a digital camera (Olympus DP 71, Tokyo, Japan).

To evaluate whether exogenous human CST3 binds to human sperm, 2 μg/ml CST3 (PRO-413; ProSpec, East Brunswick, NJ, USA) was incubated with living sperm (10^6 cells/ml, isolated using PureSperm density gradient centrifugation) in Eppendorf tubes at 37 °C for 20 min. The unbound CST3 was discarded using PBS by centrifuging at 600 *g* for 5 min at room temperature. Sperm was then transferred onto slides, fixed in 4% (*w*/*v*) paraformaldehyde for 20 min at room temperature, and air-dried.

Analysis of sperm motility

Human sperm (2×10^7 cells/ml) isolated using PureSperm density gradient centrifugation was incubated in 100 μl EBSS medium containing sodium bicarbonate (10 mM) and bovine serum albumin (BSA, 3 mg/ml) at 37 °C under 5% (*v*/*v*) CO_2 in humidified air. To analyze CST3 effect on sperm motility, the medium was supplemented with or the medium's BSA was replaced with 0.25 mg/ml CST3. Sperm motility was determined using a computer-assisted sperm analysis system with a sperm motility analyzer (IVOS version 10; Hamilton-Thorne Research, Beverly, MA, USA). A 3 μl sample was loaded into a 20 μm deep Leja slide at 37 °C for analyses at 30 min intervals up to 180 min. Motility parameters, including averaged path velocity (VAP), straight-line velocity (VSL), curvilinear velocity (VCL), percentages of sperm motility (VAP > 7 μm/s), and progressive motility [VAP > 50 μm/s and path straightness (STR) > 80%, where STR = VSL/VAP] were measured. Analyzer settings were to default values. For each assay, five fields with 100–400 sperm were analyzed.

Cholesterol efflux assay

Human spermatozoa (2×10^6 cells/ml) were preincubated with or without CST3 (0.125, 0.25, or 0.5 mg/ml) in 100 μl EBSS medium for 20 min and then supplemented with BSA (3 mg/ml) or sodium bicarbonate (10 mM) for capacitation at 37 °C for 3 h under 5% (*v*/*v*) CO_2 in humidified air. The sperm was then centrifuged at 20,000 *g* to obtain the pellet. Cholesterol on sperm plasma membrane was extracted following a previously described method [41]. Cholesterol content was measured using an Amplex Red Cholesterol Assay Kit (Invitrogen Molecular Probes) according to manufacturer instructions. A cholesterol standard curve was prepared using the cholesterol reference standard provided with the kit to calculate the cholesterol content of the samples.

Evaluating capacitation-associated sperm tyrosine phosphorylation

Capacitation-accompanied increases in 105- and 80-kDa human sperm proteins tyrosine phosphorylation were examined according to a previously described method [42]. Briefly, approximately 2×10^6 sperm/ml were incubated in 100 μl EBSS medium with or without CST3 (0.125, 0.25 or 0.5 mg/ml) at 37 °C for 20 min; BSA and sodium bicarbonate were then added as described for in vitro capacitation. After 3 h of incubation, the soluble sperm protein extract fractions were subjected to 10% SDS-PAGE. Proteins on the gel were electrotransferred onto nitrocellulose. Western blots were performed using anti-phosphotyrosine (clone 4G10; Upstate Biotechnology, Lake Placid, NY, USA) and α-tubulin antibody (Sigma-Aldrich). Relative expression levels were normalized by the loading control levels, i.e., α-tubulin protein.

Evaluation of the acrosome reaction

PureSperm-isolated sperm (2×10^6 sperm/ml) were incubated with or without CST3 (0.0625, 0.125, 0.25, or 0.5 mg/ml); subsequently, capacitation was performed as described above. The capacitated sperm was then treated with or without 10 μM A23187 in 0.1% (*v*/*v*) dimethyl sulfoxide at 37 °C for 30 min and was collected by centrifugation at 600 *g* for 5 min, smeared onto slides, and air-dried. The slides were immersed in methanol for 1 min, washed thrice in PBS for 5 min each, and stained with 10 μg/ml tetramethylrhodamine isothiocyanate-conjugated peanut agglutinin lectin (PNA; Sigma-Aldrich) in the dark for

30 min. After washing the slides thrice in PBS for 5 min each, sperm was counterstained with Hoechst 33,258 (5 μg/ml) for 30 s, mounted with Prolong Gold antifade medium (Invitrogen Molecular Probes), and examined with a fluorescence microscope (BX 40, Olympus). A random sample of 500 sperm cells per group was evaluated.

Statistical analysis

Data are presented as mean ± SD. Differences were analyzed by one-way ANOVA followed by the Bonferroni post-hoc test using GraphPad software (GraphPad, San Diego, CA, USA). $p < 0.05$ was considered statistically significant.

Results

CST3 expression in the female reproductive tract

The cellular localization of CST3 in the female reproductive tract was observed using immunohistochemical staining. Contrary to control antiserum (Fig. 1A), CST3 was prominently detected in the endocervical canal during mid- (Fig. 1B) and late-proliferative phases (Fig. 1C) of the menstrual cycle. CST3 was detected in cervical epithelial cells, glands, and mucus (Figs 1D and E), particularly during the late-proliferative phase (Fig. 1E). In the uterus, CST3 was expressed in the luminal and glandular endometrial epithelial cells throughout the proliferative and luteal menstrual cycle phases. CST3 was also detected in uterine fluid, indicating that it could be expressed and secreted by the endometrium (Fig. 2A) and in the fallopian tube epithelial cells, although its expression levels were lower there (Fig. 2B).

Binding of CST3 to human sperm

To examine whether CST3 binds to human sperm, sperm isolated from liquefied semen using the swim-up method was immunostained using anti-CST3 antibody or control antiserum. Contrary to control slides stained using control antiserum (Fig. 3A), CST3 was primarily detected on the post-acrosomal head region and the mid and principal piece of the tail (Fig. 3B). When sperm was isolated using PureSperm density gradient centrifugation, CST3 staining

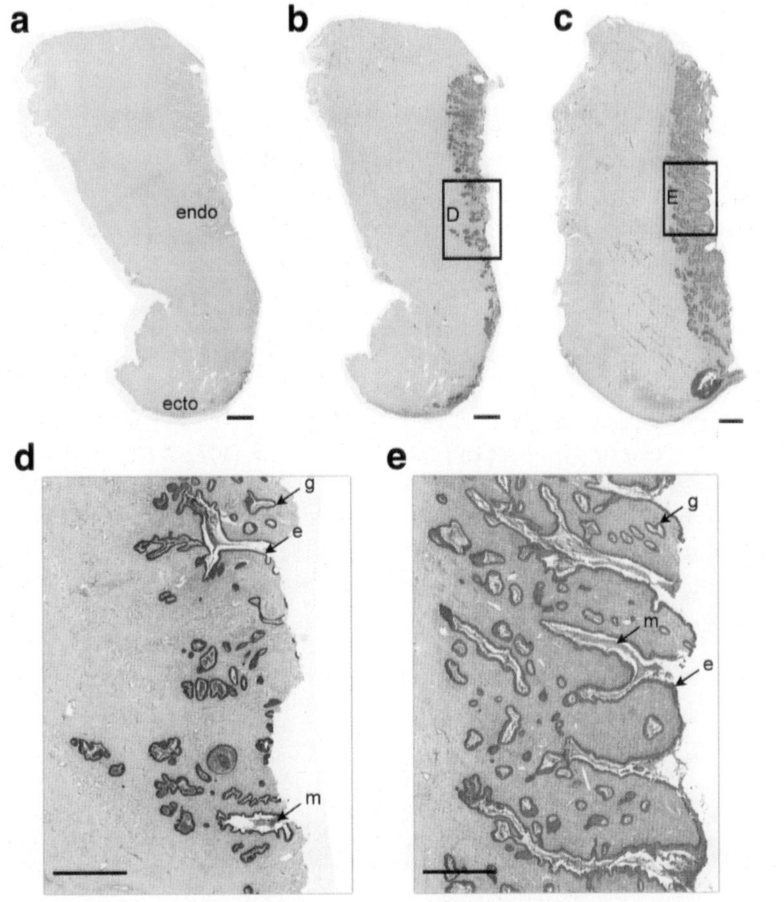

Fig. 1 CST3 immunolocalization in the cervix. Paraffin sections of the cervix at early (**a** and **b**) and late (**c**) proliferative phases of the menstrual cycle were immunostained using control antibody (**a**) or anti-CST3 antibody (**b** and **c**). The selected region in **b** and **c** was enlarged for clarity (**d** and **e**). The staining signals were colored brown by the HRP substrate DAB. Symbols: ecto, ectocervix; endo, endocervix; e, cervical epithelium; g, cervical gland; m, cervical mucus. Bars: A–C, 2 mm; D and E, 1 mm

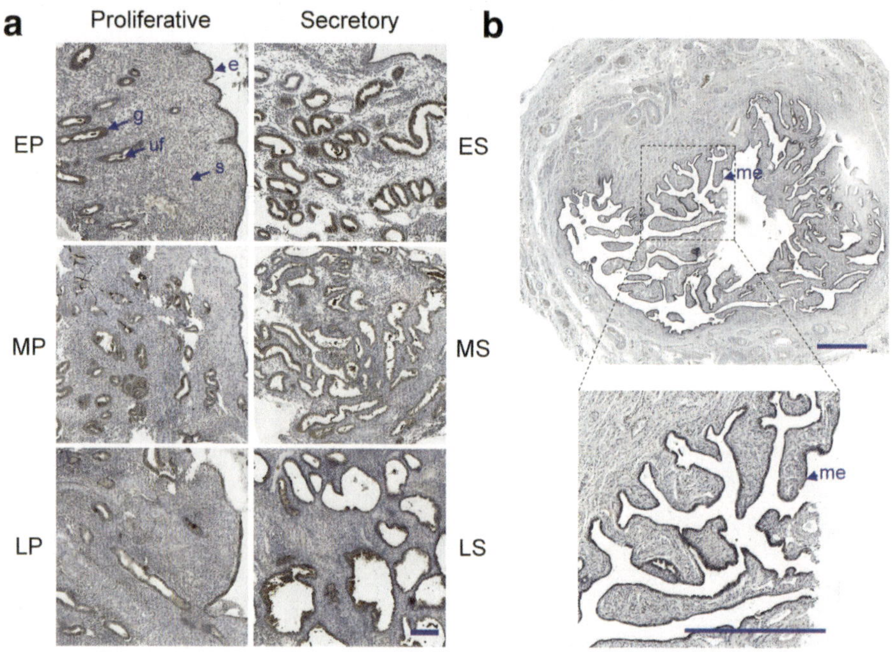

Fig. 2 CST3 expression and localization in the cyclic endometrium and fallopian tube. Paraffin sections prepared by the endometrial curettage during various proliferative and secretory phases (**a**) and the fallopian tube (**b**) were incubated with anti-CST3 antibody as stated in the text. Symbols: e, epithelium; g, gland; me, mucosal epithelium; s, stroma; uf, uterine fluid. The menstrual cycle is divided into six subphases: EP, early proliferative; MP, mid-proliferative; LP, late-proliferative; ES, early secretory; MS, mid-secretory; and LS, late-secretory phase. Bar: 200 μm in A, 1 mm in B

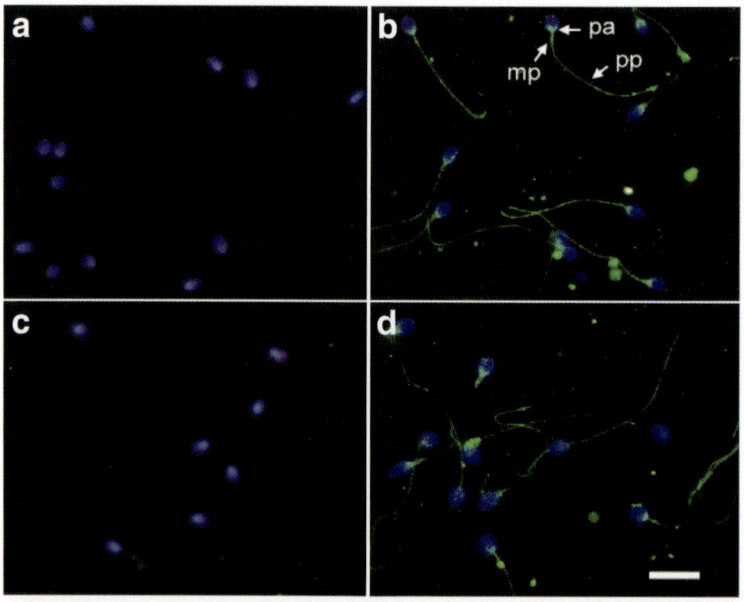

Fig. 3 CST3 binding to human sperm. Sperm isolated using the swim-up method was smeared onto slides for immunohistochemical staining (**a** and **b**). Sperm isolated using PureSperm density gradient were incubated without (**c**) or with (**d**) CST3. After washing off unbound CST3, sperm was transferred onto slides and fixed with 4% (*w/v*) paraformaldehyde. Slides were incubated with control antiserum (**a**) or anti-CST3 antibody (**b–d**) diluted 1:250, treated with FITC-conjugated goat anti-rabbit IgG, and then counterstained with Hoechst dye to localize the nuclei for contrast. Symbols: mp, midpiece; pa, post-acrosome; pp., principal piece. Bar: 10 μm

was very weak with only a faint signal on the sperm tail (Fig. 3C). However, CST3 was prominently stained on sperm with the same binding pattern when human sperm was incubated with exogenous CST3 (Fig. 3D), indicating that CST3 can bind to human sperm.

Enhancement of sperm motility by CST3

Human sperm isolated using density gradient centrifugation was mobile with a visibly beating tail in EBSS medium with sodium bicarbonate (the control group). When the medium was supplemented with BSA, a higher percentage of motile sperm was observed than in the control group. Interestingly, when supplementing the medium with 0.125 mg/ml CST3, the motile sperm percentage was comparable with the BSA group (not shown). However, 0.25 mg/ml CST3 resulted in a relatively higher motile sperm percentage than medium with BSA (Fig. 4A). Increasing CST3 concentration to 0.6 mg/ml had similar results (not shown). Also, co-incubation with CST3 and BSA showed an increased level similar to the CST3-treated group (Fig. 4A). The percentage of progressively motile sperm showed a similar tendency, with relatively higher percentages in the CST3 or in the CST3 and BSA co-treated group (Fig. 4B). A higher VCL was found in the BSA group than in the other three groups, with the CST3 group showing a relatively lower VCL (Fig. 4C). Additionally, STR is higher in sperm treated with CST3, and a considerable STR percentage is still maintained even by co-treatment with BSA (Fig. 4D). Taken together, CST3 can enhance sperm motility and maintain linear motility.

Inhibition of sperm capacitation by CST3

We assessed CST3 effects on sperm capacitation because of its sperm-binding ability and its effect on sperm motility, which was still linear even in the presence of BSA. Cholesterol efflux is a key event initiating sperm capacitation. Thus, we examined CST3 influence on albumin-induced capacitation-associated cholesterol efflux. As expected, BSA induced cholesterol efflux from the capacitated sperm; thus, lower cholesterol contents were retained on capacitated sperm rather than uncapacitated control sperm. However, CST3 suppressed cholesterol efflux in a dose-dependent, statistically insignificant manner (Fig. 5A), suggesting that CST3 might suppress sperm capacitation by blocking cholesterol efflux from the sperm plasma membrane.

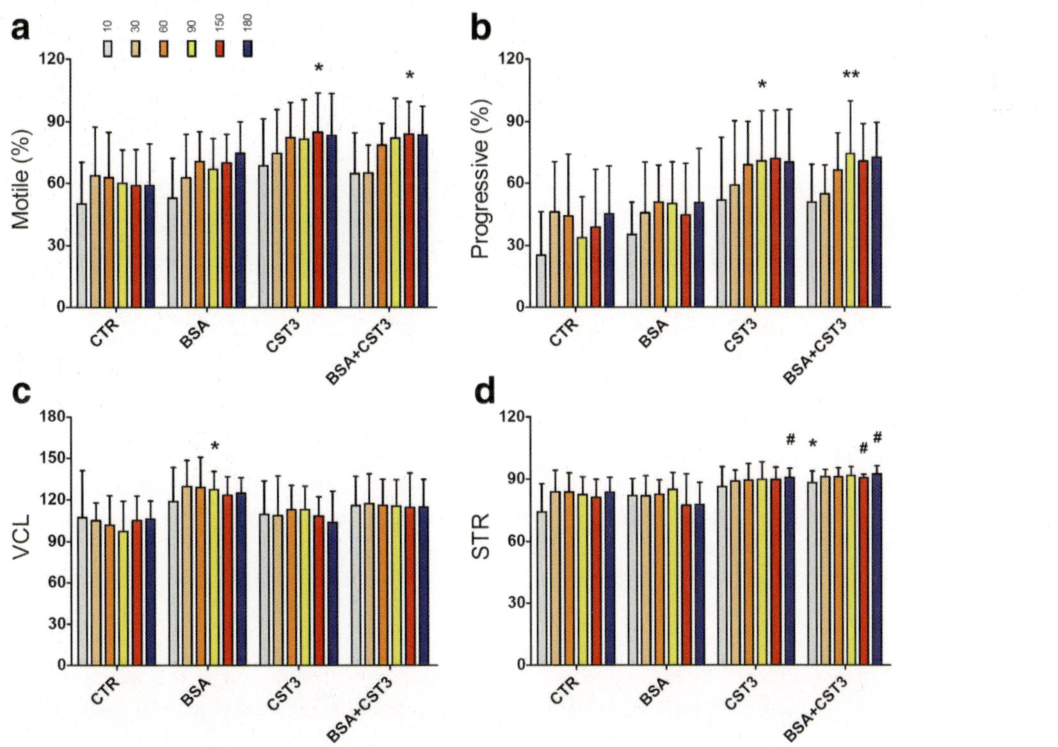

Fig. 4 Effects of CST3 on human sperm motility. Sperm isolated by density gradient was incubated in EBSS medium, or the medium was supplemented with BSA, CST3, or BSA and CST3 (see text for details) at 37 °C under 5% (*v/v*) CO_2 for 3 h. Motility parameters, including motile sperm percentage (**a**), progressively motile sperm percentage (**b**), VCL (**c**), and STR (**d**), at each specified incubation time were determined. Points are expressed as mean ± SD of eight independent determinations. *$p < 0.05$ and **$p < 0.01$ vs. the control (CTR) group; #$p < 0.05$ vs. the BSA group at corresponding time points

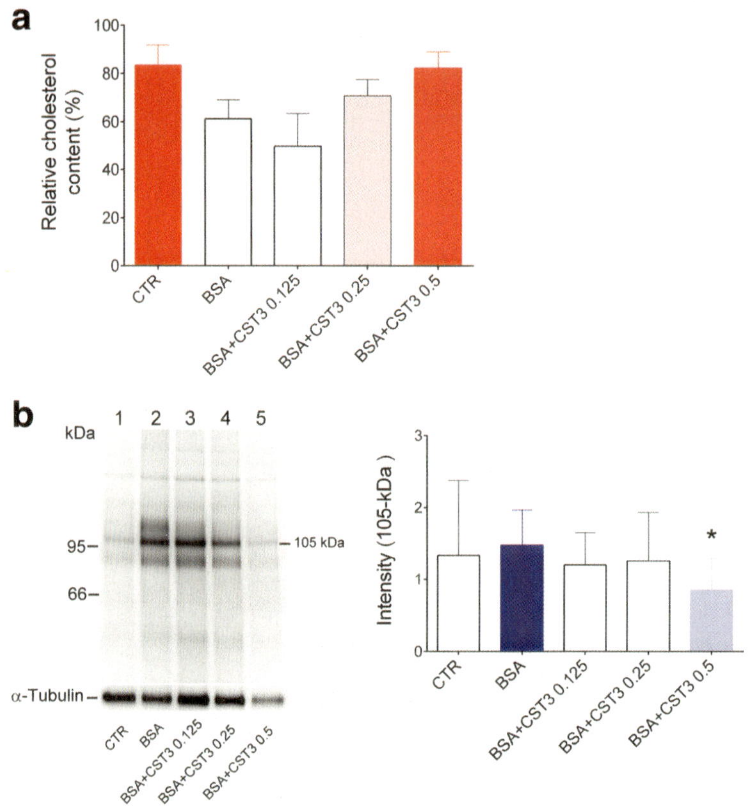

Fig. 5 CST3 inhibits sperm capacitation. Human sperm cultured in EBSS medium was preincubated with or without CST3 (0.125, 0.25, or 0.5 mg/ml) for 20 min, followed by incubation with BSA (3 mg/ml) and sodium bicarbonate (10 mM) for 3 h to induce sperm capacitation. **a** Cholesterol retained on the sperm was measured. Data are expressed as mean ± SD of three independent experiments. **b** Phosphorylation levels of sperm protein's tyrosine residues. A representative anti-phosphotyrosine western blot, out of six experiments, is shown. The relative intensity of the 105-kDa band was quantified using ImageJ, and all values were normalized to the loading control, α-tubulin. *$p < 0.05$ vs. medium supplemented with BSA and bicarbonate

To evaluate CST3 effects on downstream sperm capacitation signaling, the characteristic sperm protein tyrosine phosphorylation pattern was examined. Both bicarbonate and BSA are required for sperm protein tyrosine phosphorylation induction [43]. As expected, the control medium showed basal phosphorylation levels, while BSA remarkably increased the phosphorylation levels. CST3 significantly attenuated the induction at a concentration of 0.5 mg/ml (Fig. 5B).

CST3 inhibits sperm acrosome reaction

Only capacitated sperm can be induced to undergo acrosome reaction [13]; thus, if CST3 inhibits sperm capacitation, it might suppress the acrosome reaction. We therefore examined whether CST3 has inhibitory effects on sperm acrosome reaction induced by the calcium ionophore A23187. As shown in Fig. 6, BSA-capacitated sperm showed remarkable enhancements in acrosome reaction after A23187 induction; contrarily, the percentage of acrosome-reacted sperm gradually attenuated with significant inhibition when sperm was co-incubated with CST3 and BSA at a concentration of 0.5 mg/ml. These findings suggest that CST3 can inhibit sperm capacitation induced in vitro.

Discussion

CST3 is highly expressed in the male genital tract and semen [4, 5]. Although CST3 is expressed in the uterus of rats, sheep, and pigs [36–38], its expression in the human female genital tract is not explored. Here, we reveal the CST3 expression and localization in the cervix, uterus, and fallopian tube. CST3 was prominently expressed in the cervix and endometrium epithelia cells; however, CST3 detection in the cervical mucus and uterine fluid near ovulation is more important. The elevated serum estrogen concentration during the mid- and late-proliferative phases of the menstrual cycle leads to the cervical mucus becoming clear and slippery [44], allowing sperm to enter the cervix. CST3 expression in the cervix creates conditions for interaction between the protein and sperm.

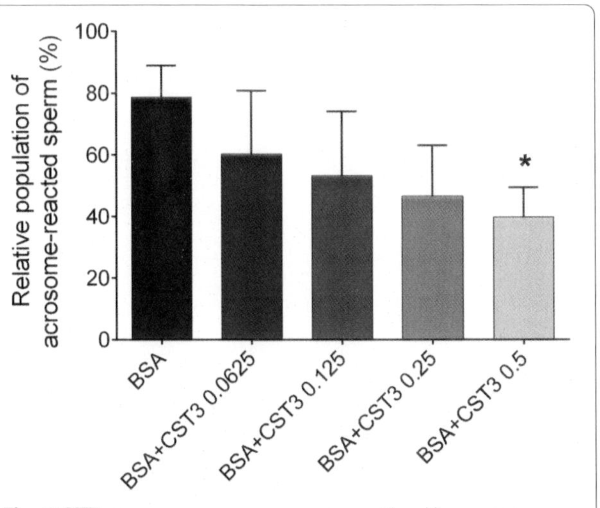

Fig. 6 CST3 suppresses sperm acrosome reaction. Human sperm was capacitated as stated in the text. The sperm acrosome reaction induced by the calcium ionophore A23187 was evaluated using PNA staining. Minimum 500 sperm cells were evaluated per trial. Data are expressed as mean ± SD of five independent experiments. $^{*}p < 0.05$ vs. medium supplemented with BSA and bicarbonate

Seminal proteins may be removed from sperm surface during transit into the cervix [31, 45]. Only sperm with a normal morphology and progressive motility can penetrate the cervix [45, 46]. It is guided into the cervical crypts by cervical mucus strands [39], retained up to several days [35], and gradually released into the upper female reproductive tract.

PureSperm density gradient centrifugation removed immature, less mobile, damaged sperm, and seminal plasma [47, 48]; thus, more morphologically normal and progressively motile sperm can be prepared [49]. Sperm isolated using PureSperm density gradient centrifugation may be similar to sperm entering the cervix and can be used to evaluate interactions between sperm and cervical mucus and/or uterine fluid.

CST3 originating from seminal plasma might bind to human sperm, as demonstrated by immunostaining sperm isolated from semen using the swim-up method; however, seminal CST3 is removed from sperm surface after PureSperm density gradient centrifugation. CST3 might bind to sperm again, as exogenous CST3 was incubated with sperm isolated using density gradient separation. These results indicate that CST3 is a sperm-binding protein and can be stripped from PureSperm-isolated sperm. Thus, PureSperm-isolated sperm was used to mimic sperm that entered the cervix for evaluating cervical CST3 effects on sperm physiology. CST3 tended to inhibit sperm capacitation initiation signaling, i.e., cholesterol efflux from the sperm plasma membrane and a late sperm capacitation event, i.e., increase in sperm protein tyrosine phosphorylation.

Cervical secretions provide hospitable environments for sperm accommodation [45]. Sperm can remain fertile in the cervix for up to several days after ejaculation [35]. Proteins in cervical secretions may protect sperm from premature capacitation. Once sperm capacitation occurs, the plasma membrane becomes unstable and easily undergoes acrosome reaction [13]. The sperm must reside at the right site, i.e., the fallopian tube ampulla, and undergo appropriate changes, i.e., successful capacitation, acrosome reaction, and fertilization, so that it can successfully fertilize [13, 45, 50]. Therefore, premature capacitation results in fertility loss. To preserve sperm fertility, secretory proteins in the lower reproductive tract may play an uncapacitation role and protect sperm from precocious capacitation.

Here, we demonstrated CST3 presence in cervical crypt and endometrium secretions during ovulation. Serum CST3 may enter the uterus by transudation because the endometrium permeability increases with elevated serum estrogen during the ovulation stage. CST3 with the ability to enhance motility may be helpful for sperm entering the upper female reproductive tract.

Ejaculated sperm cannot fertilize an egg after it has resided in the lower female reproductive tract for some duration; thus, the cervix and/or the uterus may secrete some proteins to stabilize the sperm plasma membrane and to thus prevent premature capacitation until sperm enters the fallopian tube. The cervical secretome, apart from CST3, may also contain other cervical secretory proteins with similar inhibitory effects on sperm capacitation. Cervical CST3 may be coupled with these secretory proteins to prevent sperm capacitation, and thus preserve sperm fertility until sperm reaches the fallopian tubes.

CST3 is extensively expressed in the endometrial epithelium, secretions of several animal species [36–38], and also in humans; progesterone was suggested to regulate CST3 expression levels [36–38]. Higher CST3 levels were detected in the endometrium during the mid- and late-secretory phase of the menstrual cycle, suggesting that CST3 expression in the human uterus may also be regulated by progesterone.

Because it inhibits protease's activity, CST3 may be involved in endometrial remodeling and may also play a role in inhibiting sperm capacitation. Previous studies have demonstrated that several serine protease inhibitors, including HongrES1 [26], PEBP1 [27], and SERPINE2 [25], are involved in suppressing sperm capacitation.

This in vitro study makes it difficult to assess the effects of the female tract CST3 on sperm function in vivo; however, at least the potential effect of the female tract CST3 on human sperm function can be assessed. There may be one potential application for this study. In assisted reproductive technology, the fertilization rate because of intrauterine insemination (IUI) is < 20% [51]; however, the technique is less expensive and invasive than in vitro fertilization. If some protein factors with inhibitory effects on premature capacitation and acrosome reaction can be added, e.g., CST3, to protect sperm from precocious capacitation, IUI fertilization rates might improve.

Conclusion

In conclusion, we have demonstrated that CST3 is expressed in epithelial cells lining the cervix, endometrium, fallopian tube, and in cervical mucus and uterine fluid, particularly during the late-proliferative phase around the time of ovulation. The cellular CST3 localization allows its interaction with sperm. It might bind to human sperm, enhance sperm motility, and potentially inhibit sperm capacitation.

Acknowledgements
Not applicable

Funding
This study was supported by grants from the Ministry of Science and Technology (NSC99–2314-B-195-006-MY3 and MOST105–2314-B-195-014), Taiwan, and the Mackay Memorial Hospital (MMH 10203 and 10622), Taipei, Taiwan. The funding bodies had no role in designing the study and in the collection, analysis, and interpretation of data, and in writing the manuscript.

Authors' contributions
RKKL and SHL planned and designed the experiments. HCT, JJY, and LYY conducted the experiments. YMH and MHL performed sample collection and data analysis. RKKL and SHL prepared and edited the manuscript; MHL, YMH, and RKKL provided professional consultation. All authors read and approved the final manuscript.

Authors' information
Not applicable

Competing interests
The authors declare that they have no competing interests.

Author details
[1]Department of Medical Research, Mackay Memorial Hospital, Tamsui District, New Taipei City 251, Taiwan. [2]Department of Obstetrics and Gynecology, Mackay Memorial Hospital, Taipei City 104, Taiwan. [3]Department of Obstetrics and Gynecology, Taipei Medical University, Taipei City 110, Taiwan. [4]Mackay Medical College, Sanzhi District, New Taipei City 252, Taiwan. [5]Mackay Junior College of Medicine, Nursing, and Management, Beitou District, Taipei City 112, Taiwan. [6]Office of Superintendent, Mackay Memorial Hospital, Taipei City, Taiwan. [7]Department of Medical Laboratory Science and Biotechnology, Yuanpei University, Hsinchu 300 Taiwan.

References

1. Abrahamson M, Olafsson I, Palsdottir A, Ulvsback M, Lundwall A, Jensson O, Grubb A. Structure and expression of the human cystatin C gene. The Biochemical journal. 1990;268(2):287–94.
2. Corrao AM, Lisi G, Di Pasqua G, Guizzardi M, Marino N, Ballone E, Chiesa PL. Serum cystatin C as a reliable marker of changes in glomerular filtration rate in children with urinary tract malformations. J Urol. 2006;175(1):303–9.
3. Perkins BA, Nelson RG, Ostrander BE, Blouch KL, Krolewski AS, Myers BD, Warram JH. Detection of renal function decline in patients with diabetes and normal or elevated GFR by serial measurements of serum cystatin C concentration: results of a 4-year follow-up study. Journal of the American Society of Nephrology : JASN. 2005;16(5):1404–12.
4. Abrahamson M, Barrett AJ, Salvesen G, Grubb A. Isolation of six cysteine proteinase inhibitors from human urine. Their physicochemical and enzyme kinetic properties and concentrations in biological fluids. J Biol Chem. 1986; 261(24):11282–9.
5. Jiborn T, Abrahamson M, Wallin H, Malm J, Lundwall A, Gadaleanu V, Abrahamsson PA, Bjartell A. Cystatin C is highly expressed in the human male reproductive system. J Androl. 2004;25(4):564–72.
6. Aalberts M, Stout TA, Stoorvogel W. Prostasomes: extracellular vesicles from the prostate. Reproduction. 2014, 147(1):R1–14.
7. Aalberts M, Sostaric E, Wubbolts R, Wauben MW, Nolte-'t Hoen EN, Gadella BM, Stout TA, Stoorvogel W. Spermatozoa recruit prostasomes in response to capacitation induction. Biochim Biophys Acta. 2013;1834(11):2326–35.
8. Pons-Rejraji H, Artonne C, Sion B, Brugnon F, Canis M, Janny L, Grizard G. Prostasomes: inhibitors of capacitation and modulators of cellular signalling in human sperm. Int J Androl. 2011;34(6 Pt 1):568–80.
9. Carlsson L, Ronquist G, Eliasson R, Egberg N, Larsson A. Association of cystatin C with prostasomes in human seminal plasma. Int J Androl. 2011; 34(4):363–8.
10. Austin CR. The capacitation of the mammalian sperm. Nature. 1952; 170(4321):326.
11. Chang MC. Fertilizing capacity of spermatozoa deposited into the fallopian tubes. Nature. 1951;168(4277):697–8.
12. Florman HM, Ducibella T: Fertilization in mammals. In: Knobil and Neill's Physiology of Reproduction Edited by Neill JD, Third edn San Diego: Elsevier Academic Press; 2006: 55–112.
13. Yanagimachi R: Mammalian fertilization. In: The Physiology of Reproduction. Edited by Knobil E, Neill JD. New York: Raven Press; 1994: 189–317.
14. Cross NL. Role of cholesterol in sperm capacitation. Biol Reprod. 1998;59(1):7–11.
15. Martinez P, Morros A. Membrane lipid dynamics during human sperm capacitation. Frontiers in bioscience : a journal and virtual library. 1996; 1:d103–17.
16. Visconti PE, Bailey JL, Moore GD, Pan D, Olds-Clarke P, Kopf GS. Capacitation of mouse spermatozoa. I. Correlation between the capacitation state and protein tyrosine phosphorylation. Development. 1995;121(4):1129–37.
17. Visconti PE, Kopf GS. Regulation of protein phosphorylation during sperm capacitation. Biol Reprod. 1998;59(1):1–6.
18. Chang MC. A detrimental effect of seminal plasma on the fertilizing capacity of sperm. Nature. 1957;179(4553):258–9.
19. de Lamirande E, Yoshida K, Yoshiike TM, Iwamoto T, Gagnon C. Semenogelin, the main protein of semen coagulum, inhibits human sperm capacitation by interfering with the superoxide anion generated during this process. J Androl. 2001;22(4):672–9.
20. Martins SG, Miranda PV, Brandelli A. Acrosome reaction inhibitor released during in vitro sperm capacitation. Int J Androl. 2003;26(5):296–304.
21. Zhu J, Massey JB, Mitchell-Leef D, Elsner CW, Kort HI, Roudebush WE. Platelet-activating factor acetylhydrolase activity affects sperm motility and serves as a decapacitation factor. Fertil Steril. 2006;85(2):391–4.
22. Fraser LR, Harrison RA, Herod JE. Characterization of a decapacitation factor associated with epididymal mouse spermatozoa. J Reprod Fertil. 1990;89(1): 135–48.
23. Kawano N, Yoshida M. Semen-coagulating protein, SVS2, in mouse seminal plasma controls sperm fertility. Biol Reprod. 2007;76(3):353–61.
24. Lin MH, Lee RK, Hwu YM, Lu CH, Chu SL, Chen YJ, Chang WC, Li SH. SPINKL, a Kazal-type serine protease inhibitor-like protein purified from mouse seminal vesicle fluid, is able to inhibit sperm capacitation. Reproduction. 2008;136(5):559–71.

25. Lu CH, Lee RK, Hwu YM, Chu SL, Chen YJ, Chang WC, Lin SP, Li SH. SERPINE2, a serine protease inhibitor extensively expressed in adult male mouse reproductive tissues, may serve as a murine sperm decapacitation factor. Biol Reprod. 2011;84(3):514–25.
26. Ni Y, Zhou Y, Chen WY, Zheng M, Yu J, Li C, Zhang Y, Shi QX. HongrES1, a cauda epididymis-specific protein, is involved in capacitation of guinea pig sperm. Mol Reprod Dev. 2009;76(10):984–93.
27. Nixon B, MacIntyre DA, Mitchell LA, Gibbs GM, O'Bryan M, Aitken RJ. The identification of mouse sperm-surface-associated proteins and characterization of their ability to act as decapacitation factors. Biol Reprod. 2006;74(2):275–87.
28. Tseng HC, Lee RK, Hwu YM, Lu CH, Lin MH, Li SH. Mechanisms underlying the inhibition of murine sperm capacitation by the seminal protein, SPINKL. J Cell Biochem. 2013;114(4):888–98.
29. Zhou Y, Zheng M, Shi Q, Zhang L, Zhen W, Chen W, Zhang Y. An epididymis-specific secretory protein HongrES1 critically regulates sperm capacitation and male fertility. PLoS One. 2008;3(12):e4106.
30. Katz DF, Drobnis EZ, Overstreet JW. Factors regulating mammalian sperm migration through the female reproductive tract and oocyte vestments. Gamete research. 1989;22(4):443–69.
31. Tollner TL, Yudin AI, Treece CA, Overstreet JW, Cherr GN. Macaque sperm coating protein DEFB126 facilitates sperm penetration of cervical mucus. Hum Reprod. 2008;23(11):2523–34.
32. Rodriguez-Martinez H. Role of the oviduct in sperm capacitation. Theriogenology. 2007;68(Suppl 1):S138–46.
33. Lapointe J, Bilodeau JF. Antioxidant defenses are modulated in the cow oviduct during the estrous cycle. Biol Reprod. 2003;68(4):1157–64.
34. Seppala M, Koistinen H, Koistinen R, Chiu PC, Yeung WS. Glycosylation related actions of glycodelin: gamete, cumulus cell, immune cell and clinical associations. Hum Reprod Update. 2007;13(3):275–87.
35. Zinaman M, Drobnis EZ, Morales P, Brazil C, Kiel M, Cross NL, Hanson FW, Overstreet JW. The physiology of sperm recovered from the human cervix: acrosomal status and response to inducers of the acrosome reaction. Biol Reprod. 1989;41(5):790–7.
36. Song G, Spencer TE, Bazer FW. Progesterone and interferon-tau regulate cystatin C in the endometrium. Endocrinology. 2006;147(7):3478–83.
37. Quinn CE, Simmons DG, Kennedy TG. Expression of cystatin C in the rat endometrium during the peri-implantation period. Biochem Biophys Res Commun. 2006;349(1):236–44.
38. Song G, Bailey DW, Dunlap KA, Burghardt RC, Spencer TE, Bazer FW, Johnson GA. Cathepsin B, cathepsin L, and cystatin C in the porcine uterus and placenta: potential roles in endometrial/placental remodeling and in fluid-phase transport of proteins secreted by uterine epithelia across placental areolae. Biol Reprod. 2010;82(5):854–64.
39. Cooper TG, Noonan E, von Eckardstein S, Auger J, Baker HW, Behre HM, Haugen TB, Kruger T, Wang C, Mbizvo MT, et al. World Health Organization reference values for human semen characteristics. Hum Reprod Update. 2010;16(3):231–45.
40. Lee RK, Fan CC, Hwu YM, Lu CH, Lin MH, Chen YJ, Li SH. SERPINE2, an inhibitor of plasminogen activators, is highly expressed in the human endometrium during the secretory phase. Reprod Biol Endocrinol. 2011;9:38.
41. Bligh EG, Dyer WJ. A rapid method of total lipid extraction and purification. Can J Biochem Physiol. 1959;37(8):911–7.
42. Leclerc P, de Lamirande E, Gagnon C. Cyclic adenosine 3',5'monophosphate-dependent regulation of protein tyrosine phosphorylation in relation to human sperm capacitation and motility. Biol Reprod. 1996;55(3):684–92.
43. Osheroff JE, Visconti PE, Valenzuela JP, Travis AJ, Alvarez J, Kopf GS. Regulation of human sperm capacitation by a cholesterol efflux-stimulated signal transduction pathway leading to protein kinase A-mediated up-regulation of protein tyrosine phosphorylation. Mol Hum Reprod. 1999;5(11):1017–26.
44. Bigelow JL, Dunson DB, Stanford JB, Ecochard R, Gnoth C, Colombo B. Mucus observations in the fertile window: a better predictor of conception than timing of intercourse. Hum Reprod. 2004;19(4):889–92.
45. Brannigan R, Lipshultz L: Sperm transport and capacitation. In: Women's Medicine. The global library of Women's Medicine; 2008.
46. Pretorius E, Franken DR, De Wet J, Grobler S. Sperm selection capacity of cervical mucus. Arch Androl. 1984;12(1):5–7.
47. Beydola T, Sharma RK, Lee W, Agarwal A. In: Rizk B, Aziz N, Agarwal A, editors. Sperm preparation and selection techniques. In: Male Infertility Practice. New Delhi: Jaypee Brothers Medical Publishers; 2013. p. 244–51.
48. Sakkas D, Manicardi GC, Tomlinson M, Mandrioli M, Bizzaro D, Bianchi PG, Bianchi U. The use of two density gradient centrifugation techniques and the swim-up method to separate spermatozoa with chromatin and nuclear DNA anomalies. Hum Reprod. 2000;15(5):1112–6.
49. Claassens OE, Menkveld R, Harrison KL. Evaluation of three substitutes for Percoll in sperm isolation by density gradient centrifugation. Hum Reprod. 1998;13(11):3139–43.
50. Suarez SS, Pacey AA. Sperm transport in the female reproductive tract. Hum Reprod Update. 2006;12(1):23–37.
51. Group ECW. Intrauterine insemination. Hum Reprod Update. 2009;15(3):265–77.

12

Smoke, alcohol and drug addiction and male fertility

Andrea Sansone[1*], Carla Di Dato[1], Cristina de Angelis[2,3], Davide Menafra[3], Carlotta Pozza[1], Rosario Pivonello[3], Andrea Isidori[1] and Daniele Gianfrilli[1]

Abstract

In recent decades, the decline in human fertility has become increasingly more worrying: while therapeutic interventions might help, they are vexing for the couple and often burdened with high failure rates and costs. Prevention is the most successful approach to fertility disorders in males and females alike. We performed a literature review on three of the most common unhealthy habits – tobacco, alcohol and drug addiction – and their reported effects on male fertility. Tobacco smoking is remarkably common in most first-world countries; despite a progressive decline in the US, recent reports suggest a prevalence of more than 30% in subjects of reproductive age – a disturbing perspective, given the well-known ill-effects on reproductive and sexual function as well as general health. Alcohol consumption is often considered socially acceptable, but its negative effects on gonadal function have been consistently reported in the last 30 years. Several studies have reported a variety of negative effects on male fertility following drug abuse – a worrying phenomenon, as illicit drug consumption is on the rise, most notably in younger subjects. While evidence in these regards is still far from solid, mostly as a result of several confounding factors, it is safe to assume that cessation of tobacco smoking, alcohol consumption and recreational drug addiction might represent the best course of action for any couple trying to achieve pregnancy.

Background

Almost 15% of all couples trying to conceive are affected by infertility, and in almost half of these cases male infertility is the sole or a contributing factor [1]. The decline of male fertility is not an empty threat: evidence points at a steadily progressive decline of sperm concentration over the past 35 years [2]. These reports have rekindled the interest in the potential impact of environmental factors and lifestyle on fertility: in order to decrease the social costs of male infertility and the resulting burdens on public health, identifying preventable factors is of the utmost importance. Sedentary behavior and obesity have both been associated with impaired male fertility [3, 4] and have often been addressed as potentially preventable factors; a more detailed review on the effects of sports and physical activity on male fertility is included in this *Special Issue*. The role of other unhealthy lifestyles, such as smoking and alcohol consumption, and environmental stressors on general health is universally recognized, but their effects on male fertility are less known [5]. Indeed, male reproductive health may be a sensitive marker of pollution [6] and environmental exposures [7, 8]. For ethical reasons, interventional studies in regards to the effects of tobacco use, second-hand smoking, recreational drug abuse and alcohol consumption are generally not feasible in humans. The vast majority of studies on these topics are therefore retrospective [8]. Sadly, this leads to a wide array of confounders, for which control is limited. A partial solution comes from animal studies; however, exposure in these models is significantly higher than in humans, and as such results should be interpreted with caution.

In order to provide an up-to-date and reliable reference in regards to the possible role of alcohol, tobacco and recreational drugs on male fertility, we performed a thorough review of existing literature and gathered all necessary data.

* Correspondence: andrea.sansone@uniroma1.it
[1]Department of Experimental Medicine, Section of Medical Pathophysiology, Food Science and Endocrinology, Sapienza - University of Rome, Viale Regina Elena 324, 00161 Rome, Italy
Full list of author information is available at the end of the article

Causes of male infertility

Couple infertility is defined by the failure to achieve pregnancy after at least 12 months of regular, unprotected intercourse. On the other hand, providing a fitting definition for male infertility is a more difficult task: diagnosis is traditionally based on semen analysis results, compared to the World Health Organization reference values [9].

Successful spermatogenesis is the result of the complex interaction between endocrine, paracrine and autocrine factors [10]. Unsurprisingly, several acquired and congenital conditions might impair the fine mechanisms involved in spermatogenesis (Table 1). Acquired testicular failure, as often observed following testicular torsion, orchitis, or administration of cytotoxic treatment is often associated with azoospermia. Varicocele, testicular trauma, and medications might affect fertility, although in most circumstances the spermatogenesis is impaired to a lesser extent. Genetic abnormalities, such as Klinefelter Syndrome or microdeletions in the AZF *(azoospermia factor)* region on the human male Y chromosome, usually manifest with azoospermia; however, small nucleotide polymorphisms are being investigated as a possible cause of "idiopathic" oligo-azoospermia. However, despite the recent discoveries in regards to the genetics of male infertility, to the present date most causes of oligozoospermia remain unknown.

Age is significantly associated with decline in semen quality, supposedly as a result of continued replications from mutated spermatogonial stem cells [11]. DNA fragmentation and chromatin condensation might also play a role in the pathogenesis of male infertility [12]. Among non-genetic causes of male infertility, oxidative stress resulting from exaggerated production of reactive oxygen species (ROS) is perhaps the most known factor. ROS are needed for capacitation, the acrosome reaction and ultimately fertilization; however, reduced clearance and excessive production are both able to induce DNA damage and defective membrane integrity in sperm cells, therefore resulting in reduced fertility potential [13]. Semen from fertile men has a more effective antioxidant capacity than that from infertile men; furthermore, immature teratozoospermic forms produce relatively more ROS than normal, mature sperm [13]. Inflammatory processes and vascular diseases, including varicocele, can supposedly increase ROS production: a thorough evaluation aimed to assess the presence of predisposing conditions is mandatory in the evaluation of any infertile male.

Table 1 Possible acquired causes of male reproductive impairment

Hypothalamic-pituitary axis
Compressive effect (Pituitary or brain tumors)
Ablative effect (CNS surgery or radiotherapy)
Infiltrative effect (fungal infections, sarcoidosis, hemochromatosis)
Suppressive effect (exogenous AAS)
Quantitative alterations of spermatogenesis
Varicocele
Previous chemotherapy or radiotherapy
Testicular failure (torsion, orchitis, orchiectomy)
Comorbidities (liver and kidney disease)
Qualitative alterations of spermatogenesis
Oxidative stress
DNA damage
Ductal obstructions
Surgery (vasectomy, hernia repair, pelvic surgery)
Neurological disorders (Multiple Sclerosis, Spinal Cord Injury, neural tube defects)
Erectile or ejaculatory dysfunction

Abbreviations: *CNS* central nervous system, *AAS* anabolic-androgenic steroid. Edited from H Tournaye, C Krausz and RD Oates [10]

Tobacco smoking and male fertility

More than 60% of noncommunicable diseases list smoking among their risk factors, and every year more than six million deaths result from tobacco consumption and second-hand smoke [14]. Despite the growing body of evidence supporting its deleterious effects, smoking is still a widespread phenomenon, as proven by recent reports from the World Health Organization. More than one-third of all male adults worldwide use tobacco [15]; similarly, approximately 30% of women of reproductive age smoke cigarettes [16]. Europe is still the leading continent in regards to tobacco use, whereas smoking rates have gradually declined in the United States in recent years [17].

Clinical studies

The deleterious effects of smoking on fertility have been described since 1983: Olsen and colleagues identified tobacco use as one of the causes of otherwise unexplained infertility in more than 1000 females [18]. To the present date, more than 4700 different chemicals have been identified in tobacco smoke [19], ranging from heavy metals to polycyclic aromatic hydrocarbons to mutagenic chemicals. A significant association between seminal plasma lead levels and lifetime smoking estimate has been reported [20]; likewise, smoking is considered the most common source of lead and cadmium exposure [21]. Some metal micronutrients involved in the pathogenesis of oxidative stress and male infertility, including arsenic and the aforementioned cadmium and lead, are routinely inhaled during combustion of tobacco or cigarette paper [21]. These metals all have mutagenic properties and are similarly associated with increased risk of male infertility, despite no significant differences in semen volume, concentration, and motility [22, 23]. On the other hand, impairments in sperm parameters have been observed in many studies in the last decades [24, 25]: in most of them, alterations in morphology and decreased concentration, motility and viability have been observed among smokers. A significant decrease in sperm concentrations of current smokers compared with those who had never smoked has been observed in a meta-analysis of more than 2500 men from five separate studies [26]. Similarly, Kunzle and colleagues have found a significant association between smoking and reduced sperm concentration in 2100 men presenting for fertility evaluation [27].

Mechanisms resulting in impaired sperm parameters have been investigated, but definite evidence is still missing. Ultra-structural abnormalities, mostly affecting axonemal microtubules and tail alterations, have been reported in heavy smokers [28, 29]; similarly, smoking impairs the acrosome reaction [30] and capacitation [31], two processes ultimately needed for fertilization. Increased oxidative stress has been suggested as a possible mechanism resulting in impaired sperm functions. Hypoxia resulting from cigarette smoking might also be responsible for impaired spermatogenesis, even more dramatically in patients with varicocele [8, 32]. Mitochondrial activity and chromatin structure in human sperm might be impaired by several toxins, therefore negatively affecting fertilization capacity both in vivo and in vitro [17, 33, 34].

Hypothetically, chronic cigarette smoking increases liver metabolism of testosterone, while at the same time inducing secretory dysfunction of Leydig and Sertoli cells [24]. However, there seems to be no general consensus on the effects of smoking on FSH and LH production: some studies have shown lower levels of both gonadotropins among smokers, whereas different researchers have observed increased concentration of LH and/or FSH following tobacco consumption [35, 36]. Considering all the possible confounding factors, testosterone concentration is remarkably difficult to ascertain among smokers: some studies have reported increased serum testosterone and dehydroepiandrosterone levels in smokers [35, 37], whereas others have suggested that mean levels of testosterone are not significantly different [38] between smokers and non-smokers.

The American Society of Reproductive Medicine in 2012 stated that "semen parameters and results of sperm function tests are 22% poorer in smokers than in non-smokers and the effects are dose-dependent" [16]. More recently, a meta-analysis study on a grand total of 5865 subjects has concluded that moderate and heavy smokers are more likely to have reduced sperm count and motility [17]. Evidence suggests a significant role for cigarette smoking on spermatogenesis, but on the other hand the impact of smoking on male fertility has yet to be fully elucidated. A preventive approach to infertility, suggesting smoking cessation and reduction of second-hand smoking in both women and men, should be suggested.

Experimental studies

Animal studies

Cigarette smoking results in accumulation of benzo(a)pyrene (B[a]P) and cotinine, ultimately leading to DNA damage and testicular cytotoxicity in rodent models. In a recent study, Esakky and colleagues [39] reported significantly decreased expression of aryl hydrocarbon receptor (*Ahr*), and enhanced expression of Fas, FasL, BCL2, and activated caspase-3 proteins in testes exposed to cigarette smoke condensate. The reduced expression of Ahr increases susceptibility of germ cells to polycyclic aromatic hydrocarbons, while the remaining proteins all induce apoptosis via extrinsic (FAS, FASL) or mitochondrial processes (BCL, caspase-3). Tobacco use is also closely associated to reduced antioxidant activity, therefore worsening the effects of oxidative stress [40].

Exposure to cigarette smoke also impairs the activity of sorbitol dehydrogenase and lactate dehydrogenase, reflecting the effects on spermatogenesis and sperm maturation in rats [41]. Most importantly, histomorphological alterations of testes, significantly increased abnormalities in epidydimal spermatozoa and sperm DNA damage have been observed in rats exposed to cigarette smoke [41, 42]. In both in vitro and in vivo studies, nicotine resulted involved in direct impairment of sperm motility and in apoptosis induction in rat Leydig cells [43]. Mice exposed to cigarette smoke also underwent alterations in cell signal pathway networks, including ERK1/2, nuclear factor-κB and several protein kinases involved in spermatogenesis; furthermore, modified DNA methylation patterns were observed near transcriptional start sites for the *PEBP1* gene. Expression of *PEBP1* results in production of phosphatidylethanolamine-binding protein 1, a protein that in humans has been shown to interact with C-Raf, MAP2K1 and MAPK1 [44].

High doses of nicotine induce a significant decrease in sperm count and motility in prepubertal and adult rats exposed to progressively increasing concentrations of nicotine [45]. Impaired testicular function is also reflected in significantly decreased testosterone levels [45, 46], although as previously suggested it's still unclear whether these findings are valid for humans as well as rodents.

Smoking cessation, on the other hand, improves indices of sexual health for long-term male smokers [47] and, based on finding in animal models, might improve sperm parameters [48]. However, to the present date, no conclusive evidence on the real improvements in male fertility following smoking cessation has been obtained.

Studies in humans

Recent genome-wide studies have identified alterations in the methylation profile of 95 sites in smokers [49]. Smoking-related DNA damage and methylation patterns are observed in several human tissues - even those who are not directly exposed to it because of indirect systemic exposure [50]. DNA adducts and DNA damage are inversely associated with sperm parameters, mostly concentration and motility, and both are transmitted to the zygote with little chance of repair by the ovum [51]. Sperm DNA fragmentation is also linked with increased rates of spontaneous abortion [52] and should therefore be carefully assessed in subjects undergoing assisted reproduction techniques. Oxidative DNA damage [53] and higher cadmium levels [54] resulting from tobacco consumption are similarly associated to impaired fertility, resulting in longer time to pregnancy for couples.

Smoking also reduces sperm creatine kinase activity, therefore impairing sperm motility and energy homeostasis [55]. In vitro studies have shown nicotine, cotinine and cadmium as possible culprits; in vivo, both smoking duration and amount of cigarettes smoked per day seem able to reduce creatine kinase activity in sperm [56, 57].

Alcohol consumption and male fertility

Clinical and experimental studies have examined alcohol consumption as a potential risk factor for male infertility, exerting a direct effect on both testosterone metabolism and spermatogenesis.

Clinical studies

The link between alcohol and fertility was investigated in 1985 for the first time. The analysis of seminal fluid samples and the hormonal evaluation of 20 men with alcohol dependence syndrome revealed a significant decrease in testosterone levels, seminal fluid volume and sperm concentration in chronic alcoholics than in controls [58]. Subsequently, a prospective autopsy study showed that a significant percentage of heavy drinkers (52.3%) had partial or complete spermatogenic arrest, and that the mean testicular weight of heavy drinkers was slightly but significantly lower compared with that of controls [59]. Muthusami et al., in 2005, found in chronic alcoholics a significant increase of FSH, LH, and E2 levels, while testosterone was significantly decreased. Semen volume, sperm count, motility, and number of morphologically normal sperm were significantly decreased [60]. In 2011 one meta-analysis including 57 studies and 29,914 subjects found a significant association between alcohol, semen volume, sperm morphology and sperm motility [61].

Therefore, chronic and excessive alcohol intake seem to have a detrimental effect on male reproductive hormones and on semen quality. Conversely, the effect of moderate alcohol intake is still under debate.

A cross sectional study from Jensen et al. on 8344 healthy men suggest that moderate alcohol intake (median weekly intake 8 units) is not adversely associated with semen quality in healthy men, whereas it was associated with higher serum testosterone levels [62]. Furthermore, chronic alcohol consumption seem to influence fertility more than acute alcohol consumption. Hansen et al. evaluated the association between last 5 days of alcohol intake, semen quality and reproductive hormones in a cross-sectional study among 347 men [63]. Alcohol intake was associated with impairment of most semen characteristics but without a coherent dose–response pattern. There was a tendency towards lower semen characteristics at higher intake of alcohol past 5 days and a hormonal shift towards higher estradiol/testosterone ratio. The importance of the timing of alcohol consumption was also established from Condorelli et al. The Authors retrospectively evaluated semen and hormonal parameters of moderate alcohol users, comparing occasional drinkers with daily drinkers. Within each group, a further comparison was made between the fertile subjects (pregnancy over the past 12 months) and the infertile patients (no evidence of pregnancy or fertilisation for at least 12 months). The results showed that infertile patients belonging to group of 'daily drinkers' have a semen quality and hormonal characteristics significantly worse compared with the other groups [64]. Time-to-pregnancy for was significantly longer in couples in which the male partner consumed more than 20 units of alcohol on a weekly basis [65], but literature is severely lacking concerning more moderate consumption of alcoholic beverages.

The mechanisms underlying the damage of alcohol on fertility are not yet fully clarified. Close and colleagues reported that current heavy alcohol users have significantly higher leukocyte concentrations in the seminal fluid compared with nonusers. After controlling for past sexually transmitted diseases and multiple substance exposures in a multivariate model, alcohol users had only a trend towards increased leukocytes in the seminal fluid [66]. Some Authors hypothesized that also maternal alcohol consumption during pregnancy can influence semen quality in the male offspring. From a cohort of Danish pregnant women established in 1984–1987, 347 young adult sons were selected for a follow-up study conducted in 2005–2006. The results of this study showed that the sperm concentration decreased with increasing prenatal alcohol exposure. No associations were found for sperm motility, sperm morphology, or any of the reproductive hormones, including testosterone [67].

Experimental studies

Animal studies

Alcohol consumption has often been associated with an increase in β-endorphin levels that could be involved in testicular damage, inducing sperm apoptosis. In 1999 Yin and colleagues showed that morphine induces the expression of the protein Fas (also known as CD95 or APO-1), a receptor on the cell surface that triggers the cell's suicide by apoptosis when it binds to its ligand, FasL [68]. Furthermore, an experimental study demonstrated that treatment with naloxone and naltrexone in adult and pubertal male rats could prevent alcohol-induced testosterone inhibition [69].

Apoptosis is one of the responsible factors for spermatozoal chromatin disorders. Several studies showed that ethanol consumption disturb nuclear maturity and DNA integrity of spermatozoa. Talebi and colleagues evaluated the effect of ethanol consumption on sperm parameters and chromatin integrity of spermatozoa aspirated from cauda epididymis of rats. Results revealed that sperm progressive and non progressive motility of ethanol-consuming rats were significantly decreased compared with control animals and an alteration of nuclear maturity and DNA integrity [70].

Therefore, spermatogenic cells undergo apoptosis when treated with ethanol but the mechanism remain unclear. In the study of Jana and colleagues, intraperitoneal injection of ethanol induced apoptotic spermatogenic cell death with a decrease in the plasma and intra-testicular testosterone in adult male mice. In this study, western blot analysis revealed that repeated ethanol treatment decreased the expression of steroidogenic acute regulatory protein (StAR), 3b-hydroxysteroid dehydrogenase (3b-HSD) and 17b-hydroxysteroid dehydrogenase (17b-HSD); increased the expression of active caspase-3, p53, Fas and Fas-L; and led to up-regulation of Bax/Bcl-2 ratio and translocation of cytochrome c from mitochondria to cytosol in testis. Moreover, repeated ethanol treatment led to upregulation of caspase-3, p53, Fas and Fas-L transcripts; increase in caspase-3 and caspase-8 activities; diminution of 3b-HSD, 17b-HSD and GPx activities; decrease in the mitochondrial membrane potential along with ROS generation and depletion of glutathione pool in the testicular tissue [71].

Studies in humans

Polycyclic aromatic hydrocarbons (PAH) are ubiquitous pollutants in the environment, which are able to form DNA adducts when they are activated to DNA reactive metabolites. Measurement of DNA adducts is a widely used marker of DNA damage induced by environmental pollutants. Gaspari and colleagues evaluated data on (PAH)-DNA adducts in 182 men with morphological abnormalities in the sperm, finding a significant negative association was between daily alcohol consumption and PAH-DNA adducts in sperm [72]; similarly, Rossi and colleagues reported that increased alcohol consumption was associated with fertilization failure and reduced live birth rates [73], with a 21% decline in couples in which both partners drank more than 4 units per week. On the contrary, in the study of Horak et al., no correlation between alcohol and sperm DNA adducts was found [74]. Finally, Loft evaluated the level of oxidative DNA damage in terms of 7-hydro-8-oxo-20-deoxyguanosine (8-oxodG) in sperm DNA among 225 first-pregnancy planners and the 8-oxodG level was not significantly associated with consumption of alcohol [53].

Finally, the genetic background may modulate the impact of alcohol on spermatogenesis. The glutathione S-transferase (GST)-M1 genotype may be associated with a greater susceptibility to develop, via direct mechanism at testicular level, alcohol-induced spermatogenesis disorders. An autopsy study comprising 271 subjects showed that among 50 moderate drinking men, 48% had partial and 10% complete spermatogenic arrest. Among the 21 men with normal spermatogenesis, 42.9% had GST M1 genotype with a frequency similar to that found in men with partial or complete spermatogenic arrest (44.8%). Among the 212 heavy-drinking men, 21.2% of the subjects had normal spermatogenesis, 36.3% had partial spermatogenic arrest, 38.2% showed complete arrest spermatogenic arrest and 4.2% showed Sertoli cell-only syndrome. Interestingly, 27 of the 45 heavy drinkers with normal spermatogenesis (60%) men had the GST M1 genotype. The finding that >20% of heavy drinkers had normal spermatogenesis suggests that the GST M1 genotype exerts a protective effects on alcohol-induced spermatogenesis disorders [75].

Drugs addiction and male fertility

Up to almost one in four men under the age of 35 years uses recreational drugs [76]. Several studies have suggested that these drugs might have adverse effects on human reproduction. Cannabis smoking has been shown to negatively impact male fertility, with an effect on hypothalamus-pituitary-gonadal axis, spermatogenesis, and sperm function, as cannabinoid receptors are expressed in the anterior pituitary, Leydig cells, Sertoli cells and in testicular tissues [77]. Similarly, negative effects on male fertility have been reported in subjects using cocaine, MDMA (ecstasy) and opioids. Cocaine use has been associated with other high-risk behaviors, such as tobacco smoking and sexually transmitted diseases, and might lead to testicular cell apoptosis; opioids act on the HPG axis, possibly resulting in hypogonadal hypogonadism; DNA damage and tubular degeneration have been described in rats treated with MDMA. Prevention of male infertility might be achieved by identifying and addressing the consequences of the "illicit drug epidemic".

Clinical studies

In literature, human data on hormone levels following marijuana exposure are conflicting. Referring to animal studies it could be possible that consuming cannabis decrease serum luteinizing hormone and testosterone levels, but in clinical studies a univocal interpretation is lacking.

A study from Kolodny et al. on 20 men who used marijuana chronically showed significantly lower levels of plasma testosterone in this group than that in the control-group. Decreased testosterone was dose related. Abstention from marijuana use or stimulation with human chorionic gonadotropin during continued marihuana use produced marked increases in testosterone [78]. These results have been later contradicted. In 66 males neither chronic nor acute intake of marijuana had a significant effect on plasma testosterone levels, but also subjects who drank cannabis as a tea were included [79]. In a study of 27 men, no statistically significant changes in plasma testosterone levels were observed during and after the smoking period as compared with the pre-smoking base-line levels [80]. In four healthy males subjects, cannabis smoking significantly depressed plasma LH, while cortisol significantly increased [81]. On the contrary, in the study from Gundersen et al. on 1215 Danish healthy young men, of whom 45% had smoked marijuana during the past 3 months, marijuana use was associated with increased serum testosterone to the same level as cigarette smoking [82].

Conversely, regarding the effect of cannabis on spermatogenesis, clinical studies showed an effect on volume, number morphology, motility, and fertilization capacity.

In the study from Gundersen et al. regular use of marijuana was found to be associated with an impairment in semen quality, while irregular use seems to be irrelevant [82]. A study from Hembree et al. showed an association between marijuana use and decreased sperm count, which persisted in the following 4-week recovery period [83]. These data were confirmed also by a case study on a multidrug addict, in which semen abnormalities were detected before and 2 years after cessation of the abuse [84]. In a recent unmatched case-referent study with 1700 participants, it was clearly reported that cannabis exposure is a risk factor for poor sperm morphology [85]. Only one study on 159 men attending an infertility clinic demonstrated a positive correlation between marijuana use and percentage of motile sperm [66].

There are no studies on the effect of cannabis on the reproductive organs of men. Only Kolodny et al. reported no change in testicular size and texture in chronic marijuana users [78]. The differing results of these reports may in part be due to study design, the ingestion of other pharmacological agents, such as narcotics, alcohol and cigarette smoking.

Cocaine intake during pregnancy severely affects fetal development; however, little is known in regards to its effects on male fertility. The same applies to MDMA (Ecstasy): animal models might help understand the specific effects of both substances on male fertility. Bracken et al. [86] reported increased use of cocaine among subjects with lower sperm counts and motility; Samplaski et al. [87] more recently suggested that the higher rates of concurrent substance abuse, tobacco use and infections among cocaine users might lead to biased results.

Opioids act on the hypothalamic-pituitary axis by inhibiting the pulsatility of GnRH secretion: the resulting suppression of FSH and LH release consequently leads to impaired spermatogenesis and reduced testosterone concentrations [76]. Vuong et al. [88] performed a lengthy review of the effects of opioids on endocrine parameters, and concluded that there is still insufficient information on the long-term effects of opioids in regards to fertility despite concrete evidence of opioid-induced hypogonadism. Recent reports suggest that both sperm concentration and quality are impaired in opioid abusers: increased rates of DNA fragmentation and reduced expression of catalase-like and superoxide dismutase-like activity were observed in addict men compared to age-matched healthy volunteers [89].

Experimental studies

Animal studies

Acute treatments with cannabinoids can decrease the fertilising capacity of sea urchin sperm [90]. In rodent studies, high THC doses caused a modest increase in abnormally formed sperm. Moreover, long-term cannabinoid exposure in male mice disrupted spermatogenesis and induced aberrations in sperm morphology [91].

Wenger and colleagues showed that THC alters pituitary LH release by inhibiting the release of LHRH, injecting THC into the third cerebral ventricle of male rats [92]. Smith et al. [93] found a significant decrease in serum testosterone concentration following acute doses of THC in rhesus monkeys. A study on adult male mice showed regressive changes in the testes and suppressed sperm count, viability and motility, caused by chronic intake of bhang. Bhang intake also caused significant

Table 2 Effects of tobacco smoking, alcohol consumption and drug addiction on spermatogenesis and sperm parameters

	Studies in humans	Animal studies
Tobacco smoking	Reduction of sperm concentration [26, 27] Impairment of sperm motility [17] Increase in ultra-structural abnormalities (axonemal microtubules and tail alterations) [28, 29] Impairment of mitochondrial activity and chromatin structure [17, 33, 34] Impairment of acrosome reaction and capacitation [30, 31] Increase of DNA methylation patterns [49] Alterations in ERK1/2, nuclear factor-κB signal pathway [44] Reduction of creatine kinase activity in sperm [55–57]	Increase in apoptosis via extrinsic (FAS, FASL) or mitochondrial processes (BCL, caspase-3) in rats [39, 40] Reduction of antioxidant activity in rats [40] Increase in DNA damage in sperm rats [41, 42]; of DNA methylation patterns *PEBP1* gene in rats [44] Reduction of sperm count and motility in rats [45]
Alcohol consumption	Reduction of seminal volume and sperm concentration [58, 61, 62] Impairment of sperm motility and morphology [60, 61] Increased sperm polycyclic aromatic hydrocarbon DNA adducts [72]	Increase in apoptosis (by upregulation of Fas) of spermatogenic cells in rats [68] Alteration of nuclear maturity and DNA integrity in sperm cells of rats [70] Increase in ROS generation and depletion of glutathione pool in testicular tissue of rats [71] Impairment of sperm motility in rats [70]
Drug addiction		
Marijuana	Decrease in sperm count [82–84] Impairment of sperm morphology and motility [85, 102, 103] Reduction of spontaneous acrosome reactions [102, 103]	Impaired sperm concentration and morphology in rats [91] Inhibition of sperm ATP production in rats [104] Reduction of fructose and citric acid contents in testis and prostate of male rats [95]
Cocaine	Impairment of sperm counts and motility [86]	Vasoconstriction of testicular blood vessels in rats resulting in ischemic and reperfusion injuries [96] Reduction of diameter of seminiferous tubules [97] Decrease in number of total germ cells [97] Increase in oxidative stress in mice [98]
Opioids	Impaired spermatogenesis [76] Increased rates of DNA fragmentation in humans [89] Reduced expression of catalase-like and superoxide dismutase-like activity [89]	Increase of rates of DNA damage and tubular degeneration in rats [100, 101]
Amphetamines and Ecstasy	No data available	Vasoconstriction of testicular blood vessels in rats [96] Increase in rates of DNA damage and tubular degeneration in rats [99]

Table 3 Effects of tobacco smoking, alcohol consumption and drug addiction on hormone levels

	Studies in humans	Animal studies
Tobacco smoking	Increase in liver metabolism of testosterone [24] Reduction of LH and/or FSH levels [34] Increase in concentration of LH and/or FSH [35] Increase in serum testosterone and DHEA levels [35, 37]	Reduction of testosterone levels in rats [45, 46]
Alcohol consumption	Decrease in testosterone levels [58, 59] Increase in FSH, LH, and E2 levels [60]	Decrease in plasma and intra-testicular testosterone in rats [71]
Drug addiction		
Marijuana	Decrease in levels of plasma testosterone [78] Decreased levels of plasma LH, and increased levels of plasma cortisol [81] Increased serum testosterone [82]	Inhibition of LHRH release in rats [92] Decrease in testosterone levels in monkeys [93]
Cocaine	Increase in LH levels without modifying testosterone following acute administration [97]	Increase in LH levels; No effects on testosterone and estradiol in rats [97]
Opioids	Inhibition of the pulsatility of GnRH secretion; reduction of LH, FSH and testosterone levels [76]	Reduction of LH, without effect on FSH and testosterone levels in rats [101]
Amphetamines and Ecstasy	No data available	No effects on LH, FSH, Testosterone levels in male rats [99]

decline in circulating testosterone level due to decline in testicular 3b HSD enzyme activity, a significant variation in the CB1 and CB2 receptors and FAAH protein levels (Fatty Acid Amide Hydrolase) in testes of mice exposed to bhang [94]. Finally, repeated subcutaneous administration of cannabis extract and delta-9-tetrahydrocannabinol reduced significantly fructose and citric acid contents of male reproductive organs of prepubertal as well as adult albino rats in a dose-related manner in the testis, prostate as well as in the epididymis [95].

Effects of cocaine and MDMA on fertility have been evaluated in animal models: in rodents, cocaine is able to induce prolonged vasoconstriction of testicular blood vessels, resulting in ischemic and reperfusion injuries [96]. In 1996, George et al. reported that in rats long-term exposure to cocaine resulted in reduced diameter of seminiferous tubules and similarly decreased number of total germ cells [97]. More recently, increased oxidative stress has been observed in mice following chronic administration of cocaine [98], suggesting a possible mechanism for testicular damage. Similar findings have been reported for Ecstasy and opioids: Barenys et al. described significantly decreased sperm concentration and motility, together with increased rates of DNA damage and tubular degeneration, in rats treated with varying dosages of MDMA [99], and similar findings have been described in mice treated with either tramadol [100] or morphine [101].

Studies in humans

Whan et al. investigated the effects of delta-9-tetrahydrocannabinol (THC) on human sperm function in vitro. Both therapeutic and recreational levels of THC determined a dose dependent reduction of sperm motility and of spontaneous acrosome reactions [102]. Subsequent studies confirmed these results [103], but the mechanism still remained not fully understood. Morgan et al. investigated the effects of WIN 55,212-2, a CB1 cannabinoid receptor agonist, and D9-tetrahydracannabinol (D9-THC) on the ATP levels and motility of murine sperm in vitro. High concentrations of WIN 55,212-2 or D9-THC inhibit ATP production in sperm; this effect of WIN 55,212-2 is CB1 receptor dependent whereas that of D9-THC is not [104].

Conclusions

Despite the lack of solid evidence from interventional studies, which are for the most part not feasible in humans, it is clear that smoking, alcohol use and recreational drug consumption are somehow able to impair male fertility, with possible synergistic, rather than addictive, effects. Impairments in spermatogenesis and sperm parameters as well as increased DNA methylation and oxidative stress have been observed in humans and animal models alike; similarly, effects on endocrine control of reproductive and sexual function have been reported in clinical and

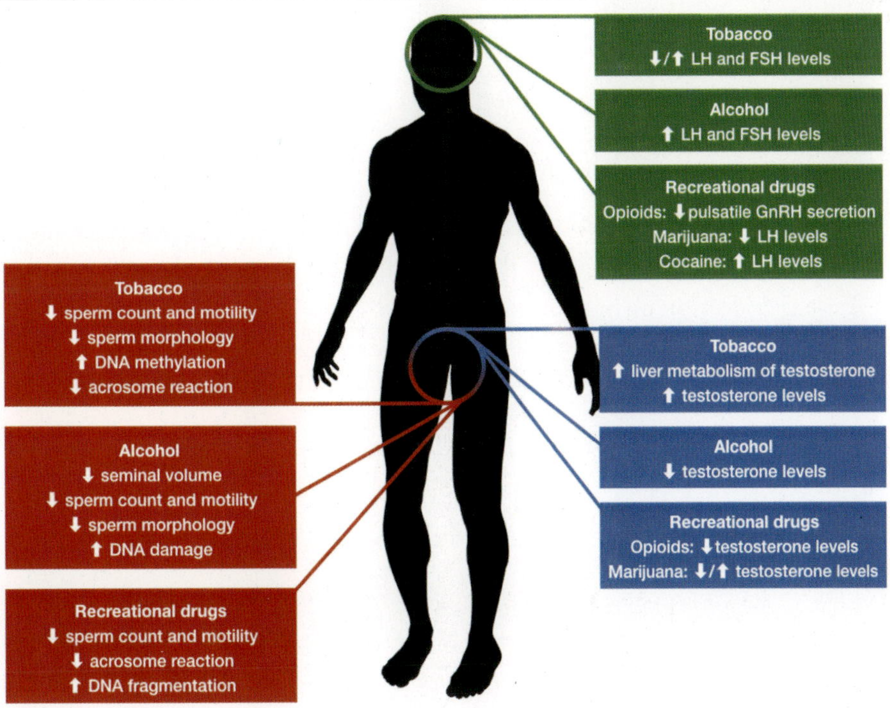

Fig. 1 Effects of smoking, alcohol and drug abuse on spermatogenesis (left) and hormonal parameters (right) in males

experimental studies (Tables 2 and 3, Fig. 1). Discontinuation of all these habits should be suggested in all patients undergoing investigation for infertility in order to provide the best outcomes, although little is known in regards to the time needed for cessation of negative effects.

Acknowledgements
None

Funding
No funding was requested for this review.

Declarations
Since Prof. Pivonello served as Guest Editor of the thematic series "The Influence of Environment and Lifestyle on Human Fertility", peer review of the present manuscript was handled by another member of the *Reproductive Biology and Endocrinology* editorial board.

Authors' contributions
AMI and DG conceived the idea. AS and CdD were involved in literature collection. All authors independently and critically reviewed the selected manuscripts. AS and CdD were involved in drafting the early manuscript and equally contributed to the first draft, which was then expanded and improved by all authors. All authors reviewed and approved the completed manuscript.

Competing interests
The authors declare that they have no competing interests.

Author details
[1]Department of Experimental Medicine, Section of Medical Pathophysiology, Food Science and Endocrinology, Sapienza - University of Rome, Viale Regina Elena 324, 00161 Rome, Italy. [2]I.O.S.& COLEMAN Srl, Naples, Italy. [3]Dipartimento di Medicina Clinica e Chirurgia, Sezione di Endocrinologia, Università "Federico II" di Napoli, Naples, Italy.

References

1. Sharlip ID, Jarow JP, Belker AM, Lipshultz LI, Sigman M, Thomas AJ, Schlegel PN, Howards SS, Nehra A, Damewood MD, et al. Best practice policies for male infertility. Fertil Steril. 2002;77(5):873–82.
2. Sengupta P, Dutta S, Krajewska-Kulak E. The disappearing sperms: analysis of reports published between 1980 and 2015. Am J Mens Health. 2017;11(4): 1279–304.
3. Gaskins AJ, Afeiche MC, Hauser R, Williams PL, Gillman MW, Tanrikut C, Petrozza JC, Chavarro JE. Paternal physical and sedentary activities in relation to semen quality and reproductive outcomes among couples from a fertility center. Hum Reprod. 2014;29(11):2575–82.
4. Eisenberg ML, Kim S, Chen Z, Sundaram R, Schisterman EF, Buck Louis GM. The relationship between male BMI and waist circumference on semen quality: data from the LIFE study. Hum Reprod. 2014;29(2):193–200.
5. Barazani Y, Katz BF, Nagler HM, Stember DS. Lifestyle, environment, and male reproductive health. The Urologic clinics of North America. 2014;41(1): 55–66.
6. Moline JM, Golden AL, Bar-Chama N, Smith E, Rauch ME, Chapin RE, Perreault SD, Schrader SM, Suk WA, Landrigan PJ. Exposure to hazardous substances and male reproductive health: a research framework. Environ Health Perspect. 2000;108(9):803–13.
7. Nordkap L, Joensen UN, Blomberg Jensen M, Jorgensen N. Regional differences and temporal trends in male reproductive health disorders: semen quality may be a sensitive marker of environmental exposures. Mol Cell Endocrinol. 2012;355(2):221–30.
8. Gabrielsen JS, Tanrikut C. Chronic exposures and male fertility: the impacts of environment, diet, and drug use on spermatogenesis. Andrology. 2016; 4(4):648–61.
9. Cooper TG, Noonan E, von Eckardstein S, Auger J, Baker HW, Behre HM, Haugen TB, Kruger T, Wang C, Mbizvo MT, et al. World Health Organization reference values for human semen characteristics. Hum Reprod Update. 2010;16(3):231–45.
10. Tournaye H, Krausz C, Oates RD. Novel concepts in the aetiology of male reproductive impairment. Lancet Diabetes Endocrinol. 2017;5(7):544–53.
11. Johnson SL, Dunleavy J, Gemmell NJ, Nakagawa S. Consistent age-dependent declines in human semen quality: a systematic review and meta-analysis. Ageing Res Rev. 2015;19:22–33.
12. Valenti D, La Vignera S, Condorelli RA, Rago R, Barone N, Vicari E, Calogero AE. Follicle-stimulating hormone treatment in normogonadotropic infertile men. Nat Rev Urol. 2013;10(1):55–62.
13. Lombardo F, Sansone A, Romanelli F, Paoli D, Gandini L, Lenzi A. The role of antioxidant therapy in the treatment of male infertility: an overview. Asian J Androl. 2011;13(5):690–7.
14. Yao DF, Mills JN. Male infertility: lifestyle factors and holistic, complementary, and alternative therapies. Asian J Androl. 2016;18(3):410–8.
15. Prevalence of tobacco use [http://www.who.int/topics/tobacco/en/].
16. Practice Committee of the American Society for Reproductive. M: smoking and infertility: a committee opinion. Fertil Steril. 2012;98(6): 1400–6.
17. Sharma R, Harlev A, Agarwal A, Esteves SC. Cigarette smoking and semen quality: a new meta-analysis examining the effect of the 2010 World Health Organization Laboratory methods for the examination of human semen. Eur Urol. 2016;70(4):635–45.
18. Olsen J, Rachootin P, Schiodt AV, Damsbo N. Tobacco use, alcohol consumption and infertility. Int J Epidemiol. 1983;12(2):179–84.
19. Borgerding M, Klus H. Analysis of complex mixtures–cigarette smoke. Exp Toxicol Pathol. 2005;57(Suppl 1):43–73.
20. Benoff S, Centola GM, Millan C, Napolitano B, Marmar JL, Hurley IR. Increased seminal plasma lead levels adversely affect the fertility potential of sperm in IVF. Hum Reprod. 2003;18(2):374–83.
21. Jurasovic J, Cvitkovic P, Pizent A, Colak B, Telisman S. Semen quality and reproductive endocrine function with regard to blood cadmium in Croatian male subjects. Biometals. 2004;17(6):735–43.
22. Wang X, Zhang J, Xu W, Huang Q, Liu L, Tian M, Xia Y, Zhang W, Shen H. Low-level environmental arsenic exposure correlates with unexplained male infertility risk. Sci Total Environ. 2016;571:307–13.
23. de Angelis C, Galdiero M, Pivonello C, Salzano C, Gianfrilli D, Piscitelli P, Lenzi A, Colao A, Pivonello R. The environment and male reproduction: the effect of cadmium exposure on reproductive functions and its implication in fertility. Reprod Toxicol. 2017;73:105–27.
24. Dai JB, Wang ZX, Qiao ZD. The hazardous effects of tobacco smoking on male fertility. Asian J Androl. 2015;17(6):954–60.
25. Asare-Anane H, Bannison SB, Ofori EK, Ateko RO, Bawah AT, Amanquah SD, Oppong SY, Gandau BB, Ziem JB. Tobacco smoking is associated with decreased semen quality. Reprod Health. 2016;13(1):90.
26. Ramlau-Hansen CH, Thulstrup AM, Aggerholm AS, Jensen MS, Toft G, Bonde JP. Is smoking a risk factor for decreased semen quality? A cross-sectional analysis. Hum Reprod. 2007;22(1):188–96.
27. Kunzle R, Mueller MD, Hanggi W, Birkhauser MH, Drescher H, Bersinger NA. Semen quality of male smokers and nonsmokers in infertile couples. Fertil Steril. 2003;79(2):287–91.
28. Zavos PM, Correa JR, Karagounis CS, Ahparaki A, Phoroglou C, Hicks CL, Zarmakoupis-Zavos PN. An electron microscope study of the axonemal ultrastructure in human spermatozoa from male smokers and nonsmokers. Fertil Steril. 1998;69(3):430–4.

29. Yeung CH, Tuttelmann F, Bergmann M, Nordhoff V, Vorona E, Cooper TG. Coiled sperm from infertile patients: characteristics, associated factors and biological implication. Hum Reprod. 2009;24(6):1288–95.
30. Zalata AA, Ahmed AH, Allamaneni SS, Comhaire FH, Agarwal A. Relationship between acrosin activity of human spermatozoa and oxidative stress. Asian J Androl. 2004;6(4):313–8.
31. Shrivastava V, Marmor H, Chernyak S, Goldstein M, Feliciano M, Vigodner M. Cigarette smoke affects posttranslational modifications and inhibits capacitation-induced changes in human sperm proteins. Reprod Toxicol. 2014;43:125–9.
32. Taha EA, Ezz-Aldin AM, Sayed SK, Ghandour NM, Mostafa T. Smoking influence on sperm vitality, DNA fragmentation, reactive oxygen species and zinc in oligoasthenoteratozoospermic men with varicocele. Andrologia. 2014;46(6):687–91.
33. Calogero A, Polosa R, Perdichizzi A, Guarino F, La Vignera S, Scarfia A, Fratantonio E, Condorelli R, Bonanno O, Barone N, et al. Cigarette smoke extract immobilizes human spermatozoa and induces sperm apoptosis. Reprod BioMed Online. 2009;19(4):564–71.
34. Sharma R, Biedenharn KR, Fedor JM, Agarwal A. Lifestyle factors and reproductive health: taking control of your fertility. Reproductive biology and endocrinology : RB&E. 2013;11:66.
35. Blanco-Munoz J, Lacasana M, Aguilar-Garduno C. Effect of current tobacco consumption on the male reproductive hormone profile. Sci Total Environ. 2012;426:100–5.
36. Ochedalski T, Lachowicz-Ochedalska A, Dec W, Czechowski B. Examining the effects of tobacco smoking on levels of certain hormones in serum of young men. Ginekol Pol. 1994;65(2):87–93.
37. Lotti F, Corona G, Vitale P, Maseroli E, Rossi M, Fino MG, Maggi M. Current smoking is associated with lower seminal vesicles and ejaculate volume, despite higher testosterone levels, in male subjects of infertile couples. Hum Reprod. 2015;30(3):590–602.
38. Pasqualotto FF, Sobreiro BP, Hallak J, Pasqualotto EB, Lucon AM. Cigarette smoking is related to a decrease in semen volume in a population of fertile men. BJU Int. 2006;97(2):324–6.
39. Esakky P, Hansen DA, Drury AM, Felder P, Cusumano A, Moley KH. Paternal exposure to cigarette smoke condensate leads to reproductive sequelae and developmental abnormalities in the offspring of mice. Reprod Toxicol. 2016;65:283–94.
40. Pasqualotto FF, Umezu FM, Salvador M, Borges E, Jr., Sobreiro BP, Pasqualotto EB: Effect of cigarette smoking on antioxidant levels and presence of leukocytospermia in infertile men: a prospective study. Fertil Steril 2008, 90(2):278-283.
41. Abdul-Ghani R, Qazzaz M, Dabdoub N, Muhammad R, Abdul-Ghani AS. Studies on cigarette smoke induced oxidative DNA damage and reduced spermatogenesis in rats. J Environ Biol. 2014;35(5):943–7.
42. La Maestra S, De Flora S, Micale RT. Effect of cigarette smoke on DNA damage, oxidative stress, and morphological alterations in mouse testis and spermatozoa. Int J Hyg Environ Health. 2015;218(1):117–22.
43. Kim KH, Joo KJ, Park HJ, Kwon CH, Jang MH, Kim CJ. Nicotine induces apoptosis in TM3 mouse Leydig cells. Fertil Steril. 2005;83(Suppl 1):1093–9.
44. Yeung K, Janosch P, McFerran B, Rose DW, Mischak H, Sedivy JM, Kolch W. Mechanism of suppression of the Raf/MEK/extracellular signal-regulated kinase pathway by the raf kinase inhibitor protein. Mol Cell Biol. 2000;20(9): 3079–85.
45. Aprioku JS, Ugwu TC. Tobacco smoke exposure induces irreversible alteration of testicular function in prepubertal rats. J Basic Clin Physiol Pharmacol. 2016;27(6):577–84.
46. Oyeyipo IP, Raji Y, Bolarinwa AF. Nicotine alters male reproductive hormones in male albino rats: the role of cessation. J Hum Reprod Sci. 2013; 6(1):40–4.
47. Harte CB, Meston CM. Association between smoking cessation and sexual health in men. BJU Int. 2012;109(6):888–96.
48. Oyeyipo IP, Raji Y, Emikpe BO, Bolarinwa AF. Effects of nicotine on sperm characteristics and fertility profile in adult male rats: a possible role of cessation. J Reprod Infertil. 2011;12(3):201–7.
49. Shenker NS, Ueland PM, Polidoro S, van Veldhoven K, Ricceri F, Brown R, Flanagan JM, Vineis P. DNA methylation as a long-term biomarker of exposure to tobacco smoke. Epidemiology. 2013;24(5):712–6.
50. Cui X, Jing X, Wu X, Wang Z, Li Q. Potential effect of smoking on semen quality through DNA damage and the downregulation of Chk1 in sperm. Mol Med Rep. 2016;14(1):753–61.
51. Harlev A, Agarwal A, Gunes SO, Shetty A, du Plessis SS. Smoking and male infertility: an evidence-based review. The world journal of men's health. 2015;33(3):143–60.
52. Agarwal A, Majzoub A, Esteves SC, Ko E, Ramasamy R, Zini A. Clinical utility of sperm DNA fragmentation testing: practice recommendations based on clinical scenarios. Transl Androl Urol. 2016;5(6):935–50.
53. Loft S, Kold-Jensen T, Hjollund NH, Giwercman A, Gyllemborg J, Ernst E, Olsen J, Scheike T, Poulsen HE, Bonde JP, Oxidative DNA. Damage in human sperm influences time to pregnancy. Hum Reprod. 2003;18(6):1265–72.
54. Sapra KJ, Barr DB, Maisog JM, Sundaram R, Buck Louis GM. Time-to-pregnancy associated with Couples' use of tobacco products. Nicotine Tob Res. 2016;18(11):2154–61.
55. Ghaffari MA, Rostami M. The effect of cigarette smoking on human sperm creatine kinase activity: as an ATP buffering system in sperm. Int J Fertil Steril. 2013;6(4):258–65.
56. Sofikitis N, Takenaka M, Kanakas N, Papadopoulos H, Yamamoto Y, Drakakis P, Miyagawa I. Effects of cotinine on sperm motility, membrane function, and fertilizing capacity in vitro. Urol Res. 2000;28(6):370–5.
57. Oyeyipo IP, Maartens PJ, du Plessis SS. In vitro effects of nicotine on human spermatozoa. Andrologia. 2014;46(8):887–92.
58. Kucheria K, Saxena R, Mohan D. Semen analysis in alcohol dependence syndrome. Andrologia. 1985;17(6):558–63.
59. Pajarinen JT, Karhunen PJ. Spermatogenic arrest and 'Sertoli cell-only' syndrome–common alcohol-induced disorders of the human testis. Int J Androl. 1994;17(6):292–9.
60. Muthusami KR, Chinnaswamy P. Effect of chronic alcoholism on male fertility hormones and semen quality. Fertil Steril. 2005;84(4):919–24.
61. Li Y, Lin H, Li Y, Cao J. Association between socio-psycho-behavioral factors and male semen quality: systematic review and meta-analyses. Fertil Steril. 2011;95(1):116–23.
62. Jensen TK, Gottschau M, Madsen JO, Andersson AM, Lassen TH, Skakkebaek NE, Swan SH, Priskorn L, Juul A, Jorgensen N. Habitual alcohol consumption associated with reduced semen quality and changes in reproductive hormones; a cross-sectional study among 1221 young Danish men. BMJ Open. 2014;4(9):e005462.
63. Hansen ML, Thulstrup AM, Bonde JP, Olsen J, Hakonsen LB, Ramlau-Hansen CH. Does last week's alcohol intake affect semen quality or reproductive hormones? A cross-sectional study among healthy young Danish men. Reprod Toxicol. 2012;34(3):457–62.
64. Condorelli RA, Calogero AE, Vicari E, La Vignera S. Chronic consumption of alcohol and sperm parameters: our experience and the main evidences. Andrologia. 2015;47(4):368–79.
65. Hassan MA, Killick SR. Negative lifestyle is associated with a significant reduction in fecundity. Fertil Steril. 2004;81(2):384–92.
66. Close CE, Roberts PL, Berger RE. Cigarettes, alcohol and marijuana are related to pyospermia in infertile men. J Urol. 1990;144(4):900–3.
67. Ramlau-Hansen CH, Toft G, Jensen MS, Strandberg-Larsen K, Hansen ML, Olsen J. Maternal alcohol consumption during pregnancy and semen quality in the male offspring: two decades of follow-up. Hum Reprod. 2010; 25(9):2340–5.
68. Yin D, Mufson RA, Wang R, Shi Y. Fas-mediated cell death promoted by opioids. Nature. 1999;397(6716):218.
69. Gianoulakis C. Characterization of the effects of acute ethanol administration on the release of beta-endorphin peptides by the rat hypothalamus. Eur J Pharmacol. 1990;180(1):21–9.
70. Talebi AR, Sarcheshmeh AA, Khalili MA, Tabibnejad N. Effects of ethanol consumption on chromatin condensation and DNA integrity of epididymal spermatozoa in rat. Alcohol. 2011;45(4):403–9.
71. Jana K, Jana N, De DK, Guha SK. Ethanol induces mouse spermatogenic cell apoptosis in vivo through over-expression of Fas/Fas-L, p53, and caspase-3 along with cytochrome c translocation and glutathione depletion. Mol Reprod Dev. 2010;77(9):820–33.
72. Gaspari L, Chang SS, Santella RM, Garte S, Pedotti P, Taioli E. Polycyclic aromatic hydrocarbon-DNA adducts in human sperm as a marker of DNA damage and infertility. Mutat Res. 2003;535(2):155–60.
73. Rossi BV, Berry KF, Hornstein MD, Cramer DW, Ehrlich S, Missmer SA. Effect of alcohol consumption on in vitro fertilization. Obstet Gynecol. 2011;117(1): 136–42.
74. Horak S, Polanska J, Widlak P. Bulky DNA adducts in human sperm: relationship with fertility, semen quality, smoking, and environmental factors. Mutat Res. 2003;537(1):53–65.

75. Pajarinen J, Savolainen V, Perola M, Penttila A, Karhunen PJ. Polymorphism in the cytochrome P450 2E1 gene and alcohol-induced disorders of human spermatogenesis. Int J Androl. 1996;19(5):314–22.
76. Fronczak CM, Kim ED, Barqawi AB. The insults of illicit drug use on male fertility. J Androl. 2012;33(4):515–28.
77. du Plessis SS, Agarwal A, Syriac A. Marijuana, phytocannabinoids, the endocannabinoid system, and male fertility. J Assist Reprod Genet. 2015; 32(11):1575–88.
78. Kolodny RC, Masters WH, Kolodner RM, Toro G. Depression of plasma testosterone levels after chronic intensive marihuana use. N Engl J Med. 1974;290(16):872–4.
79. Friedrich G, Nepita W, Andre T. Serum testosterone concentrations in cannabis and opiate users. Beitr Gerichtl Med. 1990;48:57–66.
80. Mendelson JH, Kuehnle J, Ellingboe J, Babor TF. Plasma testosterone levels before, during and after chronic marihuana smoking. N Engl J Med. 1974; 291(20):1051–5.
81. Cone EJ, Johnson RE, Moore JD, Roache JD. Acute effects of smoking marijuana on hormones, subjective effects and performance in male human subjects. Pharmacol Biochem Behav. 1986;24(6):1749–54.
82. Gundersen TD, Jorgensen N, Andersson AM, Bang AK, Nordkap L, Skakkebaek NE, Priskorn L, Juul A, Jensen TK. Association between use of marijuana and male reproductive hormones and semen quality: a study among 1,215 healthy young men. Am J Epidemiol. 2015;182(6):473–81.
83. Hembree WC 3rd, Nahas GG, Zeidenberg P, Huang HF. Changes in human spermatozoa associated with high dose marihuana smoking. Adv Biosci. 1978;22-23:429–39.
84. Singer R, Ben-Bassat M, Malik Z, Sagiv M, Ravid A, Shohat B, Livni E, Mamon T, Segenreich E, Servadio C. Oligozoospermia, asthenozoospermia, and sperm abnormalities in ex-addict to heroin, morphine, and hashish. Arch Androl. 1986;16(2):167–74.
85. Pacey AA, Povey AC, Clyma JA, McNamee R, Moore HD, Baillie H, Cherry NM, Participating Centres of Chaps-UK. Modifiable and non-modifiable risk factors for poor sperm morphology. Hum Reprod. 2014;29(8):1629–36.
86. Bracken MB, Eskenazi B, Sachse K, McSharry JE, Hellenbrand K, Leo-Summers L. Association of cocaine use with sperm concentration, motility, and morphology. Fertil Steril. 1990;53(2):315–22.
87. Samplaski MK, Bachir BG, Lo KC, Grober ED, Lau S, Jarvi KA. Cocaine use in the infertile male population: a marker for conditions resulting in subfertility. Current urology. 2015;8(1):38–42.
88. Vuong C, Van Uum SH, O'Dell LE, Lutfy K, Friedman TC. The effects of opioids and opioid analogs on animal and human endocrine systems. Endocr Rev. 2010;31(1):98–132.
89. Safarinejad MR, Asgari SA, Farshi A, Ghaedi G, Kolahi AA, Iravani S, Khoshdel AR. The effects of opiate consumption on serum reproductive hormone levels, sperm parameters, seminal plasma antioxidant capacity and sperm DNA integrity. Reprod Toxicol. 2013;36:18–23.
90. Schuel H, Chang MC, Berkery D, Schuel R, Zimmerman AM, Zimmerman S. Cannabinoids inhibit fertilization in sea urchins by reducing the fertilizing capacity of sperm. Pharmacol Biochem Behav. 1991;40(3): 609–15.
91. Zimmerman AM, Zimmerman S, Raj AY. Effects of cannabinoids on spermatogenesis in mice. Adv Biosci. 1978;22-23:407–18.
92. Wenger T, Rettori V, Snyder GD, Dalterio S, McCann SM. Effects of delta-9-tetrahydrocannabinol on the hypothalamic-pituitary control of luteinizing hormone and follicle-stimulating hormone secretion in adult male rats. Neuroendocrinology. 1987;46(6):488–93.
93. Smith C, Moore C, Besch N, Besch P. Effect of marihuana (delta-9 tetrahydrocannabinol) on secretion of sex-hormones in mature male rhesus-monkey. In: Clinical Chemistry: 1976: AMER ASSOC CLINICAL CHEMISTRY 2101 L STREET NW, SUITE 202, WASHINGTON, DC 20037-1526; 1976. p. 1184.
94. Banerjee A, Singh A, Srivastava P, Turner H, Krishna A. Effects of chronic bhang (cannabis) administration on the reproductive system of male mice. Birth Defects Res B Dev Reprod Toxicol. 2011;92(3):195–205.
95. Chakravarty I, Ghosh JJ. Influence of cannabis and delta-9-tetrahydrocannabinol on the biochemistry of the male reproductive organs. Biochem Pharmacol. 1981;30(4):273–6.
96. Li H, George VK, Crawford SC, Dhabuwala CB. Effect of cocaine on testicular blood flow in rats: evaluation by percutaneous injection of xenon-133. J Environ Pathol Toxicol Oncol. 1999;18(1):73–7.
97. George VK, Li H, Teloken C, Grignon DJ, Lawrence WD, Dhabuwala CB. Effects of long-term cocaine exposure on spermatogenesis and fertility in peripubertal male rats. J Urol. 1996;155(1):327–31.
98. Li H, Jiang Y, Rajpurkar A, Tefilli MV, Dunbar JC, Dhabuwala CB. Lipid peroxidation and antioxidant activities in rat testis after chronic cocaine administration. Urology. 1999;54(5):925–8.
99. Barenys M, Gomez-Catalan J, Camps L, Teixido E, de Lapuente J, Gonzalez-Linares J, Serret J, Borras M, Rodamilans M, Llobet JM. MDMA (ecstasy) delays pubertal development and alters sperm quality after developmental exposure in the rat. Toxicol Lett. 2010;197(2):135–42.
100. Abdellatief RB, Elgamal DA, Mohamed EE. Effects of chronic tramadol administration on testicular tissue in rats: an experimental study. Andrologia. 2015;47(6):674–9.
101. Ahmadnia H, Akhavan Rezayat A, Hoseyni M, Sharifi N, Khajedalooee M, Akhavan Rezayat A. Short-period influence of chronic morphine exposure on serum levels of sexual hormones and spermatogenesis in rats. Nephrourol Mon. 2016;8(4):e38052.
102. Whan LB, West MC, McClure N, Lewis SE. Effects of delta-9-tetrahydrocannabinol, the primary psychoactive cannabinoid in marijuana, on human sperm function in vitro. Fertil Steril. 2006;85(3):653–60.
103. Amoako AA, Marczylo TH, Marczylo EL, Elson J, Willets JM, Taylor AH, Konje JC. Anandamide modulates human sperm motility: implications for men with asthenozoospermia and oligoasthenoteratozoospermia. Hum Reprod. 2013;28(8):2058–66.
104. Morgan DJ, Muller CH, Murataeva NA, Davis BJ, Mackie K. Delta9-Tetrahydrocannabinol (Delta9-THC) attenuates mouse sperm motility and male fecundity. Br J Pharmacol. 2012;165(8):2575–83.

13

Lactate promotes specific differentiation in bovine granulosa cells depending on lactate uptake thus mimicking an early post-LH stage

Anja Baufeld and Jens Vanselow*

Abstract

Background: The LH-induced folliculo-luteal transformation is connected with alterations of the gene expression profile in cells of the granulosa layer. It has been described that hypoxic conditions occur during luteinization, thus favoring the formation of L-lactate within the follicle. Despite being a product of anaerobic respiration, L-lactate has been shown to act as a signaling molecule affecting gene expression in neuronal cells. During the present study, we tested the hypothesis that L-lactate may influence differentiation of follicular granulosa cells (GC).

Methods: In a bovine granulosa cell culture model effects of L- and D-lactate, of increased glucose concentrations and of the lactate transport inhibitor UK5099 were analyzed. Steroid hormone production was analyzed by RIA and the abundance of key transcripts was determined by quantitative real-time RT-PCR.

Results: L-lactate decreased the production of estradiol and significantly affected selected genes of the folliculo-luteal transition as well as genes of the lactate metabolism. *CYP19A1*, *FSHR*, *LHCGR* were down-regulated, whereas *RGS2*, *VNN2*, *PTX3*, *LDHA* and lactate transporters were up-regulated. These effects could be partly or completely reversed by pre-treatment of the cells with UK5099. The non-metabolized enantiomer D-lactate had even more pronounced effects on gene expression, whereas increased glucose concentrations did not affect transcript abundance.

Conclusions: In summary, our data suggest that L-lactate specifically alters physiological and molecular characteristics of GC. These effects critically depend on L-lactate uptake, but are not triggered by increased energy supply. Further, we could show that L-lactate has a positive feedback on the lactate metabolism. Therefore, we hypothesize that L-lactate acts as a signaling molecule in bovine and possibly other monovular species supporting differentiation during the folliculo-luteal transformation.

Keywords: Bovine, Granulosa cells, L-lactate, Expression

Background

The pre-ovulatory LH surge induces massive changes within the follicle, including morphological, physiological and molecular alterations [1, 2]. The reorganization of the follicle is accompanied by a tremendous shift of the gene expression profile particularly in cells of the granulosa layer [3, 4]. The aromatase-encoding gene *CYP19A1*, and the gonadotropin receptors, *FSHR* and *LHCGR*, are significantly down-regulated immediately after the pre-ovulatory LH surge in vivo [5, 6]. In contrast, *RGS2*, encoding the regulator of G protein signaling 2, and the inflammatory-related genes *VNN2*, encoding the vascular non-inflammatory molecule 2, and *PTX3*, encoding pentraxin 3, were highly up-regulated [4, 7, 8]. It was hypothesized that hypoxic conditions occur during folliculogenesis and support ovulation [9, 10]. However, it is still unclear whether hypoxia is an essential signal during the folliculo-luteal transition [11]. As for granulosa cells (GC) it was proposed that pericellular hypoxia present under high cell density conditions may induce differentiation [12]. Likewise,

* Correspondence: vanselow@fbn-dummerstorf.de
Institute of Reproductive Biology, Leibniz Institute for Farm Animal Biology (FBN), Wilhelm-Stahl-Allee 2, 18196 Dummerstorf, Germany

we showed that high cell density induces specific changes of the gene expression and steroid hormone profiles in cultured GC mimicking an early post-LH status of GC differentiation [13]. Furthermore, applying a whole-genome approach we could demonstrate in GC cultured at high plating density, that genes connected to hypoxia are affected [14]. In particular *LDHA* transcripts encoding L-lactate dehydrogenase were remarkably up-regulated. It was demonstrated also by others that *LDHA* expression is regulated by hypoxia [15]. In addition, a binding site for HIF1/2α could be identified in the *LDHA* promotor explaining the hypoxia-related expression [16, 17]. On the other hand Lee et al. [18] proposed a HIF-independent mechanism of lactate accumulation under hypoxic conditions. Hence, L-lactate might play a role during the folliculo-luteal transition. Reports from different species demonstrated higher L-lactate concentrations within the follicular fluid than in the respective serum, ranging from 6 mM in human up to 27 mM in rats [19–21]. Generated even during adequate oxygen provision L-lactate might represent an important regulator of metabolism [22]. A study in L6 cells revealed that L-lactate may be involved in the delivery of oxidative and gluconeogenic substrates thus leading to the cell-cell and intracellular lactate shuttle hypothesis [23, 24]. In this context L-lactate is also described as a metabolic signal. L-lactate affects its own metabolism by stimulating the expression of the lactate transporter MCT1 in rat muscle cells [25]. In mouse granulosa cells MCTs were identified regulating the transport of L-lactate within the female reproductive tract [26]. Moreover, in neuronal cells L-lactate affects the expression of genes linked to neuronal plasticity during establishment of the long-term memory [27, 28]. In this study we therefore tested the hypothesis that L-lactate is a signaling molecule in the bovine follicle. To that end, we analyzed the effects of L-lactate in a serum-free estradiol (E2)-producing GC culture model [13, 29, 30] on specific morphological, physiological and molecular parameters.

Methods

Tissue collection and cell culture

Bovine ovaries were obtained from a local abattoir and transported in cold 1× PBS containing penicillin (100 IU), streptomycin (0.1 mg/ml) and amphotericin (0.5 μg/μl). By aspirating small to medium sized follicle (< 6 mm) with a syringe and 18 G needle a nearly pure population of granulosa cells was recovered [5]. GC were collected in 1× PBS (with antibiotics) and pooled from 30 to 50 ovaries with 15 to 30 follicles per ovary. Accordingly, samples from at least 15 different cows with non-defined cyclicity status were included in each preparation. To determine the amount of living cells GC were counted in a hemocytometer by trypan blue exclusion method and cryo-preserved in freezing media (fetal calf serum containing 10% DMSO; Roth, Karlsruhe, Germany). The cryo-preserving procedure did not alter general characteristics of GC in culture as we could detect equal levels of marker gene expression as compared with cultures from freshly isolated GC (Additional file 1: Figure S1). All experiments were performed in technical and biological replicates (at least 3) using different cell preparations. Shortly before the onset of cell culture 24-well plates were coated with collagen R (0.02%; Serva, Heidelberg, Germany) to improve the cell attachment [13]. Frozen GC were immediately separated from the freezing media by centrifugation (500 x *g* for 3 min) and re-suspended in culture media with supplements as described previously [13]. Briefly, cells of a total cell number of 1.0×10^5 cells/well were cultured under serum-free conditions in α-MEM containing L-Glutamin (2 mM), sodium bicarbonate (0.084%), BSA (0.1%), HEPES (20 mM), sodium selenite (4 ng/ml), transferrin (5 μg/ml), insulin (10 ng/ml), non-essential amino acids (1 mM), penicillin (100 IU/ml) and streptomycin (0.1 mg/ml), FSH (20 ng/ml; Sigma Aldrich, Steinheim, Germany), R^3 IGF-1 (50 ng/ml; Sigma Aldrich), and androstenedione (2 μM; Sigma Aldrich). The cells were additionally treated over the complete culture period with sodium L-lactate (7.5 mM – 30 mM), D-lactate (30 mM, both Sigma-Aldrich), or sodium chloride as vehicle control (7.5 mM – 30 mM; Sigma Aldrich). For inhibitory studies cells were initially pre-treated with inhibitor UK5099 (50 μM; Sigma Aldrich) for 48 h and subsequently treated with L-lactate or the vehicle control. The L-lactate transporters were inhibited with UK5099 (50 μM; Sigma Aldrich). All reagents were purchased from Merck Millipore (Berlin, Germany) if not stated otherwise. GC were maintained for 8 days at 37 °C and 5% CO_2 to allow the cells to completely recover from plating stress and to resume E2 production [31]. Two thirds of the spent culture medium was replaced every other day. Also in previous studies it has been repeatedly shown that GC obtained from small follicles (< 6 mm) require several days in vitro to develop an estradiol-active status that mimics the in vivo GC state shortly before the LH surge [13, 32].

Measurements of cell viability and hormone production

The cell viability test was performed using the CellTiter 96 AQueous One Solution Cell Proliferation Assay (Promega, Mannheim, Germany). The one compound solution contains a MTS tetrazolium salt which is converted into a colored formazan product by NAD(P)H that is only present in viable cells. Therefore, the quantitative detection of the formazan product by absorbance measurement represents the number of viable cells in culture. The assay was performed according to the manufacturer's protocol. Therefore, cells were cultured in collagen R coated 96-well plates. The absorbance was measured in a 96-well plate reader (FLUOstar Omega, BMG Labtech, Ortenberg, Germany) at a wavelength of 490 nm. Progesterone (P4) and E2 concentrations were measured using competitive ^{3}H–radioimmunoassay (RIA) as described previously [33]. For P4 the tracer [1,2,6,7-3H(N)]progesterone was purchased from PerkinElmer (Boston, USA) and the E2 tracer [2,4,6,7-3H]estradiol-17β was purchased from GE Healthcare (Freiburg, Germany). Radioactivity measurement was performed in a liquid scintillation counter (LSC) with an integrated RIA-calculation program (TriCarb 2900 TR, PerkinElmer) and the intra- and interassay coefficients of variation (CV) for P4 were specified as 7.6% and 9.8%, whereas for E2 intra- and interassay CV were 6.9% and 9.9%, respectively. For analysis the cell culture media was diluted 1:40 in RIA-buffer for P4 measurement and was used undiluted for E2 and measured in duplicates.

RNA preparation, cDNA synthesis and quantitative Real-Time PCR

Total RNA isolation was performed with the NucleoSpin RNA Kit (Macherey-Nagel, Düren, Germany) following the protocol of the manufacturer and RNA concentration was measured using a NanoDrop 1000 Spectrophotometer (Thermo Scientific, Bonn, Germany). Subsequently, cDNA was synthesized with SensiFAST cDNA Synthesis Kit (Bioline, Luckenwalde, Germany) from 250 ng RNA. Quantitative Real-Time PCR for gene expression analysis was accomplished with SensiFast SYBR No-ROX (Bioline) and gene-specific primers (listed in Table 1). Complementary DNA samples were amplified in duplicate from 0.2 and 0.4 μl in a total volume of 12 μl. The PCR was performed and quantified in a LightCycler 96 instrument (Roche, Mannheim, Germany) with following cycle conditions: pre-incubation at 95 °C for 5 min, 40 amplification cycles of denaturation at 95 ° C for 20 s, annealing at 60 °C for 15 s, extension at 72 °C for 15 s, and a single-point fluorescence acquisition for 10 s. Analysis of the melting point was done immediately afterwards to ensure amplification of correct products. For the same reason the length of PCR products was checked by agarose gel electrophoresis (3%, ethidium bromide stained). Cloned and sequenced PCR products were used as external standards for absolute quantification. Of these, fresh dilutions were prepared from five different concentrations of standards (5×10^{-12}-5×10^{-16} g DNA/reaction) and co-amplified in each run. The absolute quantified transcript abundance was normalized to the reference gene *RPLP0,* showing stable expression values throughout the different treatments.

Statistics

Each experiment was done with at least three biological replicates (different GC preparations) and three technical replicates (different culture wells) each. SigmaPlot 12.0 Statistical Analysis System (Jandel Scientific, San Rafael, CA, USA) was used for statistical analysis. Statistical analysis of hormone and qPCR measurement was carried out with untransformed data. Comparison of two different treatments (e.g. L-lactate vs. vehicle control) was performed with the student *t*-test or Mann-Whitney Test, when the requirements of the t-test were not fulfilled. Multiple comparisons were done with one-way analysis of variance (ANOVA, Holm-Sidak method). Limits of statistical significance were set at $P < 0.05$. For graphical presentation the ordinate was scaled in log2 (except for glucose experiment), which distributes the effects of up- and down-regulation more uniformly.

Results

Effects of L- and D-lactate on hormone production and gene expression

Initially, effects of different L-lactate concentrations on cultured GC were analyzed. Previous studies reported effective concentrations of 20 mM or 30 mM in different cell types [27, 34, 35]. In various species L-lactate concentrations in the antral fluid of growing follicles could be detected between 6 and 27 mM [19, 21]. Therefore, we treated the GC with L-lactate concentrations ranging from 7.5 mM to 45 mM and corresponding vehicle controls (NaCl). As highly sensitive parameters we determined the abundance of several marker transcripts, which are highly regulated in the GC layer during the folliculo-luteal transition [4]. The treatment with 30 mM and 45 mM L-lactate resulted in considerable changes of these molecular parameters compared to the control (Fig. 1a). We could identify a dose-dependent down-regulation of *CYP19A1, FSHR* and *LHCGR. RGS2* and *VNN2* transcripts revealed a dose-dependent up-regulation. Whereas a significant up-regulation of *RGS2* expression was already achieved with 7.5 mM L-lactate, a significant down-regulation of *CYP19A1* expression was observed with 30 mM L-lactate. We therefore considered 30 mM L-lactate as an effective concentration during the ongoing study of in vitro cultured GC.

In studies by others D-lactate, a non-metabolized and iso-osmotic enantiomer of L-lactate, was used as a control [27, 36]. However, in GC the supplementation with D-lactate led to even more pronounced and specific changes of several marker genes (Fig. 1b). The down-regulation of *CYP19A1, FSHR* and *LHCGR* by D-lactate revealed to be more prominent than with L-lactate. The same effect could be observed for the up-regulation of *RGS2* and *VNN2.* Accordingly, D-lactate could not be used as an appropriate control.

Table 1 Gene specific primers used in quantitative Real-Time PCR

Gene	dir	Sequence	Size (bp)	Accession No.
RPLPO	for	TGGTTACCCAACCGTCGCATCTGTA	142	NM_001012682
	rev	CACAAAGGCAGATGGATCAGCCAAG		
CYP19A1	for	GCTTTTGGAAGTGCTGAACCCAAGG	172	NM_174305
	rev	GGGCCCAATTCCCAGAAAGTAGCTG		
FSHR	for	TCACCAAGCTTCGAGTCATCCCAAA	189	NM_174061
	rev	TCTGGAAGGCATCAGGGTCGATGTA		
LHCGR	for	GCATCCACAAGCTTCCAGATGTTACGA	205	NM_174381
	rev	GGGAAATCAGCGTTGTCCCATTGA		
RGS2	for	AAGCCCAGCTGTGGTCAGAAGCATT	127	NM_001075596
	rev	TCTTCACAGGCCAGCCAGAATTCAA		
VNN2	for	TCCCACAGCTTGGATGAACGTTTTG	267	NM_001163920
	rev	TAGGCACTCCAATTCATGGCTGGTG		
PTX3	for	TTTGTGCGCTCTGGTCTGCAGTGT	164	NM_001076259
	rev	CATGGTGAAGAGCTTGTCCCACTCG		
LDHA	for	GGGTTGGTGCTGTTGGCATGGCCT	232	NM_174099.2
	rev	TCTCCCTCTTGCTGACGTGCCCCA		
SLC16A1	for	GGTGGAGGTCCTATCAGCAGTGTCCT	236	NM_001037319.1
	rev	AGTCCATTTGCCAGCGGTCGTCTC		
SLC16A7	for	ACCCAGTGCCGGAGACCAGCAGTT	182	NM_001076336.2
	rev	GGATGTGGTGGTGGGGTGCCTCCT		

dir, direction; for, forward primer; rev, reverse primer

Further on we analyzed whether L-lactate or the vehicle control (NaCl) compromised the viability of cultured GC. Although the viability tended to be slightly affected in L-lactate treated cells, these effects were not statistically significant (Table 2). As a paradigm for differentiation-specific changes of cultured GC the morphology, hormone concentrations as well as the expression of GC-specific marker genes were analyzed in L-lactate-treated GC. As shown in Fig. 2a and b the morphology of cultured GC was not considerably altered. GC displayed the typical fibroblast-like phenotype with occasional cluster formation under both experimental conditions. In contrast, the estradiol production was clearly affected showing considerably lower concentration (Fig. 2c). Additionally, the abundance of several selected marker transcripts revealed a significant regulation upon L-lactate treatment (Fig. 2d). The abundance of *CYP19A1* transcripts encoding the key enzyme of estradiol synthesis, aromatase P450, was significantly lower in L-lactate treated GC than in the controls (dashed line). This is also reflected by the observed decrease of E2 production. Similarly, the amounts of *FSHR* and *LHCGR* transcripts were significantly down-regulated. In contrast, *RGS2*, *VNN2* and *PTX3* transcripts were considerably up-regulated by L-lactate.

In addition to these long-term effects of L-lactate, we were interested whether a short-term treatment is sufficient to induce these massive physiological and molecular changes. Thus, the cultured GC were treated with 30 mM L-lactate during the final 24 h of the culture period. Under these conditions no significant alterations of marker transcripts as well as of hormone concentrations could be observed (Table 3). This indicates that L-lactate has only long-term effects on GC differentiation. Additionally, because increased L-lactate concentrations might be used as an additional source of energy by the cultured GC, we analyzed whether an increased energy supply suggestively resulting in higher metabolic activity of the cells, could be responsible for the effects of L-lactate. Therefore we increased the glucose concentration of the basal media from 1 g/l up to 4 g/l. The 4-fold increase of glucose concentration however, did not lead to any changes in the expression of the selected marker genes (Fig. 3).

Effects of specific inhibition of L-lactate transporters

As a first approach to elucidate molecular mechanisms that are involved in the observed effects of L-lactate we pre-treated GC with specific inhibitor of lactate transporters (MCTs). Inhibition of MCTs with UK5099 could partly reverse the L-lactate effect (Figs. 4a and b). Negative effects of L-lactate on E2 production could be abolished (Fig. 4a). The inhibition of MCTs also resulted in a recovery of the

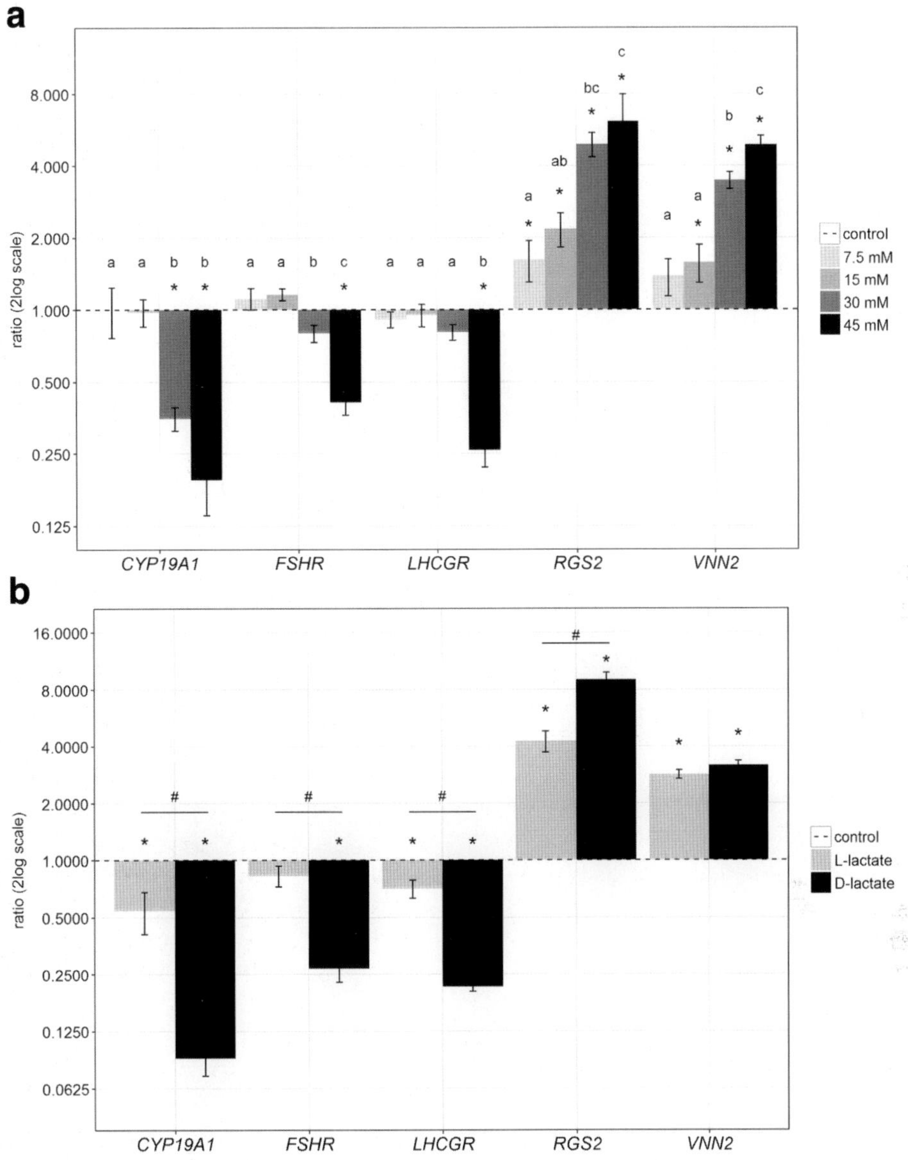

Fig. 1 Effects of different L-lactate concentrations and of the steric enantiomer D-lactate on cultured bovine GC. (**a**) Increasing L-lactate concentrations progressively decreased or increased the abundance of selected marker gene transcripts. Transcript abundance was normalized to *RPLP0* as a reference gene. The values (means ± SEM) are shown as ratio relatively to the vehicle control (dashed line). For statistical testing of the L-lactate effect the *RPLP0*-normalized values were compared using the student *t*-test or Mann-Whitney test, $n = 3$, $*P < 0.05$. To test for effects of increasing L-lactate concentration an ANOVA was performed and letters indicate significant differences between treatment groups, $n = 3$, $P < 0.05$. (**b**) The supplementation with D-lactate (30 mM) elicited more prominent effects on gene expression than L-lactate (30 mM) compared to the vehicle control (dashed line). The student's *t*-test or Mann-Whitney test was used for analyzing the L- and D-lactate effects compared to the respective control (*) and between L- and D-lactate treatment (#), $n = 3$, $P < 0.05$.

Table 2 Effects of lactate and NaCl control on the viability of cultured bovine GC

treatment	untreated	lactate	NaCl
OD	0.997	0.640	1.291
SEM	0.245	0.177	0.165

The cells were cultured for 8 days under serum-free, E2-active conditions, with L-lactate or the vehicle control NaCl (both 30 mM) supplementation. The mean OD (optical density) of $n = 4$ replicates is shown with SEM (standard error of means), no significant differences between treatment groups were observed, $P = 0.108$ (ANOVA)

transcript abundance levels of *CYP19A1* and *FSHR* (Fig. 4b). Also in case of *PTX3, RGS2* and *VNN2* the L-lactate-induced increment was reduced, although the transcript abundance was still significantly higher than in the control, except for *VNN2*. The treatment with the inhibitor alone resulted in no obvious changes compared to the vehicle control.

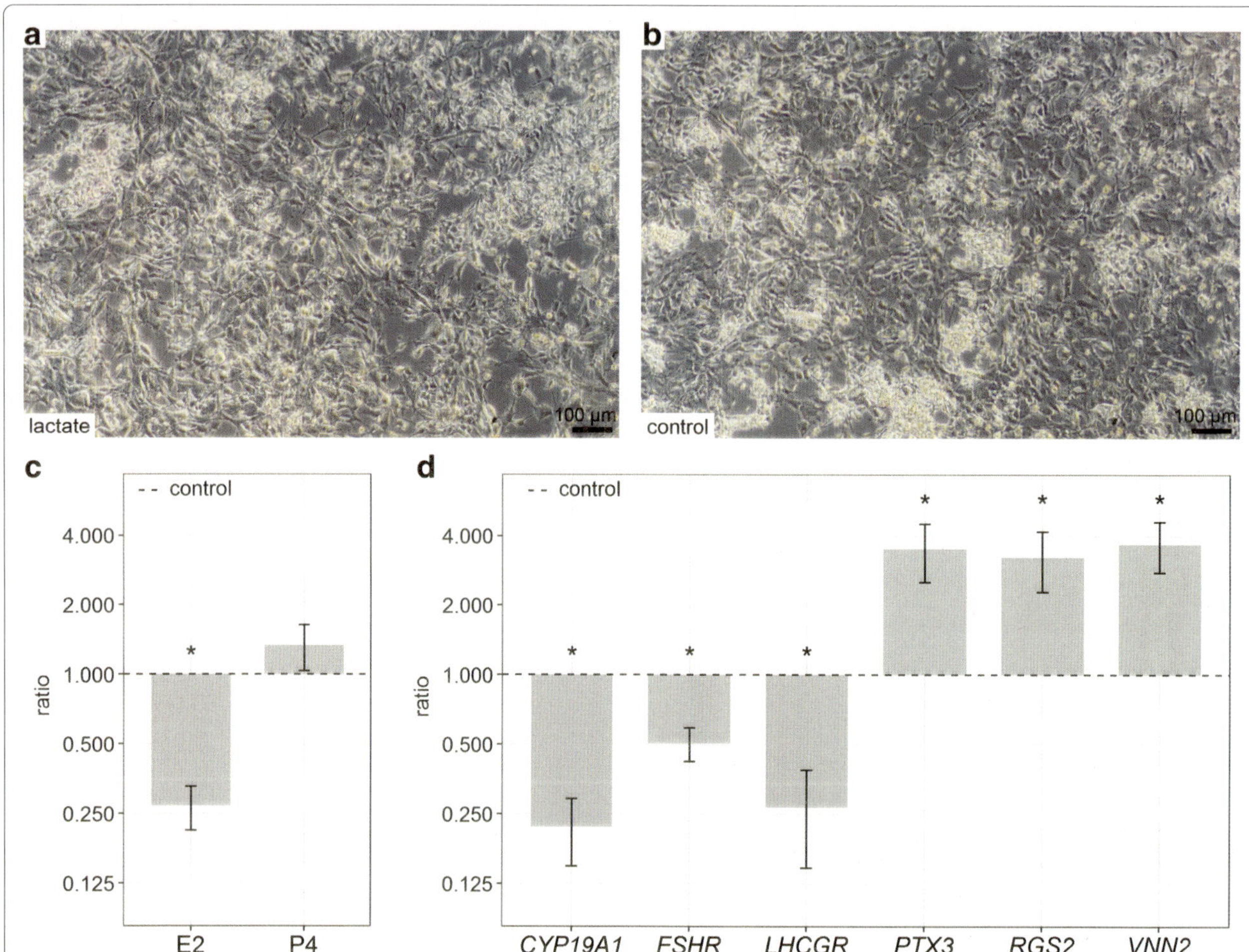

Fig. 2 Effects of L-lactate on the morphology, hormone concentration and gene expression. GC were cultured with L-lactate (30 mM) supplementation compared to the corresponding vehicle control in a standardized serum-free culture system for 8 days. (**a-b**) Cultured cells displayed a typical GC-like morphology and tended to form clusters. (**c**) Hormone profiles of L-lactate treated cells indicated relatively to the control (dashed line). The concentration of E2 (in ng/ml) was significantly decreased relative to the vehicle control (dashed line). (**d**) The expression of selected marker genes was specifically regulated in L-lactate treated cells as compared to the vehicle control (dashed line). The transcript abundance was normalized to the reference gene *RPLPO*. Means and SEM are shown of $n = 3$ replicates, $^*P < 0.05$, student *t*-test or Mann-Whitney test.

Effects of L-lactate and specific MCT inhibitor on genes related to L-lactate metabolism

It was recently reported that L-lactate can influence genes related to the L-lactate metabolism resulting in a positive feedback mechanism [25]. Therefore, we were interested whether the genes encoding L-lactate dehydrogenase, *LDHA*, or L-lactate transporters, *SLC16A1* and *SLC16A7*, were affected. The *LDHA* transcript abundance was strongly increased upon L-lactate treatment (Fig. 5), but also the L-lactate transporters *SLC16A1* and *SLC16A7* showed a significant upregulation. After pre-treatment with UK5099, the L-lactate effects on the expression of *LDHA* and *SLC16A1* could be nearly reversed.

Table 3 Effects of short-term lactate treatment on gene expression of selected marker genes and steroid hormone production

Gene / hormone	*CYP19A1*	*FSHR*	*LHCGR*	*RGS2*	*VNN2*	E2	P4
Control	3.12 (± 0.31)	34.70 (± 4.41)	3.29 (± 0.46)	5.56 (± 0.29)	6.26 (± 0.39)	23.72 (± 1.57)	824.61 (± 84.99)
L-lactate	3.78 (± 0.85)	49.10 (± 8.33)	3.18 (± 0.94)	5.78 (± 0.32)	7.39 (± 1.11)	32.31 (± 5.26)	905.01 (± 47.03)
P	0.50	0.20	0.92	0.63	0.39	0.19	0.45

GC were stimulated with 30 mM L-lactate or the vehicle control NaCl 24 h prior to the end of the culture period of 8 days. Transcript abundance ($\times10^{-3}$, normalized to the reference gene *RPLPO*) and hormone concentrations (in ng/ml) are shown as means (± SEM) of $n = 3$ replicates, *P*-values were calculated using the student's *t*-test or Mann-Whitney Test

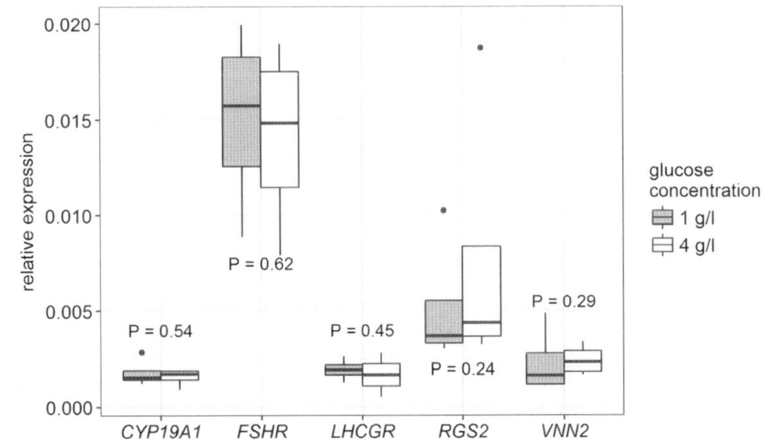

Fig. 3 Effects of different glucose concentration in media. GC were cultured in basal media with 1 g/l glucose (grey) or increased concentration of 4 g/l glucose (black). No change in the expression of selected genes could be detected. Transcript abundance was normalized to reference gene *RPLP0*. Box plots with medians of $n = 4$ replicates are shown; dots indicate outliers, student *t*-test or Mann-Whitney test with no statistical significance.

Discussion

Initial experiments with different lactate concentrations revealed significant effects on *RGS2* expression with 7.5 mM and on *CYP19A1* or *FSHR* expression with 30 mM. *LHCGR* was significantly affected only with 45 mM. However, this might be due to the generally observed greater variance of *LHCGR*, of which the very low abundance levels were close to the detection limit. Nonetheless, based on these data, an L-lactate concentration of 30 mM was used as an effective concentration throughout the following experiments. Interestingly, the non-metabolized enantiomer D-lactate elicited more prominent effects on gene expression than L-lactate. An effect of D-lactate was also described by Latham et al. [35] and Wagner et al. [37], analyzing HDAC activity. However, it must be considered that the concentrations of D-lactate in mammalian species has been shown to be three orders of magnitude lower than those of L-lactate [38], thus raising the question whether D-lactate plays any important role after all. But nonetheless, our data on increased effects of the non-metabolized D-lactate support our hypothesis that L-lactate can act as a signaling molecule apart from being metabolized. Moreover, it is reasonable that the enhanced effects of D-lactate are due to the non-metabolized status in mammalian cells. At this point we cannot exclude the possibility that a part of L-lactate is metabolized, which in turn leads to a reduction of L-lactate concentration and hence results in minor effects than the non-metabolized D-lactate. This leads to the suggestion that chirality might not be the primary

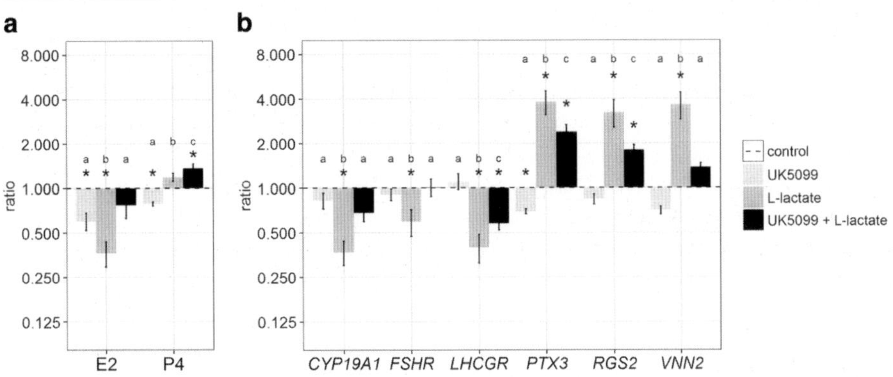

Fig. 4 Effects of L-lactate transport inhibitors on L-lactate induced changes of hormone and gene expression profile. GC were cultured as described before and additionally pre-treated for two days with the inhibitor for L-lactate transporters, UK5099 (50 μM). (**a**) Inhibition of L-lactate transporters (black bars) resulted in the reversal of the L-lactate effect (dark grey bars) on E2 production. (**b**) The gene expression levels of selected transcripts nearly regained control levels (dashed line) after inhibition of L-lactate transporters, whereas the inhibitor alone showed nearly no effects (light grey bars). Transcript abundance was normalized to the reference gene *RPLP0*. Means and SEM of the hormone concentration and gene expression are shown of $n = 4$ replicates. The student's *t*-test or Mann-Whitney test was used for analyzing the effects compared to the vehicle control (*) and between different treatments the ANOVA testing was used (indicated by letters), $n = 4$, $P < 0.05$.

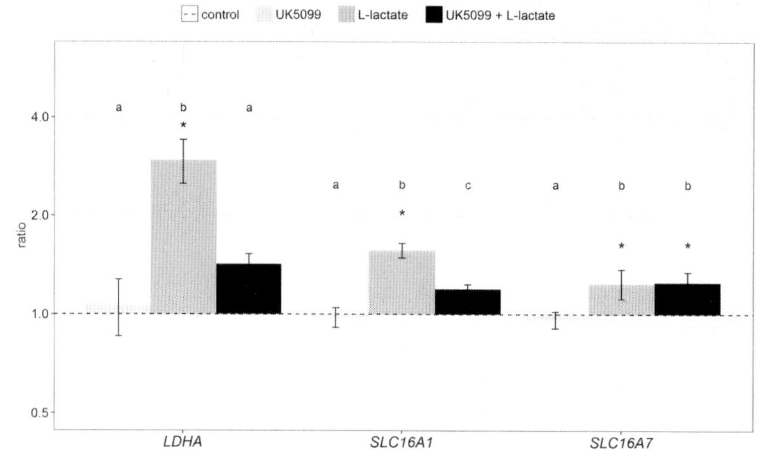

Fig. 5 Effect of L-lactate and specific inhibitor of L-lactate transport on genes involved in L-lactate metabolism. The abundance of *LDHA* and *SLC16A1* transcripts was up-regulated in L-lactate treated GC (grey bars) compared to the control (dashed line; *). When the cells were pre-incubated with the inhibitors UK5099 the L-lactate induced changes of expression levels were largely abolished. No effect was observed with the inhibitor alone (light grey bars). Transcript abundance was normalized to *RPLP0* as a reference gene. Means and SEM are shown of $n = 4$ replicates, *$P < 0.05$, student's *t*-test or Mann-Whitney test was uses to test treatment effects compared to the vehicle control (*) and between different treatments the ANOVA was used (indicated by letters).

parameter for signaling efficiency. This hypothesis has to be further taken into account in subsequent studies.

Interestingly, our results of different glucose concentration in GC media revealed no alterations in the gene expression. This indicates that an increased energy supply and thus higher metabolic activity alone is not sufficient to induce differentiation of bovine GCs in culture, which was shown in a previous work in sheep GC [39].

In follicular fluids of rats L-lactate concentrations of 27 mM had been detected at the time of the expected LH surge, when the serum concentration of L-lactate remained considerably low at 5 mM [21]. Studies in humans showed concentrations of 6.2 mM L-lactate at the time of oocyte recovery from women undergoing IVF [19]. In the bovine different values have been reported ranging from 5 mM up to 14.4 mM depending on the size or stage of the follicle [20, 40, 41]. Until now, effects of L-lactate on the cell physiology and gene expression have been only studied in rat L6 cells, human mesenchymal stem cells, human HCT116 cells or mouse neurons, where effective concentrations ranged from 10 to 30 mM lactate [27, 34, 35, 42]. To our knowledge the present study is the first one that aims at clarifying the effects of L-lactate on GC differentiation in any species.

Short-term treatment of cultured bovine GC at the end of the culture period did not lead to considerable alterations. Neither hormone production nor gene expression profiles were significantly affected. Interestingly, this observation is in line with a conclusion by others that short-term exposure to L-lactate does not affect gene expression, but may already have some effects on the cell metabolism [23]. Furthermore, it was suggested that effects on gene expression potentially require long-term exposure to L-lactate [23]. This is clearly supported by our data showing that only long-term treatment could induce significant changes of physiological and molecular parameters in cultured GC, although the typical GC-like morphology and formation of cell clusters [13, 30, 32] was not affected by L-lactate. Estradiol production clearly decreased whereas progesterone production was nearly unaffected compared to the controls. Estradiol down-regulation can be easily attributed to the remarkable down-regulation of the aromatase coding gene *CYP19A1*. Besides *CYP19A1* we also analyzed additional marker genes of an early LH-dependent differentiation, which have been shown to be highly regulated following the pre-ovulatory LH-surge in vivo [4, 5, 7]. In particular, *FSHR* and *LHCGR* were found down-regulated and *RGS2, VNN2* and *PTX3* clearly up-regulated upon L-lactate treatment. These data together with the alterations of the hormone production suggest that L-lactate can induce a stage of differentiation in cultured GC that is similar to the early post-LH stage in vivo. Previous studies identified increased L-lactate concentrations after hCG stimulation in human GC culture or in the antral fluid of follicles in macaques thus supporting our conclusion [43, 44]. L-lactate is well known as a product of anaerobic respiration, but may also play a role as regulatory molecule even during adequate oxygen provision [22, 24]. Interestingly, it was described in several studies that L-lactate can act as a signaling molecule in fibroblasts [45], macrophages [46] and even neuronal cells [27, 28]. Yang and colleagues showed that in neurons L-lactate affected the expression of genes involved in the establishment of long-term memory [27]. In another recent study L-lactate exhibited neuroprotective properties against excitotoxicity by coordinating specific cellular pathways [47]. The results of our study indicate for the first time a specific role of L-lactate as a signaling molecule in bovine GC.

As a next approach we tested if L-lactate uptake is an essential prerequisite to induce the observed effects. The inhibition of L-lactate uptake was accomplished with UK5099, a potent MCT inhibitor of L-lactate transport [27]. This inhibitor is characterized to target the group of MCT 1–4 that are responsible for lactate as well as pyruvate transport. Accordingly, the transport of L-lactate into the cells should be completely inhibited by UK5099. Our results showed that the estradiol concentrations as well as the expression of selected marker genes nearly regained control levels after inhibiting the MCTs. This clearly suggests that the observed effects are vitally dependent upon L-lactate uptake into GC. It has been shown in neurons, that transport of L-lactate into the cells and K_{ATP} channels [48] or NMDA receptor activation [27] is necessary to promote the observed changes. In contrast to our data demonstrating strong effects of the non-metabolized D-lactate, the conversion of L-lactate to pyruvate is a crucial prerequisite in both cases. Whereas the rise of ATP production is essential for K_{ATP} channel actions, the increase in the NADH/NAD ratio leads to the modulation of NMDA receptor activity [28]. Here we can only speculate on mechanisms occurring in bovine GC. But in human ovaries functional ATP-sensitive potassium channels could be identified and moreover it was shown that blocking of these ion channels negatively influences progesterone production [49]. In ovarian tissue and granulosa cells expression of specific subunits of the NMDA receptor, the subunits 1 and 2B, had been identified [50] thus supporting the view that this receptor might be involved in these cells as well. Expression of NMDAR subunits, especially of *GRIN2D* and *GRINA* has been found in vivo in GC (see database GranulosaIMAGE [51]) as well as in vitro (own GC culture microarray dataset [14]). Whether these receptor subunits can actually form functional receptors to be modulated by L-lactate in bovine GC has to be investigated in further studies. However, our data clearly show that L-lactate uptake is mandatory for most of the observed effects thus excluding the possibility that a G-protein coupled receptor for lactate, coded by *HCAR1*, might be necessary to carry the L-lactate signal across the cell membrane [52]. In addition, *HCAR1* transcripts were not detectable in our GC culture system (data not shown) thus indicating that *HCAR1* is not expressed in cultured GC. This is further supported by in vivo data demonstrating that *HCAR1* expression could not be detected in GC [51]. The mode of action of L-lactate within bovine GC, however, is still an open question and has to be further elucidated.

At present, we cannot completely exclude the possibility that endogenous L-lactate production by the cultured cells might contribute to the observed effects. However, in an initial study without any lactate treatment we measured lactate concentrations in the media of approximately 7 mM (not shown), which is far from the effective concentrations used during the presented study. Therefore, it is reasonable to assume that endogenously produced lactate did not significantly interfere with our experimental settings.

The present results demonstrate that L-lactate has positive effects on the expression of *LDHA*, the enzyme regulating the L-lactate-pyruvate-ratio as well as on the expression of its transporters, *SLC16A1* and *SLC16A7*. This is in accordance with earlier observations by others that L-lactate directly stimulates the expression of the MCT1 protein (encoded by *SLC16A1*) in L6 cells [34]. Another study showed that endurance training, leading to a higher L-lactate production, increased MCT1 expression in rats and humans [23]. This suggests that also in bovine GC L-lactate can stimulate its own metabolism and transport, thus being part of a positive feedback loop. Supportively, in skeletal muscle cells it was shown that MCT1 expression and L-lactate uptake is dependent on the activation of PKA and PKC signaling [53]. This is an interesting hypothesis, having in mind that the PKA signaling is one pathway involved in inducing luteinization of GC [54].

Conclusions

The presented data on hormone production and expression of marker genes clearly suggest that L-lactate treatment of cultured bovine GC results in a differentiation similar to early LH-induced alterations in vivo. Furthermore, the data suggest that L-lactate is involved in a positive feedback mechanism regulating its own transport and metabolism. The accumulation of L-lactate within the follicular fluid [19–21, 40] suggests that L-lactate also plays a role in vivo as a differentiation factor during late folliculogenesis and the folliculo-luteal transition in monovular species. In subsequent studies this hypothesis of the impact of lactate on GC differentiation has to be proven in in vivo models as well.

Abbreviations

BSA: Bovine serum albumin; CV: Coefficient of variation; *CYP19A1*: Aromatase; DMSO: Dimethyl sulfoxide; E2: Estradiol; FSH: Follicle stimulating hormone; *FSHR*: FSH receptor; GC: Granulosa cells; *GRIN2D*: Glutamate ionotropic receptor NMDA type subunit 2D; *GRINA*: Glutamate ionotropic receptor NMDA type subunit associated protein 1; *HCAR1*: Hydroxycarboxylic acid receptor 1; hCG: Human choriogonadotropin; HDAC: Histone deacetylase; HIF1/2α: hypoxia-inducible factors 1/2 alpha; IGF-1: Insulin-like growth factor 1; *LDHA*: Lactate dehydrogenase; LH: Luteinizing hormone; *LHCGR*: LH/choriogonadotropin receptor; MCT: Monocarboxylate transporter; MEM: Minimal essential media; NMDAR: N-methyl-D-aspartate receptor; P4: Progesterone; PBS: Phosphate buffered saline; PKA: Protein kinase A; PKC: Protein kinase C; *PTX3*: Pentraxin 3; qPCR: quantitative PCR; RIA: Radioimmunoassay; *RGS2*: Regulator of G protein signaling 2; *SLC16A1*: Solute carrier family 16 member 1; *SLC16A7*: Solute carrier family 16 member 7; UK5099: 2-Cyano-3-(1-phenyl-1H-indol-3-yl)-2-propenoic acid; *VNN2*: Vanin 2

Acknowledgments

We thank Veronica Schreiter and Maren Anders for excellent technical assistance.

Funding

This study was funded by the core budget of the Leibniz Institute for Farm Animal Biology (FBN).

Authors' Contributions

A.B. executed and analyzed the data, wrote the manuscript draft and created the figures; J.V. designed the study, analyzed data and contributed to the final version of the manuscript. Both authors read and approved the final manuscript.

Competing interests

The authors declare that there is no conflict of interest that could be perceived as prejudicing the impartiality of the research reported.

References

1. Bao B, Garverick HA. Expression of steroidogenic enzyme and gonadotropin receptor genes in bovine follicles during ovarian follicular waves: a review. J Anim Sci. 1998;76:1903–21.
2. Adams GP, Jaiswal R, Singh J, Malhi P. Progress in understanding ovarian follicular dynamics in cattle. Theriogenology. 2008;69:72–80.
3. Gilbert I, Robert C, Dieleman S, Blondin P, Sirard MA. Transcriptional effect of the LH surge in bovine granulosa cells during the peri-ovulation period. Reproduction. 2011;141:193–205.
4. Christenson LK, Gunewardena S, Hong X, Spitschak M, Baufeld A, Vanselow J. Research resource: preovulatory LH surge effects on follicular theca and granulosa transcriptomes. Mol Endocrinol. 2013;27:1153–71.
5. Nimz M, Spitschak M, Schneider F, Fürbass R, Vanselow J. Down-regulation of genes encoding steroidogenic enzymes and hormone receptors in late preovulatory follicles of the cow coincides with an accumulation of intrafollicular steroids. Domest Anim Endocrinol. 2009;37:45–54.
6. Bao B, Garverick HA, Smith GW, Smith MF, Salfen BE, Youngquist RS. Changes in messenger ribonucleic acid encoding luteinizing hormone receptor, cytochrome P450 side chain cleavage, and aromatase are associated with recruitment and selection of bovine ovarian follicles. Biol Reprod. 1997;56:1158–68.
7. Ujioka T, Russell DL, Okamura H, Richards JS, Espey LL. Expression of regulator of G-protein signaling protein-2 gene in the rat ovary at the time of ovulation. Biol Reprod. 2000;63:1513–7.
8. Varani S, Elvin JA, Yan C, DeMayo J, DeMayo FJ, Horton HF, Byrne MC, Matzuk MM. Knockout of pentraxin 3, a downstream target of growth differentiation factor-9, causes female subfertility. Mol Endocrinol. 2002; 16:1154–67.
9. Fadhillah YS, Nishimura R, Okuda K. Hypoxia promotes progesterone synthesis during luteinization in bovine granulosa cells. J Reprod Dev. 2014;60:194–201.
10. Kim J, Bagchi IC, Bagchi MK. Signaling by hypoxia-inducible factors is critical for ovulation in mice. Endocrinology. 2009;150:3392–400.
11. Thompson JG, Brown HM, Kind KL, Russell DL. The ovarian antral follicle: living on the edge of hypoxia or not? Biol Reprod. 2015;92:153.
12. Marsters P, Alhamdan R, Campbell BK. Cell density-mediated pericellular hypoxia and the local dynamic regulation of VEGF-a splice variants in ovine ovarian granulosa cells. Biol Reprod. 2014;91:35.
13. Baufeld A, Vanselow J. Increasing cell plating density mimics an early post-LH stage in cultured bovine granulosa cells. Cell Tissue Res. 2013;354:869–80.
14. Baufeld A, Koczan D, Vanselow J. Induction of altered gene expression profiles in cultured bovine granulosa cells at high cell density. Reprod Biol Endocrinol. 2017;15:3.
15. Cui XG, Han ZT, He SH, Wu XD, Chen TR, Shao CH, Chen DL, Su N, Chen YM, Wang T, et al. HIF1/2alpha mediates hypoxia-induced LDHA expression in human pancreatic cancer cells. Oncotarget. 2017;8:24840–52.
16. Firth JD, Ebert BL, Ratcliffe PJ. Hypoxic regulation of lactate dehydrogenase a. Interaction between hypoxia-inducible factor 1 and cAMP response elements. J Biol Chem. 1995;270:21021–7.
17. Semenza GL, Jiang BH, Leung SW, Passantino R, Concordet JP, Maire P, Giallongo A. Hypoxia response elements in the aldolase a, enolase 1, and lactate dehydrogenase a gene promoters contain essential binding sites for hypoxia-inducible factor 1. J Biol Chem. 1996;271:32529–37.
18. Lee DC, Sohn HA, Park ZY, Oh S, Kang YK, Lee KM, Kang M, Jang YJ, Yang SJ, Hong YK, et al. A lactate-induced response to hypoxia. Cell. 2015;161: 595–609.
19. Leese HJ, Lenton EA. Glucose and lactate in human follicular fluid: concentrations and interrelationships. Hum Reprod. 1990;5:915–9.
20. Leroy JL, Vanholder T, Delanghe JR, Opsomer G, Van SA, Bols PE, de Kruif A. Metabolite and ionic composition of follicular fluid from different-sized follicles and their relationship to serum concentrations in dairy cows. Anim Reprod Sci. 2004;80:201–11.
21. Zeilmaker GH, Verhamme CM. Lactate concentrations in pre-ovulatory follicles of pro-oestrous rats before and after onset of oocyte maturation. Acta Endocrinol. 1977;86:380–3.
22. Philp A, Macdonald AL, Watt PW. Lactate–a signal coordinating cell and systemic function. J Exp Biol. 2005;208:4561–75.
23. Brooks GA. Cell-cell and intracellular lactate shuttles. J Physiol. 2009;587: 5591–600.
24. Brooks GA. Lactate shuttles in nature. Biochem Soc Trans. 2002;30:258–64.
25. Hashimoto T, Masuda S, Taguchi S, Brooks GA. Immunohistochemical analysis of MCT1, MCT2 and MCT4 expression in rat plantaris muscle. J Physiol. 2005;567:121–9.
26. Kuchiiwa T, Nio-Kobayashi J, Takahashi-Iwanaga H, Yajima T, Iwanaga T. Cellular expression of monocarboxylate transporters in the female reproductive organ of mice: implications for the genital lactate shuttle. Histochem Cell Biol. 2011; 135:351–60.
27. Yang J, Ruchti E, Petit JM, Jourdain P, Grenningloh G, Allaman I, Magistretti PJ. Lactate promotes plasticity gene expression by potentiating NMDA signaling in neurons. Proc Natl Acad Sci U S A. 2014;111:12228–33.
28. Mosienko V, Teschemacher AG, Kasparov S. Is L-lactate a novel signaling molecule in the brain? J Cereb Blood Flow Metab. 2015;35:1069–75.
29. Silva JM, Price CA. Effect of follicle-stimulating hormone on steroid secretion and messenger ribonucleic acids encoding cytochromes P450 aromatase and cholesterol side-chain cleavage in bovine granulosa cells in vitro. Biol Reprod. 2000;62:186–91.
30. Gutierrez CG, Campbell BK, Webb R. Development of a long-term bovine granulosa cell culture system: induction and maintenance of estradiol production, response to follicle- stimulating hormone, and morphological characteristics. Biol Reprod. 1997;56:608–16.
31. Yenuganti VR, Vanselow J. Cultured bovine granulosa cells rapidly lose important features of their identity and functionality, but partially

recover under long term culture conditions. Cell & Tissue Research. 2017;368(2):397–403.
32. Hamel M, Vanselow J, Nicola ES, Price CA. Androstenedione increases cytochrome P450 aromatase messenger ribonucleic acid transcripts in non-luteinizing bovine granulosa cells. Mol Reprod Dev. 2005;70:175–83.
33. Yenuganti VR, Viergutz T, Vanselow J. Oleic acid induces specific alterations in the morphology, gene expression and steroid hormone production of cultured bovine granulosa cells. Gen Comp Endocrinol. 2016;232:134–44.
34. Hashimoto T, Hussien R, Oommen S, Gohil K, Brooks GA. Lactate sensitive transcription factor network in L6 cells: activation of MCT1 and mitochondrial biogenesis. FASEB J. 2007;21:2602–12.
35. Latham T, Mackay L, Sproul D, Karim M, Culley J, Harrison DJ, Hayward L, Langridge-Smith P, Gilbert N, Ramsahoye BH. Lactate, a product of glycolytic metabolism, inhibits histone deacetylase activity and promotes changes in gene expression. Nucleic Acids Res. 2012;40:4794–803.
36. Oh MS, Uribarri J, Alveranga D, Lazar I, Bazilinski N, Carroll HJ. Metabolic utilization and renal handling of D-lactate in men. Metabolism. 1985;34:621–5.
37. Wagner W, Ciszewski WM, Kania KD. L- and D-lactate enhance DNA repair and modulate the resistance of cervical carcinoma cells to anticancer drugs via histone deacetylase inhibition and hydroxycarboxylic acid receptor 1 activation. Cell Commun Signal. 2015;13:36.
38. Ewaschuk JB, Naylor JM, Zello GA. D-lactate in human and ruminant metabolism. J Nutr. 2005;135:1619–25.
39. Campbell BK, Onions V, Kendall NR, Guo L, Scaramuzzi RJ. The effect of monosaccharide sugars and pyruvate on the differentiation and metabolism of sheep granulosa cells in vitro. Reproduction. 2010;140:541–50.
40. Nishimoto H, Hamano S, Hill GA, Miyamoto A, Tetsuka M. Classification of bovine follicles based on the concentrations of steroids, glucose and lactate in follicular fluid and the status of accompanying follicles. J Reprod Dev. 2009;55:219–24.
41. Orsi NM, Gopichandran N, Leese HJ, Picton HM, Harris SE. Fluctuations in bovine ovarian follicular fluid composition throughout the oestrous cycle. Reproduction. 2005;129:219–28.
42. Zieker D, Schafer R, Glatzle J, Nieselt K, Coerper S, Kluba T, Northoff H, Konigsrainer A, Hunt TK, Beckert S. Lactate modulates gene expression in human mesenchymal stem cells. Langenbeck's Arch Surg. 2008;393:297–301.
43. Richardson MC, Cameron IT, Simonis CD, Das MC, Hodge TE, Zhang J, Byrne CD. Insulin and human chorionic gonadotropin cause a shift in the balance of sterol regulatory element-binding protein (SREBP) isoforms toward the SREBP-1c isoform in cultures of human granulosa cells. J Clin Endocrinol Metab. 2005;90:3738–46.
44. Brogan RS, MacGibeny M, Mix S, Thompson C, Puttabyatappa M, Vandevoort CA, Chaffin CL. Dynamics of intra-follicular glucose during luteinization of macaque ovarian follicles. Mol Cell Endocrinol. 2011;332:189–95.
45. Trabold O, Wagner S, Wicke C, Scheuenstuhl H, Hussain MZ, Rosen N, Seremetiev A, Becker HD, Hunt TK. Lactate and oxygen constitute a fundamental regulatory mechanism in wound healing. Wound Repair Regen. 2003;11:504–9.
46. Constant JS, Feng JJ, Zabel DD, Yuan H, Suh DY, Scheuenstuhl H, Hunt TK, Hussain MZ. Lactate elicits vascular endothelial growth factor from macrophages: a possible alternative to hypoxia. Wound Repair Regen. 2000;8:353–60.
47. Jourdain P, Allaman I, Rothenfusser K, Fiumelli H, Marquet P, Magistretti PJ. L-lactate protects neurons against excitotoxicity: implication of an ATP-mediated signaling cascade. Sci Rep. 2016;6:21250.
48. Parsons MP, Hirasawa M. ATP-sensitive potassium channel-mediated lactate effect on orexin neurons: implications for brain energetics during arousal. J Neurosci. 2010;30:8061–70.
49. Kunz L, Richter JS, Mayerhofer A. The adenosine 5′-triphosphate-sensitive potassium channel in endocrine cells of the human ovary: role in membrane potential generation and steroidogenesis. J Clin Endocrinol Metab. 2006;91:1950–5.
50. Tachibana N, Kinoshita M, Kametani F, Tanaka K, Une Y, Komatsu Y, Kobayashi Y, Ikeda S. Expression of N-methyl-D-aspartate receptor subunits in the bovine ovum: ova as a potential source of autoantigens causing anti-NMDAR encephalitis. Tohoku J Exp Med. 2015;235:223–31.
51. Khan DR, Fournier E, Dufort I, Richard FJ, Singh J, Sirard MA. Meta-analysis of gene expression profiles in granulosa cells during folliculogenesis. Reproduction. 2016;151:R103–10.
52. Cai TQ, Ren N, Jin L, Cheng K, Kash S, Chen R, Wright SD, Taggart AK, Waters MG. Role of GPR81 in lactate-mediated reduction of adipose lipolysis. Biochem Biophys Res Commun. 2008;377:987–91.
53. Narumi K, Furugen A, Kobayashi M, Otake S, Itagaki S, Iseki K. Regulation of monocarboxylate transporter 1 in skeletal muscle cells by intracellular signaling pathways. Biol Pharm Bull. 2010;33:1568–73.
54. Morris JK, Richards JS. Luteinizing hormone induces prostaglandin endoperoxide synthase-2 and luteinization in vitro by A-kinase and C-kinase pathways. Endocrinology. 1995;136:1549–58.

14

Melatonin inhibits 17β-estradiol-induced migration, invasion and epithelial-mesenchymal transition in normal and endometriotic endometrial epithelial cells

Shasha Qi[1,2,3], Lei Yan[1,2,3], Zhao Liu[4], Yu-lan Mu[5], Mingjiang Li[5], Xingbo Zhao[5], Zi-Jiang Chen[1,2,3,6,7] and Hui Zhang[5*]

Abstract

Background: Melatonin is a potential therapeutic agent for endometriosis, but its molecular mechanism is unclear. Here, we investigated the effect of melatonin on the epithelial-mesenchymal transition (EMT) in endometriotic endometrial epithelial cells and explored the pathway that might be involved.

Methods: This hospital-based study included 60 women of reproductive age using the endometrium for immunohistochemistry, 6 women of reproductive age undergoing bilateral tubal ligation and 6 patients with endometriosis for isolation of endometrial epithelial cells or subsequent analysis, respectively. We examined the expression of Notch1/Numb signaling and EMT markers by immunohistochemistry analysis and western blot analysis, the invasion and migration of endometrial epithelial cells by transwell assays, and the cell proliferation by CCK8 assays.

Results: Compared with normal endometrium, the endometriotic eutopic endometrium showed increased expression of Notch1, Slug, Snail, and N-cadherin, and decreased expression of E-cadherin and Numb. Melatonin or Notch inhibition by specific inhibitor blocked 17β-estradiol-induced cell proliferation, invasion, migration and EMT-related markers in both normal and endometriotic epithelial cells.

Conclusions: Our data suggest that aberrant expression of Notch1/Numb signaling and the EMT is present in endometriotic endometrium. Melatonin may block 17β-estradiol-induced migration, invasion and EMT in normal and endometriotic epithelial cells by upregulating Numb expression and decreasing the activity of the Notch signaling pathway.

Keywords: Endometrial epithelial cells, Melatonin, 17β-estradiol, Migration and invasion, Epithelial-mesenchymal transition

Background

Endometriosis is a chronic disease that affects approximately 10% of reproductive-age women and is characterized by chronic pelvic pain and infertility [1]. Endometriosis is a benign disease, but its tendency to progression and recurrence causes disability and distress [2]. In recent decades, much effort has been focused on developing new drugs to relieve the clinical symptoms and prevent the recurrence of the disease.

Epithelial-mesenchymal transition (EMT), which is characterized by an increased rate of cellular migration, invasion properties and increased resistance to apoptosis, is also considered essential for the formation and progression of endometriosis [3–5]. Key transcription factors including Snail, Slug and Twist drive the EMT process, which along with cleaved and then degraded E-cadherin and increased expression of mesenchymal-related

* Correspondence: huizhang1218@126.com
[5]Department of Obstetrics and Gynecology, Shandong Provincial Hospital Affiliated to Shandong University, 324 Jingwu Road, Jinan 250021, People's Republic of China
Full list of author information is available at the end of the article

proteins, including N-cadherin, Vimentin [6]. Snail also represses E-cadherin transcription by binding to the E-box site in the promoter of E-cadherin [7]. In previous studies, we found that the expression of both Notch1, a key signaling factor involved in EMT regulation, and EMT-related proteins was upregulated in the ectopic endometrium of adenomyosis compared with those in normal endometrium [8].

Melatonin (N-acetyl-5-methoxy-tryptamine), a scavenger of free radicals and a broad-spectrum antioxidant, is the main pineal hormone synthesized from tryptophan in response to darkness [9]. A series of studies have shown that melatonin has a potential therapeutic effect on endometriosis [10–16]. In experimental rat models, melatonin causes the regression and atrophy of endometriotic lesions [11], and the combination of letrozole and melatonin causes a significant regression in lesion volumes but not in the histopathological scores of endometriotic lesions [15]. Higher doses of melatonin treatment have been reported to be more effective in inducing the regression of implants and in improving histologic scores [10]. Moreover, compared with letrozole, melatonin causes a more pronounced regression of endometriotic foci and lower recurrence [16]. It was reported that pinealectomy increased the progression of endometriosis explants, and that melatonin reversed the effects of pinealectomy [12]. Melatonin is effective in treating experimental endometriosis induced by implanting human endometriotic cells in SCID mice [14]. Kocadal et al. [13] reported that melatonin caused a regression of endometriotic lesions and an improvement in their histopathological scores in an oophorectomized rat endometriosis model.

Melatonin has been proved to be involved in the modulation of EMT. Lipopolysaccharide- induced EMT was inhibited by melatonin in peritoneal mesothelial cells via the inactivation of the Toll-like receptor (TLR) 4/c-Jun N-terminal kinase and TLR4/NFκB-Snail signaling pathways [17]. It has also been reported that melatonin inhibits TGFβ1-induced EMT in human lung alveolar epithelial cells [18]. In the process of bleomycin-induced pulmonary fibrosis, melatonin significantly attenuated endoplasmic reticulum stress-mediated EMT [19]. However, the effects of melatonin on the EMT in endometriosis are unclear.

In the current study, we assumed that melatonin might be involved in the EMT regulation of endometriosis. We investigated the effect of melatonin on the migration, invasion and EMT of normal and endometriotic epithelial cells, and explored the possible signaling pathways that might be involved.

Methods

Materials

CollagenaseIA, trypsin, Melatonin and Matrigel were obtained from Sigma-Aldrich (St. Louis, MO, USA). Penicillin, DMEM/F12 (1:1) media were obtained from HyClone (Logan, Utah, USA). Charcoal-stripped fetal bovine serum (FBS) was obtained from GIBCO (Invitrogen, NY, USA). Rabbit anti-human E-Cadherin, N-Cadherin and Vimentin primary antibodies were obtained from Abcam (Cambridge, MA, USA). Rabbit anti-human Notch, Numb, Slug and Snail primary antibodies were obtained from Cell Signaling Technology (Danvers, MA, USA) for western blot and obtained from Abcam (Cambridge, MA, USA) for immunohistochemistry. Mouse anti-human β-Actin primary antibody and Goat anti-rabbit and Goat anti-mouse HRP-conjugated secondary antibodies were obtained from ZSGB-BIO (Beijing, China). Mammalian Cell Protein Extraction Kit was purchased from Beyotime (Shanghai, China). ECL Plus Western Blotting Detection System was obtained from Millipore Corporation (Billerica, MA, USA).

Tissue collection and immunohistochemistry analysis

Normal endometria were obtained from 30 women of reproductive age undergoing bilateral tubal ligation (proliferative phase: $n = 15$; secretory phase: $n = 15$). Endometriotic eutopic endometria were obtained from 30 patients with endometriosis undergoing hysterectomy or subtotal hysterectomy (proliferative phase: $n = 15$; secretory phase: $n = 15$). Normal and endometriotic endometrial tissues were collected during the surgery. The diagnosis of endometriosis was confirmed by histological examination. No patients had received any hormonal therapy in the 3 months prior to their surgery. Immunohistochemistry analysis was performed on normal and endometriotic endometria as previously reported [8]. The primary antibodies used in this study included Rabbit anti-human E-Cadherin(4 μg/ml), N-Cadherin(2 μg/ml), Notch1(400 μg/ml), Numb(7 μg/ml), Slug(7 μg/ml), and Snail(5 μg/ml) antibodies. Immunostaining was expressed as the immunoscore, i.e., the H-score, which was a semi quantitative product of the quantity score and staining intensity. The quantity score was estimated as reported previously [8].

Tissue collection and cells culture

Eutopic endometria were obtained from 6 patients with endometriosis. Normal endometria obtained from 6 women of reproductive age undergoing bilateral tubal ligation were used as controls. All participants had regular menstrual cycles and had not received any hormonal therapy in the 3 months prior to their surgery. Diagnoses were confirmed by histological examination. Endometriotic eutopic epithelial cells (EEC) and normal endometrial epithelial cells (NEC) were isolated from fresh tissues. Isolation and culture of endometrial cells were conducted as reported previously [20]. Briefly, specimens obtained during surgery were placed immediately in ice-cold sterile PBS and transported to the laboratory. Tissues were washed twice with sterile PBS to remove the blood, minced into small pieces, and incubated with 0.25% collagenase type IA in a shaking water bath for 1 h at 37 °C. The collagenase activity was terminated by adding three volumes of pre-warmed medium containing 10% FBS. The cell suspension was sequentially filtered through a 154 μm monofilament nylon mesh and then through a 38.5 μm monofilament nylon mesh. The 38.5 μm monofilament was washed thoroughly upside down with medium to obtain epithelial cells. The resulting cell suspension was collected and centrifuged at 110 g for 10 min. The pellet was re-suspended in DMEM/F12 (1:1) medium containing 10% FBS and was incubated in cell culture dishes for 2 h at 37 °C in 95% air and 5% CO_2. The medium was then replaced with fresh medium; non-attached cells were discarded, and the attached epithelial cells were cultured further. The culture medium was changed every 2–3 days. The cultured cells were characterized by immunocytochemical staining with mouse anti-human Cytokeratin antibodies, the purified epithelial cells were positive for Cytokeratin [21]. The purity for cells of 1 passage was more than 98%. The primary cultured cells were used in the western blot and morphology experiments. The cells of passage 1 were used in the CCK-8 and transwell experiments.

Cell treatments

The cells were initially cultured without any estradiol, and were cultured about 48 h until passage. The culture media was changed every 2 to 3 days. The cells were about 50% confluent before treatment. Melatonin was dissolved in ethanol at a stock concentration of 100 mM and was stored at – 20 °C. 17β-estradiol was dissolved in ethanol at a stock concentration of 10 mM and stored at – 20 °C. DAPT, a specific Notch inhibitor, was dissolved in DMSO at a stock concentration of 10 mM and stored at – 20 °C. The concentrations chosen for the used treatments were determined according to published literatures. The cells were treated with 1 mM melatonin [22, 23], 10 μM DAPT [24, 25] or/and 10 nM 17β-estradiol [26, 27]. Mock treatments with an identical volume of ethanol or DMSO were used as controls.

Transwell assays

The transwell assays were performed using 24-well plates with 8-μm pore size inserts (Corning Life Sciences, NY, USA) according to the manufacturer's instructions. The cells were treated with various agents at the indicated concentration for 48 h before they were seeded into the inserts. The migration and invasion assays were performed as reported previously [6].

In the migration assay, the cells (normal and endometriotic epithelial cells 10^5cells/well) were added to the upper chamber in 200 μL of serum-free DMEM medium and were allowed to migrate to the bottom compartment, which contained DMEM medium with 10% FBS, for 24 h. Then, the non-migrated cells were wiped off with a cotton swab.

For the invasion assay, Matrigel (1 mg/ml, BD Biosciences) was prepared in serum-free cold cell culture medium, placed in the upper chamber, and incubated for 5 h at 37 °C. Next, the cells (normal and endometriotic epithelial cells 2×10^5cells/well) were placed in the upper chamber of each insert in 200 μL of serum-free medium, and were allowed to invade to the bottom compartment, which contained medium with 10% FBS, for 36 h. Then, the non-invaded cells were wiped off with a cotton swab.

For quantification, transwell filters were fixed in 4% paraformaldehyde for 15 min, stained with haematoxylin for 15 min, and mounted on a glass slide. The results were expressed as the number of cells migrated per field, as viewed under a microscope (× 200 magnification), and the numbers of cells in three randomly selected fields were counted. All experiments were performed three times.

Cell proliferation assay

Cell proliferation was assessed using the Cell Counting Kit (CCK)-8 (Dojindo, Japan). Briefly, the cells (normal and endometriotic epithelial cells 8×10^3 cells /well) were plated on 96-well plates in 100 μL of medium and were allowed to attach overnight for 24 h. Then, they were exposed to the indicated concentrations of melatonin and DAPT, with or without 17β-estradiol, and were cultured for an additional 0, 24, 48 and 72 h, respectively. After treatments, 10 μL of CCK-8 reagent was added to each well, and the plates were incubated at 37 °C for 4 h. The cell confluence was about 50–60% confluence at 0 h, and allowed to grow to about 90% confluence at 72 h. The optical density (OD) at 450 nm was measured in each well using a microplate reader. The measurements were performed at the density of 90% confluence approximately. The data were shown as fold change of control (Day 0). The experiments were repeated three times, and each assay was performed in triplicate.

Total protein extraction and western blot analysis

Cells were harvested by trypsinization and centrifugation. Total protein was extracted, and western blot analysis was performed as reported previously [20]. 50 μg of total protein extracted from cells after 72 h treatments was applied to a 10% polyacrylamide gel, and PageRuler Prestained Protein Ladder (Fermentas) was used as the size marker. After the proteins were transferred to membranes and the membranes were blocked, the membranes were incubated overnight at 4 °C with the primary antibodies. The primary antibodies used in this study included Rabbit anti-human E-Cadherin (0.3 μg/ml), N-Cadherin(1 μg/ml), Vimentin(0.2 μg/ml), Notch1(0.85 μg/ml), Numb(0.26 μg/ml), Slug(0.25 μg/ml), Snail(0.2 μg/ml) and β-actin (0.5 μg/ml). After incubation with the Goat anti-rabbit HRP-conjugated secondary antibody (0.1 μg/ml) for 1 h at room temperature, the protein bands were detected using the ECL detection system (BD Biosciences). β-actin was used as the loading control.

Statistical analysis

The statistical analyses were performed using SPSS 19.0 (SPSS, Chicago, USA). The values are expressed as the means ± SD. The differences between the two groups were determined by one-way ANOVA. A p value < 0.05 was considered statistically significant.

Results

Aberrant expression of notch/numb signaling and EMT markers in endometriotic endometrium

The expression of Notch/Numb signaling and EMT markers in normal endometria and in endometriotic eutopic endometria were determined by immunohistochemical analysis. We take Notch1 as the representative of Notch family. As shown in Fig. 1, in normal endometria, the staining of Notch1 (NICD) (Fig. 1A), N-cadherin (Fig. 1B), and Slug (Fig. 1C) were weakly positive or positive and were concentrated in the cytoplasm of endometrial epithelial cells. In stromal cells, the immunostainings of Notch1, N-cadherin, and Slug were very weak. In endometriotic eutopic endometria, the immunostaining of Notch1 (Fig. 1D), N-cadherin (Fig. 1E), and Slug (Fig. 1F) was strongly positive and was restricted to the cytoplasm of epithelial cells, whereas weak immunostaining patterns were observed in stromal cells. Endometriotic eutopic endometria showed significantly increased Notch1 (Fig. 1a, $p< 0.05$), N-cadherin (Fig. 1b, $p < 0.05$), and Slug (Fig. 1c, $p < 0.05$) expression levels compared to normal endometria. No significant differences in Notch1 (Fig. 1d, $p > 0.05$), N-cadherin (Fig. 1e, $p > 0.05$), or Slug (Fig. 1f, $p > 0.05$) expression were observed between endometriotic endometria in the proliferative and secretory phases.

In normal endometria, the staining of Snail was weakly positive or positive and was restricted to the nucleus of endometrial epithelial cells (Fig. 1G). In stromal cells, the immunostaining of Snail was very weak. In endometriotic eutopic endometria, the immunostaining of Snail was strongly positive and was restricted to the nucleus of epithelial cells (Fig. 1H), whereas weak immunostaining was observed in stromal cells. Endometriotic eutopic endometria showed significantly increased Snail expression compared to normal endometria (Fig. 1g, $p < 0.05$). No significant difference of Snail expression was observed between endometriotic endometria in the proliferative and secretory phases (Fig. 1h, $p > 0.05$).

In normal endometria, the immunostaining of Numb (Fig. 1I) and E-cadherin (Fig. 1J) was strongly positive, and the staining was concentrated in the cytoplasm of endometrial epithelial cells. In stromal cells, the immunostaining of Numb and E-cadherin was very weak. In endometriotic eutopic endometria, the immunostaining of Numb (Fig. 1K) and E-cadherin (Fig. 1L) was weakly positive and was restricted to the cytoplasm of epithelial cells. Endometriotic eutopic endometria showed significantly decreased Numb (Fig. 1i, $p < 0.01$) and E-cadherin (Fig. 1j, $p < 0.01$) expression compared to normal endometria. No significant difference in Numb (Fig. 1k, $p > 0.05$) and E-cadherin (Fig. 1l, $p > 0.05$) expression was observed between endometriotic endometria in the proliferative and secretory phases.

Melatonin abolished 17β-estradiol-induced proliferation in normal and endometriotic epithelial cells

CCK-8 assays were performed to determine the proliferation of EEC and NEC. 17β-estradiol significantly increased the growth of EEC and NEC on days 2–3 (Fig. 2a, b, $p < 0.05$). DAPT, a specific inhibitor of Notch signaling, significantly decreased the growth of both EEC and NEC (Fig. 2a, b, $p < 0.05$). DAPT also abolished 17β-estradiol-induced cell growth (Fig. 2a, b, $p < 0.05$).

In CCK-8 assays, melatonin significantly decreased the growth of EEC and NEC at day 3 (Fig. 2a, b, $p < 0.05$). Melatonin also abolished 17β-estradiol-induced cell growth in both cells (Fig. 2a, b, $p < 0.05$).

Melatonin abolished 17β-estradiol-induced migration and invasion in normal and endometriotic epithelial cells

The migration and invasion of EEC (Fig. 3) and NEC (Fig. 4) were determined using transwell assays. In migration assays, 17β-estradiol significantly increased the migration of EEC ($p < 0.01$) and NEC ($p < 0.01$) after treatment for 24 h. DAPT significantly decreased the migration of EEC ($p < 0.05$) and NEC ($p < 0.05$). DAPT also abolished 17β-estradiol-induced cell migration ($p < 0.01$). Similar data were obtained in invasion assays. 17β-estradiol significantly increased the invasion of EEC ($p < 0.01$) and NEC ($p < 0.01$) after treatment for 36 h, whereas DAPT significantly decreased the invasion and 17β-estradiol-induced invasion in EEC ($p < 0.01$) and NEC ($p < 0.01$).

In migration and invasion assays, melatonin significantly decreased the migration and invasion of EEC (Fig. 3, $p < 0.05$) and NEC (Fig. 4, $p < 0.05$).

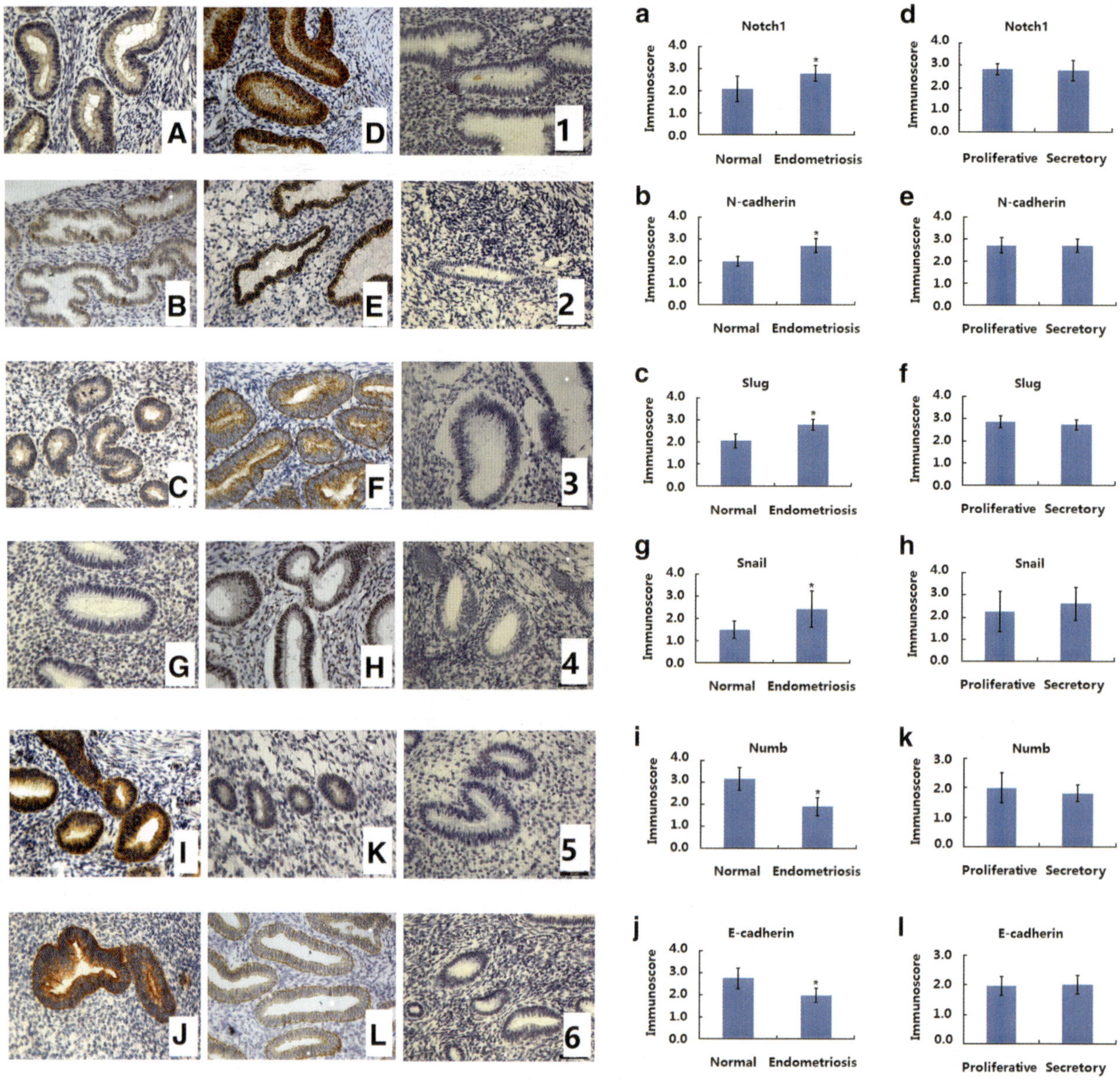

Fig. 1 Aberrant expressions of Notch1/Numb signaling and EMT markers in endometrium of endometriosis. **A, B, C, G, I, J**: The expression of Notch1, N-Cadherin, Slug, Snail, Numb and E-Cadherin in normal endometrium ($n = 15$); **D, E, F, H, K, L**: The expression of Notch1, N-Cadherin, Slug, Snail, Numb and E-Cadherin in eutopic endometria of endometriosis ($n = 15$); **a, b, c, g, i, j**: Immunoscore of Notch1, N-Cadherin, Slug, Snail, Numb and E-Cadherin in normal endometrium ($n = 30$) and eutopic endometria of endometriosis ($n = 30$); **d, e, f, h, k, l**: Immunoscore of Notch1, N-Cadherin, Slug, Snail, Numb and E-Cadherin in the proliferative phases ($n = 15$) and secretory phases ($n = 15$) of endometriotic endometria; **1,2,3,4,5,6:** negative controls. Magnification: × 200. $^*p < 0.05$

Melatonin also abolished 17β-estradiol-induced cell migration and invasion ($p < 0.05$).

Melatonin abolished 17β-estradiol-induced EMT in normal and endometriotic epithelial cells

The expression of EMT markers was determined using western blot analysis. As shown in Fig. 5, 17β-estradiol significantly increased the expression of N-cadherin, Slug and Snail, and decreased the expression of Numb and E-cadherin in EEC ($p < 0.05$). In NEC, 17β-estradiol significantly increased the expression of N-cadherin and decreased the expression of Numb (Fig. 6, $p < 0.05$), but showed no significant effect on the expression of Notch1 (NICD), Vimentin, E-cadherin, Slug, or Snail (Fig. 6, $p > 0.05$). In EEC, DAPT significantly decreased the expression of Notch1 (NICD), Vimentin, Slug, and Snail and increased the expression of Numb and E-cadherin (Fig. 5, $p < 0.05$). DAPT also abolished 17β-estradiol-induced expression of Notch1 (NICD), Vimentin, Slug, and Snail and the downregulation

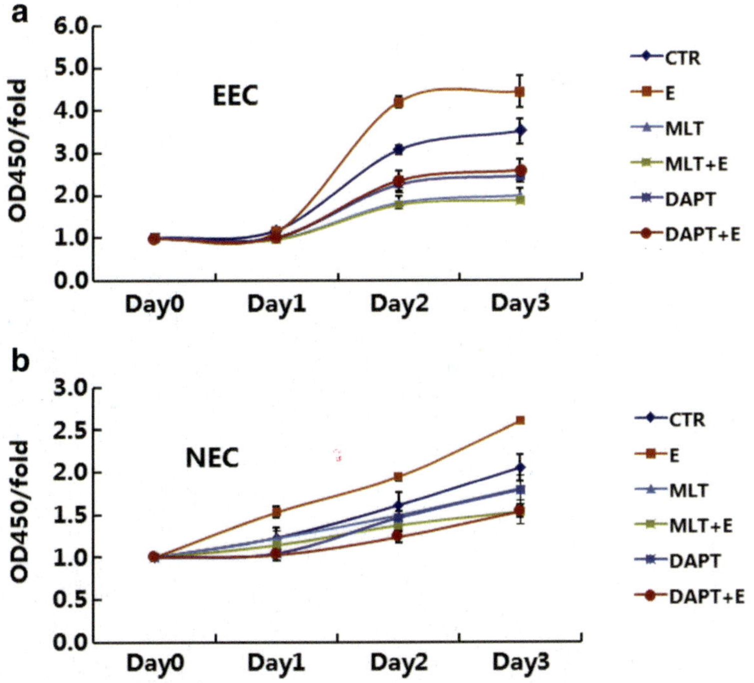

Fig. 2 Melatonin abolishes 17β-estradiol-induced proliferation in EEC and NEC. **a**: EEC were treated with MLT, DAPT, or E2 with or without MLT/DAPT, cell numbers were measured by CCK-8 assays at the indicated times. **b**: NEC were treated with MLT, DAPT, or E2 with or without MLT/DAPT, cell numbers were measured by CCK-8 assays at indicated times. Data are presented as the mean ± SD. E2: 17β-estradiol; MLT: melatonin

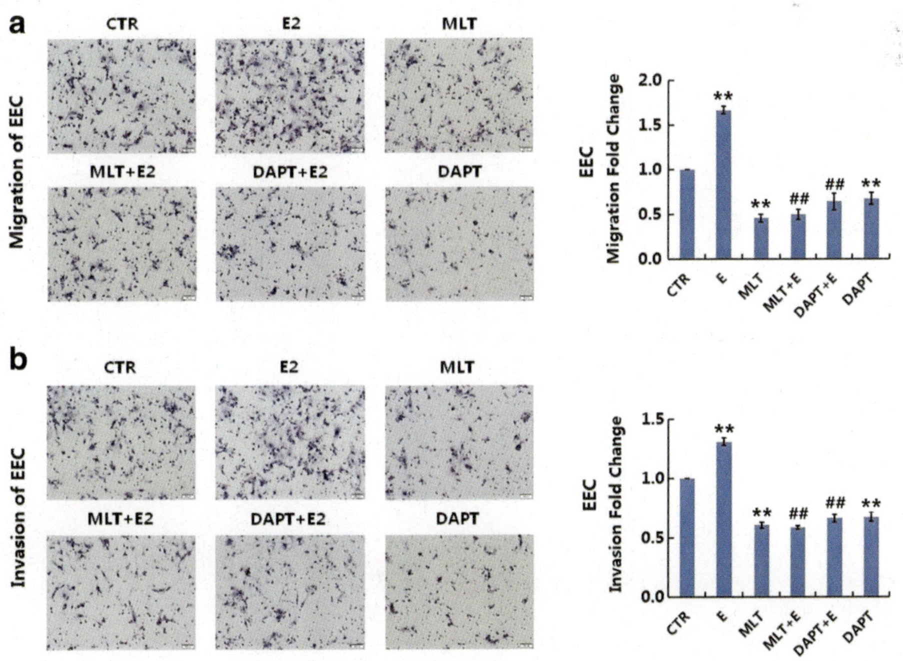

Fig. 3 Melatonin abolishes 17β-estradiol-induced migration and invasion in EEC. **a**: Transwell migration assays of EEC after treatment. EEC were treated with MLT, DAPT, or E2 with or without MLT/DAPT **b**: Transwell invasion assays of EEC after treatment. Representative images were obtained at 200× magnification. Graphs show the relative number of migrating and invading cells for each treatment group (averaged across four random images). Scale bar: 50 μm. Data are presented as the mean ± SD. E2: 17β-estradiol; MLT: melatonin. *$p < 0.05$, ** $p < 0.01$ vs. untreated cells. #$p < 0.05$, ##$p < 0.01$ vs. E2-treated cells

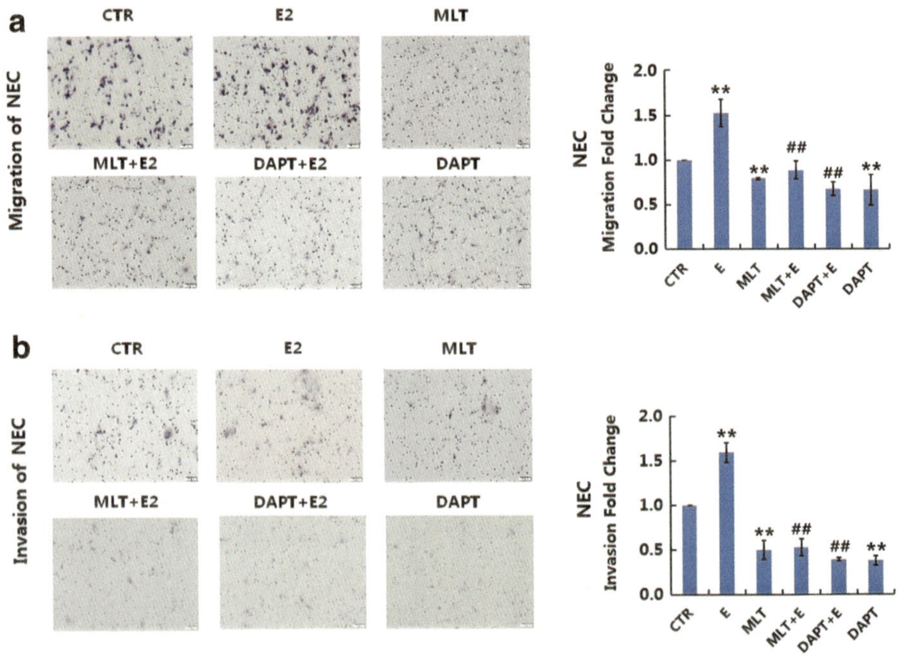

Fig. 4 Melatonin abolishes 17β-estradiol-induced migration and invasion in NEC. **a**: Transwell migration assays of NEC after treatment. NEC were treated with MLT, DAPT, or E2 with or without MLT/DAPT **b**: Transwell invasion assays of NEC after treatment. Representative images were obtained at 200× magnification. Graphs show the relative number of migrating and invading cells for each treatment group (averaged across four random images). Scale bar: 50 μm. Data are presented as the mean ± SD. E2: 17β-estradiol; MLT: melatonin. *$p < 0.05$, ** $p < 0.01$ vs. untreated cells. #$p < 0.05$, ##$p < 0.01$ vs. E2-treated cells

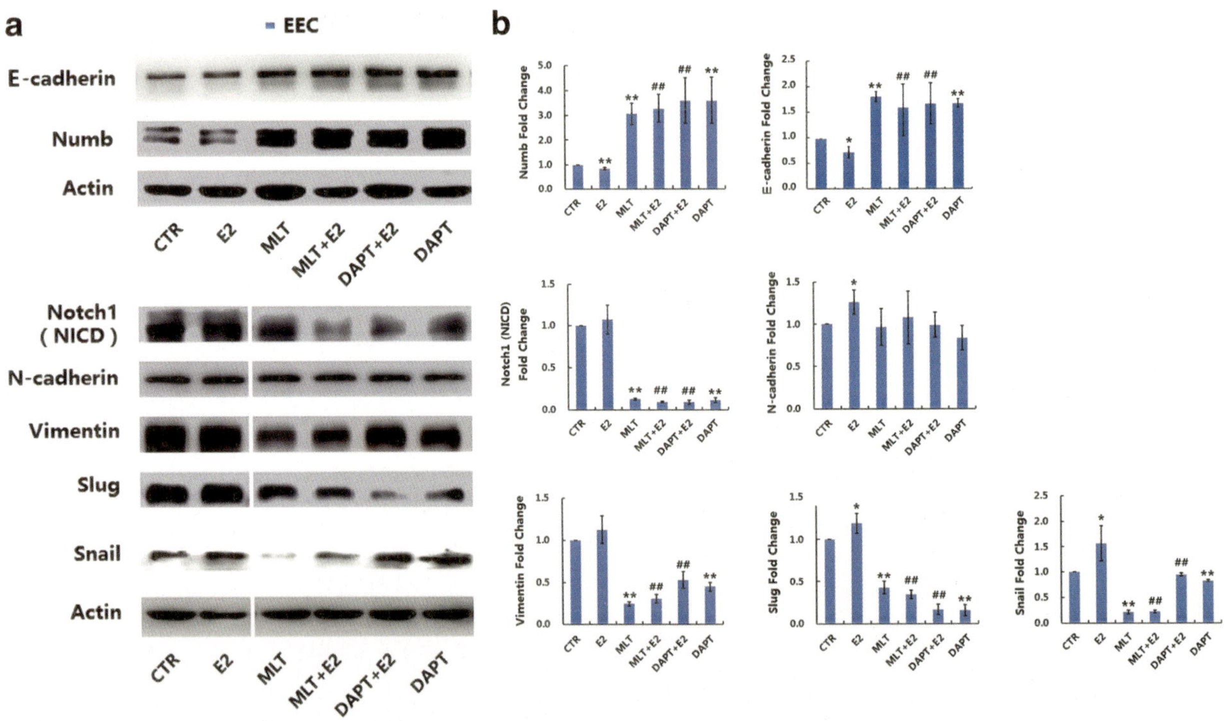

Fig. 5 Melatonin reverses 17β-estradiol-induced EMT in EEC involving Notch1 signaling pathway. EEC were treated with different drugs for 72 h. **a** The protein expression levels of Notch1 (NICD), E-cadherin, N-cadherin, Vimentin, Slug, Snail, Numb and Actin were determined by western blot. β-actin was used as a loading control. **b** The ratios of Notch1/E-cadherin/N-cadherin/Vimentin/Slug/Snail/Numb to β-actin were analyzed. Data are presented as the mean ± SD. E2: 17β-estradiol; MLT: melatonin. *$p < 0.05$, ** $p < 0.01$ vs. untreated cells. #$p < 0.05$, ##$p < 0.01$ vs. E2-treated cells

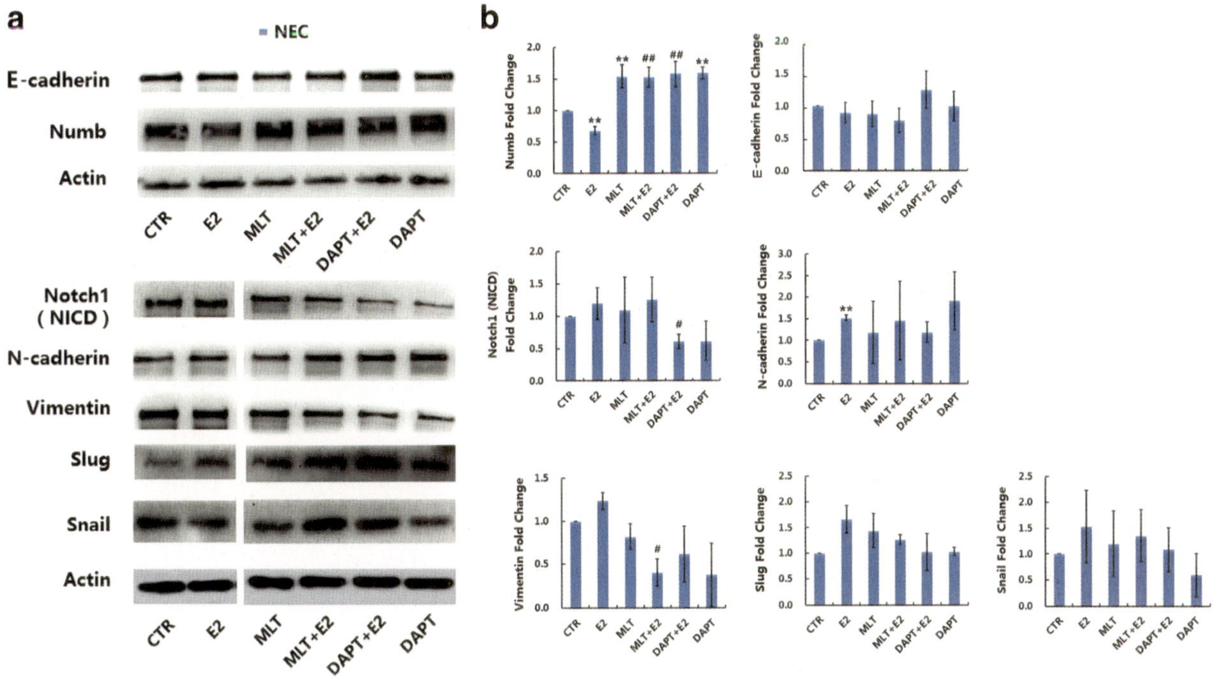

Fig. 6 The expression of EMT and Notch signaling pathway-related markers in NEC. NEC were treated with different drugs for 72 h. **a** The protein expression of Notch1 (NICD), E-cadherin, N-cadherin, Vimentin, Slug, Snail, Numb and Actin were determined by western blot. β-actin was used as a loading control. **b** The ratios of Notch1/ E-cadherin/ N-cadherin/Vimentin/Slug/ Snail/Numb to β-actin were analyzed. Data are presented as the mean ± SD. E2: 17β-estradiol; MLT: melatonin. *$p < 0.05$, ** $p < 0.01$ vs. untreated cells. #$p < 0.05$, ##$p < 0.01$ vs. E2-treated cells

of Numb and E-cadherin (Fig. 5, $p < 0.05$). In NEC, Notch inhibition by DAPT significantly increased the expression of Numb, and 17β-estradiol-caused downregulation of Numb (Fig. 6, $p < 0.05$).

In western blot analyses, melatonin significantly decreased the expression of Notch1 (NICD), Vimentin, Slug, and Snail and increased the expression of Numb and E-cadherin in EEC (Fig. 5, $p < 0.05$). Melatonin also abolished the 17β-estradiol-induced expression of Notch1 (NICD), Vimentin, Slug, and Snail and the downregulation of Numb and E-cadherin in EEC (Fig. 5, $p < 0.05$). In NEC, melatonin significantly increased the expression of Numb (Fig. 6, $p < 0.05$) but had no significant effect on the expression of Notch1 (NICD), Vimentin, N-cadherin, E-cadherin, Slug or Snail. Melatonin also abolished the 17β-estradiol-induced expression of Vimentin and downregulation of Numb in NEC (Fig. 6, $p < 0.05$).

We then examined the effect of 17β-estradiol and melatonin on the morphology of normal and endometriotic epithelial cells. The cells were treated with recombinant transforming growth factor-β1 (TGF-β1), which is known to be an EMT inducer. As expected, after stimulation with 0.78 nM of recombinant TGF-β1 for

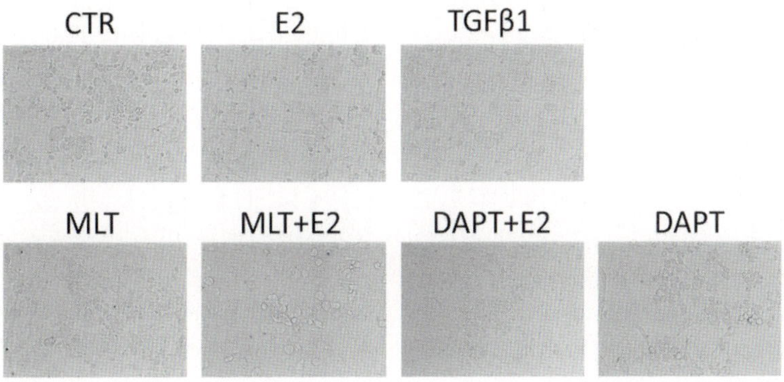

Fig. 7 The morphology of EEC treated with E2, TGF-β1, Melatonin, DAPT, a combination of E2 and Melatonin, or a combination of E2 and DAPT for 48 h. The cells were observed using phase contrast microscopy at 400x magnification. Scale bar: 20 μm.E2: 17β-estradiol; MLT: Melatonin

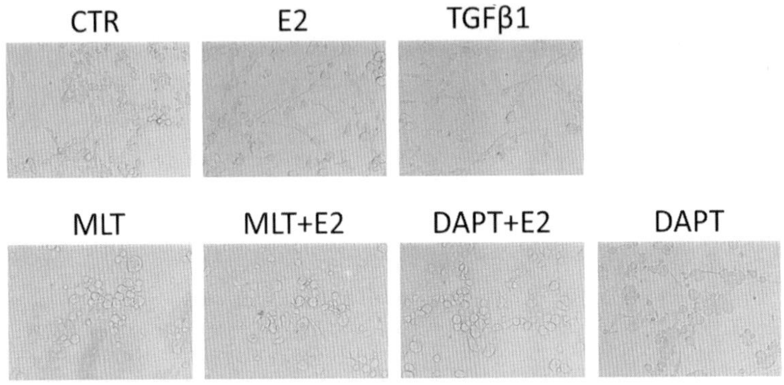

Fig. 8 The morphology of NEC treated with E2, TGF-β1, Melatonin, DAPT, a combination of E2 and Melatonin, or a combination of E2 and DAPT for 48 h. The cells were observed using phase contrast microscopy at 400× magnification. Scale bar: 20 μm.E2: 17β-estradiol; MLT: Melatonin

48 h, both EEC (Fig. 7) and NEC (Fig. 8) showed reduction of the epithelial "cobblestone" morphology, became scattered, acquired a spindle-shaped morphology, and lost cell-cell contacts, all of which are characteristics of a mesenchymal-like morphology. 17β-estradiol exhibited similar effects as TGF-β1 in the cells. Treatment with 1 mM melatonin or 10 μM DAPT for 48 h abolished the TGF-β1 or 17β-estradiol-induced morphological changes in EEC and NEC.

Discussion

Although endometriosis is a benign disease, it exhibits a series of biological behaviors similar to malignant tumors, including adhesion, invasion, and implantation [28]. In the current study, we found that aberrant expression of EMT-related markers existed in endometriotic eutopic endometrium, and estrogen promoted the migration, invasion and EMT phenotype in normal and endometritic eutopic epithelial cells, while melatonin and the blocking of Notch signaling inhibited 17β-estradiol-induced migration, invasion and epithelial-mesenchymal transition in normal and endometriotic endometrial epithelial cells.

The Notch signaling pathway is thought to be critical for the induction of EMT and is involved in the progression of a series of diseases [29, 30]. Notch signaling can promote TGF-β1-induced EMT via the induction of Snail [30]. Jagged1-mediated Notch signaling activation can elevate the expression of Snail and Slug, resulting in the repression of E-cadherin in various disease models [29]. Numb is an inhibitory regulator of Notch1 signaling that acts by promoting the ubiquitination and degradation of the Notch1 intracellular domain [31]. In the current study, decreased epithelial marker expression and elevated mesenchymal marker expression indicate that the phenotype of EMT exists in endometriosis. In addition, elevated expression of EMT inducer, Snail and Slug, was also noted in endometriotic eutopic endometrium, suggesting an essential role of EMT in the development and pathogenesis of endometriosis. Immunohistochemistry analysis also showed increased Notch1 (NICD) expression and decreased Numb expression in endometriotic eutopic epithelial cells, indicating that Notch1/Numb signaling might be involved in the regulation of EMT in the endometriotic eutopic endometrium. Furthermore, there is no significant difference between proliferative and secretory phases observed in endometriosis. In our previous studies, we found that the expression of Numb, Slug and E-cadherin showed no significant difference, but Snail, N-cadherin and Notch1 showed cycle changement between proliferative and secretory phases in normal endometria. This might be due to the aberrant level of hormones in endometriosis.

Vimentin is a mesenchymal cell marker and is increased in cells that undergo EMT as known. In immunochemistry assays, cytokeratin immunostaining is positive in normal and endometriotic epithelial cells, while Vimentin immunostaining was negative [20]. In western blot experiments, we found that Vimentin showed bands in both cells and showed differences in drug intervention. Then, we searched other literature and found that Vimentin was also determined in endometrial epithelial cells by western blot [32, 33]. We cannot explain this phenomenon and will continue to explore it in follow-up studies.

Endometriosis is an estrogen-dependent disease [34]. Considerable biochemical evidence demonstrates that aromatase activity and P450 aromatase mRNA expression were noted in endometrial tissues from endometriosis [35], suggesting that endometriotic tissues are able to produce estrogens locally. It has been reported that estrogen receptor (ERα) signaling regulates E-cadherin and EMT through slug, and estrogen is proved to be involved in the process of EMT [36]. In human ovarian and breast cancer cells, 17β-estradiol can induce EMT via the activation of the PI3K/AKT pathway by enhancing the expression of snail and slug [37, 38]. In prostate epithelium, the ERα-mediated enhanced estrogenic effect is a crucial inductive factor of epithelial dedifferentiation, giving rise to the activation of an EMT program [39]. However, the role of estrogen in the EMT of endometriosis is rarely reported. In the current study, we found that estrogen promoted the migration, invasion and mesenchymal phenotype in normal and endometritic eutopic epithelial cells, suggesting that estrogen plays a role in the regulation of EMT in endometrial epithelial cells. What's more, 17β-estradiol activated the Notch pathway, which is a key signaling pathway in EMT regulation, and downregulated the expression of Numb, an inhibitory regulator of Notch signaling. In addition, DAPT, a specific Notch inhibitor, abolished the effect of 17β-estradiol in endometrial epithelial cells, suggesting that Notch signaling might participate in the effect of 17β-estradiol on migration, invasion and EMT-related markers.

Reversing the migration and invasion of eutopic endometrium should be meaningful for the prevention and treatment of endometriosis. In in-vivo studies, melatonin showed potential therapeutic effects on endometriosis in animal models [40–42]. However, the molecular mechanism of the melatonin effect remains unclear. In animal studies, melatonin significantly inhibits ovarian aromatase expression and increases the levels of uterine ERα and progesterone receptor [43]. The genotoxic changes in the uterus caused by estrogen might be prevented by giving melatonin [44]. The addition of melatonin to estrogen replacement treatment is associated with a decrease in endometrial proliferation and prevents the appearance of cellular atypia [45]. In non-photoperiodic animals such as rats, melatonin positively affects the endometrial morphology and improves embryo implantation [46]. These data indicate that the effect of 17β-estradiol can be modified by melatonin. In the current study, melatonin abolished the 17β-estradiol-induced proliferation, migration, invasion and EMT phenotype in both normal and endometriotic epithelial cells, demonstrating the protective effect of melatonin on the endometrium, especially on endometriotic endometrium, which has locally elevated estrogen levels [35].

In the current in-vitro study, melatonin showed a similar effect on normal and endomotriotic epithelial cells. However, in the local high estrogen microenvironment of endometriosis in vivo, melatonin may show anti-estrogen effects and therefore has a potential therapeutic effect.

Notch signaling pathway is a key signaling pathway for EMT regulation. Here, we found that Notch signaling pathway is also involved in EMT regulation in endometriosis. We showed that a specific inhibitor of Notch signaling pathway inhibited the proliferation, migration, invasion and in endometriotic epithelial cells and normal endometrial cells, but EMT-like phenotype was not inhibited in normal endometrial cells. The data suggested that Notch signaling plays a key role in the regulation of EMT in endometriosis. Melatonin can inhibit the activity of Notch1 signaling pathway in endometriotic epithelial cells, which is reflected in the decrease of NICD expression. This phenomenon was absent in normal endometrial epithelial cells. There is insufficient evidence that the Notch signaling pathway is a direct pathway for melatonin action or that it is the only downstream pathway for melatonin action in endometriosis. However, the data suggest that Notch signaling pathway may be a potential therapeutic target in endometriosis.

Studies have reported that Numb completely prevents EMT by antagonizing Notch signaling [47, 48]. In the present study, Melatonin and Notch-specific inhibitor promotes the expression of Numb in both normal and endometriotic endometrium, indicating that the effect of melatonin on Notch signaling might be mediated by Numb upregulation. We also proved that Numb expression was decreased in endometrium of endometriosis, implying that Numb might be a potent therapeutic target in endometriosis.

Conclusions

In summary, we confirm that aberrant expression of Notch1/Numb signaling and an active EMT process are present in eutopic endometrium of endometriosis, and we provide an experimental basis for considering melatonin as a potential treatment for endometriosis. In addition, we observed that Notch signaling pathway might be involved in the progression of endometriosis. The role of Notch signaling pathway in the effect of estrogen and melatonin in endometriosis need further investigation in future studies.

Abbreviations

CCK-8: Cell Counting Kit-8; EEC: Endometriotic eutopic epithelial cells; EMT: Epithelial-mesenchymal transition; ERα: Estrogen receptor alpha; FBS: Charcoal-stripped fetal bovine serum; MMPs: Matrix metalloproteinases; NEC: Normal endometrial epithelial cells; NFκB: Nuclear factor-κB; NICD: Notch1 intracellular domain; NSC: Normal stromal cells; OD: Optical density; TLR: Toll-like receptor

Acknowledgements

We are grateful to all the participants involved in this study. We thank American Journal Experts for the language editing.

Funding

This research was supported by grants from the National Natural Science Foundation of China (No.81300468; NO. 81671433), a grant from Shandong Province key research and development projects (No. 2016GSF201086), a grant from Shandong Province medical and health technology development project (2016WS0442), a grant from Science and Technology Development Program of Jinan (No. 201506012), and a grant from Shandong Province Natural Science Foundation (No. ZR2014HM008).

Authors' contributions

HZ participated in the study design and coordination, and edited the manuscript for submission. SQ carried out the experiments, participated in the interpretation of the data and drafted the manuscript. LY and ZL helped to revise the manuscript and performed the statistical analysis. XZ, ML and ZC participated in the design of the study, supervised the study and critically helped to draft the manuscript. All authors read and approved the final manuscript.

Competing interests

The authors declare that they have no competing interests.

Author details

[1]Center for Reproductive Medicine, Shandong Provincial Hospital Affiliated to Shandong University, Jinan 250021, People's Republic of China. [2]National Research Center for Assisted Reproductive Technology and Reproductive Genetics, Jinan 250021, People's Republic of China. [3]The Key laboratory for Reproductive Endocrinology, Shandong University, Ministry of Education, Jinan 250021, People's Republic of China. [4]Department of Urology, Qilu Hospital of Shandong University, 107 Wenhua Xi Road, Jinan 250012, People's Republic of China. [5]Department of Obstetrics and Gynecology, Shandong Provincial Hospital Affiliated to Shandong University, 324 Jingwu Road, Jinan 250021, People's Republic of China. [6]Shanghai Key Laboratory for Assisted Reproduction and Reproductive Genetics, Shanghai 200030, People's Republic of China. [7]Center for Reproductive Medicine, Ren Ji Hospital, School of Medicine, Shanghai Jiao Tong University, Shanghai 200030, People's Republic of China.

References

1. Giudice LC. Clinical practice. Endometriosis N Engl J Med. 2010;362:2389–98.
2. Simoens S, Dunselman G, Dirksen C, Hummelshoj L, Bokor A, Brandes I, et al. The burden of endometriosis: costs and quality of life of women with endometriosis and treated in referral centres. Hum Reprod. 2012;27:1292–9.
3. Giudice LC, Kao LC. Endometriosis. Lancet. 2004;364:1789–99.
4. Matsuzaki S, Darcha C. Epithelial to mesenchymal transition-like and mesenchymal to epithelial transition-like processes might be involved in the pathogenesis of pelvic endometriosis. Hum Reprod. 2012;27:712–21.
5. Santamaria X, Massasa EE, Taylor HS. Migration of cells from experimental endometriosis to the uterine endometrium. Endocrinology. 2012;153: 5566–74.
6. Liu Z, Qi S, Zhao X, Li M, Ding S, Lu J, et al. Metformin inhibits 17beta-estradiol-induced epithelial-to-mesenchymal transition via betaKlotho-related ERK1/2 signaling and AMPKalpha signaling in endometrial adenocarcinoma cells. Oncotarget. 2016;7:21315–31.
7. Dong C, Wu Y, Yao J, Wang Y, Yu Y, Rychahou PG, et al. G9a interacts with snail and is critical for snail-mediated E-cadherin repression in human breast cancer. J Clin Invest. 2012;122:1469–86.
8. Qi S, Zhao X, Li M, Zhang X, Lu Z, Yang C, et al. Aberrant expression of Notch1/numb/snail signaling, an epithelial mesenchymal transition related pathway, in adenomyosis. Reprod Biol Endocrinol. 2015;13:96.
9. Reiter RJ. Pineal melatonin: cell biology of its synthesis and of its physiological interactions. Endocr Rev. 1991;12:151–80.
10. Cetinkaya N, Attar R, Yildirim G, Ficicioglu C, Ozkan F, Yilmaz B, et al. The effects of different doses of melatonin treatment on endometrial implants in an oophorectomized rat endometriosis model. Arch Gynecol Obstet. 2015;291:591–8.
11. Guney M, Oral B, Karahan N, Mungan T. Regression of endometrial explants in a rat model of endometriosis treated with melatonin. Fertil Steril. 2008;89:934–42.
12. Koc O, Gunduz B, Topcuoglu A, Bugdayci G, Yilmaz F, Duran B. Effects of pinealectomy and melatonin supplementation on endometrial explants in a rat model. Eur J Obstet Gynecol Reprod Biol. 2010;153:72–6.
13. Kocadal NC, Attar R, Yildirim G, Ficicioglu C, Ozkan F, Yilmaz B, et al. Melatonin treatment results in regression of endometriotic lesions in an ooferectomized rat endometriosis model. J Turk Ger Gynecol Assoc. 2013;14:81–6.
14. Yesildaglar N, Yildirim G, Yildirim OK, Attar R, Ozkan F, Akkaya H, et al. The effects of melatonin on endometriotic lesions induced by implanting human endometriotic cells in the first SCID-mouse endometriosis-model developed in Turkey. Clin Exp Obstet Gynecol. 2016;43:25–30.
15. Yildirim G, Attar R, Ficicioglu C, Karateke A, Ozkan F, Kilic E, et al. The combination of letrozole and melatonin causes regression in size not histopathological scores on endometriosis in an experimental rat model. J Turk Ger Gynecol Assoc. 2009;10:199–204.
16. Yildirim G, Attar R, Ozkan F, Kumbak B, Ficicioglu C, Yesildaglar N. The effects of letrozole and melatonin on surgically induced endometriosis in a rat model: a preliminary study. Fertil Steril. 2010;93:1787–92.
17. Shi S, Zhang Y, Wen W, Zhao Y, Sun L. Molecular mechanisms of melatonin in the reversal of LPS-induced EMT in peritoneal mesothelial cells. Mol Med Rep. 2016;14:4342–8.
18. Yu N, Sun YT, Su XM, He M, Dai B, Kang J. Melatonin attenuates TGFbeta1-induced epithelial-mesenchymal transition in lung alveolar epithelial cells. Mol Med Rep. 2016;14:5567–72.
19. Zhao H, Wu QQ, Cao LF, Qing HY, Zhang C, Chen YH, et al. Melatonin inhibits endoplasmic reticulum stress and epithelial-mesenchymal transition during bleomycin-induced pulmonary fibrosis in mice. PLoS One. 2014;9:e97266.
20. Zhang H, Li M, Zheng X, Sun Y, Wen Z, Zhao X. Endometriotic stromal cells lose the ability to regulate cell-survival signaling in endometrial epithelial cells in vitro. Mol Hum Reprod. 2009;15:653–63.
21. Zhang H, Li M, Wang F, Liu S, Li J, Wen Z, et al. Endometriotic epithelial cells induce MMPs expression in endometrial stromal cells via an NFkappaB-dependent pathway. Gynecol Endocrinol. 2010;26:456–67.
22. Wu SM, Lin WY, Shen CC, Pan HC, Keh-Bin W, Chen YC, et al. Melatonin set out to ER stress signaling thwarts epithelial mesenchymal transition and peritoneal dissemination via calpain-mediated C/EBPbeta and NFkappaB cleavage. J Pineal Res. 2016;60:142–54.
23. Prieto-Dominguez N, Ordonez R, Fernandez A, Mendez-Blanco C, Baulies A, Garcia-Ruiz C, et al. Melatonin-induced increase in sensitivity of human hepatocellular carcinoma cells to sorafenib is associated with reactive oxygen species production and mitophagy. J Pineal Res. 2016;61:396–407.
24. Gao W, Sweeney C, Walsh C, Rooney P, McCormick J, Veale DJ, et al. Notch signalling pathways mediate synovial angiogenesis in response to vascular endothelial growth factor and angiopoietin 2. Ann Rheum Dis. 2013;72:1080–8.
25. Song BQ, Chi Y, Li X, Du WJ, Han ZB, Tian JJ, et al. Inhibition of notch signaling promotes the Adipogenic differentiation of mesenchymal stem cells through autophagy activation and PTEN-PI3K/AKT/mTOR pathway. Cell Physiol Biochem. 2015;36:1991–2002.
26. Ray S, Pollard JW. KLF15 negatively regulates estrogen-induced epithelial cell proliferation by inhibition of DNA replication licensing. Proc Natl Acad Sci U S A. 2012;109:E1334–43.
27. Meng YG, Han WD, Zhao YL, Huang K, Si YL, Wu ZQ, et al. Induction of the LRP16 gene by estrogen promotes the invasive growth of Ishikawa human endometrial cancer cells through the downregulation of E-cadherin. Cell Res. 2007;17:869–80.
28. Leyendecker G, Wildt L, Mall G. The pathophysiology of endometriosis and adenomyosis: tissue injury and repair. Arch Gynecol Obstet. 2009;280:529–38.
29. Leong KG, Niessen K, Kulic I, Raouf A, Eaves C, Pollet I, et al. Jagged1-mediated notch activation induces epithelial-to-mesenchymal transition through slug-induced repression of E-cadherin. J Exp Med. 2007;204:2935–48.
30. Matsuno Y, Coelho AL, Jarai G, Westwick J, Hogaboam CM. Notch signaling mediates TGF-beta1-induced epithelial-mesenchymal transition through the induction of Snai1. Int J Biochem Cell Biol. 2012;44:776–89.
31. McGill MA, McGlade CJ. Mammalian numb proteins promote Notch1 receptor ubiquitination and degradation of the Notch1 intracellular domain. J Biol Chem. 2003;278:23196–203.
32. Xiong Y, Liu Y, Xiong W, Zhang L, Liu H, Du Y, et al. Hypoxia-inducible factor 1alpha-induced epithelial-mesenchymal transition of endometrial

epithelial cells may contribute to the development of endometriosis. Hum Reprod. 2016;31:1327–38.

33. Zheng QM, Lu JJ, Zhao J, Wei X, Wang L, Liu PS. Periostin facilitates the epithelial-mesenchymal transition of endometrial epithelial cells through ILK-Akt signaling pathway. Biomed Res Int. 2016;2016:9842619.
34. Yang YM, Yang WX. Epithelial-to-mesenchymal transition in the development of endometriosis. Oncotarget. 2017;8:41679–89.
35. Bulun SE, Zeitoun KM, Takayama K, Sasano H. Estrogen biosynthesis in endometriosis: molecular basis and clinical relevance. J Mol Endocrinol. 2000;25:35–42.
36. Ye Y, Xiao Y, Wang W, Yearsley K, Gao JX, Shetuni B, et al. ERalpha signaling through slug regulates E-cadherin and EMT. Oncogene. 2010;29:1451–62.
37. Chimge NO, Baniwal SK, Little GH, Chen YB, Kahn M, Tripathy D, et al. Regulation of breast cancer metastasis by Runx2 and estrogen signaling: the role of SNAI2. Breast Cancer Res. 2011;13:R127.
38. Jeon SY, Hwang KA, Choi KC. Effect of steroid hormones, estrogen and progesterone, on epithelial mesenchymal transition in ovarian cancer development. J Steroid Biochem Mol Biol. 2016;158:1–8.
39. Shao R, Shi J, Liu H, Shi X, Du X, Klocker H, et al. Epithelial-to-mesenchymal transition and estrogen receptor alpha mediated epithelial dedifferentiation mark the development of benign prostatic hyperplasia. Prostate. 2014;74: 970–82.
40. Paul S, Bhattacharya P, Das Mahapatra P, Swarnakar S. Melatonin protects against endometriosis via regulation of matrix metalloproteinase-3 and an apoptotic pathway. J Pineal Res. 2010;49:156–68.
41. Paul S, Sharma AV, Mahapatra PD, Bhattacharya P, Reiter RJ, Swarnakar S. Role of melatonin in regulating matrix metalloproteinase-9 via tissue inhibitors of metalloproteinase-1 during protection against endometriosis. J Pineal Res. 2008;44:439–49.
42. Schwertner A, Conceicao Dos Santos CC, Costa GD, Deitos A, de Souza A, de Souza IC, et al. Efficacy of melatonin in the treatment of endometriosis: a phase II, randomized, double-blind, placebo-controlled trial. Pain. 2013;154: 874–81.
43. Bondi CD, Alonso-Gonzalez C, Clafshenkel WP, Kotlarczyk MP, Dodda BR, Sanchez-Barcelo E, et al. The effect of estradiol, progesterone, and melatonin on estrous cycling and ovarian aromatase expression in intact female mice. Eur J Obstet Gynecol Reprod Biol. 2014;174:80–5.
44. Berstein L, Tsyrlina E, Poroshina T, Bychkova N, Kalinina N, Gamajunova V, et al. Switching (overtargeting) of estrogen effects and its potential role in hormonal carcinogenesis. Neoplasma. 2002;49:21–5.
45. Ciortea R, Costin N, Braicu I, Haragas D, Hudacsko A, Bondor C, et al. Effect of melatonin on intra-abdominal fat in correlation with endometrial proliferation in ovariectomized rats. Anticancer Res. 2011;31:2637–43.
46. Dair EL, Simoes RS, Simoes MJ, Romeu LR, Oliveira-Filho RM, Haidar MA, et al. Effects of melatonin on the endometrial morphology and embryo implantation in rats. Fertil Steril. 2008;89:1299–305.
47. Zhang J, Shao X, Sun H, Liu K, Ding Z, Chen J, et al. NUMB negatively regulates the epithelial-mesenchymal transition of triple-negative breast cancer by antagonizing notch signaling. Oncotarget. 2016;7:61036–53.
48. Bocci F, Jolly MK, Tripathi SC, Aguilar M, Hanash SM, Levine H, et al. Numb prevents a complete epithelial-mesenchymal transition by modulating notch signalling. J R Soc Interface. 2017;14

15

The enigmatic seminal plasma: a proteomics insight from ejaculation to fertilization

Luna Samanta[1,2], Rajeshwari Parida[2], Tania R. Dias[1,3,4,5] and Ashok Agarwal[1*]

Abstract

Background: The 'omics' approach for a noninvasive diagnosis of male reproductive system disorders has gained momentum during the last decade, particularly from a screening and prognosis point of view. Due to the rapid development in assisted reproductive technologies (ART) over the years, the major focus of proteomic studies has been around the ejaculated spermatozoa. Although seminal plasma is not a requirement for ART, the question arose whether the role of seminal plasma is merely to transport spermatozoa.

Main body: Seminal plasma (SP) contains a large diversity of proteins that are essential not only for sperm transport, but also for sperm protection and maturation. Most of the proteins bind to sperm surface through exosomes (epididymosomes and prostasomes), modulating sperm function, interaction with the female reproductive tract and finally fertilization. This review focuses on the state-of-art discoveries regarding SP proteome and its role in fertilization.

Conclusion: Tissue-specific proteins in the SP have emerged as fundamental contributors for protein biomarker discovery. This is important for a noninvasive diagnosis of male infertility and development of new therapeutic approaches. Moreover, ART success rates may be improved by taking into account the critical role of seminal proteome in fertilization.

Keywords: Seminal plasma, Exosomes, Prostasomes, Epididymosomes, Cytokines, Female reproductive tract, Male infertility, Proteomics, Assisted reproductive technologies

Background

Semen comprises about 5% of testicular secretions containing spermatozoa and 95% of seminal plasma (SP), which includes secretions from accessory sex glands. The use of assisted reproductive technologies (ART) facilitated the direct involvement of sperm in fertilization, specifically for the delivery of paternal genetic content and embryo development. Consequently, the role of SP in the regulation of reproductive processes to achieve a successful birth has been largely neglected. Although SP components have a potential diagnostic value, such as measurement of fructose levels for abnormalities in seminal vesicles [1] and measurement of prostatic acid phosphatase for the presence of prostatic secretions in SP [2], they have been given little clinical consideration. SP plays a key role in natural fertilization as it contributes to a timely capacitation, acrosome reaction and sperm-oocyte interaction [3, 4]. Its complex proteomic composition, growth factors and transcription factors, nourishes and protects spermatozoa as they travel throughout the male and female reproductive tracts. As a result, it ensures the interaction of spermatozoa with the oocyte to undergo fertilization [5]. The presence of tissue-specific proteins in the SP can serve as potential biomarkers for the assessment of male fertility. One comprehensive review by Drabovich et al. [6] reported the role of SP proteins as markers of male fertility evaluation with special reference to prostate cancer and azoospermia. The various milestones in our understanding of SP proteome (Table 1) have prompted many investigators to gain further insights into its function and role in human reproduction, as well

* Correspondence: agarwaa@ccf.org; http://www.ClevelandClinic.Org/ReproductiveResearchCenter
[1]American Center for Reproductive Medicine, Cleveland Clinic, 10681 Carnegie Avenue, Desk X11, Cleveland, OH 44195, USA
Full list of author information is available at the end of the article

Table 1 Major breakthroughs in the development of proteomic biomarkers through proteomic analysis of human seminal plasma

Year	Technique used	Outcome	Reference
1888	Acetic acid precipitation	Detection of propeptone	[16]
1942	Electrophoresis (Tiselius apparatus)	First electrophoretic separation that identified 4 protein fractions	[18]
1942	Electrophoresis (Tiselius apparatus)	Electrophoretically separated 4 protein fractions correspond to albumin, α-, β- and γ-globulins	[17]
1978	2DE	Separated 40 peptides and identified p30 as a marker for semen in forensic samples (vaginal swabs). Established the idea that semen proteins can act as biomarkers	[19]
1981	2DE	Detected > 200 peptides and reported the absence of many glycoproteins in vasectomized men	[20]
2003	2DE-MALDI-TOF-MS	Detected impaired spermatogenesis-associated markers by narrow immobilized pH gradients in azoospermic men	[21]
2007	2DE-LC-MS/MS	Reported candidate marker proteins for non-obstructive and obstructive azoospermia	[26]
2009	1DE-LC-MS/MS	Proposed that downregulation of DJ-1 is responsible for oxidative stress and thereby affects the quality of the semen in asthenozoospermia	[27]
2011	N-linked glycosylated peptide enrichment, combined with LC-MS/MS	N-glycosylated prostate-specific antigen is known to be an efficient biomarker that can distinguish benign prostate hyperplasia from prostate cancer	[30]
2012	2DE-LC-MS/MS	Identified 59 proteins in seminal plasma as candidate biomarkers of prostatitis	[28]
2013	LC-MS/MS	Testis-specific TKTL1, LDHC and PGK2 could distinguish semen from fertile and infertile men	[23]
2013	1DE-LC-MS/MS	Identified proteins that are over- or underexpressed in the seminal plasma of teratozoospermic, oligozoospermic and oligoteratozoospermic men	[29]
2014	LC-MS/MS followed by MS-based multiplex SRM assay	ECM1 and TEX101 levels can distinguish OA from NOA and circumvent testicular biopsies for prediction of outcome of sperm retrieval in azoospermic patients	[6]
2015	1DE-LC-MS/MS	MME and FAM3D along with ROS levels in the seminal plasma may serve as good markers for diagnosis of male infertility	[24]
2016	LC-MS/MS	Cab45/SDF4, protein lefty-1, DNase I, PAP2-alpha, IBP-7, HDC, and CRISP-3 are proposed as putative biomarkers in adolescents with varicocele	[25]

Abbreviations: *1DE* one-dimensional electrophoresis, *2DE* two-dimensional electrophoresis, *Cab45/SDF4* 45 kDa calcium-binding protein, *CRISP-3* Cysteine- rich secretory protein 3, *ECM1* extracellular matrix protein 1, *HDC* Histidine decarboxylase, *FAM3D* family with sequence similarity 3 member D, *IBP-7* Insulin-like growth factor-binding protein 7, *LC* liquid chromatography, *LDHC* lactate dehydrogenase C, *MALDI* matrix-assisted laser desorption/ionization, *MME* membrane metalloendopeptidase, *MS* mass spectrometry, *MS/MS* tandem mass spectrometry, *NOA* non-obstructive azoospermia, *OA* obstructive azoospermia, *PAP2* Prostatic acid phosphatase type 2, *PGK2* Phosphoglycerate kinase 2, *ROS* reactive oxygen species, *SRM* selected reaction monitoring, *TEX101* Testis-expressed protein 101, *TKTL1* Transketolase-like protein 1, *TOF* time-of-flight

as its potential as a screening, diagnostic and prognostic tool in male fertility assessment. Therefore, this review focuses on the role of SP proteins in different reproductive processes including the modulation of spermatozoa functions and fertilization.

Review criteria

PUBMED and Google Scholar databases were explored for relevant literature (1942–2017) on the proteomics study of SP using the following keywords: "seminal fluid proteins", "semen proteins", "seminal plasma proteins", "proteomics and biomarker discovery", "seminal plasma proteomics", "seminal plasma biomarkers", "seminal plasma and sperm", "seminal plasma and male fertility", "seminal plasma and inflammation", "seminal plasma and immune tolerance", "seminal plasma and ovarian function", "seminal plasma and female reproductive tract events", "seminal plasma and endometrial tissue remodeling", "seminal plasma and uterine receptivity" and "seminal plasma and embryotrophic cytokines". All full-text articles published in peer-reviewed journals in English were selected, total of 262 articles. Many review articles and animal studies were not considered either due to poor relevance to our topic or repeated information in more recent studies. A total of 99 references were included (97 articles and two book chapters). Nine references with more than 20 years were considered either due to historical importance or as supportive evidence. The majority of the references (61) are from the last 10 years.

Composition of seminal plasma

SP is constituted by secretions derived from testes (~ 2–5%; sperm cells), epididymides and prostate (~ 20–30%), seminal vesicles (~ 65–75%), as well as bulbouretheral and periurethral gland (~ 1%) (Fig. 1) [7]. It is rich in sugars, oligosaccharides, glycans [8], lipids [9], inorganic ions, small molecule metabolites [10], cell-free DNA [11], RNA, microRNAs [12], peptides and proteins [10]. The average protein

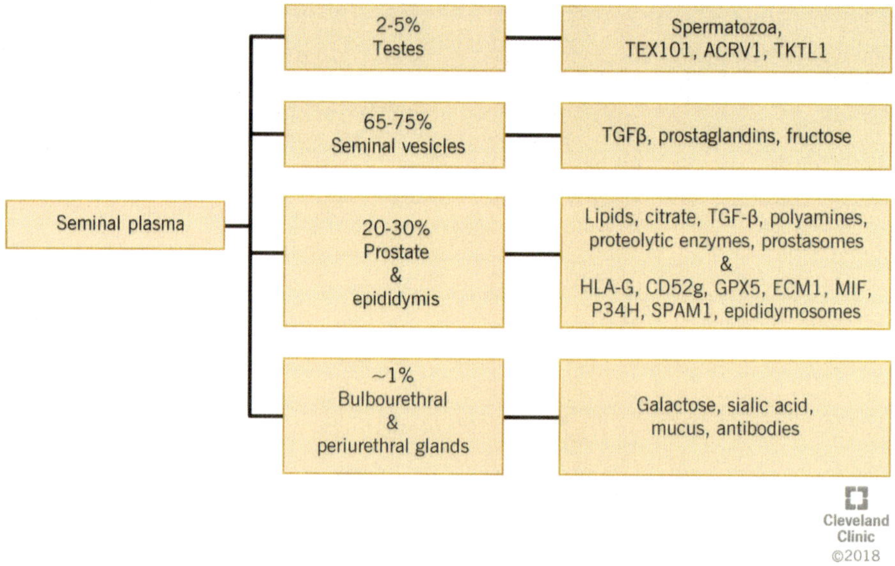

Fig. 1 Composition of seminal plasma including the secretions from testes, epididymis, seminal vesicles, prostate, and bulbourethral and periurethral glands

concentration in SP is about 35–55 g/L. These components mediate the interaction between SP and spermatozoa, regulating their function and facilitating their transit through the female reproductive tract [13, 14]. The alkaline secretions of seminal vesicles and prostate counteract the vaginal acidity for optimal sperm survival. The overall contribution of seminal vesicles to SP is the highest in terms of molecular content and includes cytokines, prostaglandins and fructose [15], while the prostate gland secretions are rich in lipids, citrate and proteolytic enzymes [2]. Basic polyamines, namely, spermine, spermidine and putrescine maintain the alkalinity of the semen. Galactose, sialic acid and mucus secreted by the bulbourethral glands act as lubricants for efficient sperm transfer (Fig. 1) [7].

History and evolution of the study of seminal plasma proteome

In 1888, a report by C. Posner regarding the presence of proteose or propeptone (cocktail of proteolytic digested products) in SP, marked the beginning of seminal plasma proteomics (Table 1) [16, 17]. However, the first electrophoretic separation of SP proteins was in 1942 using a Tiselius apparatus, where two water-soluble fractions including one non-heat-coagulable proteose and a glycoprotein, and two water-insoluble fractions were identified. They also confirmed the content of albumin in seminal plasma to be less than 0.02% and that of nucleoprotein to be less than 0.04% [18]. In the same year, Gray and Huggins [17] reported that the 4 fractions yielded by electrophoretic separation of SP correspond to albumin, α-globulin, β-globulin, and γ-globulin of normal serum. Sensabaugh [19] was able to separate 40 peptides by SDS-PAGE, purify and characterize the semen specific protein p30, which could be used as an alternative test for the forensic identification of semen based on the detection of this protein. Thus, the foundation for the use of seminal proteins as biomarkers was established. Over the years, there has been a tremendous advance in the analytical tools used to decipher the proteome profile of human samples. These advances also enabled the identification of a large number of proteins at a much faster pace (Table 1). More than 200 peptides were detected in the SP of normal fertile men using 2D-electrophoresis, while their vasectomized counterparts lacked a series of glycoproteins. Besides, immunodetection revealed the presence of a number of serum proteins as well as prostatic acid prosphatase and creatine kinase [20]. Subsequently, Starita-Geribaldi et al. [21] developed a narrow immobilized pH gradient covering one pH unit for human SP proteomic analysis, which was followed by matrix-assisted laser desorption ionization (MALDI) and tandem mass spectrometry (MS-MS). These techniques increased the accuracy of differential expression analysis and identification of markers associated with impaired spermatogenesis. Separation of SP proteins from a pool of five samples by gel electrophoresis (1D and 2D) and identification either by matrix-assisted laser desorption ionization-time-of-flight-mass spectrometry (MALDI-TOF-MS) or capillary liquid chromatography tandem mass spectrometry (LC-MS/MS) revealed 100 peptides and proteins [22]. A total of 923 SP proteins including proteases of extracellular origin and other proteins originating from male accessory glands were identified by LC-MS/MS from a single sample [14]. Rolland et al. [23] identified 699 proteins in SP and predicted the presence of a total of 2545 distinctive proteins by comparing their results with previous studies. From their data, the authors also confirmed the presence of proteins from testes (83), epididymis (42), seminal vesicles (7) and prostate (17). Beginning with a moving boundary electrophoresis using a Tiselius apparatus, proteomic research has undergone remarkable evolution over time with the development of high throughput technologies such as LC-MS/MS and with the inclusion of targeted proteomics and possibility to detect post-translational modifications (PTMs) in proteins to assess their functionality. Studies by various groups have recorded thousands of proteins in SP and these were consolidated by Drabovich et al. [6], amounting to 3200 in total. These studies and the advances in proteomic technologies contributed to the recent discovery of key proteins associated with male infertility [24, 25], which may be used as biomarkers for clinical application.

Proteomic signatures of seminal plasma in evaluation of male infertility

The past decade witnessed an enormous rise in the number of reports on comparative proteomics of SP to identify putative protein markers for various reproductive conditions such as infertility in general [23], obstructive and non-obstructive azoospermia [6, 26], asthenozoospermia [27], prostatitis [28], oxidative-induced infertility [24, 29], varicocele [25], and prostate cancer and benign prostate hyperplasia [30] (Table 2).

A member of the lipocalin superfamily, prostaglandin-D synthase (PGDS) is an extracellular transport protein that includes retinol-binding protein and shows high binding affinity for specific cell receptors and small hydrophobic ligands. PGDS was reported to be associated with poor semen parameters such as decreased sperm count, percentage of motility, and percentage of normal morphology. The expression of this protein showed a gradual decrease from normal to oligospermic, azoospermic and patients who underwent vasectomy [31]. Upon further investigation, PGDS was proposed as a biomarker of obstructive azoospermia [32]. The same group developed a multiplex selected reaction monitoring (SRM) assay to detect the level of testis-expressed protein 101 (TEX101) and epididymis-expressed extracellular matrix protein 1 (ECM1) to distinguish men with obstructive azoospermia from those with non-obstructive azoospermia (Table 2). This technique circumvented the clinical evaluation using the invasive technique of testicular biopsy [33].

A comparative proteomic study by Davalieva et al. [13] using two-dimensional differential gel electrophoresis (2D-DIGE) showed overexpression of 8 proteins: fibronectin, prostatic acid phosphatase (PAP), prolactin-inducible protein (PIP), beta-2-microglobulin (B2M), proteasome subunit alpha type-3 (PSMA3), cytosolic nonspecific dipeptidase (CNDP2), and galectin-3-binding protein (LGALS3BP) in the SP of azoospermic men when compared with at least one of the other studied groups (normozoospermic, asthenozoospermic and oligozoospermic). In particular, PAP was significantly overexpressed in azoospermic patients relative to all the other groups. Milardi et al. [3] evaluated the seminal proteomic profile among a pool of five men with proven fertility and proposed a panel of proteins of importance for male fertility such as semenogelin I, semenogelin II, olfactory receptor 5R1, lactoferrin, human cationic antimicrobial protein (hCAP18), spindling 1, and clusterin. Semenogelins are the main proteins responsible for the formation of a gel matrix that entraps spermatozoa into a seminal coagulum right after ejaculation. This has a particular importance for sperm function because semenogelins act as natural regulators of sperm capacitation as they prevent its premature occurrence [34]. High concentrations of semenogelins were also suggested as a biomarker in asthenozoospermic men [35]. The hCAP18 is

Table 2 Potential protein markers in seminal plasma under altered pathophysiology

Condition	Identified protein markers	Reference
Poor semen parameters/azoospermia	PGDS	[31, 32]
Obstructive and non-obstructive azoospermia	TEX101, ECM1	[33]
Azoospermia vs normo-, astheno- and oligozoospermia	Fibronectin, PAP, PIP, B2M, PSMA3, LGALS3BP, CNDP2	[13]
Infertility	Semenogelin I/II, olfactory receptor 5R1, Lactoferin, hCAP18, Spindling 1, Clusterin	[3]
Abnormal semen parameters, ROS and asthenozoospermia	DJ-1	[27, 29]
ROS and prostate cancer	LGALS3BP	[37]
Different levels of ROS and infertility	MME, FAM3D	[24]
Fertile vs infertile	TKTL1, LDHC, PGK2	[23]

Seminal plasma proteins as potential biomarkers in several infertile conditions. These biomarkers can be targeted for seminal analysis in clinical research for male fertility evaluation

Abbreviations: *B2M* beta-2-microglobulin, *CNDP2* cytosolic nonspecific dipeptidase, *ECM1* extracellular matrix protein 1, *FAM3D* family with sequence similarity 3 member D, *hCAP18* human cationic antimicrobial protein, *LDHC* lactate dehydrogenase C, *LGALS3BP* galectin 3 binding protein, *MME* membrane metalloendopeptidase, *PAP* prostatic acid phosphatase, *PGK2* phosphoglycerate kinase 2, *PIP* prolactin-inducible protein, *PSMA3* proteasome subunit alpha type-3, *PGDS* prostaglandin-D synthase, *ROS* reactive oxygen species, *TEX101* testis-expressed protein 101, *TKTL1* transketolase-like protein 1 also expressed by the epididymal epithelium and in seminal plasma at high concentrations and has a key role in the innate immunity of the male reproductive system [36].

Stress proteins such as DJ-1 were found to be differentially regulated and expressed in men with: (1) normal sperm count and abnormal morphology, (2) oligozoospermia and normal morphology, and (3) oligozoospermia and abnormal morphology, when compared to normozoospermic samples. These proteins may serve as a potential biomarkers to identify the underlying mechanisms that lead to poor sperm quality in these men [37]. Wang et al. [27] proposed that the downregulation of DJ-1 induces oxidative stress, thereby affecting the quality of semen in asthenozoospermic men. A comparative proteomics study using semen samples with normal or high levels of reactive oxygen species (ROS) indicated that the LGALS3BP, which is responsible for host defense against viruses and tumor cells, was exclusively detected in the group with normal ROS levels. Thus, LGALS3BP could be a candidate marker for the diagnosis and treatment of patients with cancer of the reproductive tract [29]. Further in-depth investigation involving SP from fertile and infertile men with varying levels of ROS (low, medium and high) showed that the expression profile of proteins involved in PTMs, protein folding and transport were severely altered in the infertile group. Furthermore, two proteins were identified as putative markers: the membrane metalloendopeptidase (MME) and family with sequence similarity 3 member D (FAM3D).The former was consistently overexpressed in all three groups of infertile men, whereas the latter was uniquely expressed in the fertile group [24]. A combined sample pre-fractionation using peptide ligand library columns followed by shotgun nano-LC-MS/MS analysis of the tryptic peptides corresponding to each elution fraction, enabled the identification of 669 proteins. Among those, three important proteins: transketolase-like protein 1 (TKTL1), L-lactate dehydrogense C chain (LDHC) and phosphoglycerate kinase 2 (PGK2), were also proposed as biomarkers of fertility [23].

SP has also a high expression of cytokines that are associated with male infertility [38]. In the male genital tract, there is a tissue-specific secretion of cytokines and chemokines into the SP. The epididymis mainly secretes soluble HLA-G and CD52g, whereas the seminal vesicles are the principal source of prostaglandins and transforming growth factor β (TGF-β). The prostate also produces TGF-β and other bioactive components including small RNAs. The penile urethra is primarily responsible for the production of local antibodies in the male genital tract [5, 39, 40].

The studies presented in our review provide an evidence that SP proteome is vast and may have a role beyond spermatozoa transport. Although these mechanisms are not completely understood, the identified proteins may serve as biomarkers for the development of new diagnostic and therapeutic tools. For instance, a testis-secreted acrosomal vesicle protein 1 (ACRV1, SP-10) associated with sperm-zona binding and penetration [41] has been the basis for the development of an immunodiagnostic home test, SpermCheck Fertility® (Bio-Rad Laboratories, Hercules, CA), to detect the sperm concentration in semen. In this qualitative test, the number of sperm is directly proportional to the signal strength of ELISA assays for the measurement of SP-10 [42]. Similar approaches can be used to develop new technologies for the clinical evaluation of male infertility.

Seminal exosomal proteins and their role in sperm function

SP contains a heterogeneous population of microvesicles called exosomes. Seminal exosomes include mainly tetraspanin CD9-positive epididymosomes and prostasomes (Fig. 2), which account for 3% of the total protein complement of SP [43]. Transcription and translation are almost silent in mature spermatozoa due to DNA packaging during spermatogenesis. Besides the PTMs that occur during sperm maturation along the male reproductive tract, exosomes play an important role in supporting sperm functions [44]. Exosomes are RNA and protein containing microvesicles, which like viruses, originate from inside the cells and are released into the extracellular compartment. This is in contrast to other microvesicles that are pinched off from the plasma membrane [45]. Genetic material can be delivered into target cells via exosomes including protein-encoding mRNAs and small noncoding RNAs involved in regulation of gene expression [46–48]. A recent comprehensive proteomic analysis by Yang et al. [49] reported a total of 1474 proteins in human seminal exosome samples. Through gene ontology (GO) analysis, the authors showed that seminal exosomes-associated proteins were mostly linked to 'exosomes,' 'cytoplasm,' and 'cytosol,' which are involved in biologic processes such as metabolism, energy pathways, protein metabolism, cell growth and maintenance, and transport [49]. SP transmits a plethora of proteins to the spermatozoa via exosomal-binding that are important for maturation and protection of the male gametes, as well as for the maintenance of their function.

Epididymosomes have a complex proteome and their composition changes along the epididymis. Moreover, the epididymosomes present in the ejaculate do not significantly contribute to the population of exosomes present in the ejaculate. These suggests that epididymosomes transfer their contents to the spermatozoa during their transit through the epididymis. Proteins associated to epididymosomes are not processed through the endoplasmic reticulum–Golgi apparatus secretory vesicles, have unusual

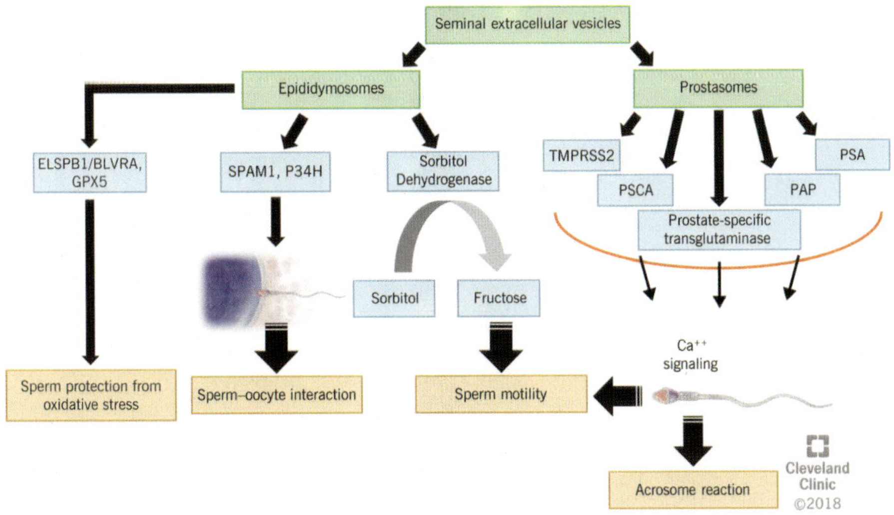

Fig. 2 Role of seminal extracellular vesicles, epididymosomes and prostasomes, and their proteome on spermatozoa function

glycosylation and lack N-terminal signal peptides. Additionally, some of them are strongly glycosylphosphatidylinositol (GPI)-anchored to these membranous vesicles. There are basically two subpopulations of epididymosomes, those enriched with epididymal sperm binding protein 1 (ELSPBP1) and the CD9-positive epididymosomes (Fig. 2). ELSPBP1, first described as HE12 in humans, was associated with dead and dying spermatozoa in the ejaculated semen. This protein in association with biliverdin reductase A (BLVRA) uses NADPH as a proton donor to reduce biliverdin to bilirubin. Bilirubin then uses ROS to regenerate biliverdin in the presence of Zn^{2+}. Thus, the binding of ELSPBP1/BLVRA complex to dying spermatozoa acts as a scavenger of ROS generated by dying spermatozoa, thereby protecting the surviving spermatozoa from oxidative damage [50, 51]. CD9-positive epididymosomes preferentially bind to or fuse with live spermatozoa and are involved in epididymal sperm maturation. HE5, which is specifically expressed by the human epididymis, is also a human lymphocyte surface protein (CD52) and is GPI-anchored to the sperm surface during the epididymal transit. It is proposed that this protein is transferred to the sperm surface by epididymosomes and is thought to be associated with human immunological infertility [50, 52]. Other epididymosome-associated proteins that are also transferred to sperm surface during epididymal maturation include: enzymes of the polyol pathway, macrophage migration inhibitory factor (MIF), type 5 glutathione peroxidase (GPX5), the sperm adhesion molecule 1 (SPAM1 or PH-20), and the zona pellucida binding protein P34H. Two enzymes of polyol pathway, aldose reductase and sorbitol dehydrogenase are responsible for the generation of fructose by oxidation of sorbitol to fuel sperm motility. MIF is a cytokine that modulates sperm motility during the transit along the male reproductive tract and GPX5 might protect the transiting epididymal spermatozoa against OS. Finally, SPAM1 and P34H play a key role in sperm-egg binding [53].

Prostasomes are well-characterized markers of SP function. Examples of prostasomes in human SP include PAP, prostate specific antigen (PSA), type 2 transmembrane serine protease (TMPRSS2), prostate-specific transglutaminase (pTGase) and prostate stem cell antigen (PSCA) (Fig. 2) [54, 55]. These seminal exosomes transfer Ca^{2+} signaling tools namely, progesterone receptors, cyclic adenosine diphosphoribose (cADPR)-synthesizing enzymes, ryanodine receptors (RyRs), and other related molecules to the sperm neck, thus triggering sperm motility and acrosome reaction [56]. By binding to sperm cells, these proteins are able to control the timing of early and late capacitation events to avoid premature induction of the acrosome reaction. Studies have reported that prostasomes help to increase intracellular cAMP which then stimulates protein kinase A (PKA) to indirectly induce tyrosine phosphorylation to activate capacitation and reorganization of plasma membrane in the spermatozoon [57–61]. In vitro studies have shown that prostasomes can be responsible for transferring cholesterol to spermatozoa during end-stage capacitation [60, 62]. In addition, interactions of prostasomes within the female reproductive tract cause local modulation of the immune system and hence, prevent spermatozoa from being phagocytosed, damaged or killed by the attacks of neutrophil granulocytes [62].

Protective role of seminal plasma molecules in fertilization

In semen, both leukocytes and immature/abnormal spermatozoa are intracellular sources of ROS. If uncontrolled, ROS can lead to damages in spermatozoa proteins, lipids and DNA. Spermatozoa are particularly susceptible to oxidative damage due to the high content of polyunsaturated fatty acids (PUFAs) in their plasma membrane and also the limited inner antioxidant system [24, 63, 64]. However, SP has an efficient antioxidant defense system that protects spermatozoa during ejaculation and the first steps of their journey through the female reproductive tract [65]. SP has a great repertoire of inflammatory molecules obtained from the testes, including macrophages, somatic cells (Leydig and Sertoli cells), spermatogonia, leukocytes and mesenchymal cells [66, 67]. The secretion of seminal cytokines is also carried out by immunocompetent cells in various pathogenic conditions including leukocytospermia [68]. Cytokines are small proteins that are important in cell signaling and play a key role in the regulation of fertilization. The accumulation of cytokines and their soluble receptors such as interleukins (IL-1, IL-2, IL-4, IL-6, IL-8, IL-10, IL-12, IL-13, IL-17, IL-18), tumor necrosis factor-alpha (TNF-α), tumor necrosis factor receptor 1 and 2 (TNFR1/2), interferon-gamma (IFN-γ) and granulocyte colony-stimulating factor (G-CSF) in the SP has been observed in semen samples of both fertile and infertile men [38, 66, 67, 69]. A study by Seshadri et al. [69] confirms that cytokines seldom act in isolation and may affect sperm function directly or indirectly by acting as members of a network with other cytokines. Their results also suggest that the cytokines may not originate from the testis as their level is observed to be augmented in the obstructed azoospermic group.

SP can modulate immune responses in the male and female reproductive tracts (Table 3). During intercourse, a normal influx of leukocytes is important for the interaction of spermatozoa with the female tract [70]. This early leukocyte attack allows the female reproductive system to eliminate spermatozoa with poor fertilizing capacity based on poor DNA integrity [71]. However, the most capable spermatozoa to fertilize have to escape these harsh uterine conditions very quickly to avoid immune opposition by the female reproductive tract after their detachment from the SP microenvironment [71–73]. TGF-β in human seminal plasma plays a key role in inducing proinflammatory cytokine synthesis and leukocyte recruitment by the cervical cells [74]. Some of the proinflammatory cytokines produced by human cervical and vaginal epithelial cells after interaction with SP include granulocyte-macrophage colony-stimulating factor (GM-CSF), IL-1, IL-6 and IL-8. They also produce some chemokines, such as the monocyte chemoattractant protein-1 (MCP-1) [75, 76]. These molecules contribute to the recruitment of macrophages, dendritic cells and lymphocytes into the epithelial layers and deeper stromal tissues [5, 70, 76].

Additional studies have shown that the role of SP is not only restricted to the cervix, but it also extends to the uterus [76, 77]. Uterine receptivity is entirely dependent on a healthy uterine environment to encourage embryonic implantation [78]. Seminal constituents bound to the post-acrosomal region of the sperm head are carried in conjunction with the sperm to the higher parts of the female tract. Along with the peristaltic contractions transporting macromolecular materials, unique vascular connections facilitate the transport of progesterone and inflammatory mediators from the cervix to the endometrial tissue [40]. IL-1 and TNF-α have been found to stimulate progesterone and prostaglandin synthesis to regulate gonadotropin secretion for corpus luteum function [79]. Seminal fluid helps in the regulation of endometrial tissue remodeling and uterine

Table 3 Seminal plasma proteins in spermatozoa protection, transport and interaction with the female reproductive tract

Proteins involved	Site of Action	Mechanism of action	Reference
FOXP3	Uterine regulatory T cells	Immunosuppression and improved tolerance towards paternal antigens	[96–98]
GM-CSF	Embryo	Blastocyst stage development	[72]
IL-6	Embryo	Protection from apoptosis by secreting anti-apoptotic micro RNAs	[72]
LIF	Inner cell mass	Blastocyst development	[72]
IGF-1	Germ cells	Maturation of spermatozoa	[27, 28]
α_2-macroglobulin	Germ cells	Progressive motility	[27, 28]
Enkephalin	Sperm cells	Sperm motility	[27, 28]
VEGF, MMPs	Endometrium	Embryo implantation	[40, 99]
TGF-β, PGE	Female reproductive epithelial tissues	Inflammatory signaling response	[40, 99]
GM-CSF, IL-1A, IL-6, IL-8, MCP-1 (CCL2), MIP3A (CCL20)	Female epithelial layers and deeper stromal tissues	Immediate and rapid influx of inflammation to cause fertilization	[5, 65, 74, 99]

Several studies showing the importance of seminal plasma proteins in the regulation of male and female reproductive mechanisms. However, some of the studies were conducted with animal samples and still need validation by studies with human samples

Abbreviations: *FOXP3* forkhead box P3, *GM-CSF* granulocyte-macrophage colony stimulating factor, *IL* interleukin, *LIF* leukemia inhibitory factor, *IGF* insulin like growth gactor, *VEGF* vascular endothelial growth factor, *MMPs* matrix metalloproteinases, *TGF-β* transforming growth factor beta, *PGE* prostaglandin E synthase, *MCP-1* monocyte chemoattractant protein-1, *MIP-3A* macrophage inflammatory protein 3, *CCL* chemokine ligand receptivity by recruiting leukocytes, especially macrophages. These are further mediated by adhesion ligands such as integrins, selectins, cadherins and immunoglobulins, thereby losing the inhibitory components that may act as a barrier to an attaching embryo [40, 76, 80]. The expression of epididymal protein, E-cadherin in the SP was found to be responsible for sperm-oocyte adhesion [81]. Clinical studies on SP insemination in couples undergoing in vitro fertilization (IVF) or intracytoplasmic sperm injection (ICSI) have shown a significant improvement in embryo transfer after exposure to SP [82, 83]. Human studies indicated that when embryos were cultured in the presence of GM-CSF, blastocyst development rate was increased, leading to increased cell numbers both in the inner cell mass and trophectoderm [84]. Thus, SP plays a key role in spermatozoa protection from oxidative damage, spermatozoa function and interaction with the female reproductive tract. However, further studies are needed to clarify the role of SP in fertilization and contribution to a successful pregnancy using ART.

Seminal plasma as a source of biomarkers and targeted drug delivery

SP is a complex body fluid, containing a large diversity of proteins. The exact number of proteins expressed by the SP is not known, but possibly up to 10,000. SP proteomics is regarded as a great resource for the discovery of potential biomarkers to improve diagnosis or classification of a wide range of male reproductive disorders. However, the major limitations are the complexity of SP proteome, the inter- and intra-individual variation and the probability of the low abundant proteins to be masked in the presence of very high abundant proteins like semenogelins. This implies that the discovery of low abundance proteins with a critical role in reproductive functions could be facilitated by a selective removal of high abundant proteins using specific methods such as immunoprecipitation. For instance, the removal of the top high abundant proteins from blood by a single-step purification method using a mixer of high-specificity polyclonal antibodies (MARS) is commercially available [85]. Additionally, extracellular vesicles such as exosomes were isolated from small volumes of human blood plasma by Protein Organic Solvent Precipitation (PROSPR) [86]. Similar methods should be applied to SP samples to clarify the role of low abundance SP proteins in male fertility.

Seminal exosomal vesicles may be developed for targeted delivery of drugs, vaccines and anti-virals. Recent in vivo studies indicated specific cell tropism by exosomes, which based on their unique characteristics and origin, can be targeted to tissues and/or organs [87–90]. Intravenous injection of exosomes expressing a neuron-targeting protein on their surface into mice was reported to elicit specific gene knockdown in the brain [91]. Furthermore, in murine model of Parkinson's disease, administration of autologous macrophage-derived exosomes loaded with catalase, produced potent anti-inflammatory and neuroprotective effects [92]. Modification of exosomal membrane is feasible and can be developed to enhance their targeting capability and specificity [93]. It was possible to target exosomes expressing an epidermal growth factor receptor (EGFR)-binding peptide to tumor cells [94]. The major envelope of Epstein–Barr-Virus protein gp350 incorporated into the exosomal membrane target B cells and resulted in improved interaction between helper T cells and B cells [95]. Exosome-mediated therapy may ultimately lead to in vitro maturation of gametes and improvement of ART outcomes. However, more studies need to be conducted to support these early-stage discoveries and develop an interesting technique from the clinical point of view.

Conclusion

Diagnostic tools to assess male infertility are limited, particularly for investigation of idiopathic infertility. Therefore routine semen analysis is still the basis for evaluation of a subject's fertility status. However, as semen analysis offers a rough assessment of male fertility, additional diagnostic tools are needed in a clinical setting. Emerging 'omics studies' in general and high throughput proteomics of SP in particular, holds promise for the development of novel biomarkers. These biomarkers could be useful in the evaluation of natural fertility, differentiating between the various infertility etiologies, and predicting ART success. Nevertheless, a closer look into the seminal exosomes, natural nanocarriers, could bring new insights for targeted drug delivery for new therapies.

Abbreviations

2D-DIGE: Two-dimensional difference gel electrophoresis; ART: Assisted reproductive technologies; B2M: Beta-2-microglobulin; cADPR: Cyclic adenosine diphosphoribose; CNDP2: Cytosolic nonspecific dipeptidase; ECM1: Extracellular matrix protein 1; FAM3D: Family with sequence similarity 3 member D; G-CSF: Granulocyte colony-stimulating factor; GM-CSF: Granulocyte-macrophage colony-stimulating factor; GO: Gene ontology; GPI: Glycosylphosphatidylinositol; GPX5: Type 5 glutathione peroxidase; hCAP18: Human cationic antimicrobial protein; ICSI: Intracytoplasmic sperm injection; IFN-γ: Interferon-gamma; IL: Interleukin; IVF: In vitro fertilization; LC: Liquid chromatography; LDHC: Lactate dehydrogenase C; LGALS3BP: Galectin 3 binding protein; MALDI: Matrix-assisted laser desorption/ionization; MCP-1: Monocyte chemoattractant protein-1; MIF: Macrophage migration inhibitory factor; MIP: Macrophage inflammatory protein; MME: Membrane metalloendopeptidase; MS: Mass spectrometry; MS/MS: Tandem mass spectrometry; PAP: Prostatic acid phosphatase; PGDS: Prostaglandin-D synthase; PGK2: Phosphoglycerate kinase 2;

β: Transforming growth factor beta; TKTL1: Transketolase-like protein 1; TMPRSS2: Type 2 transmembrane serine protease; TNFR1/2: Tumor necrosis factor receptor 1 or 2; TNF-α: Tumor necrosis factor-alpha; TOF: Time-of-flight

Acknowledgements
Authors wish to thank Dr. Damayanthi Durairajanayagam, PhD (MARA University of Technology, Malaysia) for her help in reviewing and editing this manuscript.

Funding
Financial support for this study was provided by the American Center for Reproductive Medicine, Cleveland Clinic, Ohio, USA. RP thanks Council of Scientific and Industrial Research for the award of senior research fellowship (09/1036/0005/2016 EMR-I). Tania R. Dias was supported by "Fundação para a Ciência e a Tecnologia" (FCT, SFRH/BD/109284/2015) and Fulbright Program (E0585639).

Authors' contributions
AA conceived the idea, provided guidance and edited the article for submission. RP wrote the manuscript. LS designed the study, compiled the information, helped with the writing, reviewing and editing. TRD helped in reorganizing the structure of the manuscript and tables, edited the text and introduced new information. All authors read and approved the final manuscript.

Competing interests
The authors declare that they have no competing interests.

Author details
[1]American Center for Reproductive Medicine, Cleveland Clinic, 10681 Carnegie Avenue, Desk X11, Cleveland, OH 44195, USA. [2]Redox Biology Laboratory, Department of Zoology, School of Life Sciences, Ravenshaw University, Cuttack, Odisha 753003, India. [3]Universidade da Beira Interior, 6201-001 Covilhã, Portugal. [4]Department of Microscopy, Laboratory of Cell Biology, Institute of Biomedical Sciences Abel Salazar and Unit for Multidisciplinary Research in Biomedicine, University of Porto, 4050-313 Porto, Portugal. [5]LAQV/REQUIMTE - Laboratory of Bromatology and Hydrology, Faculty of Pharmacy, University of Porto, 4050-313 Porto, Portugal.

References
1. Gonzales GF, Villena A. True corrected seminal fructose level: a better marker of the function of seminal vesicles in infertile men. Int J Androl. 2001;24:255–60.
2. Drake RR, White KY, Fuller TW, Igwe E, Clements MA, Nyalwidhe JO, Given RW, Lance RS, Semmes OJ. Clinical collection and protein properties of expressed prostatic secretions as a source for biomarkers of prostatic disease. J Proteome. 2009;72:907–17.
3. Milardi D, Grande G, Vincenzoni F, Messana I, Pontecorvi A, De Marinis L, Castagnola M, Marana R. Proteomic approach in the identification of fertility pattern in seminal plasma of fertile men. Fertil Steril. 2012;97:67–73. e1
4. Primakoff P, Myles DG. Penetration, adhesion, and fusion in mammalian sperm-egg interaction. Sci. 2002;296:2183–5.
5. Robertson SA. Seminal plasma and male factor signalling in the female reproductive tract. Cell Tissue Res. 2005;322:43–52.
6. Drabovich AP, Saraon P, Jarvi K, Diamandis EP. Seminal plasma as a diagnostic fluid for male reproductive system disorders. Nat Rev Urol. 2014;11:278–88.
7. Verze P, Cai T, Lorenzetti S. The role of the prostate in male fertility, health and disease. Nat Rev Urol. 2016;13:379–86.
8. Ferens-Sieczkowska M, Kowalska B, Kratz EM. Seminal plasma glycoproteins in male infertility and prostate diseases: is there a chance for glyco-biomarkers? Biomarkers. 2013;18:10–22.
9. Lenzi A, Picardo M, Gandini L, Dondero F. Lipids of the sperm plasma membrane: from polyunsaturated fatty acids considered as markers of sperm function to possible scavenger therapy. Hum Reprod Update. 1996;2:246–56.
10. Owen DH, Katz DF. A review of the physical and chemical properties of human semen and the formulation of a semen simulant. J Androl. 2005;26:459–69.
11. Li HG, Huang SY, Zhou H, Liao AH, Xiong CL. Quick recovery and characterization of cell-free DNA in seminal plasma of normozoospermia and azoospermia: implications for non-invasive genetic utilities. Asian J Androl. 2009;11:703–9.
12. Wu W, Hu Z, Qin Y, Dong J, Dai J, Lu C, Zhang W, Shen H, Xia Y, Wang X. Seminal plasma microRNAs: potential biomarkers for spermatogenesis status. Mol Hum Reprod. 2012;18:489–97.
13. Davalieva K, Kiprijanovska S, Noveski P, Plaseski T, Kocevska B, Broussard C, Plaseska-Karanfilska D. Proteomic analysis of seminal plasma in men with different spermatogenic impairment. Andrologia. 2012;44:256–64.
14. Pilch B, Mann M. Large-scale and high-confidence proteomic analysis of human seminal plasma. Genome Biol. 2006;7:R40.
15. Gonzales GF. Function of seminal vesicles and their role on male fertility. Asian J Androl. 2001;3:251–8.
16. Posner C. Berl Klin Wochenschr, vol. 25; 1888. p. 416.
17. Gray S, Huggins C. Electrophoretic analysis of human semen. Proc Soc Exp Biol Med. 1942;50:351–3.
18. Ross V, Moore DH, Miller EG. Proteins of human seminal plasma. J Biol Chem. 1942;144:667–77.
19. Sensabaugh GF. Isolation and characterization of a semen-specific protein from human seminal plasma: a potential new marker for semen identification. J Forensic Sci. 1978;23:106–15.
20. Edwards JJ, Tollaksen SL, Anderson NG. Proteins of human semen. I. Two-dimensional mapping of human seminal fluid. Clin Chem. 1981;27:1335–40.
21. Starita-Geribaldi M, Roux F, Garin J, Chevallier D, Fenichel P, Pointis G. Development of narrow immobilized pH gradients covering one pH unit for human seminal plasma proteomic analysis. Proteomics. 2003;3:1611–9.
22. Fung KY, Morris C, Sathe S, Sack R, Duncan MW. Characterization of the in vivo forms of lacrimal-specific proline-rich proteins in human tear fluid. Proteomics. 2004;4:3953–9.
23. Rolland AD, Lavigne R, Dauly C, Calvel P, Kervarrec C, Freour T, Evrard B, Rioux-Leclercq N, Auger J, Pineau C. Identification of genital tract markers in the human seminal plasma using an integrative genomics approach. Hum Reprod. 2013;28:199–209.
24. Agarwal A, Ayaz A, Samanta L, Sharma R, Assidi M, Abuzenadah AM, Sabanegh E. Comparative proteomic network signatures in seminal plasma of infertile men as a function of reactive oxygen species. Clin Proteomics. 2015;12:23.
25. Del Giudice PT, Belardin LB, Camargo M, Zylbersztejn DS, Carvalho VM, Cardozo KH, Bertolla RP, Cedenho AP. Determination of testicular function in adolescents with varicocoele - a proteomics approach. Androl. 2016;4:447–55.
26. Yamakawa K, Yoshida K, Nishikawa H, Kato T, Iwamoto T. Comparative analysis of interindividual variations in the seminal plasma proteome of fertile men with identification of potential markers for azoospermia in infertile patients. J Androl. 2007;28:858–65.
27. Wang J, Wang J, Zhang HR, Shi HJ, Ma D, Zhao HX, Lin B, Li RS. Proteomic analysis of seminal plasma from asthenozoospermia patients reveals proteins that affect oxidative stress responses and semen quality. Asian J Androl. 2009;11:484–91.
28. Kagedan D, Lecker I, Batruch I, Smith C, Kaploun I, Lo K, Grober E, Diamandis EP, Jarvi KA. Characterization of the seminal plasma proteome in men with prostatitis by mass spectrometry. Clin Proteomics. 2012;9:2.
29. Sharma R, Agarwal A, Mohanty G, Du Plessis SS, Gopalan B, Willard B, Yadav SP, Sabanegh E. Proteomic analysis of seminal fluid from men exhibiting oxidative stress. Reprod Biol Endocrinol. 2013;11:85.
30. Yang L, Nyalwidhe JO, Guo S, Drake RR, Semmes OJ. Targeted identification of metastasis-associated cell-surface sialoglycoproteins in prostate cancer. Mol Cell Proteomics. 2011;M110(007294):10.
31. Diamandis EP, Arnett WP, Foussias G, Pappas H, Ghandi S, Melegos DN, Mullen B, Yu H, Srigley J, Jarvi K. Seminal plasma biochemical markers and their association with semen analysis findings. Urol. 1999;53:596–603.
32. Heshmat SM, Mullen JB, Jarvi KA, Soosaipillai A, Diamandis EP, Hamilton RJ, Lo KC. Seminal plasma lipocalin-type prostaglandin D synthase: a potential new marker for the diagnosis of obstructive azoospermia. J Urol. 2008;179:1077–80.
33. Drabovich AP, Jarvi K, Diamandis EP. Verification of male infertility biomarkers in seminal plasma by multiplex selected reaction monitoring assay. Mol Cell Proteomics. 2011;10:M110.004127.

34. Lamirande E, Yoshida K, Yoshiike M, Iwamoto T, Gagnon C. Semenogelin, the main protein of semen coagulum, inhibits human sperm capacitation by interfering with the superoxide anion generated during this process. J Androl. 2001;22:672–9.
35. Zhao C, Huo R, Wang FQ, Lin M, Zhou ZM, Sha JH. Identification of several proteins involved in regulation of sperm motility by proteomic analysis. Fertil Steril. 2007;87:436–8.
36. Malm J, Sørensen O, Persson T, Frohm-Nilsson M, Johansson B, Bjartell A, Lilja H, Ståhle-Bäckdahl M, Borregaard N, Egesten A. The human cationic antimicrobial protein (hCAP-18) is expressed in the epithelium of human epididymis, is present in seminal plasma at high concentrations, and is attached to spermatozoa. Infect Immun. 2000;68:4297–302.
37. Sharma R, Agarwal A, Mohanty G, Jesudasan R, Gopalan B, Willard B, Yadav SP, Sabanegh E. Functional proteomic analysis of seminal plasma proteins in men with various semen parameters. Reprod Biol Endocrinol. 2013;11:38.
38. Havrylyuk A, Chopyak V, Boyko Y, Kril I, Kurpisz M. Cytokines in the blood and semen of infertile patients. Cent Eur J Immunol. 2015;40:337–44.
39. Anderson DJ, Politch JA. Role of seminal plasma in human female reproductive failure: immunomodulation, inflammation, and infections. Adv Exp Med Biol. 2015;868:159–69.
40. Robertson SA, Bromfield JJ, Glynn DJ, Sharkey DJ, Jasper MJ. Actions of seminal plasma cytokines in priming female reproductive tract receptivity for embryo implantation. In: Mor G, editor. Immunology of pregnancy. New York: Springer; 2006. p. 148–58.
41. Foster JA, Klotz KL, Flickinger CJ, Thomas TS, Wright RM, Castillo JR, Herr JC. Human SP-10: acrosomal distribution, processing, and fate after the acrosome reaction. Biol Reprod. 1994;51:1222–31.
42. Coppola MA, Klotz KL, Kim KA, Cho HY, Kang J, Shetty J, Howards SS, Flickinger CJ, Herr JC. SpermCheck fertility, an immunodiagnostic home test that detects normozoospermia and severe oligozoospermia. Hum Reprod. 2010;25:853–61.
43. Aalberts M, van Dissel-Emiliani FM, van Adrichem NP, van Wijnen M, Wauben MH, Stout TA, Stoorvogel W. Identification of distinct populations of prostasomes that differentially express prostate stem cell antigen, annexin A1, and GLIPR2 in humans. Biol Reprod. 2012;86:82.
44. Machtinger R, Laurent LC, Baccarelli AA. Extracellular vesicles: roles in gamete maturation, fertilization and embryo implantation. Hum Reprod Update. 2016;22:182–93.
45. Colombo M, Raposo G, Thery C. Biogenesis, secretion, and intercellular interactions of exosomes and other extracellular vesicles. Annu Rev Cell Dev Biol. 2014;30:255–89.
46. Valadi H, Ekstrom K, Bossios A, Sjostrand M, Lee JJ, Lotvall JO. Exosome-mediated transfer of mRNAs and microRNAs is a novel mechanism of genetic exchange between cells. Nat Cell Biol. 2007;9:654–U72.
47. Nolte-'t Hoen EN, Buermans HP, Waasdorp M, Stoorvogel W, Wauben MH, Hoen PA T. Deep sequencing of RNA from immune cell-derived vesicles uncovers the selective incorporation of small non-coding RNA biotypes with potential regulatory functions. Nucleic Acids Res. 2012;40:9272–85.
48. Yanez-Mo M, Siljander PRM, Andreu Z, Zavec AB, Borras FE, Buzas EI, Buzas K, Casal E, Cappello F, Carvalho J, et al. Biological properties of extracellular vesicles and their physiological functions. J Extracell Vesicles. 2015;4:27066.
49. Yang C, Guo WB, Zhang WS, Bian J, Yang JK, Zhou QZ, Chen MK, Peng W, Qi T, Wang CY, Liu CD. Comprehensive proteomics analysis of exosomes derived from human seminal plasma. Androl. 2017;5:1007–15.
50. Sullivan R. Epididymosomes: a heterogeneous population of microvesicles with multiple functions in sperm maturation and storage. Asian J Androl. 2015;17:726–9.
51. D'Amours O, Frenette G, Bordeleau LJ, Allard N, Leclerc P, Blondin P, Sullivan R. Epididymosomes transfer epididymal sperm binding protein 1 (ELSPBP1) to dead spermatozoa during epididymal transit in bovine. Biol Reprod. 2012;87:94.
52. Aalberts M, Stout TA, Stoorvogel W. Prostasomes: extracellular vesicles from the prostate. Reprod. 2014;147:R1–14.
53. Sullivan R. Epididymosomes: a heterogeneous population of microvesicles with multiple functions in sperm maturation and storage. Asian J Androl. 2015;17:726.
54. Poliakov A, Spilman M, Dokland T, Amling CL, Mobley JA. Structural heterogeneity and protein composition of exosome-like vesicles (prostasomes) in human semen. Prostate. 2009;69:159–67.
55. Utleg AG, Yi EC, Xie T, Shannon P, White JT, Goodlett DR, Hood L, Lin B. Proteomic analysis of human prostasomes. Prostate. 2003;56:150–61.
56. Park KH, Kim BJ, Kang J, Nam TS, Lim JM, Kim HT, Park JK, Kim YG, Chae SW, Kim UH. Ca2+ signaling tools acquired from prostasomes are required for progesterone-induced sperm motility. Sci Signal. 2011;4:ra31.
57. Bailey JL. Factors regulating sperm capacitation. Syst Biol Reprod Med. 2010; 56:334–48.
58. Fraser LR. The "switching on" of mammalian spermatozoa: molecular events involved in promotion and regulation of capacitation. Mol Reprod Dev. 2010;77:197–208.
59. Harrison RA, Miller NG. cAMP-dependent protein kinase control of plasma membrane lipid architecture in boar sperm. Mol Reprod Dev. 2000;55:220–8.
60. Pons-Rejraji H, Artonne C, Sion B, Brugnon F, Canis M, Janny L, Grizard G. Prostasomes: inhibitors of capacitation and modulators of cellular signalling in human sperm. Int J Androl. 2011;34:568–80.
61. Visconti PE, Westbrook VA, Chertihin O, Demarco I, Sleight S, Diekman AB. Novel signaling pathways involved in sperm acquisition of fertilizing capacity. J Reprod Immunol. 2002;53:133–50.
62. Aalberts M, Sostaric E, Wubbolts R, Wauben MW, Nolte-'t Hoen EN, Gadella BM, Stout TA, Stoorvogel W. Spermatozoa recruit prostasomes in response to capacitation induction. Biochim Biophys Acta. 1834;2013:2326–35.
63. Henkel RR. Leukocytes and oxidative stress: dilemma for sperm function and male fertility. Asian J Androl. 2011;13:43–52.
64. Pasqualotto FF, Sharma RK, Nelson DR, Thomas AJ, Agarwal A. Relationship between oxidative stress, semen characteristics, and clinical diagnosis in men undergoing infertility investigation. Fertil Steril. 2000;73:459–64.
65. WS O, Chen H, Chow PH. Male genital tract antioxidant enzymes–their ability to preserve sperm DNA integrity. Mol Cell Endocrinol. 2006;250:80–3.
66. Maegawa M, Kamada M, Irahara M, Yamamoto S, Yoshikawa S, Kasai Y, Ohmoto Y, Gima H, Thaler CJ, Aono T. A repertoire of cytokines in human seminal plasma. J Reprod Immunol. 2002;54:33–42.
67. Politch JA, Tucker L, Bowman FP, Anderson DJ. Concentrations and significance of cytokines and other immunologic factors in semen of healthy fertile men. Hum Reprod. 2007;22:2928–35.
68. Fraczek M, Czernikiewicz A, Kurpisz M. Cytokines and oxidative stress in the germ line. In: Agarwal A, Aitken RJ, Alvarez JG, editors. Studies on Men's health and fertility. Totowa: Humana press; 2012. p. 179–205.
69. Seshadri S, Bates M, Vince G, Jones DI. The role of cytokine expression in different subgroups of subfertile men. Am J Reprod Immunol. 2009;62:275–82.
70. Sharkey DJ, Tremellen KP, Jasper MJ, Gemzell-Danielsson K, Robertson SA. Seminal fluid induces leukocyte recruitment and cytokine and chemokine mRNA expression in the human cervix after coitus. J Immunol. 2012;188:2445–54.
71. Velando A, Torres R, Alonso-Alvarez C. Avoiding bad genes: oxidatively damaged DNA in germ line and mate choice. BioEssays. 2008;30:1212–9.
72. Bromfield JJ, Schjenken JE, Chin PY, Care AS, Jasper MJ, Robertson SA. Maternal tract factors contribute to paternal seminal fluid impact on metabolic phenotype in offspring. Proc Natl Acad Sci U S A. 2014;111:2200–5.
73. Suarez SS, Pacey AA. Sperm transport in the female reproductive tract. Hum Reprod Update. 2006;12:23–37.
74. Sharkey DJ, Macpherson AM, Tremellen KP, Mottershead DG, Gilchrist RB, Robertson SA. TGF-beta mediates proinflammatory seminal fluid signaling in human cervical epithelial cells. J Immunol. 2012;189:1024–35.
75. Sharkey DJ, Macpherson AM, Tremellen KP, Robertson SA. Seminal plasma differentially regulates inflammatory cytokine gene expression in human cervical and vaginal epithelial cells. Mol Hum Reprod. 2007;13:491–501.
76. Gutsche S, von Wolff M, Strowitzki T, Thaler CJ. Seminal plasma induces mRNA expression of IL-1beta, IL-6 and LIF in endometrial epithelial cells in vitro. Mol Hum Reprod. 2003;9:785–91.
77. Robertson SA, Mau VJ, Hudson SN, Tremellen KP. Cytokine-leukocyte networks and the establishment of pregnancy. Am J Reprod Immunol. 1997;37:438–42.
78. Brosens JJ, Salker MS, Teklenburg G, Nautiyal J, Salter S, Lucas ES, Steel JH, Christian M, Chan YW, Boomsma CM, et al. Uterine selection of human embryos at implantation. Sci Rep. 2014;4:3894.
79. Pate JL. Involvement of immune cells in regulation of ovarian function. J Reprod Fertil Suppl. 1995;49:365–77.
80. Achache H, Revel A. Endometrial receptivity markers, the journey to successful embryo implantation. Hum Reprod Update. 2006;12:731–46.
81. Marin-Briggiler CI, Veiga MF, Matos ML, Echeverria MF, Furlong LI, Vazquez-Levin MH. Expression of epithelial cadherin in the human male reproductive tract and gametes and evidence of its participation in fertilization. Mol Hum Reprod. 2008;14:561–71.
82. Friedler S, Ben-Ami I, Gidoni Y, Strassburger D, Kasterstein E, Maslansky B, Komarovsy D, Bern O, Ron-El R, Raziel A. Effect of seminal plasma application to the vaginal vault in in vitro fertilization or intracytoplasmic sperm injection treatment cycles-a double-blind, placebo-controlled, randomized study. J Assist Reprod Genet. 2013;30:907–11.

83. Chicea R, Ispasoiu F, Focsa M. Seminal plasma insemination during ovum-pickup–a method to increase pregnancy rate in IVF/ICSI procedure. A pilot randomized trial. J Assist Reprod Genet. 2013;30:569–74.
84. Robertson SA, Sjoblom C, Jasper MJ, Norman RJ, Seamark RF. Granulocyte-macrophage colony-stimulating factor promotes glucose transport and blastomere viability in murine preimplantation embryos. Biol Reprod. 2001; 64:1206–15.
85. Bellei E, Bergamini S, Monari E, Fantoni LI, Cuoghi A, Ozben T, Tomasi A. High-abundance proteins depletion for serum proteomic analysis: concomitant removal of non-targeted proteins. Amino Acids. 2011;40:145–56.
86. Gallart-Palau X, Serra A, Wong ASW, Sandin S, Lai MK, Chen CP, Kon OL, Sze SK. Extracellular vesicles are rapidly purified from human plasma by PRotein organic solvent PRecipitation (PROSPR). Sci Rep. 2015;5:14664.
87. Zomer A, Maynard C, Verweij Frederik J, Kamermans A, Schäfer R, Beerling E, Schiffelers Raymond M, de Wit E, Berenguer J, Ellenbroek Saskia Inge J, et al. Vivo imaging reveals extracellular vesicle-mediated Phenocopying of metastatic behavior. Cell. 2015;161:1046–57.
88. Fruhbeis C, Frohlich D, Kuo WP, Amphornrat J, Thilemann S, Saab AS, Kirchhoff F, Mobius W, Goebbels S, Nave KA, et al. Neurotransmitter-triggered transfer of exosomes mediates oligodendrocyte-neuron communication. PLoS Biol. 2013;11:e1001604.
89. Kim MS, Haney MJ, Zhao Y, Mahajan V, Deygen I, Klyachko NL, Inskoe E, Piroyan A, Sokolsky M, Okolie O, et al. Development of exosome-encapsulated paclitaxel to overcome MDR in cancer cells. Nanomedicine. 2016;12:655–64.
90. Ridder K, Sevko A, Heide J, Dams M, Rupp AK, Macas J, Starmann J, Tjwa M, Plate KH, Sultmann H, et al. Extracellular vesicle-mediated transfer of functional RNA in the tumor microenvironment. Oncoimmunology. 2015;4:e1008371.
91. Zhang Y, Chopp M, Meng Y, Katakowski M, Xin H, Mahmood A, Xiong Y. Effect of exosomes derived from multipluripotent mesenchymal stromal cells on functional recovery and neurovascular plasticity in rats after traumatic brain injury. J Neurosurg. 2015;122:856–67.
92. Haney MJ, Klyachko NL, Zhaoa YL, Gupta R, Plotnikova EG, He ZJ, Patel T, Piroyan A, Sokolsky M, Kabanov AV, Batrakova EV. Exosomes as drug delivery vehicles for Parkinson's disease therapy. J Control Release. 2015;207:18–30.
93. Gajos-Michniewicz A, Duechler M, Czyz M. MiRNA in melanoma-derived exosomes. Cancer Lett. 2014;347:29–37.
94. Ohno S, Takanashi M, Sudo K, Ueda S, Ishikawa A, Matsuyama N, Fujita K, Mizutani T, Ohgi T, Ochiya T, et al. Systemically injected exosomes targeted to EGFR deliver antitumor microRNA to breast cancer cells. Mol Ther. 2013; 21:185–91.
95. Ruiss R, Jochum S, Mocikat R, Hammerschmidt W, Zeidler R. EBV-gp350 confers B-cell tropism to tailored exosomes and is a neo-antigen in normal and malignant B cells–a new option for the treatment of B-CLL. PLoS One. 2011;6:e25294.
96. Robertson SA, Guerin LR, Bromfield JJ, Branson KM, Ahlstrom AC, Care AS. Seminal fluid drives expansion of the CD4+CD25+ T regulatory cell pool and induces tolerance to paternal alloantigens in mice. Biol Reprod. 2009; 80:1036–45.
97. Zenclussen AC, Hammerling GJ. Cellular regulation of the uterine microenvironment that enables embryo implantation. Front Immunol. 2015;6:321.
98. Jasper MJ, Tremellen KP, Robertson SA. Primary unexplained infertility is associated with reduced expression of the T-regulatory cell transcription factor Foxp3 in endometrial tissue. Mol Hum Reprod. 2006;12:301–8.
99. Tremellen KP, Seamark RF, Robertson SA. Seminal transforming growth factor beta1 stimulates granulocyte-macrophage colony-stimulating factor production and inflammatory cell recruitment in the murine uterus. Biol Reprod. 1998;58:1217–25.

16

Effects of pelvic endometriosis and adenomyosis on ciliary beat frequency and muscular contractions in the human fallopian tube

Wei Xia[1,2†], Duo Zhang[1,2†], Jing Ouyang[1,2†], Yan Liang[1,2], Huiyu Zhang[1,2], Zhen Huang[1,2], Guiling Liang[1,2], Qian Zhu[1,2], Xiaoming Guan[3*] and Jian Zhang[1,2*]

Abstract

Background: Pelvic endometriosis (EM) and adenomyosis (AM) have different effects on the fallopian tube. This study aimed to assess the transport capability of the fallopian tube in women with pelvic EM or AM.

Methods: Twenty women with uterine leiomyoma (control group), 20 with adenomyosis without pelvic EM (AM group) and 35 with pelvic EM without AM (EM group) were included. EM cases were further divided into the tubal EM and non-tubal EM subgroups. Ciliary beat frequency (CBF), percentage of ciliated cells, and smooth muscle contraction were measured.

Results: CBFs of the ampulla in EM cases were significantly lower than those of control and AM cases; CBFs of the ampulla and isthmus in tubal EM cases were significantly lower than those of the control group and non-tubal EM subgroup. In both the ampulla and isthmus segment, percentages of ciliated cells in EM patients were significantly lower than those of AM and control patients; the tubal EM subgroup showed significantly lower values than the control group and non-tubal EM subgroup. Amplitude-to-weight ratios of longitudinal muscular contractility in EM cases were significantly lower than control values; tubal EM cases showed significantly lower values than controls and the non-tubal EM subgroup. Contraction frequencies in EM cases were significantly lower than those of control and AM cases, in both longitudinal and circular muscles; tubal EM cases showed significantly lower values than controls and the non-tubal EM subgroup.

Conclusion: EM with tubal EM damaged transport function of the fallopian tube, to varying degrees, whereas tubal function in EM without tubal EM and in AM is not altered.

Keywords: Endometriosis, Adenomyosis, Ciliary beat frequency (CBF), Muscular contraction, Percentage of ciliated cells

Background

Although the association of endometriosis (EM) with infertility is well recognized, the mechanisms that underlie this enigmatic disease remain unclear [1]. The overall prevalence of EM in infertile women in population-based studies varies from 20 to 50% [2]. It is generally admitted that infertility related to endometriosis can result from many factors affecting the reproductive process, including altered folliculogenesis or ovulation, defects in luteal phase function, mechanical distortion of female pelvic anatomy, impaired oocyte release or pickup, altered sperm function, and disturbances in uterine contractility [1–3]. Distortion of pelvic anatomy adversely affects sperm motility, egg transport, fertilization, and embryo transport.

Each human fallopian tube can be divided into the interstitial section, isthmus, ampulla, and fimbria. In a cross-section, the fallopian tube comprises four layers, including the serosa, subserosa, lamina propria, and innermost mucosa rich in cilia. In the reproductive process, the fallopian

* Correspondence: xiaoming@bcm.edu; zhangjian_ipmch@sjtu.edu.cn
†Equal contributors
3Department of Obstetrics & Gynaecology, Baylor College of Medicine, Houston, TX, USA
1Department of Obstetrics and Gynaecology, International Peace Maternity and Child Health Hospital, School of Medicine, Shanghai Jiaotong University, Shanghai, China
Full list of author information is available at the end of the article

tube plays a crucial role in gamete transport, fertilization, and early embryo development. Gamete transportation is affected by contractions of the tubal musculature, ciliary activity, and the flow of tubal secretions [4, 5]. Unlike the ovary and uterus, which have been extensively studied and relatively well understood, the oviduct is less defined for its contribution to the reproduction [6].

Recent findings have suggested new pathomechanisms of endometriosis and adenomyosis, as both result from the same physiological mechanism of "tissue injury and repair" (TIAR) [7] and can be regarded as variants of the same disease—a dislocation of basal endometrium [8]. In EM, the ectopic endometrium (including the glands and stroma) appearing outside the uterine cavity, most often affects the ovary, pelvic peritoneum, sacral ligaments, and fallopian tubes. Meanwhile, adenomyosis is considered a benign invasion of the endometrium into the myometrium.

It is increasingly evident that the mechanism of tubal transport is much more complex than originally thought and can be affected by a wide range of factors; however, the presence of lesions that may entrap the tubes in infertile women with moderate and severe EM is clearly understood [9]. To the best of our knowledge, few studies have assessed the association of fallopian tube function in pelvic EM without tubal lesions or AM with subfertility. Kissler and coworkers examined sperm utero-tubal transport by hysterosalpingoscintigraphy (HSSG) and revealed that sperm transport is significantly reduced in infertile women with AM combined with pelvic EM, with pregnancy rate diminished due to this impairment [10, 11]. Studies analyzing the effects of peritoneal fluid samples from women with endometriosis on ciliary beat frequency (CBF) concluded that CBF is significantly lower in women with endometriosis compared with fertile controls [12, 13]. Reeve and coworkers demonstrated that sperm binding to the tubal epithelium may be disrupted in women with endometriosis [14].

Currently, it is commonly admitted that the function of the fallopian tube can be precisely assessed by CBF and tubal smooth muscle contraction. However, no study simultaneously evaluating the transport capacity of cilia and muscles of the fallopian tube by the above methods in women with pelvic EM and AM is available. The present study aimed to assess the transport capability of the fallopian tube by CBF and tubal smooth muscle contraction in women with pelvic EM or AM.

Methods

Participants

This study was approved by the institutional ethics committee of the International Peace Maternity and Child Health Hospital in Shanghai, China (No. GKLW 2016-42). Written informed consent was obtained from each participant before enrolment.

Fallopian tube specimens were obtained were obtained between June 2016 and August 2017 at the Department of Obstetrics and Gynecology of the International Peace Maternity and Child Health Hospital, Shanghai. The specimens were obtained from 20 women with uterine leiomyoma (control group), 20 with adenomyosis without pelvic EM, and 35 with pelvic EM without AM according to the MRI before operation (all EM patients had ovarian endometrioma). All the patients with uterine leiomyoma and adenomyosis were treated with hysterectomy and salpingectomy. All the diagnosis were depended on the pathological examinations. All women had a regular menstrual cycle, and had not used hormonal medication within 3 months of surgery; they had no history of tubal surgery. As shown by pathological examination, all the women included in the present study were in the proliferative stage.

Before surgery, the participants were interviewed personally using a standard questionnaire on paper the day before operation for sociodemographic characteristics, reproductive history, the visual analogue scale (VAS) score, and the Mansfield-Voad-Jorgensen (MVJ) score, which ranging from 1 (spotting) to 6 (gushing) to assess the menstrual blood loss. An MVJ score equal to or > 5 is considered hypermenorrhoea [15].

Collection of human fallopian tubes

The ampulla and isthmus of the fallopian tube in each participant were placed in 50 mL tubes containing the culture medium (Dulbecco modified Eagle medium) and we transported the specimens from operation room to the lab for experiments in 10 min. The fallopian tubes were rinsed several times to remove all visible blood, and the muscular and epithelial tissues were dissected.

Hematoxylin and eosin (H&E) staining and immunohistochemistry

Specimens were fixed with paraformaldehyde for 48 h at 4 °C, dehydrated in graded ethanol, paraffin embedded, and sliced into 5-μm-thick sections using a microtome (Leica, Wetzlar, Germany). Subsequently, the sections were deparaffinized with xylene and stained with H&E. For immunohistochemistry, the sections were treated with 3% hydrogen peroxide. After three washes in phosphate-buffered saline (PBS, Goodbio technology Co., Ltd., Wuhan, China), 10% normal mouse serum was applied for 15 min, followed by incubation with mouse monoclonal anti-CD10 (clone 56C6, Thermo Scientific) antibody overnight in a humidified chamber at 4 °C. Then, the sections were incubated with goat anti-mouse secondary antibody for 30 min at room temperature, sand detected by

3,30-diaminobenzidine tetra-hydrochloride solution (DAB, Goodbio technology Co., Ltd., Wuhan, China) [16].

Diagnostic criteria of tubal endometriosis

Tubal EM diagnosis was confirmed by final postoperative pathology based on H&E staining and CD10 immunohistochemistry. Tubal EM cases were evaluated and classified as proposed by Kurman and coworkers [17]. All assessments were performed independently by two experienced pathologists, in a blinded manner. Any disagreements between the two pathologists required evaluation by a third pathologist, and the final results were determined by the two pathologists.

Measurement of CBF

Small (1–2 mm^2) pieces of oviduct epithelium were separated from the isthmus-ampulla portion of the fallopian tube. CBF was measured on an inverted bright-field microscope (Leica DMi8, Leica Co., Germany) equipped with a × 40 objective. Moving cilia were imaged and analyzed as previously described [18]. Five regions were randomly selected in each specimen, and two specimens per patient were measured. Thus, a total of 10 CBF measurements were performed per sample and averaged.

Percentage of ciliated cells

Specimens were fixed in paraformaldehyde solution for hematoxylin and eosin (H&E) staining for 48 h at 4 °C, dehydrated in a graded ethanol series, and paraffin embedded. Sections (5 μm) were cut on a microtome (Leica, Wetzlar, Germany). The morphology of the oviduct epithelium was analyzed under a microscope (DSM 2500; Leica Stereozoom, Leica Microsystems, Heerbrugg, Switzerland). Five images were randomly acquired per sample. In each image, all cells as well as ciliated cells were counted (× 400 magnification) [19, 20].

Contraction of muscle strips

The isthmus-ampulla segments of fallopian tube samples were immediately removed and placed in a glass beaker containing cooled Krebs solution. Circular and longitudinal muscle strips (2 mm × 8 mm) of human oviducts were prepared. The isolated smooth muscle strips were placed in isolated organ baths filled with Krebs solution (5.9 mM KCl, 1.2 mM NaH_2PO_4, 1.2 mM $MgCl_2$, 120. 6 mM NaCl, 15.4 mM $NaHCO_3$, 11.5 mM glucose and 2.5 mM $CaCl_2$), incubated in an environment containing 95% O_2 and 5% CO_2, and connected with tension transducers. The strips were equilibrated for 30 min, and stretched with a tension of 0.3 g.

Statistical analysis

Statistical analyses were performed with GraphPad Prism 6.0 (GraphPad Soft-ware Inc., California, USA). Data are mean ± SEM, and were compared by unpaired Student's t-test. $P < 0.05$ was considered statistically significant.

Results

Of the 35 women with pelvic endometriosis, 11 and 24 were laparoscopically diagnosed with endometriosis stage III and endometriosis stage IV, respectively, according to the revised American Society for Reproductive Medicine (ASRM) classification (ASRM, 1997).

Table 1 shows the characteristics of the recruited patients. No differences were obtained between control patients and the AM or EM group, in age, gravidity, parity, and baseline MVJ score. Compared with control values, VAS scores in the AM ($p < 0.001$) and EM ($p < 0.001$) groups were significantly higher.

According to pathological findings, 24 of the 35 women in the EM group had lesions involving the fallopian tubes, and were included in the tubal EM subgroup; the remaining 11 were included in the non-tubal EM subgroup.

The CBF of the ampulla in the EM group (3.202 ± 0.077 Hz) was significantly lower than those of the control (5.811 ± 0.021 Hz) and AM (5.725 ± 0.018 Hz) groups (both $p < 0.001$). The CBF of the isthmus segment in the EM group (2.842 ± 0.061 Hz) was also significantly lower than those of the control (5.744 ± 0.031 Hz) and AM (5.432 ± 0.034 Hz) groups (both $p < 0.001$; Fig. 1). There were no significant differences in CBF between the control and AM groups, or between the control group and non-tubal EM subgroup. CBFs of the ampulla and isthmus in the tubal EM subgroup (1.661 ± 0.102 Hz and 1.173 ± 0.093 Hz, respectively) were both significantly lower than those of the control group and non-tubal EM subgroup (5.510 ± 0.037 Hz and 5.339 ± 0.041 Hz, respectively).

Figures 2 and 3 shows the percentages of ciliated cells in ampulla and isthmus samples from the fallopian tubes. In both the ampulla and isthmus, the percentages of ciliated cells in the EM group (30.319 ± 0.359% and 25.601 ± 0.305%, respectively) were significantly lower (both $p < 0.001$) than those of the AM (65.312 ± 0.408% and 48.314 ± 0.339%, respectively) and control (68.339 ± 0.381% and 51.281 ± 0.351%, respectively) groups; the values in the tubal EM subgroup (10.561 ± 0.414% and 15.849 ± 0.407%, respectively) were both significantly lower (both $p < 0.001$) than those of the control group and non-tubal EM subgroup (59.961 ± 0.539% and 40.227 ± 0.501%, respectively); the values in the non-tubal EM subgroup were both significantly lower ($p < 0.01$ and $p < 0.001$, respectively) than those of the control group. There were no significant differences between control cases and the AM group.

Figure 4 summarize the spontaneous contractile activities of the isthmus-ampulla segments of fallopian tube strips.

Table 1 Characteristics of the recruited patients

Variables	Control group ($n = 20$)	AM group ($n = 20$)	EM group ($n = 35$)
Age[a] (year)	47.2 ± 4.8	44.4 ± 5.2	43.4 ± 5.1
BMI[a] (kg/m^2)	23.8 ± 2.2	21.0 ± 1.9	21.8 ± 2.3
Gravidity(n)	1.9 ± 1.4	1.8 ± 1.5	1.25 ± 0.9
Parity (n)	1.1 ± 0.9	0.9 ± 0.7	1.0 ± 0.5
Baseline of dysmenorrhea VAS score[a]	1.7 ± 1.6[c]	5.9 ± 2.7	5.7 ± 2.6
Baseline of MVJ score[b]	4.8 ± 0.9	4.7 ± 0.9	4.2 ± 1.0

Data are mean ± standard deviation (SD)
AM adenomyosis, *EM* endometriosis
[a]The degree of baseline pain was evaluated by the pre-surgical visual analogue scale (VAS) score (0–10 indicates no pain to severe pain)
[b]Baseline menstrual blood loss was assessed using the pre-surgical Mansfield-Voda-Jorgensen (MVJ) score, ranging from 1 (spotting) to 6 (gushing)
[c]Significant difference compared with the AM and EM groups (both $p < 0.001$)

The amplitude/weight ratio of longitudinal muscular contractility in the EM group (10.357 ± 0.269) was significantly ($p < 0.001$) lower than control values (22.061 ± 0.594). The tubal EM subgroup (7.491 ± 0.496) showed significantly lower values than the control group and non-tubal EM subgroup (14.657 ± 0.569) ($p < 0.001$ and $p < 0.05$, respectively). There were no significant differences in circular muscle contractility among groups.

Figure 5 shows the frequency of contraction in the EM group was significantly ($p < 0.001$) lower than those of the control and AM groups, both in the longitudinal (0.054 ± 0.002 Hz, 0.133 ± 0.001 Hz, and 0.13 ± 0.003 Hz, respectively) and circular (0.062 ± 0.003 Hz, 0.153 ± 0.003 Hz, and 0.187 ± 0.004 Hz, respectively) muscles. Frequencies of contraction in the tubal EM subgroup were significantly ($p < 0.001$) lower than those of the control group and non-tubal EM subgroup, both in longitudinal (0.013 ± 0.002 Hz, 0.133 ± 0.001 Hz, and 0.114 ± 0.002 Hz, respectively) and circular (0.019 ± 0.001 Hz, 0.153 ± 0.003 Hz, 0.127 ± 0.004 Hz, respectively) muscles.

Discussion

To the best of our knowledge, this is the first report assessing the effects of pelvic endometriosis, tubal endometriosis, and adenomyosis on ciliary beat frequency and contraction of tubal smooth muscle in the human fallopian tube. AM and EM without tubal EM did not affect tubal function. EM with tubal EM resulted in lower ciliary beat frequency, lower ciliated cells percentage, weaker muscular contractile activity, and lower contraction frequency.

Moderate to severe EM may cause pelvic adhesions and anatomical changes. The morphology and function of the fallopian tube are susceptible to damage because it is located between the uterus and ipsilateral ovary. As early as 1984, Schenken and coworkersshowed that pregnancy rates are lower among monkeys with moderate or severe endometriosis, which showed pelvic adhesion involving ovaries and tubes [21]. According to the TOP score [22] and endometriosis fertility index (EFI) [23, 24] to predict the reproductive outcomes of EM patients, the results are mostly affected by the function of tubal function.

Using objective measures to evaluate fallopian tube function, including CBF, percentage of ciliated cells, and smooth muscle contraction amplitude and frequency, we demonstrated for the first time that EM with tubal EM damaged transport function of the fallopian tube, to varying degrees, whereas tubal function in EM without -tubal EM is not altered. Tubal EM refers to functional endometrial glands and stroma implant involving the fallopian tube. Currently, only a few studies have assessed tubal EM prevalence, with results varying widely. Some of them are retrospective trials with small sample sizes or case reports [25–27]. Furthermore, there is no

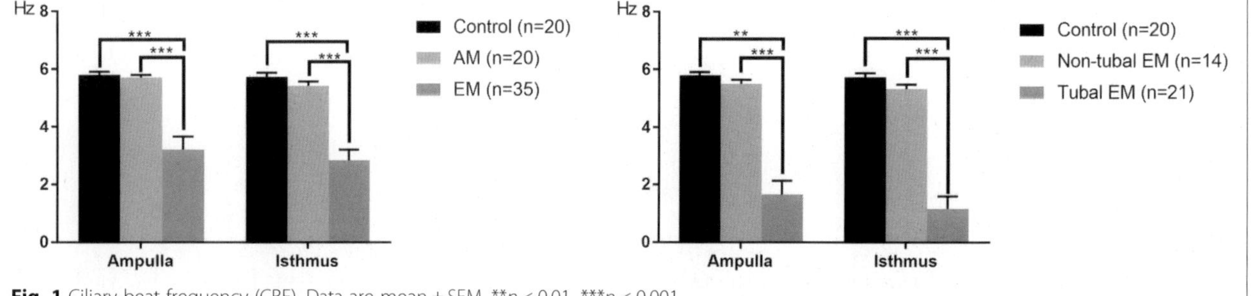

Fig. 1 Ciliary beat frequency (CBF). Data are mean ± SEM. **$p < 0.01$, ***$p < 0.001$

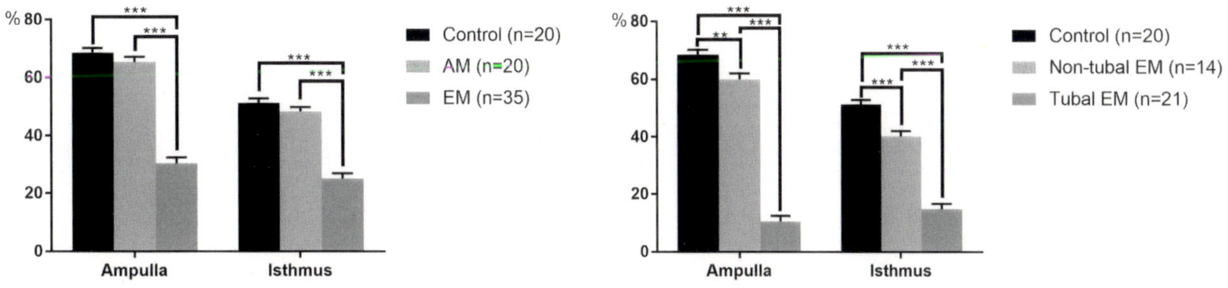

Fig. 2 Percentage of ciliated cells. Data are mean ± SEM. $^{**}p < 0.01$, $^{***}p < 0.001$

research evaluating associations of internal tubal environment, tubal muscle contraction, tubal cilia movement, and reproductive function with tubal EM. The tubal EM layer may infiltrate the serosa, muscle, and mucosa, and the ectopic endometrial tissue may give rise to a variety of lesions, including endometrial-type polyps, tubal adenomyosis (analogous to salpingitis isthmica nodosa), and intraluminal endometriosis, with occlusion of one or both tubal lumens. In this study, endometriosis lesions were found in the fallopian tubes of 60% (21/35) EM patients; therefore, tubal involvement in moderate and severe EM is common. Tubal inflammation, edema,

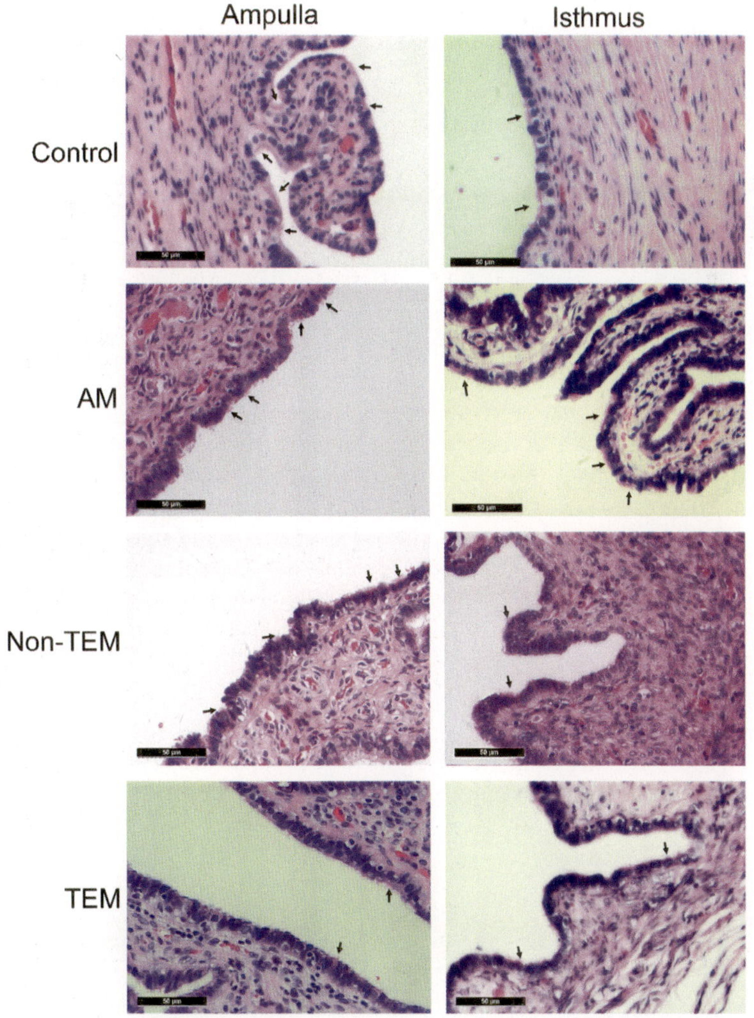

Fig. 3 Histological analysis of human fallopian tubes. Light microscopy images showing that the non-tubal EM (tubal endometriosis) and tubal EM subgroups had less ciliated cells. Arrows indicate ciliated cells

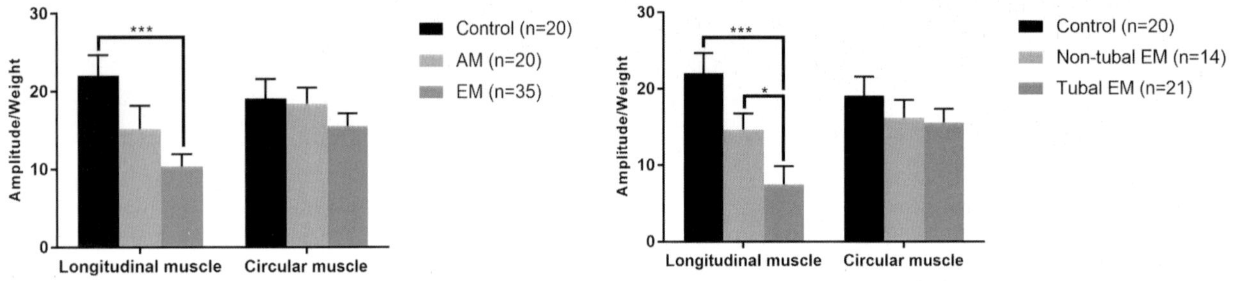

Fig. 4 Amplitude/Weight ratio of the tubal smooth muscle spontaneous contraction. Data are mean ± SEM. *$p < 0.05$, ***$p < 0.001$

damage of mucosal folds, and fibrosis hyperplasia can decrease tubal transport function in the epithelium and muscle. This study also found for the first time that AM did not affect the transport function of fallopian tubes, indicating that adenomyosis and EM differ in pathogenesis. Endometriosis lesions in AM without pelvic EM are confined to the myometrium, and the fallopian tubes are often not involved.

The abnormal local microenvironment of pelvic and tube invading by EM lesion, including immune environment, oxidative stress, high estrogen, increased local inflammatory factors, etc., can lead to cell damage and apoptosis [1]. In this study, although the CBF in non-tubal EM subgroup has not been changed, but the local cilia cells were less than the normal control group, suggesting that endometriosis, regardless of tubal involvement or not, can cause different degrees of damage of ciliated cells.

Although the importance of each of the ciliary and muscular motion mechanisms remains unclear, there is evidence that ciliary activity may play a dominant role in the transport of normal gametes and embryos. With reduced muscular activity, total transport rates through the ampulla are unchanged, suggesting that ciliary motion alone is capable of transporting ova to the site of fertilization in the absence of muscle contractility [27, 28]. Conversely, women with the 'immotile cilia syndrome', or Kartagener's syndrome, may suffer from infertility because of a dyskinetic ciliary activity in the fallopian tubes [29, 30]. We evaluated the functions of the tubal cilia and smooth muscle objectively, for the first time in the related research field studying the impact of EM on transport function in fallopian tubes. Currently, it is widely admitted that fallopian tube function can be precisely assessed by ciliary beat frequency (CBF) and smooth muscle contraction. The current findings revealed that cilia and muscle functions were impaired, indicating that EM damages the tubal epithelium and muscle layers. Considering the great importance of cilia and smooth muscle to the reproductive function of the fallopian tube, our study provide a new perspective for the research of the tubal function in AM and EM.

This study had several limitations. First, because most of the patients with mild endometriosis have operations to get pregnant, we cannot do the salpingectomy. Patients with stage I and stage II EM were not included, and whether mild EM impacts fallopian tube function was not evaluated. Secondly, other tubal segments (interstitial and fimbria) were not assessed. Thirdly, we did not observe the tubal ultrastructure, e.g. by transmission electron microscopy, which detects ultrastructural defects of cilia. Fourthly, animal experiments would have helped unveil the mechanisms. Further studies assessing the impact of mild EM on tubal function and animal experiments evaluating the impact on transport function in vivo are warranted. In addition, drugs, surgery, or other means, which can reverse the functional impairment of the fallopian tubes deserve further investigation.

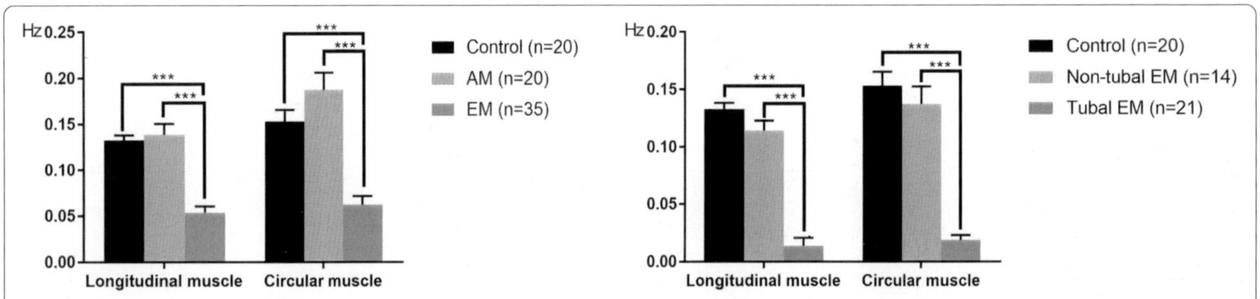

Fig. 5 Frequency of the tubal smooth muscle spontaneous contraction. Data are mean ± SEM. **$p < 0.01$, ***$p < 0.001$

Conclusion

Fallopian tubes in women with moderate and severe EM, especially EM with tubal EM, show lower ciliary beat frequency, lower ciliated cells percentage, weaker muscular contractile activity, and lower contraction frequency. These findings suggest that the fallopian tube plays an important role in EM-related infertility. AM does not affect tubal function, indicating that there are other factors responsible for AM-related infertility.

Abbreviations

AM: Adenomyosis; CBF: Ciliary beat frequency; EM: Endometriosis; MVJ: Mansfield-Voad-Jorgensen; VAS: Visual analogue scale

Acknowledgements

We thank Jason J. Chen from University of California, Irvine for providing the MATLAB program to analyze the frequency of fallopian tube.

Funding

This work was supported by the National Natural Science Foundation of China [grant number 81671482] and Shanghai Jiaotong University [grant number YG2016ZD07 and YG2017QN39].

Authors' contributions

JZ and XG conceived of the study and participated in its design, as well as supervised the study and critically revised the manuscript. WX and DZ were responsible for collecting data and writing the manuscript. HZ and ZH and were participated in the revising of the manuscript. GL and QZ contributed to statistical analysis. JO and YL contributed to the revision of the manuscript. All authors read and approved the final version of the manuscript.

Competing interests

The authors declare that they have no competing interests.

Author details

[1]Department of Obstetrics and Gynaecology, International Peace Maternity and Child Health Hospital, School of Medicine, Shanghai Jiaotong University, Shanghai, China. [2]Institute of Embryo-Fetal Original Adult Disease Affiliated to School of Medicine, Shanghai Jiaotong University, Shanghai, China. [3]Department of Obstetrics & Gynaecology, Baylor College of Medicine, Houston, TX, USA.

References

1. de Ziegler D, Borghese B, Chapron C. Endometriosis and infertility: pathophysiology and management. Lancet. 2010;376:730–8.
2. Tanbo T, Fedorcsak P. Endometriosis-associated infertility: aspects of pathophysiological mechanisms and treatment options. Acta Obstet Gynecol Scand. 2017;96:659–67.
3. Holoch KJ, Lessey BA. Endometriosis and infertility. Clin Obstet Gynecol. 2010;53:429–38.
4. Raidt J, Werner C, Menchen T, Dougherty GW, Olbrich H, Loges NT, Schmitz R, Pennekamp P, Omran H. Ciliary function and motor protein composition of human fallopian tubes. Hum Reprod. 2015;30:2871–80.
5. Lyons RA, Saridogan E, Djahanbakhch O. The reproductive significance of human fallopian tube cilia. Hum Reprod Update. 2006;12:363–72.
6. Li S, Winuthayanon W. Oviduct: roles in fertilization and early embryo development. J Endocrinol. 2017;232:R1–R26.
7. Leyendecker G, Wildt L, Mall G. The pathophysiology of endometriosis and adenomyosis: tissue injury and repair. Arch Gynecol Obstet. 2009;280:529–38.
8. Leyendecker G, Herbertz M, Kunz G, Mall G. Endometriosis results from the dislocation of basal endometrium. Hum Reprod. 2002;17:2725–36.
9. Burns WN, Schenken RS. Pathophysiology of endometriosis-associated infertility. Clin Obstet Gynecol. 1999;42:586–610.
10. Kissler S, Hamscho N, Zangos S, Gatje R, Muller A, Rody A, Dobert N, Menzel C, Grunwald F, Siebzehnrubl E, Kaufmann M. Diminished pregnancy rates in endometriosis due to impaired uterotubal transport assessed by hysterosalpingoscintigraphy. BJOG. 2005;112:1391–6.
11. Kissler S, Zangos S, Wiegratz I, Kohl J, Rody A, Gaetje R, Doebert N, Wildt L, Kunz G, Leyendecker G, Kaufmann M. Utero-tubal sperm transport and its impairment in endometriosis and adenomyosis. Ann N Y Acad Sci. 2007;1101:38–48.
12. Papathanasiou A, Djahanbakhch O, Saridogan E, Lyons RA. The effect of interleukin-6 on ciliary beat frequency in the human fallopian tube. Fertil Steril. 2008;90:391–4.
13. Lyons RA, Djahanbakhch O, Saridogan E, Naftalin AA, Mahmood T, Weekes A, Chenoy R. Peritoneal fluid, endometriosis, and ciliary beat frequency in the human fallopian tube. Lancet. 2002;360:1221–2.
14. Reeve L, Lashen H, Pacey AA. Endometriosis affects sperm-endosalpingeal interactions. Hum Reprod. 2005;20:448–51.
15. Mansfield PK, Voda A, Allison G. Validating a pencil-and-paper measure of perimenopausal menstrual blood loss. Womens Health Issues. 2004;14:242–7.
16. Groisman GM, Meir A. CD10 is helpful in detecting occult or inconspicuous endometrial stromal cells in cases of presumptive endometriosis. Arch Pathol Lab Med. 2003;127:1003–6.
17. Blaustein's Pathology of the Female Genital Tract. 2011. https://doi.org/10.1007/978-1-4419-0489-8.
18. Chen JJ, Lemieux BT, Wong BJ. A low-cost method of ciliary beat frequency measurement using iPhone and MATLAB: rabbit study. Otolaryngol Head Neck Surg. 2016;155:252–6.
19. Chen S, Einspanier R, Schoen J. In vitro mimicking of estrous cycle stages in porcine oviduct epithelium cells: estradiol and progesterone regulate differentiation, gene expression, and cellular function. Biol Reprod. 2013;89:54.
20. Zhao W, Zhu Q, Yan M, Li C, Yuan J, Qin G, Zhang J. Levonorgestrel decreases cilia beat frequency of human fallopian tubes and rat oviducts without changing morphological structure. Clin Exp Pharmacol Physiol. 2015;42:171–8.
21. Schenken RS, Asch RH, Williams RF, Hodgen GD. Etiology of infertility in monkeys with endometriosis: luteinized unruptured follicles, luteal phase defects, pelvic adhesions, and spontaneous abortions. Fertil Steril. 1984;41:122–30.
22. Fujishita A, Khan KN, Masuzaki H, Ishimaru T. Influence of pelvic endometriosis and ovarian endometrioma on fertility. Gynecol Obstet Investig. 2002;53(Suppl 1):40–5.
23. Adamson GD, Pasta DJ. Endometriosis fertility index: the new, validated endometriosis staging system. Fertil Steril. 2010;94:1609–15.
24. Tomassetti C, Geysenbergh B, Meuleman C, Timmerman D, Fieuws S, D'Hooghe T. External validation of the endometriosis fertility index (EFI) staging system for predicting non-ART pregnancy after endometriosis surgery. Hum Reprod. 2013;28:1280–8.
25. Jenkins S, Olive DL, Haney AF. Endometriosis: pathogenetic implications of the anatomic distribution. Obstet Gynecol. 1986;67:335–8.
26. Clement PB. The pathology of endometriosis: a survey of the many faces of a common disease emphasizing diagnostic pitfalls and unusual and newly appreciated aspects. Adv Anat Pathol. 2007;14:241–60.
27. Fortier KJ, Haney AF. The pathologic spectrum of uterotubal junction obstruction. Obstet Gynecol. 1985;65:93–8.
28. Halbert SA, Becker DR, Szal SE. Ovum transport in the rat oviductal ampulla in the absence of muscle contractility. Biol Reprod. 1989;40:1131–6.
29. Abu-Musa A, Nassar A, Usta I. In vitro fertilization in two patients with Kartagener's syndrome and infertility. Gynecol Obstet Investig. 2008;65:29–31.
30. Halbert SA, Patton DL, Zarutskie PW, Soules MR. Function and structure of cilia in the fallopian tube of an infertile woman with Kartagener's syndrome. Hum Reprod. 1997;12:55–8.

17

The monocyte counts to HDL cholesterol ratio in obese and lean patients with polycystic ovary syndrome

Akin Usta[1*], Eyup Avci[2], Cagla Bahar Bulbul[1], Hasan Kadi[2] and Ertan Adali[1]

Abstract

Background: Women with polycystic ovary syndrome are more likely to suffer from obesity, insulin resistance, and chronic low-grade inflammation. In fact, the excessive activation of monocytes exacerbates oxidative stress and inflammation. However, high-density lipoprotein cholesterol neutralizes the pro-inflammatory and pro-oxidant effects of monocytes. The aim of this study is to investigate whether monocyte counts to high-density lipoprotein cholesterol ratio can predict the inflammatory condition in patients with polycystic ovary syndrome.

Methods: In this cross-sectional study, a total of 124 women (61 of them with polycystic ovary syndrome and 63 age-matched healthy volunteers) were included in the study population. Obese polycystic ovary syndrome patients ($n = 30$) with a body mass index of ≥25 kg/m^2 and lean polycystic ovary syndrome patients ($n = 31$) with a body mass index of < 25 kg/m^2 were compared to age-and body mass index-matched healthy subjects (30 obese and 33 non-obese).

Results: The monocyte counts to high density lipoprotein cholesterol values in women with polycystic ovary syndrome were significantly higher than in control subjects ($p = 0.0018$). Moreover, a regression analysis revealed that body mass index, the homeostasis model assessment of insulin resistance and the high sensitivity C-reactive protein levels were confounding factors that affected the monocyte counts to high density lipoprotein cholesterol values. Additionally, a univariate and multivariate logistic regression analysis demonstrated that the increased monocyte counts to high density lipoprotein cholesterol values were more sensitive than the other known risk factors (such as increased body mass index, homeostasis model assessment of insulin resistance and high sensitive C-reactive protein levels) in the prediction of the inflammation in patients with polycystic ovary syndrome.

Conclusion: The present study demonstrated that the monocyte count to high density lipoprotein cholesterol may be a novel and useful predictor of the presence of polycystic ovary syndrome.

Keywords: PCOS, Monocyte count to HDL cholesterol ratio, Inflammation, Insulin resistance, Cardiovascular disease

Background

Polycystic ovary syndrome (PCOS) is a common endocrine disorder that affects 6-20% of women of reproductive age [1, 2]. The disorder is characterized by oligo/anovulation, hormonal and/or clinical hyperandrogenism, and the appearance of polycystic ovaries on ultrasound [1, 2].

Women with PCOS are more likely to suffer from obesity, insulin resistance, glucose intolerance, endothelial dysfunction, hyperandrogenism, and chronic low-grade inflammation than are women without the condition. Chronic low-grade inflammation seems to have a stimulatory effect on the development and progression of endothelial dysfunction and atherosclerosis [3], and long-term complications include type 2 diabetes mellitus and cardiovascular disease [1, 2]. It is therefore important to understand the underlying molecular and cellular mechanisms of this syndrome.

The high-sensitivity C-reactive protein (hsCRP) has been found to be a highly sensitive inflammatory biomarker that is commonly used in the detection of

* Correspondence: drakinusta@gmail.com
[1]Department of Obstetrics and Gynecology, School of Medicine, Balıkesir University Faculty of Medicine, Cagis Yerleskesi, Bigadic yolu 17. km, 10145 Balikesir, Turkey
Full list of author information is available at the end of the article

subclinical inflammation in patients with PCOS [4]. The hsCRP test is also used to detect future cardiovascular disease risk [5]. Moreover, increased counts of leucocytes or related subgroups have been found to be additional independent markers as well as prognostic factors in the development of inflammation and atherosclerosis [6, 7]. Regarding the initiation and progression of the atherosclerotic process, several biochemical markers (to include hsCRP and leukocyte counts) associated with inflammatory conditions, oxidative stress, and endothelial dysfunction have been shown to reflect the severity and prognosis of cardiovascular disease risk.

Monocytes constitute roughly 3-8% of circulating leukocytes and-in conjunction with other granular and agranular cells such as eosinophils, basophils, neutrophils, and lymphocytes-are essential components of the innate immune system. In tissues, circulating monocytes and their differentiated forms, known as macrophages, play central roles in the initiation and resolution of inflammation; this is principally achieved via phagocytosis, the release of inflammatory cytokines, the presence of reactive oxygen species, and the activation of the acquired immune system [8]. However, the accumulation of monocytes exacerbates oxidative stress and inflammation. Thus the excessive activation of monocytes aggravates diseases such as atherosclerosis, arthritis, and multiple sclerosis, primarily affecting platelets and endothelial cells and leading to the activation of the prothrombotic pathway [9].

In contrast, high-density lipoprotein cholesterol (HDL-C) neutralizes the pro-inflammatory and pro-oxidant effects of monocytes by hindering the oxidation of low-density lipoprotein (LDL) molecules and the migration of macrophages as well as by promoting the efflux of cholesterol from these cells [10]. In addition to outlining the well-known anti-inflammatory and anti-oxidant actions of HDL-C particles, it has recently been claimed that these molecules play a suppressive role in the control of monocyte activation and in the proliferation and differentiation of the progenitor cells of monocytes [11].

Recognised as a recently-emerged inflammation-based marker, the monocyte count to HDL-C ratio (MHR) has been reported to be a new predictor and prognostic indicator of mortality and morbidity in many diseases [12, 13]. The MHR has also been found to be correlated with hsCRP levels in diseases that are associated with chronic inflammation, such as cardiovascular disease [14], chronic kidney disease [12], abdominal aortic aneurysm [15], intracerebral hemorrhage [16], hypertension [17], and metabolic syndromes [18].

According to the Rotterdam criteria [1], the prevalence of PCOS in Turkish women is approximately 20% [2]. Thus, a considerable number of Turkish women with PCOS are at an increased risk of developing diabetes and cardiovascular disease in the future. The early diagnosis and prevention of inflammatory conditions in the PCOS population is essential to maintain the long-term wellbeing of these women and will aid in the proper utilization of public health resources. To the best of our knowledge, no study has yet examined the association between PCOS and the MHR. Therefore, we aimed to investigate whether the MHR, a readily available inflammatory and oxidative stress marker, is associated with PCOS.

Methods

A cross-sectional study was conducted at the Balikesir University, School of Medicine, Department of Obstetrics and Gynecology and Department of Cardiology between January 2017 and June 2017. The study was approved by the Ethics Committee of Balikesir University, and study protocols of were in accordance with the Helsinki Committee requirements. Informed consent was obtained from all participants.

In total, 124 women (61 with PCOS and 63 age-matched healthy volunteers) were included in the study population. Obese PCOS patients ($n = 30$) with a body mass index (BMI) of ≥25 kg/m^2 and lean PCOS patients ($n = 31$) with a BMI of < 25 kg/m^2 were compared to healthy age-and BMI-matched subjects (30 obese and 33 non-obese). All patients were aged between 18 and 40 years.

PCOS was diagnosed using the Rotterdam criteria [1]. According to these diagnostic criteria, the presence of oligomenorrhea (wherein menstrual cycles occur more than 35 days apart) or amenorrhea (wherein menstrual cycles ocur at least six months apart) was defined as oligoovulation, and the presence of at least 12 follicles measuring 2–9 mm in diameter and/or an ovarian volume greater than 10 cm^3 in per ovary indicated the existence of polycystic ovaries; additionally, the presence of hirsutism was evaluated using the Ferriman–Gallwey scoring system [19]. Areas near the lip, chin, chest, upper and lower abdomen, upper arm, forearm and thigh were visually assessed and granded a score between zero (the absence of terminal hair) and four (the presence of male-pattern terminal hair). A score greater than or equal to six was defined as hirsutism.

Patients who were diagnosed with other disorders whose clinical features are similar to those of PCOS, to include Cushing's syndrome, congenital adrenal hyperplasia and androgen-secreting tumors, were excluded from participation. Additionally, patients who took medicines, such as oral contraceptives, antilipidemic and/or antihypertensive medications, steroids, antidiabetic medications, anticoagulants, or antiplatelet drugs were excluded from the study.

Each participant's height (m) and weight (kg) were measured while the patient was dressed only in underwear clothing. Waist circumference was measured as the minimum distance between the iliac crest and the lateral costal margin. The waist-to-hip ratio (WHR) was calculated as the ratio of the waist measurement to that of the hip. BMI was calculated as the patient's mass in kilograms divided by the square of the patient's body height in meters (kg/m^2). All participant data was recorded and stored in a computer database.

All PCOS and control patients were pooled from university's gynecology clinic. Additionally, PCOS patients were reevaluated to determine whether they truly met the clinical, ultrasound scan (U/S), and biochemical criteria for PCOS based on the Rotterdam criteria. Physical and gynecological examinations, pelvic ultrasounds, and peripheral venous blood samplings were performed during Day 2 or 3 of a participant's menstrual cycles or progestogen induced early follicular phase (Day 2 or 3) in subjects with amenorrhea. All women were examined, and pelvic ultrasound scans were performed using a 7. 0 MHz vaginal transducer (Voluson 730, GE Healthcare, USA) by the same gynecologist.

During blood pressure measurements, the brachial artery was occluded by a cuff placed around the patient's upper arm; the cuff was then inflated to above systolic pressure. As the cuff gradually deflated, pulsatile blood flow was reestablished and was accompanied by sounds that were able to be detected by a stethoscope held over the artery just below the cuff. The onset of the pulsatile blood flow sound (Korotkoff I) was recorded as systolic blood pressure and the disappearance of blood flow sounds (Korotkoff V) was recorded as diastolic blood pressure. All measurements were performed by healthcare professionals, who were blinded to the clinical diagnoses of the patients.

Biochemical evaluation

After overnight fasting, blood samples were collected from the antecubital vein of patients between the hours of 9 and 10 AM. Serum was collected following centrifugation at 2500 g for 10 min, and stored in deep freeze at − 80 °C to await biochemical and hormonal assessment. To avoid possible assay variability, all patient blood samples were analyzed together.

Complete blood counts were measured via Sysmex XE-2100 (Sysmex Corp. Kobe, Japan) using either the fluorescence flow cytometry or electrical impedance method. The serum levels of follicle-stimulating hormone (FSH), luteinizing hormone (LH), estradiol (E2), thyroid-stimulating hormone (TSH), and total testosterone were determined using commercially avaliable enzyme-linked immunosorbent assay (ELISA) kits (eBioscience, Austria) on a diagnostic instrument (BioTek, ELx 800, USA). 2nd International reference preparation was used for FSH and LH measurements. The levels of glucose, total cholesterol, low-density lipoprotein (LDL) cholesterol, and high-density lipoprotein (HDL) cholesterol were measured using commercially available kits on a chemistry AutoAnalyzer (Cobas Integra 800; Roche Diagnostics GmbH; Mannheim, Germany). Serum high sensitive C-reactive protein (hs CRP) was measured with chemiluminescent immunoassay using an ADVIA Centaur XP (Siemens Healthcare Diagnostics, NY, USA). The levels of fasting insulin were determined using commercial kits and an automatic hormone analyzer (Beckman Coulter; Unicel DXI 600; Access Immunoassay System). The homeostasis model assessment for insulin resistance (HOMA-IR) was defined as (insulin x glucose) / 22.5 as previously described [6].

Statistical analysis

The MedCalc Statistical Software Program version 17.2 (MedCalc, Belgium) was used for statistical analysis. Normally distributed data are described as mean ± standard deviation, otherwise, as median (minimum-maximum). Whether the distributions of continuous variables were normal or not was determined by Kolmogorov–Smirnov test. Also, the Levene test or F test was used for the evaluation of homogeneity of variances.

The student's t test was used to compare normally distributed measurements for independent samples and the Mann–Whitney U test was applied for comparisons of the median values. The Chi-square test was used to compare categorical data. While the mean differences among more than two independent groups were analyzed by one-way ANOVA, the Kruskal–Wallis test was applied for comparisons of the median values. When the p value from one-way ANOVA or Kruskal–Wallis test statistics was statistically significant the Scheffé test or Post-Hoc analysis nonparametric multiple comparison test was used to determine which group differed from which others. The possible confounding factors that associated with MHR value were evaluated by using logistic regression analysis. In order to determine of the independent variables for presence of PCOS, the univariate and multivariate logistic regression analysis were performed. To evaluate model characteristics of fitness, Hosmer–Lemeshow tests were used. A p-value of < 0.05 was considered statistically significant.

Results

A total of 124 women—61 with PCOS (30 obese, 31 non-obese) and 63 age- and BMI matched controls (30 obese, 33 non-obese)—were included in this study. The mean age of participants was 23.9 ± 4.9 in the PCOS group and 25.2 ± 5.1 in the control group; there was no statistically significant difference ($p = 0.1566$) between the groups. The mean BMI of participants was 26.6 ± 6.1 in the PCOS group, and 24.8 ± 5.3 in the control group ($p = 0.0858$).

As compared to the control subjects, PCOS patients had significantly higher WHRs, Ferriman Gallwey scores, diastolic blood pressure levels, insuline levels, HOMA-IR readings, hsCRP scores, total leucocytes counts, neutrophil counts, monocyte counts, total cholesterol levels, LDL levels, total testosterone levels, LH levels and MHRs ($p < 0.05$). However, HDL-C levels were lower in PCOS patients than in control subjects ($p < 0.0001$). The clinical, hormonal, and biochemical characteristics of the groups are summarized in Table 1.

The biochemical parameters of obese and lean patients with or without PCOS are shown in Table 2. Obese PCOS patients had higher levels of diastolic blood pressure, HOMA-IR, hsCRP, monocytes, total cholesterol, and LDL-C but lower levels of HDL-C than did control participants ($p < 0.05$). Lean PCOS patients had higher levels of HOMA-IR, hsCRP, neutrophils, monocytes, and total testosterone but lower levels of HDL-C and lymphocytes than did control participants ($p < 0.05$).

Interestingly, we found that obese PCOS patients had higher levels of systolic blood pressure, diastolic blood pressure, HOMA-IR, hsCRP, and total leucocytes but lower HDL-C levels than did lean PCOS patients ($p < 0.05$).

Importantly, we found that MHR values were significantly higher in patients with PCOS than in control subjects ($p = 0.0018$). Moreover, subgroup analysis showed that MHR values of obese PCOS patients were significantly higher than those of lean PCOS patients. Also, MHR values of obese control patients were significantly higher than lean control subjects.

A univariate regression analysis showed that BMI, diastolic blood pressure, HOMA-IR, and hsCRP, were possible confounding factors affecting MHR values (Table 3). Furthermore, in order to identify independent variables that might predict the presence of PCOS, univariate and multivariate logistic regression analyses were performed (Table 4). During the univariate logistic regression analysis, HOMA-IR (odds ratio [OR]: 1.3133 [95% CI: 1.0543–1.6358]; $p = 0.0067$), hsCRP (OR:1.2996 [95% CI: 1.0804–1.5634]; $p = 0.0023$) and the MHR (OR:

Table 1 The clinical, hormonal, and biochemical characteristics of patients in tje PCOS and non-PCOS groups

	PCOS	Non-PCOS	*P* value
Age (year)	23.9 ± 4.9	25.2 ± 5.1	0.1566
Body mass index (kg/m^2)	26.6 ± 6.1	24.8 ± 5.3	0.0858
Waist to hip ratio (WHR) (cm)	0.80 ± 0.07	0.77 ± 0.06	0.0030
Ferriman–Gallwey score	5 (2-17)	3 (1-6)	< 0.0001
Systolic blood pressure (mmHg)	120 (90-150)	110 (90-130)	0.1195
Diastolic blood pressure (mmHg)	70 (60-110)	70 (60-80)	0.0115
Glucose (mg/dl)	88 (64-123)	81 (61-110)	0.0092
HOMA-IR	2.42 (0.6-13.8)	1.49(0.4-8.8)	0.0027
hsCRP (mg/l)	3.2 (0.3-29.0)	1.8 (0.2-7.8)	0.0074
Leucocytes (/mm^3)	7.86 ± 2.28	6.92 ± 2.19	0.0208
Neutrophil (/mm^3)	4.76 ± 1.68	4.08 ± 1.35	0.0150
Lymphocytes (/mm^3)	2.48 ± 0.76	2.29 ± 0.65	0.0820
Monocyte (/mm^3)	645.9 ± 205.8	510.9 ± 184.9	0.0002
Trigliserid (mg/dL)	95.0 (46.0-529.0)	78.0 (44.0-280.0)	0.1080
Total cholesterol (mg/dL)	180.1 ± 33.6	168.1 ± 28.5	0.0221
LDL (mg/dL)	102.1 ± 29.7	91.2 ± 25.6	0.0373
HDL (mg/dL)	47.5 ± 10.8	58.7 ± 13.4	< 0.0001
Total testosteron (ng/dl)	1.20 (0.10-4.71)	0.15 (0.07-0.90)	< 0.0001
FSH (IU/L)	5.86 ± 1.37	6.34 ± 1.68	0.0818
LH (IU/L)	9.15 (5.03-22.10)	6.40 (4.72-14.60)	< 0.0001
Estradiol (pg/ml)	45.32 ± 13.67	41.87 ± 14.21	0.1705
TSH (mIU/L)	2.15 ± 1.17	2.08 ± 1.03	0.7119
Prolaktin (ng/ml)	17.34 ± 8.17	16.27 ± 5.89	0.4072
Monocytes to HDL ratio	11.46 (3.70-30.50)	8.77 (3.31-24.19)	0.0018

Data was showed: mean ± standard deviation (SD) or median (min-max)

Table 2 The clinical and laboratory parameters of obese and lean patients with or without PCOS

	Obese PCOS $n = 30$	Lean PCOS $n = 31$	Obese Control $n = 30$	Lean Control $n = 33$	p value
Age (year)	24.6 ± 4.6	24.7 ± 4.9	23.4 ± 4.3	26.9 ± 5.3	0.059
Body mass index (kg/m^2)	29.1 ± 4.2 ^{a,c}	22.3 ± 3.7 ^{d}	31.1 ± 4.6 ^{f}	21.4 ± 2.8	< 0.001
Waist to hip ratio (WHR) (cm)	0.85 ± 0.06 ^{a,b,c}	0.75 ± 0.04 ^{d,e}	0.80 ± 0.06 ^{f}	0.73 ± 0.03	< 0.001
Ferriman–Gallwey score	7 (3-17) ^{a,b,c}	4 (2-13) ^{d,e}	2 (1-5)	1 (1-4)	< 0.001
Systolic blood pressure (mmHg)	120 (90-150) ^{a,c}	110 (90-130)	110 (100-130)	110 (90-120)	0.011
Diastolic blood pressure (mmHg)	80 (60-110) ^{a,b,c}	70 (60-80)	70 (60-80)	70 (60-80)	0.006
Glucose (mg/dl)	92 (74-123) ^{a,b,c}	83 (64-112)	85 (65-110)	78 (61-98)	0.007
HOMA-IR	3.5 (1.4-13.8) ^{a,b,c}	2.2 (0.6-9.8)^{d,e}	2.6 (1.1-8.8) ^{f}	1.2 (0.4-5.6)	< 0.001
hsCRP (mg/l)	4.1(1.2-29.1) ^{a,b,c}	1.5 (0.3-8.8) ^{e}	2.7 (0.9-7.8) ^{f}	0.9 (0.2-3.5)	< 0.001
Leucocytes (/mm^3)	8.9 ± 2.3 ^{a,c}	6.9 ± 1.8 ^{d}	7.8 ± 2.6	6.2 ± 1.4	< 0.001
Neutrophil (/mm^3)	5.1 ± 1.9 ^{c}	4.5 ± 1.3 ^{e}	4.5 ± 1.4	3.7 ± 1.2	0.005
Lymphocytes (/mm^3)	2.3 ± 0.7	2.1 ± 0.6	2.5 ± 0.8	2.5 ± 0.7	0.158
Monocyte (/mm^3)	657.7 ± 259.3 ^{b,c}	634.6 ± 139.1 ^{d,e}	517.4 ± 184.9	504.7 ± 187.9	0.005
Trigliserid (mg/dL)	145.5(46.0-529.0) ^{a,c}	69.0 (53.0-136.0) ^{d}	116.0 (58.0-280.0) ^{f}	64.0 (44.0-170.0)	< 0.001
Total cholesterol (mg/dL)	189.6 ± 32.1 ^{a,b}	164.1 ± 27.5	167.1 ± 26.2	172.2 ± 30.3	0.005
LDL (mg/dL)	110.7 ± 30.5 ^{b,c}	95.7 ± 34.6	94.9 ± 22.7	87.8 ± 26.5	0.015
HDL (mg/dL)	43.6 ± 8.9 ^{a,b,c}	51.2 ± 11.3 ^{e}	54.5 ± 9.9 ^{f}	62.8 ± 14.6	< 0.001
Total testosteron (ng/dl)	1.40 (0.32-4.71) ^{a,b,c}	1.04 (0.12-2.80) ^{d,e}	0.58 (0.07-0.98) ^{f}	0.11 (0.07-0.25)	< 0.001
FSH (IU/L)	5.75 ± 1.24	5.97 ± 1.49	6.22 ± 1.60	6.46 ± 1.77	0.302
LH (IU/L)	9.80 (5.03-22.1) ^{b,c}	9.15 (5.50-14.5) ^{d,e}	6.88 (4.76-14.6) ^{f}	5.70 (4.72-10.01)	< 0.001
Estradiol (pg/ml)	47.37 ± 22.64	43.35 ± 18.44	43.26 ± 21.03	41.60 ± 19.47	0.297
TSH (mIU/L)	2.03 ± 1.27	2.27 ± 1.07	1.92 ± 0.91	2.22 ± 1.13	0.564
Prolaktin (ng/ml)	16.42 ± 7.68	18.22 ± 8.42	15.65 ± 6.72	17.15 ± 6.10	0.442
Monocytes to HDL ratio	15.6 (3.7-30.5) ^{a,b,c}	9.6 (5.4-24.7) ^{e}	9.9 (3.8-20.9) ^{f}	7.9 (3.3-24.2)	< 0.001

Data was present: mean ± standard deviation (SD) or median (min-max)
[a] Obese PCOS vs. Nonobese PCOS ($p < 0.05$)
[b] Obese PCOS vs. Obese Control ($p < 0.05$)
[c] Obese PCOS vs. Nonobese Control ($p < 0.05$)
[d] Nonobese PCOS vs. Obese Control ($p < 0.05$)
[e] Nonobese PCOS vs Nonobese Control ($p < 0.05$)
[f] Obese Control vs. Nonobese Control ($p < 0.05$)

1.1006 [95% CI: 1.0314–1.1745]; $p = 0.0020$) reached statistical significance. In the multivariate logistic regression analysis, only the MHR (OR: 1.0755 [95% CI: 1. 0010–1.1556]; $p = 0.0470$) was found to be an independent marker for the prediction of PCOS.

Discussion

In the present study, we evaluated multiple clinical and biochemical variables in PCOS patients and compared them with those of age- and BMI-matched non-PCOS subjects. Our clinical and biochemical parameters confirmed that women with PCOS, had higher scores in terms of WHR, hirsutism, diastolic blood pressure, insulin, HOMA-IR, hsCRP, total cholesterol, LDL-C, total testosterone, and LH but also lower HDL-C values. Additionally, a subgroup analysis revealed that obese PCOS patients had higher levels of diastolic blood pressure, insulin, HOMA-IR, hsCRP, and monocytes, while members of the lean PCOS group had higher levels of diastolic blood pressure, insulin, HOMA-IR, hsCRP, neutrophils, lymphocytes, monocytes, and total testosterone as compared to age- and BMI-matched controls; notably, these findings were consistent with those of many previous studies [3, 20–24]. Importantly, we found that the MHR was significantly higher in women with PCOS than in women in the control group. To the best of our knowledge, this is the first study to investigate the association between the MHR and PCOS.

PCOS is a complex endocrine and metabolic disease that is associated with obesity, insulin resistance, compensatory hyperinsulinemia, and chronic low-grade inflammation [3]. Previous studies have shown that various biomarker alterations are associated with insulin resistance and low-grade inflammation in patients with PCOS [21, 22]. Therefore, PCOS is linked to a combination of risk factors that may lead to the development of cardiovascular disease and type 2 diabetes mellitus.

Table 3 Possible confounding factors associated with monocyte counts to HDL-C ratio

Variables	Univariate logistic regression analysis		
	OR	95% CI	*P* value
Age (year)	1.0566	0.9818 to 1.1370	0.1368
Body mass index (kg/m^2)	1.1600	1.0758 to 1.2509	< 0.0001
Systolic blood pressure (mmHg)	1.0209	0.9930 to 1.0496	0.1370
Diastolic blood pressure (mmHg)	1.0986	1.0525 to 1.1468	< 0.0001
HOMA-IR	1.9183	1.3913 to 2.6449	< 0.0001
Glucose (mg/dl)	1.0033	0.9738 to 1.0336	0.8296
hsCRP (mg/l)	1.2107	1.0181 to 1.4396	0.0211
Leucocytes (/mm^3)	1.4282	1.1749 to 1.7361	0.0001
Neutrophil (/mm^3)	1.6002	1.1971 to 2.1389	0.0004
Lymphocytes (/mm^3)	1.8149	1.0584 to 3.1119	0.0238
Trigliserid (mg/dL)	1.0020	0.9965 to 1.0074	0.4713
Total cholesterol (mg/dL)	1.0093	0.9968 to 1.0220	0.1406
LDL (mg/dL)	1.0192	1.0053 to 1.0333	0.0041
Total testosteron (ng/dl)	1.9936	1.2264 to 3.2408	0.0024
FSH (IU/L)	1.0346	0.8252 to 1.2972	0.7681
LH (IU/L)	1.3157	1.1552 to 1.4985	< 0.0001
Estradiol (pg/ml)	1.0203	0.9934 to 1.0480	0.1297
TSH (mIU/L)	0.9632	0.6983 to 1.3286	0.8192
Prolaktin (ng/ml)	0.9889	0.9407 to 1.0395	0.6599

Indeed, low-grade inflammation, impaired glucose tolerance, central obesity, dyslipidemia, and hypertension in PCOS patients are associated with an increase in cardiovascular disease risk [20].

The activation of monocytes and their differentiated forms into lipid-laden macrophages plays a significant role in the promotion of immune defenses in patients with chronic inflammatory conditions; these actions also drive inflammation and cardiovascular disease. Johnsen et al. demonstrated that an elevated monocyte count can be used as an independent predictor of future plaque development in previously plaque-free arteries [25]. Moreover, the activation of monocytes and their differentiated forms into macrophages can be modulated by inflammatory cytokines [26]. However, HDL-C molecules have the ability to counteract macrophage migration and eliminate cholesterol from these cells. Classically known as an antiatherogenic lipoprotein, HDL-C promotes reverse cholesterol transport from the arterial wall-specifically from lipid-laden macrophages [27]. It has been suggested that HDL-C may play a protective role in atherogenesis via the regulation of endothelial adhesion molecule expression, thereby preventing the generation of oxidatively modified LDL-C and the stimulation of endothelial nitric oxide synthases [27]. Additionally, HDL-C has anti-inflammatory, anti-oxidant, and anti-thrombotic effects [10, 27]. The anti-inflammatory effect of HDL-C results from its interaction with both circulating cells, which have the ability to inhibit both leukocyte and platelet activations. HDL-C is highly effective in inhibiting the endothelial expression of adhesion molecules and in preventing monocyte recruitment to the artery wall [28]. As briefly mentioned above, higher monocyte counts and lower HDL-C levels seem to be indirect indicators of inflammation and of the development of atherosclerosis [26]. Indeed, the relationship between these two parameters provides a better understanding of concomitant inflammation.

Relevant literature contains a limited number of studies on the MHR and its role in predicting inflammation. A recent study conducted by Cetin et al. found that the MHR was a novel inflammation-based marker that could be used as an independent predictor of both the severity of coronary artery disease and the likelihood of future cardiovascular events in patients with acute coronary syndrome [14]. Similarly, increases in the MHR have been associated with more severe cardiovascular prognoses in patients with chronic kidney disease [12]. Additionally, the MHR was an independent variable for cardiovascular events within this population [28]. Cockerill et al. indicated that the MHR may be a predictor of stent thrombosis and mortality in ST elevated myocardial infarction (STEMI) patients [29]. Moreover, a recent study conducted by Vahit et al. demonstrated that an increased MHR score may be a useful indicator of metabolic syndromes [18]. Consistent with these

Table 4 Univariate and multivariate logistic regression analysis showing the predictors for the presence of polycystic ovary syndrome

Variables	Univariate logistic regression analysis			Multivariate logistic regression analysis		
	OR	95% CI	*P* value	OR	95% CI	*P* value
Age (year)	0.9863	0.9199 to 1.0575	0.6977	–	–	–
Body mass index (kg/m^2)	1.0594	0.9934 to 1.1298	0.0744	0.9838	0.9077 to 1.0663	0.6904
HOMA-IR	1.3133	1.0543 to 1.6358	0.0067	1.1212	0.8660 to 1.4515	0.3854
hsCRP (mg/l)	1.2996	1.0804 to 1.5634	0.0023	1.2271	0.9970 to 1.5102	0.0534
Leucocytes (/mm^3)	1.1091	0.9481 to 1.2973	0.1894	–	–	–
MHR	1.1006	1.0314 to 1.1745	0.0020	1.0755	1.0010 to 1.1556	0.0470

studies, we found that the average MHR value of patients with PCOS was substantially higher than that of patients without PCOS. Moreover, the univariate regression analysis showed that BMI, diastolic blood pressure, HOMA-IR, and CRP, were possible confounding factors affecting MHR values in our study population. Also, in an effort to identify independent variables for the prediction of PCOS, univariate and multivariate logistic regression analyses were conducted; these analyses showed that the MHR was the only independent variable for women with PCOS. These results indicated that higher MHR values may be associated with ongoing inflammation in the pathophysiology of PCOS. In their entirely, these findings signaled the importance of the MHR with regard to systemic inflammatory conditions and endothelial dysfunction, both of which play crucial roles in the development of future cardiovascular disease.

Insulin resistance is a cornerstone of PCOS. Insulin resistance and compensatory hyperinsulinemia in PCOS patients seem to have a stimulatory effect on chronic low-grade inflammation. It is known that obesity is associated with insulin resistance and low-grade inflammation in the PCOS population [24]. Fat tissues, such as those found in endocrine organs, engage in metabolic and endocrinological activities whereby cytokines and other messenger proteins called adipokines are produced and secreted. Cytokines mediate many physiological and pathological metabolic processes, such as satiety and energy balance, inflammation, insulin resistance/sensitivity, angiogenesis, lipid metabolism, and atherosclerosis. Many previous studies have shown that early atherogenesis and subclinical atherosclerosis are more common in patients with PCOS than in control subjects [30]. In line with the existing literature, we found that obese PCOS patients had higher HOMA-IR, hsCRP, and total leucocyte counts but lower HDL-C levels than did lean PCOS patients [3, 20–24]. Moreover, the MHR values of obese PCOS patients were significantly higher than those of lean PCOS patients. Additionally, the HOMA-IR and total leucocyte counts were significantly higher in obese control patients than lean control patients. As expected, the MHR values in obese control patients were higher than in lean control patients in our study population. These results clearly indicated that obese PCOS patients tend to be at a higher risk for the development of future cardiovascular disease than are other patients.

Limitations

The main limitations of this study concerns its cross-sectional study design and its relatively small population size. Moreover, monocyte and lymphocyte counts were calculated automatically using peripheric blood samples. The absence of other inflammation and oxidation parameters, in conjunction with the lack of a comparison to other inflammation biomarkers, was another limitation of this study. Data regarding patients' alcohol intake and smoking habits to include frequency of use and years of smoking history, both of which may affect the development of PCOS, were not included in our study due to the absence of records.

Conclusions

This study was the first to investigate the significance of the MHR in patients with PCOS. Our study demonstrated that patients with PCOS have higher MHR values than do women without the condition. The MHR may be used as a simple, low-cost, reproducible biochemical marker to be used in the detection of cardiovascular disease risk in PCOS patients; notably, it is also beneficial in the diagnosis of PCOS using other diagnostic criteria. The present study suggests that further prospective randomized studies be conducted in order to fully evaluate the association between the MHR and PCOS.

Abbreviations

BMI: Body mass index; CVD: Cardiovascular disease; DM: Diabetes mellitus; E2: Estradiol; ELISA: Enzyme-linked immunosorbent assay; FSH: Follicle-stimulating hormone; HDL: High-density lipoprotein; HOMA-IR: Homeostatic model assessment for insulin resistance; hsCRP: High-sensitivity C-reactive protein; LDL: Low-density lipoprotein cholesterol; LH: Luteinizing hormone; MHR: Monocyte counts to high-density lipoprotein cholesterol ratio; OR: Odds ratio; PCOS: Polycystic ovary syndrome; SD: Standard deviation; STEMI: ST-segment elevation myocardial infarction; TSH: Thyroid-stimulating hormone

Acknowledgments

The authors have no relevant affiliations or financial involvement with any organization or entity with a financial interest in or financial conflict with the subject matter or materials discussed in the manuscript. This includes employment, consultancies, honoraria, stock ownership or options, expert testimony, grants or patents received or pending, or royalties.

Funding

Authors do not have any funds for this study.

Financial disclosure

The authors have no connection to any companies or products mentioned in this article.

Authors'contributions

AU, EA and HK designed the study. AU, EA, HK and CBB conducted the sample collection and compiled the data. AU, EA, CBB and EA analyzed the data. AU and EA performed statistical analysis and AU, EA, HK and EA generated the manuscript. EA: Critical review, control/supervision. All authors read and approved the final manuscript.

Competing interests
The authors declare that they have no competing interests.

Author details
[1]Department of Obstetrics and Gynecology, School of Medicine, Balıkesir University Faculty of Medicine, Cagis Yerleskesi, Bigadic yolu 17. km, 10145 Balikesir, Turkey. [2]Department of Cardiology, School of Medicine, Balikesir University, Balikesir, Turkey.

References

1. Fauser BCJM, Tarlatzis BC, Rebar RW, Legro RS, Balen AH, Lobo R, et al. Consensus on women's health aspects of polycystic ovary syndrome (PCOS): the Amsterdam ESHRE/ASRM-sponsored 3rd PCOS consensus workshop group. Fertil Steril. 2012;97:28–38. e25
2. Yildiz BO, Bozdag G, Yapici Z, Esinler I, Yarali H. Prevalence, phenotype and cardiometabolic risk of polycystic ovary syndrome under different diagnostic criteria. Hum Reprod Oxf Engl. 2012;27:3067–73.
3. Puder JJ, Varga S, Kraenzlin M, De Geyter C, Keller U, Müller B. Central fat excess in polycystic ovary syndrome: relation to low-grade inflammation and insulin resistance. J Clin Endocrinol Metab. 2005;90:6014–21.
4. Kim JW, Han JE, Kim YS, Won HJ, Yoon TK, Lee WS. High sensitivity C-reactive protein and its relationship with impaired glucose regulation in lean patients with polycystic ovary syndrome. Gynecol Endocrinol. 2012; 28:259–63.
5. Toulis KA, Goulis DG, Mintziori G, Kintiraki E, Eukarpidis E, Mouratoglou S-A, et al. Meta-analysis of cardiovascular disease risk markers in women with polycystic ovary syndrome. Hum Reprod Update. 2011;17:741–60.
6. Keskin Kurt R, Okyay AG, Hakverdi AU, Gungoren A, Dolapcioglu KS, Karateke A, et al. The effect of obesity on inflammatory markers in patients with PCOS: a BMI-matched case-control study. Arch Gynecol Obstet. 2014; 290:315–9.
7. Margolis KL, Manson JE, Greenland P, Rodabough RJ, Bray PF, Safford M, et al. Leukocyte count as a predictor of cardiovascular events and mortality in postmenopausal women: the Women's health initiative observational study. Arch Intern Med. 2005;165:500–8.
8. Auffray C, Sieweke MH, Geissmann F. Blood monocytes: development, heterogeneity, and relationship with dendritic cells. Annu Rev Immunol. 2009;27:669–92.
9. Linker R, Gold R, Luhder F. Function of neurotrophic factors beyond the nervous system: inflammation and autoimmune demyelination. Crit Rev Immunol. 2009;29:43–68.
10. Parthasarathy S, Barnett J, Fong LG. High-density lipoprotein inhibits the oxidative modification of low-density lipoprotein. Biochim Biophys Acta. 1990;1044:275–83.
11. Westerterp M, Gourion-Arsiquaud S, Murphy AJ, Shih A, Cremers S, Levine RL, et al. Regulation of hematopoietic stem and progenitor cell mobilization by cholesterol efflux pathways. Cell Stem Cell. 2012;11:195–206.
12. Kanbay M, Solak Y, Unal HU, Kurt YG, Gok M, Cetinkaya H, et al. Monocyte count/HDL cholesterol ratio and cardiovascular events in patients with chronic kidney disease. Int Urol Nephrol. 2014;46:1619–25.
13. Canpolat U, Çetin EH, Cetin S, Aydin S, Akboga MK, Yayla C, et al. Association of Monocyte-to-HDL cholesterol ratio with slow coronary flow is linked to systemic inflammation. Clin Appl Thromb. 2016;22:476–82.
14. Cetin MS, Ozcan Cetin EH, Kalender E, Aydin S, Topaloglu S, Kisacik HL, et al. Monocyte to HDL cholesterol ratio predicts coronary artery disease severity and future major cardiovascular adverse events in acute coronary syndrome. Heart Lung Circ. 2016;25:1077–86.
15. Cagli K, Tok D, Turak O, Gunertem E, Yayla C, Lafci G, et al. Monocyte count-to-high-density lipoprotein-cholesterol ratio is associated with abdominal aortic aneurysm size. Biomark Med. 2016;10:1039–47.
16. You S, Zhong C, Zheng D, Xu J, Zhang X, Liu H, et al. Monocyte to HDL cholesterol ratio is associated with discharge and 3-month outcome in patients with acute intracerebral hemorrhage. J Neurol Sci. 2017;372:157–61.
17. Aydin E, Ates I, Fettah Arikan M, Yilmaz N, Dede F. The ratio of monocyte frequency to HDL cholesterol level as a predictor of asymptomatic organ damage in patients with primary hypertension. Hypertens Res. 2017;40:758–64.
18. Vahit D, Mehmet KA, Samet Y, Hüseyin E. Assessment of monocyte to high density lipoprotein cholesterol ratio and lymphocyte-to-monocyte ratio in patients with metabolic syndrome. Biomark Med. 2017;11:535–40.
19. Ferriman D, Gallwey JD. Clinical assessment of body hair growth in women. J Clin Endocrinol Metab. 1961;21:1440–7.
20. Samy N, Hashim M, Sayed M, Said M. Clinical significance of inflammatory markers in polycystic ovary syndrome: their relationship to insulin resistance and body mass index. Dis Markers. 2009;26:163–70.
21. Diamanti-Kandarakis E, Alexandraki K, Piperi C, Protogerou A, Katsikis I, Paterakis T, et al. Inflammatory and endothelial markers in women with polycystic ovary syndrome. Eur J Clin Investig. 2006;36:691–7.
22. Bayram F, Kocer D, Ozsan M, Muhtaroglu S. Evaluation of endothelial dysfunction, lipid metabolism in women with polycystic ovary syndrome: relationship of paraoxonase 1 activity, malondialdehyde levels, low-density lipoprotein subfractions, and endothelial dysfunction. Gynecol Endocrinol. 2012;28:497–501.
23. Türkçüoğlu I, Kafkasli A, Meydanli MM, Ozyalin F, Taşkapan C. Independent predictors of cardiovascular risk in polycystic ovarian syndrome. Gynecol Endocrinol. 2011;27:915–9.
24. Repaci A, Gambineri A, Pasquali R. The role of low-grade inflammation in the polycystic ovary syndrome. Mol Cell Endocrinol. 2011;335:30–41.
25. Johnsen SH, Fosse E, Joakimsen O, Mathiesen EB, Stensland-Bugge E, Njølstad I, et al. Monocyte count is a predictor of novel plaque formation: a 7-year follow-up study of 2610 persons without carotid plaque at baseline the Tromsø study. Stroke. 2005;36:715–9.
26. Akboga MK, Balci KG, Maden O, Ertem AG, Kirbas O, Yayla C, et al. Usefulness of monocyte to HDL-cholesterol ratio to predict high SYNTAX score in patients with stable coronary artery disease. Biomark Med. 2016;10:375–83.
27. Murphy AJ, Chin-Dusting JPF, Sviridov D, Woollard KJ. The anti inflammatory effects of high density lipoproteins. Curr Med Chem. 2009;16:667–75.
28. Açıkgöz SK, Açıkgöz E, Şensoy B, Topal S, Aydoğdu S. Monocyte to high-density lipoprotein cholesterol ratio is predictive of in-hospital and five-year mortality in ST-segment elevation myocardial infarction. Cardiol J. 2016;23:505–12.
29. Cockerill GW, Rye KA, Gamble JR, Vadas MA, Barter PJ. High-density lipoproteins inhibit cytokine-induced expression of endothelial cell adhesion molecules. Arterioscler Thromb Vasc Biol. 1995;15:1987–94.
30. Guleria AK, Syal SK, Kapoor A, Kumar S, Tiwari P, Dabadghao P. Cardiovascular disease risk in young Indian women with polycystic ovary syndrome. Gynecol Endocrinol. 2014;30:26–9.

18

Decreased MUC1 in endometrium is an independent receptivity marker in recurrent implantation failure during implantation window

Fangrong Wu[1], Xiaoyan Chen[1], Yingyu Liu[1], Bo Liang[1], Hui Xu[1], Tin Chiu Li[1] and Chi Chiu Wang[1,2,3*]

Abstract

Background: It is postulated that women suffered from recurrent implantation failure (RIF) have different endometrial receptivity compared to those who experienced with idiopathic recurrent miscarriage (RM). In this study, expression of common endometrial markers Leukemia inhibitor factor (LIF), mucin 1 (MUC1) and integrin β3 were studied and compared.

Methods: Fourteen women with RIF, 25 with RM and 20 fertile controls were recruited for endometrial biopsy during implantation window on day LH + 7. Spatial and temporal expression of MUC1, LIF and Integrin β3 were compared using semi-quantitative immunohistochemistry. Association of MUC1, LIF and integrin β3 expression levels with demographic and clinical characteristics were determined.

Results: MUC1 expression in both luminal and glandular epithelium in women with RIF were significantly lower than that in women with RM and fertile controls. There were no differences in LIF and Integrin β3 expression in endometrial epithelium among three groups. Decreased MUC1 expression were not significantly associated with age, BMI, gravidity, parity, cycle length, progesterone level and previous miscarriage.

Conclusions: Deceased expression of MUC1 is an independent marker for endometrial receptivity in RIF women, suggesting MUC1 may contribute to the reproductive failure in RIF women.

Keywords: Implantation, Endometrium, Receptivity markers, Reproductive failure

Introduction

Endometrium is critical for a successful implantation [1]. For only a short period of time during mid-luteal phase, the endometrium becomes receptive to the embryo to implant. This specific period has been referred as implantation window around 7 days after surge of luteinizing hormone (LH + 7) [2]. During this implantation window, endometrium will equip with adhesion ligands but remove inhibitory factors to facilitate the implantation process [3]. Many molecules have been proposed as markers for endometrial receptivity, but there is as yet no consensus on which marker is the best. Most of previous studies only focused on a single marker; often the endometrial specimens were not precisely timed; few studies compared the RIF and RM with fertile control at the same time. These may be the potential reasons of the contrasting observation. In addition, the effects of various confounding factors on the result were not examined as well.

Some endometrial receptivity markers expressed in epithelium and others expressed in stroma of the endometrium. Mucin 1(MUC1) is a member-associated protein, highly expressed in luminal and glandular epithelium on LH + 7 day [4, 5]. Fertile women showed a higher level of

* Correspondence: ccwang@cuhk.edu.hk
Paper presentation information: Part of this work was presented at the 7th congress of the Asia Pacific Initiative on Reproduction (ASPIRE 2017) held in Kuala Lumper, Malaysia, 30 March-2 April 2017
[1]Department of Obstetrics and Gynaecology, The Chinese University of Hong Kong, Shatin, Hong Kong
[2]Li Ka Shing Institute of Health Sciences, Faculty of Medicine, The Chinese University of Hong Kong, Shatin, Hong Kong
Full list of author information is available at the end of the article

endometrium MUC1 expression than infertile patients [6]. LIF belongs to interleukin-6 family and has complex regulatory roles in implantation [7]. Animal study showed that blastocysts from LIF knock-out mice failed to implant, however, they were viable when transferred to wild-type recipients with normal endometrium [8]. Integrin is a family of transmembrane glycoprotein that regulates cell-cell and cell-matrix interaction. Integrin isoform β3 expression in endometrium coexists with the period of implantation window [9]. Women underwent IVF treatment with normal Integrin β3 in endometrium had twice pregnancy rate than women with low Integrin β3 level [10]. Abnormal endometrial receptivity may contribute to the reproductive failure. It is postulated that different aspects of endometrial receptivity are disrupted in recurrent implantation failure (RIF) compared with idiopathic recurrent miscarriage (RM). In this study, we studied the expression of three endometrial receptivity markers, MUC1, LIF and Integrin β3 in the same endometrium specimens precisely collected at LH + 7 day and compared among women with RIF, RM and fertile control.

Materials and methods

Participants and endometrial biopsy

This study was approved by the ethics committee of The Chinese University of Hong Kong, and informed consent has been obtained from all the participants. Inclusion criteria included women less than 40 years old, with regular menstrual cycle and normal body mass index (BMI), and had no use of hormonal contraception or intrauterine devices for at least 3 months preceding the study. Exclusion criteria included endometrial or uterine pathology such as adenomyosis, fibroids, endometrial polyps and hyperplasia, endometriosis, endometritis, as well as anovulation and polycystic ovary syndrome (PCOS).

RIF was defined as failure to achieve a clinical pregnancy after at least 4 good-quality embryos have been transferred in 3 or more transfer cycles [11]. RM was defined as 3 or more consecutive pregnancy losses before 20-week gestation. All patients were idiopathic with normal uterine cavity examined by ultrasonography and hysterosalpingogram, normal thyroid function, tested negative for lupus anticoagulant and anticardiolipin antibodies, with normal parental karyotype results. Women who had at least one previous live birth within 1–2 years and no history of infertility, implantation failure and miscarriage were included as control.

All participants underwent daily urine test from day 9 of the cycle onwards to identify the LH surge. Endometrial biopsy was obtained using a Pipelle sampler (Prodimed) or Pipet Curet (Cooper Surgical) precisely at LH + 7 day. The endometrial specimens were washed immediately in phosphate-buffered saline (PBS, pH = 7.4) and divided into two parts. One part was fixed in 10% neutral buffered formalin for immunohistochemistry, the other part was sent to pathology examination for endometrial dating by qualified gynecological pathologist blinded to the clinical diagnosis. If the endometrial dating results were not coincident with the endometrium at mid-secretary phase and have been diagnosed as chronic endometritis, the samples were excluded from the study. Chronic endometritis was defined by presence and diagnostic criteria of CD138 plasma cells as described before [12].

Immunohistochemistry

After overnight formalin fixation and a serial ethanol dehydration, the endometrial specimens were embedded into paraffin wax and sectioned to a thickness of 4 μm. Spatial expression of MUC1, LIF and Integrin β3 in endometrial specimens were determined by standard immunohistochemistry. In brief, sections were dewaxed in xylene, rehydrated through descending ethanol to PBS, and then quenched in 3% hydrogen peroxide in methanol for 20 min. Antigen retrieval was performed in microwave oven with 10 mmol/L sodium citrate buffer (pH = 6.0). Sections were then washed in PBS and blocked in 1% BSA (bovine serum albumin) buffer for 1 h at room temperature, then incubated at 4 °C overnight with primary antibody (goat polyclonal anti-human LIF antibody (1:20, R&D system, AF-250-NA), mouse monoclonal anti-human MUC1 antibody (1:50, abcam, ab8949), or rabbit polyclonal anti-human β3 antibody, (1:50, abcam, ab197662). Then the sections were washed in 0.5% PBST and incubated in appropriate secondary antibody for 1 h at room temperature. The specific antibody binding was visualized by peroxidase substrate 3,3′-diaminobenzidene tetrahydrochloride (DAB, Dako) and counterstained with hematoxylin. Sections were then dehydrated and mounted in synthetic resin DPX. The expression of MUC1, LIF and Integrin β3 in luminal and glandular epithelium were examined under light microscopy (Leica, Germany). Five visual fields were selected under magnification of 400 for analysis. A qualified field was defined as endometrial tissue occupied ≥90% area with both luminal and glandular epithelium.

H-score analysis

The intensity of LIF, MUC1 and Integrin β3 expression in the endometrial sections were quantified according to the equation: H-score = $\sum P_i$, where i was referred as staining intensity (0 = negative; 1 = weak; 2 = moderate; 3 = strong) and P_i was referred as percentage of cells stained at each intensity (0–100%). H-score of MUC1, LIF and Integrin β3 in luminal epithelium and glandular epithelium were obtained in 5 qualified 400× visual fields per sample, respectively. Each section was scored independently by two observers both were blinded to the clinical diagnosis. In the event of differences in the score obtained, slides were reexamined until the H-score for the section agreed by both observers. The final scores were averaged from 5 fields for each sample.

Statistical analysis

Data were analyzed with SPSS 19.0 (IBM, USA). Quantitative data were compared by Mann-Whitney test, and qualitative data were compared by Chi's square test. H-sores of LIF, MUC1 and Integrin β3 were compared by one-way ANOVA, and then post-hoc LSD test for the multiple-pairwise comparisons. Multivariate linear regression was used to test the association between the receptive markers. A value of $P < 0.05$ was considered to be significant.

Results

A total of 78 participants were recruited in this study. Of the 78 endometrial specimens, 8 were excluded due to the histological dating not consistent with mid-secretary phase, and another 11 were excluded due to diagnosed of chronic endometritis and history of endometriosis. Immunohistochemistry study was performed on the remained 59 endometrial specimens, including 20 from fertile controls, 14 from RIF women and 25 from RM. Demographic details are summarized in Table 1. Age, number of previous pregnancy, number of live birth and previous miscarriage were significantly different among three study groups, but not BMI and menstrual cycle length. Women in RIF and RM group were older than control fertile women (both $P < 0.001$). However, there was no significant correlation between age and expression of LIF, MUC1 and integrin β3 in both luminal and glandular epithelium (Additional file 1: Table S1).

MUC1, LIF and Integrin β3 expression were identified in both luminal and glandular epithelium, but LIF and Integrin β3 can also be found in stromal cells (Fig. 1). MUC1 showed strong immunoreactivity in both luminal and glandular epithelial cells in control group, but less intense in RM group and very low in RIF group. LIF showed positive immunoreactivity in the glandular epithelium than that in the luminal epithelium and stromal cells, but overall the immunoreactivity was not as strong as MUC1. Integrin β3 showed positive immunoreactivity in both luminal and glandular epithelium in both RIF and RM groups but less in control group.

The H-score analysis showed that expression of MUC1 in both luminal and glandular epithelium in RIF group was significantly lower than those in control and RM group (Fig. 2). No significant differences in LIF and Integrin β3 expression in either luminal or glandular epithelium among and between the three groups were

Table 1 Demographic characteristics of participants

Variables	Control ($N = 20$)	RIF ($N = 14$)	RM ($N = 25$)	P-value[a]
Age (y)	28.9 ± 3.0	35.2 ± 3.3	36.1 ± 3.2	< 0.001
BMI (kg/m^2)	21.7 ± 1.9	21.9 ± 2.4	22.9 ± 3.9	0.43
Smoking (n)	0/20 (0%)	0/14 (0%)	3/25 (12.0%)	0.12[a]
Cycle length (d)	29.4 ± 1.7	29.1 ± 2.0	29.8 ± 4.8	0.89
Abnormal karyotype (n)	0/20 (0%)	0/14 (0%)	0/25 (0%)	NA[a]
Progesterone level (nmol/L)	–	62.4 ± 33.5	47.3 ± 20.9	0.31[b]
No. of previous pregnancy				
0	0/20 (0%)	10/14 (71.4%)	0/25 (0%)	< 0.001
1	12/20 (60.0%)	3/14 (21.4%)	0/25 (0%)	< 0.001
≥ 2	8/20 (40.0%)	1/14 (7.1%)	25/25 (100%)	< 0.001
No. of live birth				
0	0/20 (0%)	13/14 (92.9%)	23/25 (92.0%)	< 0.001
1	14/20 (70.0%)	1/14 (7.1%)	2/25 (8.0%)	< 0.001
≥ 2	6/20 (30.0%)	0/14 (0%)	0/25 (0%)	< 0.001
No. of previous miscarriage				
0	20/20 (100%)	10/14 (71.4%)	0/25 (0%)	< 0.001
1	0/20 (0%)	3/14 (21.4%)	0/25 (0%)	< 0.001
2	0/20 (0%)	1/14 (7.1%)	0/25(0%)	< 0.001
≥ 3	0/20 (0%)	0/14 (0%)	25/25 (100%)	< 0.001

Data are presented as mean ± SD or n/N (%). *RIF*, recurrent implantation failure; *RM*, recurrent miscarriage. [a]Chi square test compared among 3 groups when indicated; [b] Mann-Whitney test compared between RIF and RM groups only; NA: not available

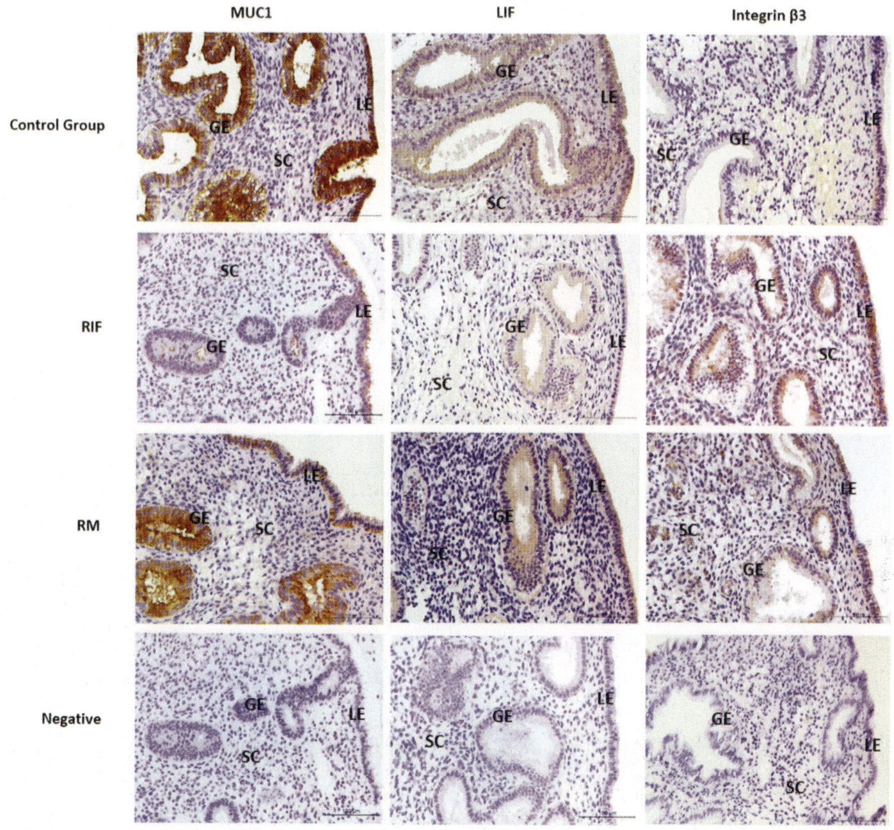

Fig. 1 MUC1, LIF and integrin β3 staining in endometrium. *LE*, luminal epithelium, *GE*, glandular epithelium, *SC*, stromal cell. Magnification: X 200. Scale bar: 100μm

found, although the expression of LIF in luminal and glandular epithelium in RIF group was slightly lower and expression of Integrin β3 were slightly higher than other groups. Although chronic endometritis and endometriosis were excluded, there were no significant differences in MUC1, LIF and Integrin β3 expressions in the endometrium between women with and women without chronic endometritis and endometriosis (Additional file 1: Table S2).

In multivariate linear regression analysis (Table 2), age, BMI, cycle length, progesterone level, gravidity, parity and previous miscarriage were not significantly associated with endometrial MUC1, LIF and Integrin β3 expression levels. The association remained not significant when the multivariate regression analysis was adjusted by the clinical diagnosis.

Discussion

Recurrent implantation failure and idiopathic recurrent miscarriage present two major challenges of reproductive failure to clinicians providing care for patients who wish to start or extend their family [13, 14]. The luminal epithelium is the first point of contact between the endometrium and blastocyst, which acts as both barrier and receptor at the same time. In the present study, expression of endometrial receptivity markers LIF, MUC1 and Integrin β3 in luminal and glandular epithelium during the implantation window in women with RIF and RM were examined and compared.

MUC1, LIF and Integrin β3 have long been proposed as biomarkers for endometrial receptivity. Many studies have been carried out; however, the results were inconsistent (Table 3). A special strength of our study is the precise timing of the specimens; all specimens were obtained precisely 7 days after the LH surge. It is particularly important as endometrial morphology and function change rapidly in the peri-implantation period, so that a difference of only one or two days could have introduced significant variance to the results. It also explains why there was significant controversy regarding the observations reported in the literature. One reason for these discrepancies is the different time point of collecting endometrium biopsy for examination, especially if the biopsy specimens were obtained over a period of several days.

MUC1 has been proposed as an anti-adhesive protein because of its physiochemical hindrance mediated by its long ectodomain, which may inhibit the attachment between blastocyst and endometrium. Animal studies

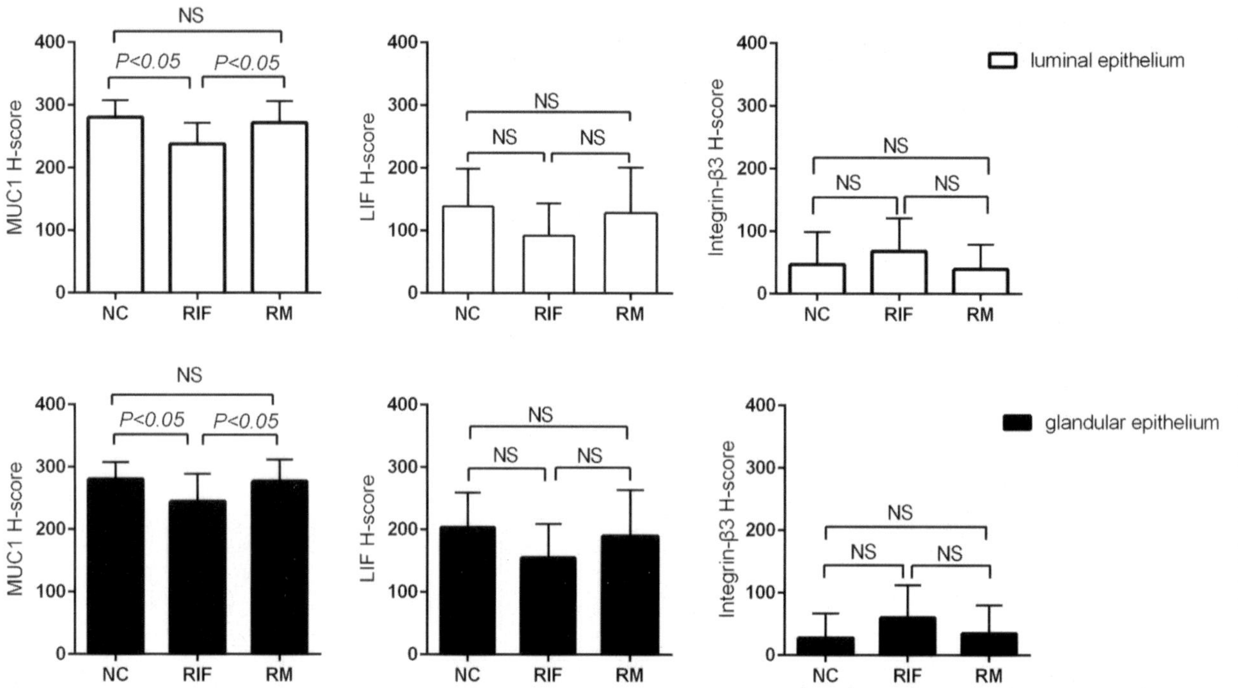

Fig. 2 Differentiated expression of MUC1, LIF and integrin β3. H-sores of LIF, MUC1 and integrin β3 expression in luminal (upper panels) and glandular (lower panels) epithelium were compared by one-way ANOVA among groups, and post-hoc LSD test has been used to test the multiple-pairwise comparisons. *NC*, control group; *RIF*, recurrent implantation failure; *RM*, recurrent miscarriage. *NS*, no significant.

have showed that MUC1 is down-regulated before implantation [15, 16], but human studies found that MUC1 is up-regulated during implantation window [4]. Although the precise role of MUC1 in implantation is still unclear, many studies showed low level of MUC1 was associated with impaired receptivity of endometrium [6, 17–19]. Women with RM had reduced endometrial MUC1 expression when compared to fertile women on days LH + 7 and 8 [17]. They proposed that decreased expression of MUC1 may induce endometrial super-fertility and interrupt embryo selection, which allows defective blastocysts to implant but leads to increase miscarriage rate. However, our data did not show significantly decrease of MUC1 in RM group, suggesting MUC1 may not be a reliable receptivity marker for RM. In contrast, MUC1 was significantly decreased in RIF group and multivariate linear regression analysis showed MUC1 was independent of demographic and clinical characteristics of the subjects, regardless of RM, RIF or control. It suggests that decreased endometrium MUC1 expression is an independent receptivity marker in RIF during implantation window.

As for Integrin β3 in endometrium, we found no significant difference among three study groups. Many investigators like us also failed to find significant change in Integrin β3 expression between fertile and RM

Table 2 Multivariate linear regression model of demographic and clinical characteristics

Dependent variables	Post-hoc statistical power ($P < 0.05$)	Model summary				Coefficients (constant)		
		R	R^2	Adjusted R^2	*P*	B	95%CI	*P*
MUC1 H-score in luminal epithelium	0.99	0.61	0.37	−0.64	0.90	235.52	– 370.43-841.48	0.36
MUC1 H-score in glandular epithelium	0.97	0.57	0.32	−0.77	0.94	226.85	– 402-48-856.19	0.40
LIF H-score in luminal epithelium	0.45	0.34	0.12	−1.29	0.99	257.86	– 1026.67-1542.39	0.63
LIF H-score in glandular epithelium	0.25	0.28	0.07	−1.40	1.00	384.53	– 973.02-1742.07	0.50
Integrin β3 H-score in luminal epithelium	0.99	0.68	0.50	−0.39	0.79	−45.99	– 721.89-629.92	0.87
Integrin β3 H-score in luminal epithelium	0.96	0.55	0.31	−0.81	0.95	54.47	– 745.01-853.95	0.87

Independent variables include age, *BMI*, cycle length, gravidity, parity, number of previous miscarriage and progesterone level on biopsy day. With or without adjustment of clinical conditions: control, RIF and RM; *R*, residual; R^2, R square *B*, beta coefficient *SE*, standard error. 95% *CI*, 95% confidence interval for B

Table 3 Summary of previous inconsistent studies of MUC1, LIF and integrin β3 expression in endometrium

Source		Study (n)	Fertile control (n)	Timing of biopsy	Methods	MUC1	LIF	Integrin αvβ3/β3
RPL/RM	Xu et al. 2011	30	26	LH + 7–8 day	Immunohistochemistry	↓	↔	↔
	Banerjee et al. 2012	36	30	LH + 5–10 day	Immunohistochemistry Flow cytometric analysis	↓	↓	↓
	Germeyer et al. 2014	21	29	LH + 5–7 day	Immunohistochemistry	NA	NA	↓
	Karaer et al. 2014	30	30	LH + 6–11 day	RT-PCR	NA	↑	NA
	WU et al.2018 [a]	25	20	LH+ 7 day	Immunohistochemistry	↔	↔	↔
RIF	Mariee et al. 2012	45	15	LH + 7–9 day	Immunohistochemistry	NA	↓	NA
	Coughlan et al. 2013	45	6	LH + 7–9 day	Immunohistochemistry	NA	NA	↔
	Bastu et al. 2015	26	23	LH + 7–9 day	ELISA & Western-blot	↓	NA	NA
	Comba et al. 2015	21	20	LH + 6–10 day	ELISA	NA	↓	NA
	WU et al. 2018 [a]	14	20	LH + 7 day	Immunohistochemistry	↓	↔	↔

RPL, recurrent pregnancy loss *RM*, recurrent miscarriage *RIF*, recurrent implantation failure *RT-PCR*, quantitative real-time *PCR*, *ELISA*, enzyme-linked immunosorbent assay. ↓ expression significantly reduced; ↔ expression no significant difference; ↑ expression significantly increased when compared with control. *NA*, not available; [a] present study

women [17, 20, 21], although Germeyer et al. observe that women with unexplained pregnancy loss had significantly reduced Integrin β3 expression compared with health control [22]. Coughlan et al. demonstrated that RIF was not associated with abnormal endometrial Integrin expression, and the expression of Integrins α1, α4, and αvβ3 have no prognostic value in subsequent IVF treatment [20]. In this study, we also did not find any significant difference in Integrin β3 among RM, RIF and fertile control and nor any significant correlation between MUC1, LIF and Integrin β3.

In agreement with others, we observed a stronger endometrium staining of LIF in epithelial cells compared with stromal cells. Comba et al. found that both blood and tissue levels of LIF were statistically lower in patients with RPL [23]. Decreased LIF expression level has been demonstrated in RIF patients by other study, when endometrium biopsy was obtained on days LH + 7 to LH + 9 [24]. However, the results of our study showed no significant difference in expression of LIF among three study groups in both luminal and glandular epithelium, even though H-scores showed a tendency of reduced expression in RIF patients.

There are some limitations of our study. First, the total number of participants included in the study is relatively small. The relative small sample size in each of the three groups studies may result small or subtle differences. Nevertheless, the demonstration of significant reduction of MUC1 expression in this suggests that the difference is likely to be of significant biological relevance. Our current sample size allowed us to show a difference of mean H score at least 30 with SD 15 with Power 99% and Type I error of 0.01. Second, the use of immunohistochemistry to examine the expression of various markers is rather semi-quantitative but it has the advantage of obtaining information of spatial expression of the protein markers in different tissue compartments. In our study, we were able to show that the expression of MUC1 in women with RIF was significantly reduced in the both luminal and glandular epithelium. The use of alternative methods such as quantitative real-time polymerase chain reaction or Western blot will not be able to demonstrate the expression of the protein markers in specific cellular components. Thirdly, although MUC1, LIF and Integrin β3 had been separately investigated in different studies, we studied 3 markers simultaneously in the serial sections of same sample; the endometrial specimens were collected precisely during implantation window; and RIF and RM were compared with fertile control in the same study.

Conclusions

In summary, our study showed MUC1, but not LIF and Integrin β3, was significantly decreased in both luminal and glandular epithelium in women with RIF, but not in women with RM. Both LIF and Integrin β3 do not appear to be sensitive receptivity markers for RIF or RM. In addition, the reduction in MUC1 expression was an independent marker of endometrial receptivity in women with RIF. It suggests MUC1 contributes to the unexplained reproductive failure in RIF. Further in-depth functional and interventional studies of MUC1 in RIF are needed.

Acknowledgments
We sincerely thank the women who participated in the study. We also thank the medical and nursing staff of the Reproductive Medical Center of The Price of Wales Hospital for their assistance in patient recruitment and management.

Authors' contributions
CCW and TCL designed the study. FW performed the experiments and the statistical analysis with help from HX and BL. XC and YL provided clinical advice and managed the biopsy. FW and CCW wrote the manuscript. All authors reviewed the manuscript. All authors read and approved the final manuscript.

Competing interests
The authors declare that they have no competing interests.

Author details
[1]Department of Obstetrics and Gynaecology, The Chinese University of Hong Kong, Shatin, Hong Kong. [2]Li Ka Shing Institute of Health Sciences, Faculty of Medicine, The Chinese University of Hong Kong, Shatin, Hong Kong. [3]School of Biomedical Sciences, Faculty of Medicine, The Chinese University of Hong Kong, Shatin, Hong Kong.

References
1. Simón C, Martín JC, Pellicer A. Paracrine regulators of implantation. Bailliere's Best Pract Res Clin Obstet Gynaecol. 2000;14:815–26.
2. Psychoyos A. Hormonal control of Ovoimplantation. Vitam Horm. 1974;31: 201–56.
3. Aplin JD. The cell biological basis of human implantation. Baillieres Best Pr Res Clin Obs Gynaecol [Internet]. 2000;14:757–64.
4. Hey NA, Li TC, Devine PL, Graham RA, Saravelos H, Aplin JD. MUC1 in secretory phase endometrium: expression in precisely dated biopsies and flushings from normal and recurrent miscarriage patients. Hum Reprod. 1995;10:2655–62.
5. Aplin JD, Hey NA, Graham RA. Human endometrial MUC! Carries keratin sulphate: characteristic glycoforms in the luminal epithelium at receptivity. Glycobiol. 1998;8:269–76.
6. Margarit L, Taylor A, Roberts MH, Hopkins L, Davies C, Brenton AG, et al. MUC1 as a discriminator between endometrium from fertile and infertile patients with PCOS and endometriosis. J Clin Endocrinol Metab. 2010;95: 5320–9.
7. Kimber SJ. Leukaemia inhibitory factor in implantation and uterine biology. Reproduction. 2005;130:131–45.
8. Stewart CL, Kaspar P, Brunet LJ, Bhatt H, Gadi I, Köntgen F, et al. Blastocyst implantation depends on maternal expression of leukaemia inhibitory factor. Nature [Internet]. 1992;359:76–9.
9. Lessey BA, Castelbaum AJ, Wolf L, Greene W, Paulson M, Meyer WR, et al. Use of integrins to date the endometrium. Fertil Steril. 2000;73:779–87.
10. Thomas K, Thomson A, Wood S, Kingsland C, Vince G, Lewis-Jones I. Endometrial integrin expression in women undergoing in vitro fertilization and the association with subsequent treatment outcome. Fertil Steril. 2003;80:502–7.
11. Coughlan C, Ledger W, Wang Q, Liu F, Demirol A, Gurgan T, et al. Recurrent implantation failure: definition and management. Reprod BioMed Online. 2014;28:14–38.
12. Liu Y, Chen X, Huang J, Wang CC, Yu MY, Laird S, et al. A comparison of the prevalence of chronic endometritis determined by the use of different diagnostic methods in women with and without reproductive failure. Fertil Steril. 2018; *in press*
13. Teklenburg G, Salker M, Heijnen C, Macklon NS, Brosens JJ. The molecular basis of recurrent pregnancy loss: impaired natural embryo selection. Mol Hum Reprod. 2010;16:886–95.
14. Orlando J, Coulam C. Is Superfertility associated with recurrent pregnancy loss? Am J Reprod Immunol. 2014;72:549–54.
15. Surveyor GA, Gendler SJ, Pemberton L, Das SK, Chakraborty I, Julian J, et al. Expression and steroid hormonal control of muc-1 in the mouse uterus. Endocrinology. 1995;136:3639–47.
16. DeSouza MM. Reduction of mucin-1 expression during the receptive phase in the rat uterus [in process citation]. Biol Reprod [Internet]. 1998;58:1503–7.
17. Xu B, Sun X, Li L, Wu L, Zhang A, Feng Y. Pinopodes, leukemia inhibitory factor, integrin-β3, and mucin-1 expression in the peri-implantation endometrium of women with unexplained recurrent pregnancy loss. Fertil Steril. 2012;98:389–95.
18. Horne AW, Lalani EN, Margara RA, Ryder TA, Mobberley MA, White JO. The expression pattern of MUC1 glycoforms and other biomarkers of endometrial receptivity in fertile and infertile women. Mol Reprod Dev. 2005;72:216–29.
19. Bastu E, Mutlu MF, Yasa C, Dural O, Aytan AN, Celik C, et al. Role of Mucin 1 and Glycodelin A in recurrent implantation failure. Fertil Steril [Internet]. 2015;103:1059–1064.e2.
20. Coughlan C, Sinagra M, Ledger W, Li TC, Laird S. Endometrial integrin expression in women with recurrent implantation failure after in vitro fertilization and its relationship to pregnancy outcome. Fertil Steril. 2013;100:825–30.
21. Tuckerman EM, Laird SM, Prakash A, Li TC. Expression of integrins in the endometrium of women with recurrent miscarriage. Fertil Steril. 2006;86:755–7.
22. Germeyer A, Savaris RF, Jauckus J, Lessey B. Endometrial beta3 integrin profile reflects endometrial receptivity defects in women with unexplained recurrent pregnancy loss. Reprod Biol Endocrinol. 2014;12:1–5.
23. Comba C, Bastu E, Dural O, Yasa C, Keskin G, Ozsurmeli M, et al. Role of inflammatory mediators in patients with recurrent pregnancy loss. Fertil Steril. 2015;104:1467–1474.e1.
24. Mariee N, Li TC, Laird SM. Expression of leukaemia inhibitory factor and interleukin 15 in endometrium of women with recurrent implantation failure after IVF; correlation with the number of endometrial natural killer cells. Hum Reprod. 2012;27:1946–54.

19

Role of L-carnitine in female infertility

Ashok Agarwal[1*], Pallav Sengupta[2] and Damayanthi Durairajanayagam[3]

Abstract

Background: L-carnitine (LC), and its acetylated form, acetyl L-carnitine (ALC), have immense functional capabilities to regulate the oxidative and metabolic status of the female reproductive system. The vulnerability of this system to free radicals demand for advanced strategies to combat them. For this purpose, the 'quasi vitamins' LC and ALC can be used either individually, or in combination with each other or with other antioxidants.

Main body: This review (a) summarizes the effects of carnitines on female fertility along with the findings from various in vivo and in vitro studies involving human, animal and assisted reproductive technology, and (b) proposes their mechanism of actions in improving female fertility through their integrated actions on reducing cellular stress, maintaining hormonal balance and enhancing energy production. They reportedly aid β-oxidation in oocytes, maintain its cell membrane stability by acetylation of phospholipids and amphiphilic actions, prevent free radical-induced DNA damage and also stabilize acetyl Co-A/Co-A ratio for adequate acetyl storage as energy supply to maintain the robustness of reproductive cells.

Conclusion: While both LC and ALC have their applications in improving female fertility, ALC is preferred for its better antioxidant properties and LC for amelioration of energy supply to the cells. These beneficial effects show great promise in its application as a treatment option for women facing infertility disorders.

Keywords: Assisted reproductive technology, Acetyl-L-carnitine, Antioxidants, Female fertility, In vitro fertilization, L-carnitine, Oocyte quality

Background

The revolution of modern day reproductive biology research and assisted reproductive technology (ART) are promising to provide a more exhaustive description of the effects of metabolic supplementation on infertility. To date, thousands of supplements have been proposed to mitigate the outcomes of reproductive disorders, but most of them have ended up having several side-effects on other systems [1]. In order to combat this, reproductive biologists are currently searching for some supplements, or combination of supplements to fight against the problems of infertility. In this aspect, mitochondrial metabolism of both the male and female germ cells exert a crucial role [2]. Mitochondrial nutrient supplementation is also reported to be effective in many cases [3].

Levocarnitine or L-carnitine (LC) is a biologically active stereoisomer of 3-carboxy-2-hydroxy-N, N, N-trimethyl-1-propanaminium. It exists as a highly polar, small zwitterion (an ion that while electrically neutral, carries both a positive and a negative electrical charge in different parts of the molecule, as seen in certain amino acids and protein molecules) [4]. LC is reported to have benefits in the management of infertility [5, 6]. The impact of LC on male infertility is now well documented. It has been reported to be concerned with epididymal maturation of spermatozoa [7]. LC serves as an intra-mitochondrial vehicle for the acyl group, which in the form of acyl-CoA acts as a substrate for the oxidation process, producing energy for sperm respiration and motility [7, 8]. It has also been reported to ameliorate the effects of reactive oxygen species (ROS) and free radical-induced oxidative stress (OS) and minimizing pathological disorders of sperm, like adenosine triphosphate (ATP) depletion leading to insufficient axonemal phosphorylation, lipid peroxidation as well as loss of motility and viability [9, 10]. As LC has been reported to act as a potent antioxidant with very less side-effects, researchers are now considering its implementation as a treatment for female infertility [5, 11, 12]. It is well known that OS also affects female reproduction in

* Correspondence: agarwaa@ccf.org
[1]American Center for Reproductive Medicine, Cleveland Clinic, Glickman Urological and Kidney Institute, Mail Code X-11, 10681 Carnegie Avenue, Cleveland, OH 44195, USA
Full list of author information is available at the end of the article

various ways, including lipid peroxidation of oocytes [13], fertilization and embryo development in animals [14].

Similarly, acetyl-L-carnitine (ALC), the primary acetyl ester of LC has been reported to have beneficial impacts on reproductive functions through its antioxidative effects [7, 8, 15]. ALC plays an essential role in intermediary metabolism, acting as a donor of acetyl groups and facilitating the transfer of fatty acids from cytosol to mitochondria during beta-oxidation in animals [15]. ALC has also been reported to exert cholinomimetic effects and to modulate the gamma-amino butyric acid (GABA) system. Since it is abundant in hypothalamus, it can affect the neuronal activity and thus hypothalamo-pituitary gonadal (HPG) axis to exert its impact on female reproduction [16].

To date, many research studies have already been carried out in human [11, 12, 17, 18] and animal models [16, 19–21] using carnitines to treat female infertility as well as to improve reproductive performance. It has also been used in ART in an attempt to solve similar problems [22, 23].

This review summarizes the effects of both LC and acetyl-L-carnitine (ALC) on female fertility with detailed scrutiny of the reports published till date. It provides a glimpse of human, animal and in vitro experimental studies carried out to solve the problems of female infertility. It also provides its possible mechanism of actions when supplemented individually or in combination with other nutrients.

L-carnitine and acetyl L-carnitine: Physiological actions

LC is a small water-soluble molecule that plays an enormous role in normal physiology. It was first isolated from bovine muscle in 1905 by two Russian scientists [24], and only the L-isomer was found to be bioactive [4]. In mammals, ingested LC is absorbed from the small intestine via active transport and passive diffusion [25]. LC is then incorporated into the total body carnitine pool that includes uncharged LC, and short chain carnitine esters (acylcarnitines) such as ALC and propionyl L-carnitine (PLC). LC is also synthesized in the liver and kidneys via methylation of L-lysine [26]. A strict vegetarian diet may lead to deficiency of LC since red meat is the richest source of lysine. The accumulation of LC occurs in liver, skeletal muscle, heart, brain and testis [27]. The body tissue distribution studies show a very high concentration of LC in mature spermatozoa and luminal fluid of cauda epididymis [26]. Under physiological conditions, the carnitine pool (LC and ALC) remains in equilibrium because of the actions of local transferases and tubular reabsorption in the kidney [28].

Carnitines belong to one of the special classes of nutrients called 'quasi-vitamins' or 'conditionally-essential' nutrients [29]. LC intake is widely regarded as one of the most effective ways to promote endurance, burn fat, and shorten post-workout recovery [27]. In peripheral tissues, it helps in β-oxidation by transporting medium and long chain fatty acids into the mitochondria [30]. It is also important in maintaining cell membrane stability through its involvement in acetylation of membrane phospholipids and amphiphilic actions [31, 32]. LC also prevents DNA damage induced by the detrimental actions of free radicals [33]. It also functions as a stabilizer of a low acetyl CoA/CoA concentration ratio and as an acetyl store to supply energy in carbohydrate and lipid metabolic pathways [34] (Fig. 1).

L-carnitine and acetyl L-carnitine in female fertility

Several research studies have been carried out till date in human patients, animal models and in ART settings to investigate the effectiveness of LC and ALC in the improvement of female fertility [5, 22].

L-carnitine or acetyl L-carnitine - which carnitine is suitable for the treatment of female infertility?

Though a minute functional difference between LC and ALC has been reported, both are used in reproductive biology research to improve mitochondrial functions to treat infertility [5, 8, 9]. ALC is used most often associated with the improvement of antioxidant/anti-aging effects, while LC is commonly used to improve the body's ability to oxidize fat cells which assists in the production of energy and burning fat [27]. During oocyte development, it has been reported that the cumulus-oocyte complex (COC) plays an essential role in lipid metabolism and energy production. Thus, in oocytes, maintenance of proper lipid oxidation with/without a minimum production of free radicals is crucial to preserve its quality [30]. Though it is well documented that both forms of carnitine possess antioxidant properties [10], it has been suggested in some reports that ALC is more effective in combating ROS-induced oxidative damage compared to LC [15]. Thus, studies focusing on antioxidant defense-mediated improvement of female fertility preferentially utilize ALC, whereas, studies demonstrating improved lipid metabolism-induced enhancement of oocyte quality, and thereby fertility, tend to use LC. Other acylcarnitines are also used in reproductive biology research, but to a lesser extent [35]. In 2013, Varnagy et al. reported the profiling of several acylcarnitines in the serum and follicular fluids of women undergoing IVF. They provided suggestive evidence that in IVF patients with better reproductive potential (higher number of oocytes and/or viable embryos), the LC/acylcarnitine pathway appears to be upregulated while the endogenous carnitine pool is diminished, which consequently improves oocyte quality [35]. In the following sections,

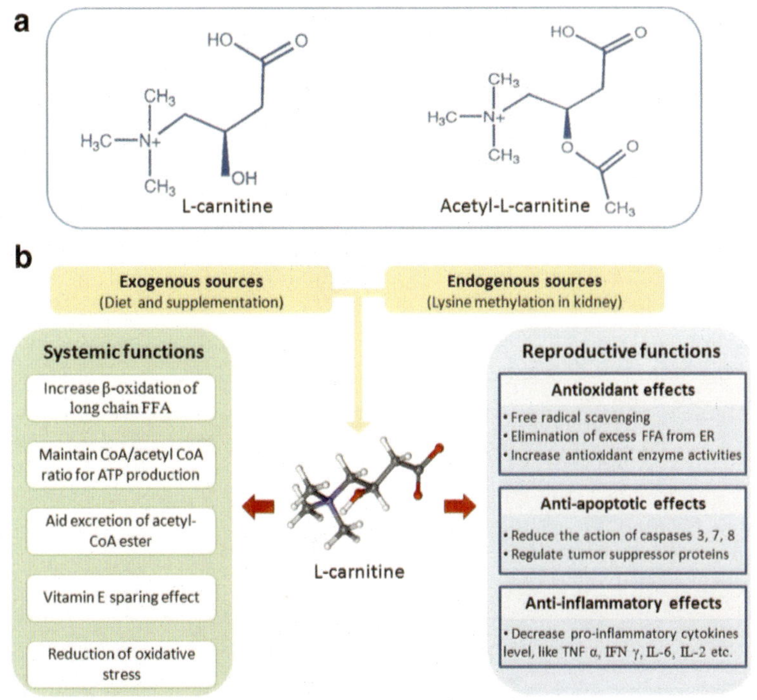

Fig. 1 (**a**) Molecular structures of L-carnitine and acetyl-L-carnitine, (**b**) systemic and reproductive functions of L-carnitine. CoA, coenzyme A; ER, endoplasmic reticulum; FFA, free fatty acid; IFN, interferon; IL, interleukin; TNF, tumor necrosis factor

we will provide evidence of LC and/or ALC supplementation and their role in female fertility.

Human studies

Most of the human experiments were carried out using LC as a supplement to alleviate/combat the problem of female infertility [11, 18, 36] (Table 1). Several studies found that both LC and ALC supplementation improves disorders such as polycystic ovary syndrome [12], endometriosis [19] and amenorrhea [17]. Carnitines are reported to increase gonadotropins and sex hormone levels as well as improve oocyte health [17]. However, the effects of LC on endometriosis are still a matter of debate [19, 29, 37, 38]. The possible mechanistic pathways through which LC could exert its effects on endometriosis will be discussed in a subsequent section.

Carnitine and PCOS

Polycystic ovary syndrome (PCOS) is a common female reproductive endocrinopathy. The main pathophysiological mechanisms underlying this syndrome include obesity, insulin resistance and hyperinsulinemia. Samimi and colleagues found that LC supplementation (250 mg per day orally for 12 weeks) lead to significant reduction in body weight, BMI, waist and hip circumference respectively as well as improved glycemic control in women with PCOS (mean age 24.8 ± 5.5 years) [12]. This study indicated that LC supplementation improves PCOS by decreasing blood glucose levels and opposing insulin resistance [12], which could perhaps be attributed to LC-induced increase in beta-oxidation of fatty acids and basal metabolic rates [39].

Women with PCOS also have an imbalance between male and female hormones as their ovaries tend to produce androgens in excessive amounts. One study suggested that hyperandrogenism and/or insulin resistance in the non-obese women with PCOS may be associated with decreased total serum LC levels [36]. Fenkci's group had measured the serum total LC levels in non-obese women with PCOS ($n = 27$; aged between 16 to 37 years) in comparison to that of healthy adult women ($n = 30$). They demonstrated these PCOS patients have significantly lower total LC (40.5 ± 5.7 μmol/L; in control: 91.1 ± 15.2 μmol/L), but higher levels of dehydroepiandrosterone (DHEA), testosterone, luteinizing hormone (LH), low-density lipoproteins (LDL) and fasting insulin compared to healthy women [36].

Another common feature of PCOS is chronic anovulation. The standard approach to treat women with anovulatory infertility, secondary to PCOS, is to administer clomiphene citrate to induce ovulation. However, some women do not ovulate despite receiving increasing doses of clomiphene citrate, and are therefore considered to be clomiphene citrate-resistant. In a single center, double blinded, randomized controlled clinical trial, Ismail et al. studied the effect of LC

Table 1 Human and animal studies involving carnitine supplementation to improve female fertility/reproductive status

Study aim	Carnitine(s) supplementation (dose and duration)	Study design/Subjects	Outcomes relevant to reproduction	Reference
Human Studies				
Single center, prospective study to evaluate whether ALC modulates opiatergic pathway in a group of patients with stress-induced amenorrhea	1 g/day ALC orally for 16 weeks	24 patients (aged 21–32 years) with FHA for the last 6 months were subdivided into 2 groups: Group A (hypogonadotropic patients, plasma LH levels ≤3 mIU/ml, $n = 16$) Group B (normogonadotropic patients, plasma LH levels > 3 mIU/ml, $n = 8$)	• ALC administration significantly modulates GnRH and LH secretion in hypothalamic amenorrhea in hypogonadotropic patients • ALC probably affects neuroendocrine control of gonadotropin secretion by modulating opiatergic control of GnRH-LH secretion • Data support the use of ALC as a therapeutic drug for stress-induced reproductive disorders with low LH levels or hypogonadotropic condition	[17]
Single center, double blinded, randomized controlled clinical trial to evaluate the effectiveness of LC on improving the ovulation and pregnancy rates as well as adverse metabolic indices in clomiphene-resistant PCOS women	3 g/day LC orally from day three until day seven of the cycle	170 clomiphene resistant PCOS women (aged less than 35 years) were randomly allocated into 2 groups: Group A ($n = 85$) received 250 mg clomiphene citrate plus LC Group B ($n = 85$) received 250 mg clomiphene citrate with placebo	• The combination of LC and CC significantly improved both the ovulation and the pregnancy rates in clomiphene-resistant PCOS women • The number of stimulated follicles reaching ≥17 mm diameter was significantly higher in Group A as compared to Group B • Endometrium at the time of hCG administration was significantly thicker in Group A • Serum E2, on the day of hCG administration, was significantly higher in the LC group • Pregnancy occurred in 42/85 cycles in Group A (54.5%) and 5/85 cycles in Group B (5.8%) and the difference was statistically significant. • The miscarriage rate was lower in Group A (2/85; 2.3%) than in Group B (4/85; 4.7%) ($p = 0.67$)	[11]
Before-after clinical trial to examine the effect of adding LC to PCOS patients who were resistant to clomiphene citrate and gonadotropin	2 g LC orally every 12 h, given from the third day of treatment with clomiphene citrate and gonadotropin until the hCG injection	50 PCOS patients (aged 20–35 years) either received LC or did not receive LC	• LC-treated women experienced the growth of dominant follicles (64%, 32/50 therapeutic cycles) and displayed a positive pregnancy test (20%, 10/50 therapeutic cycles) • LC-supplemented women had increased left ovarian follicle size compared to those without LC, however right ovarian follicle size was not significantly different between both groups • LC supplementation increased the mean endometrial thickness compared to those without LC.	[18]
Prospective, randomized, double-blind, placebo-controlled trial to determine the effects of oral LC supplementation on weight loss, and glycemic and lipid profiles in women with PCOS	250 mg LC orally for 12 weeks	60 overweight PCOS (aged 18–40 years) were randomized to receive either LC ($n = 30$) or placebo ($n = 30$)	• LC supplementation reduced body weight, body mass index, waist circumference and hip circumference and improved glycemic control in PCOS patients compared with placebo. • LC supplementation did not affect lipid profiles or free testosterone levels compared with placebo	[12]

Table 1 Human and animal studies involving carnitine supplementation to improve female fertility/reproductive status *(Continued)*

Study aim	Carnitine(s) supplementation (dose and duration)	Study design/Subjects	Outcomes relevant to reproduction	Reference
Oral LC supplementation on mental health and biomarkers of OS in women with PCOS	250 mg LC for 12 weeks	60 patients: randomized, double-blind, placebo-controlled study	• LC supplementation improved general and mental health parameters • LC supplementation improved TAC, MDA/TAC ratio and decreased lipid peroxidation	[40]
Animal Studies				
LC supplementation on endometriosis in BALB/c mice	25 mg/ml/d LC for 7 days	Young female BALB/c mice of 4–8 weeks of age	• Increased concentration of LC in serum • Decreased levels of IFN-γ, TNF-α, IL-6, IL-2	[19]
LC on reproductive hormones and organs of pregnant mice	0.5 and 1.0 mg/kg LC from day-1 until parturition	Female Swiss albino mice of 12–14 weeks of age	• Significantly increased FSH, LH and estradiol levels • Increased litter size, weight of reproductive organs and thickness of endometrium	[42]
ALC on HPG axis of female Sprague-Dawley rats	50 mg/kg/d ALC for 2 consecutive estrous cycles	Female Sprague-Dawley rats of 3 months of age	Improved hormonal secretions through HPG axis: increased GnRH, LH, estradiol and progesterone levels	[16]
LC on OS parameters in oophorectomized rats	100 mg/kg/d LC during post-castration day-21 to -35 (14 consecutive days)	Female adult Wistar rats	Decreased MDA, and NO levels, and improved TAC and OS index	[49]
Reproductive performance of sows on LC-supplementation	125 mg/d LC (pregnancy), 250 mg/d LC (lactation)	300 sows (Leicoma)	Improved litter size and piglets' body weight gain, decreased number of stillborn piglets	[51]
LC in gestating sow diet on fetal development	50 ppm in diet for 3 reproductive cycles, until day-110 of gestation	232 gestating sows	Increased leanness and muscle density in offspring	[52]
Dietary LC on laying hen performance and egg quality	500 mg/kg LC diet for 84 days	180 Isabrown laying hens of 27-weeks of age	Improved egg quality parameters including albumin content	[50]
LC on reproductive traits of white leghorns	125 ppm LC until 37-week of age	720 White leghorns	Improved total lipid and LC content in yolk	[43]
LC in cows during transition and high lactation period	2 g/d LC for 5 weeks	262 dairy cows (German Holstein)	Improved metabolic status during lactation period, increased milk protein content	[53]

ALC, Acetyl-L-carnitine, *FHA*, Functional hypothalamic amenorrhea, *HPG* Hypothalamo-pituitary-gonadal axis, *LC* L-Carnitine, *MDA* Malondialdehyde, *NO* Nitric oxide, *OS* Oxidative stress, *PCOS* Polycystic ovary syndrome, *SCC* Somatic cell count, *TAC* Total antioxidant capacity supplementation on clomiphene-resistant women with PCOS. All subjects received 250 mg clomiphene citrate daily from day-3 until day-7 of the cycle. In addition, women in the treatment arm ($n = 85$) were supplemented daily with 3 g of LC orally (day-3 until day of first positive pregnancy test), while those in the control arm (n = 85) received a placebo. Follicular maturation was monitored using transvaginal ultrasonography on all patients on day-7 and day-9,. and subsequently adjusted according to individual response [11].

Ismail's group found that LC supplementation along with clomiphene citrate treatment improved both ovulation (64.4% vs.17.4%; < 0.0001) and pregnancy (51.5% vs. 5.8%; $p < 0.0001$) rates in clomiphene-resistant women with PCOS. LC supplementation seemed to improve the number and rate at which the stimulated follicles developed (to a diameter of ≥17 mm for induction of ovulation), increase beta-oxidation and oocyte maturation as well as increase serum levels of both estradiol (E_2) and progesterone. LC supplementation not only improved reproductive health, but also enhanced the patients' lipid profile and body mass index (BMI) [11].

A typical alternative treatment to induce ovulation in clomiphene citrate-resistant PCOS patients is gonadotropin therapy. However, some women with PCOS fail to respond to both these treatments. Latifian et al. studied the effects of LC on 50 infertile women with PCOS who were both clomiphene- and gonadotropin-resistant. These women (mean age 27.98 ± 4.61 years) showed improvement following LC supplementation, which was given 2 g orally every 12 h (from the third day of the ovarian stimulation cycle onwards until the HCG injection). The LC-treated women in this study experienced the growth of dominant follicles (64%, $n = 32$) and displayed a positive pregnancy test (20%, $n = 10$). Moreover, LC was observed to increase the mean endometrium thickness as well as to inculcate positive changes in the left ovarian follicle size [18].

Not only does LC supplementation improve reproductive parameters in PCOS patients, but it can also confer positive effects on other health parameters in these women. This was demonstrated in a recent study whereby oral LC supplementation (250 mg for 12 weeks) among patients with PCOS improved total antioxidant capacity (TAC), decreased lipid peroxidation and enhanced general and mental health parameters [40].

Carnitine and functional hypothalamic amenorrhea

Functional hypothalamic amenorrhea (FHA) is a form of hypogonadotropic hypogonadism that results from an aberration in the pulsatile release of hypothalamic gonadotropin-releasing hormone (GnRH), which causes decreased gonadotropin release leading to reduced estradiol production in the ovary [41]. ALC administration (1 g/day orally for 16 weeks) in patients suffering from FHA ($n = 24$, age range 21 to 32 years) was found to increase LH levels by counteracting certain neuroendocrine pathways that have an inhibitory effect on the reproductive axis [17]. Genazzani and co-workers proposed that ALC acts through the opioidergic pathway and alters protein/hormone functions by acetylating -OH groups in amino acids like serine, threonine or tyrosine, thereby improving their functions. They concluded that ALC has positive therapeutic effects on the reproductive axis in hypogonadotropic women with FHA and improves the condition by acting through the HPG axis [17].

Animal studies

Numerous research studies have been carried out in animal models (murine and farm animals) to investigate how LC and ALC improve female reproductive functions [16, 19, 21, 42–44] (Table 1). Carnitines have been showed to have beneficial impacts in most of the studies involving PCOS, endocrine disorders and other cases of infertility. However, as alluded earlier, carnitines appear to possibly exert mixed effects on endometriosis [19, 29, 37, 38].

a) Mice and rat models

Carnitine, cytokines and immune response

Despite the aforementioned beneficial effects of LC and ALC treatment on female fertility, Dionyssopoulou et al. found that carnitine supplementation modified the production of various cytokines, such as interferon-γ, tumor necrosis factor-α, interleukins-2, – 4, – 6, vascular endothelial growth factor, granulocyte-macrophage colony stimulating factor, and insulin-like growth factor-1 in serum and peritoneal fluid as tested using the immunofluorescence or ELISA technique [19]. Furthermore, carnitine treatment altered the percentage of immune cells (macrophages, T cells, $CD4^+$ and $CD8^+$ cells) in peritoneal exudates and uterine cells. Immune modifications such as these as well as the presence of cytokines and growth factors in the peritoneal cavity may contribute to the development of endometriosis. The potential role of prostaglandins (PG), including that of PGE_1 and PGE_2, are directly associated with inflammation and could affect the function of immune cells. It was found that while inhibition of PGE_1 further increased the levels of certain cytokines in serum and peritoneal fluid [45], inhibition of PGE_2 reversed these values toward that of control [46]. Thus in presence of LC, it was suggested that PGE_2 plays a role in the mechanistic pathway leading to endometriosis, while PGE_1 may potentially be involved in suppressing the production of immune cells and inflammatory response [29].

Carnitine and the HPG axis

In 1992, Krsmanovic et al. examined the impact of ALC (50 mg/kg/day for a month) on the HPG axis in female rats and found that serum LH and prolactin levels were increased during the proestrous and estrous phases, while serum E_2 levels were increased during the estrous phase of the cycle. They have also noted an increase in uterine weight during both the proestrous and estrous phases of ALC-treated animals. Release of basal GnRH was found to be increased during the proestrous and diestrous I in hypothalamic slices of ALC-treated rats, which could mean that ALC stimulates the secretory activity of GnRH-producing hypothalamic neurons. In contrast, no alteration in pituitary functions was detected following ALC treatment in vitro. From these results, it was concluded that ALC may act through the HPG axis and cause gonadotropin release and this action is dependent on the cycle stage [16].

Carnitine and oocyte quality

Virmani et al. reported in 2015 that treatment of mice with both LC (0.4 mg/mouse) and ALC (0.12 mg/mouse) resulted in increased number of mature oocytes and less degradation of oocytes. They concluded that LC and ALC co-treatment showed better response in maintaining the quality and quantity of oocytes in mice. In females, an age-related decline in the number and quality of follicles and oocytes have already been documented [47]. Aging and ROS affects many biochemical pathways of developing oocytes that may produce a deleterious impact on oocyte health and in this aspect, LC supplementation has showed some beneficial roles. Christiana's group investigated another potential effect of LC through their study in which young BALB/c mice were given LC supplementation (2.5 mg/day/mouse for 7 days), superovulated and then mated with healthy males. They showed that 7 day-LC administration alters the lipid body content in pre-implantation embryos and did not result in live births in these females. This is because lipid body content is an important contributory factor towards healthy oocyte and embryo development and therefore its alteration may lead to infertility [37]. Conversely, a recent report by Virmani et al. (2017) showed that supplementation of carnitines (LC 0.4 mg/mouse + ALC 0.12 mg/mouse) to 8-week-old female CD1 mice not only improved oocyte formation but also increased the number of live birth in superovulated mice [48].

Carnitine and pregnancy-related parameters

Fakhrildin and Flayyih reported an improvement in weight of the reproductive organs (ovaries, uterine horns, vagina) and endometrial thickness, litter sizes as well as serum LH, FSH and E2 levels in pregnant mice (Swiss albino strain females aged between 12 to 14 weeks) given 0.5 and 1.0 mg/kg LC compared to the control group. As the parameters measured did not differ significantly between the two LC doses used, the study concluded that a low dose of LC was sufficient to render positive effects on pregnancy and offspring outcomes in pregnant mice [42].

Carnitine and oxidative stress

Canbolat and co-worker's study investigated the antioxidant property of LC (100 and 500 mg/kg/day) on oxidative stress parameters (nitric oxide (NO), malondialdehyde, total antioxidant status, total oxidative stress (OS), and OS index in the kidney, liver and heart, as well as sera of bilateral oophorectomized rats. They have reported LC exhibits antioxidant effects in different tissues with less NO production, lipid peroxidation and OS index when supplemented with 500 mg/kg/day LC intraperitoneally for 14 consecutive days in surgically menopausal rats [49].

b) Farm animal models

Several studies have also looked into the effects of carnitine supplementation on improving the rate of ovulation and fertilization [20], egg quality [44, 50], number of litters born [20, 51] etc., of farm animals such as pigs, chickens and cows.

Carnitine and ovulation and fertilization rates

Samland et al. examined the effect of dietary supplementation of LC (200 ppm) on the ovulation and fertilization rate of gilts (young female adult breeding pigs that have not yet farrowed). After two weeks, the gilts fed with added carnitine were found to have increased rate of ovulation, but decreased fertilization rate of the recovered embryos. However, the report did not offer an explanation as to the possible cause of decreased fertilization rates despite increased ovulation rates in this group of gilts [20].

Carnitine, embryo development and post-natal growth

Zhai and co-workers examined the effect of dietary supplementation of LC (125 ppm) on the reproductive traits of male and female White Leghorn chicken. They reported that the yolk of fresh eggs retrieved from LC-hens that were inseminated with semen from roosters consuming either the control or the LC-diet contained higher concentrations of LC but decreased hatchling yolk sac weights and yolk sac lipid content compared to that of control hens. This suggests that LC encourages fat utilization in the developing embryos [43].

In another study using gestating sows (mature female pigs that have farrowed at least once before the current gestation), Musser et al. demonstrated that a 50 ppm LC supplementation in gestation sow diet improved muscle fiber development by increasing the leanness and muscling of the fetal piglet. These changes could perhaps improve postnatal growth in the piglets [52].

Carnitine and egg quality

In another study on the performance and egg quality parameters of Brown egg-type laying hens, Corduk and Sarica reported that supplementation of 500 mg LC per kg of low energy diets containing either sunflower or palm oil increases the eggshell breaking strength. Moreover, the addition of LC into normal diet containing palm oil increased the albumen index (calculated from the albumen height, length and weight) of the eggs [50]. Greater eggshell breaking strength and a higher albumen index indicates higher egg quality.

Carnitine and milk production and quality

Pirestani and colleagues evaluated the effect of LC supplementation (50 g/day/cow) for 40 days on milk somatic cell count (SCC) (as a measure of the milk quality) and several reproductive indices in Holstein dairy cattle. They reported a significant reduction in milk SCC (indicating less mastitis or enhanced udder immunity and therefore better quality of milk) and improvement in the reproductive indices. In addition, the study found that a combination of LC and a vitamin-like essential macronutrient, choline (60 g/day/cow) further reduced milk SCC and improved the reproductive indices [21].

In another study on German Holstein dairy cows, Scholz's group showed that supplementation with 2 g of LC/cow (contained in 10 g of a rumen-protected product) for three months improved metabolic health during the critical periods of transition and high lactation and showed a trend of improving milk production during the initial 2-months after calving. Furthermore, LC-supplemented cows had a lower insemination index and increased conception rate compared to controls [53].

In vitro studies and assisted reproduction

Following reports on the antioxidant properties of LC and ALC and its beneficial effects on female fertility, carnitines have been used in in vitro studies focusing on the improvement of oocyte health and maturation, embryo development as well as in assisted reproduction [54, 55] (Table 2). In the last two decades, a good number of studies have been published that showcase the impact of carnitine supplementation on female fertility. Of late, it has been used to minimize ROS-mediated delayed embryonic development in culture medium, high DNA fragmentation and development of morphologically abnormal blastocysts after prolonged culture [6, 23, 56].

During in vitro fertilization (IVF) procedures, embryo fragmentation due to apoptosis is a common occurrence that is well documented. Nonetheless, supplementation of culture medium with LC may confer protection to the developing immature cells. Pillich et al. have shown that ALC supplementation (0.3, 0.6 and 1.2 mM for 5 h and 24 h) in mouse fibroblast culture media stabilizes the mitochondrial membrane, increases energy supply to the organelle and protects the developing cell from apoptosis through the mitochondrial pathway [57]. In another laboratory, Abdelrazik and colleagues looked into the optimal dose of LC that is required for blastocyst development of mouse embryos. They have showed that 0.3 and 0.6 mg/mL of LC possesses anti-apoptotic effects as well as increased the rate of blastocyst development [33].

A marked increase in TNF-α concentration in granulosa cell cultures of women with endometriosis has been demonstrated [58–61]. Studies have also shown that increased levels of TNF-α restrict inner cell mass and trophectoderm proliferation in mouse blastocyst. At a concentration of 50 ng/mL, TNF-α was found to affect protein synthesis in mouse embryos in both morula and blastocyst stages [62, 63]. However, LC at the doses of 0.3 and 0.6 mg/mL were able to neutralize the anti-proliferative effects on TNF-α. LC supplementation in embryo culture medium also decreased DNA damage during development [6].

These observations were reaffirmed by Zare and coworkers who used the same doses (0.3 and 0.6 mg/mL) of LC supplementation during in vitro maturation of immature BCB+ (Brilliant Cresyl Blue positive) oocytes. LC-treated oocytes demonstrated an improved pre-implantation developmental competence (quality) after IVF, which is probably due to LC-induced improvement in the cytoplasmic and nuclear maturation of immature oocytes. LC at the doses used also exhibited an antioxidative effect during embryo development by reducing ROS levels in the maturation medium [64].

In another study, Mansour et al. used the same dose (0.6 mg/mL) of LC to demonstrate the protective effects of LC on oocytes and embryos against the toxic effects of peritoneal fluid in women with endometriosis. They have showed that peritoneal fluid of patients with endometriosis which was supplemented with LC had decreased apoptosis levels in the embryos and improved oocyte microtubular and chromosomal structure [38]. Bareh has also reported that LC-induced improvements in cytoskeleton could lead to reduced aneuploidy rates in an animal model [65].

In 2013, Phongmitr et al. added LC (0.3, 0.6 and 1.2 mg/mL) to culture media containing swamp buffalo oocytes and noted an improved nuclear maturation rate with a maximum number of metaphase II (MII) oocytes in the 0.3 mg/mL LC-supplemented group [66]. Moawad's group later showed that LC supplementation (0.6 mg/ml or 3.72 mM) during vitrification/warming and in vitro maturation of germinal vesicle stage-oocytes increased the proportions of oocytes with normal MII spindles. They also reported that LC supplementation causes increased oxidative activity of mitochondria in

Table 2 In vitro studies with carnitine supplementation to improve oocyte quality, maturation and embryo development

Study aim	Carnitine dose	Study design/Subjects	Outcomes	Reference
LC on antagonizing the harmful effect of TNF-α, apoptosis, and oxidative stress on mouse embryo development.	LC was dissolved in HTF culture medium in concentrations of 0.3 and 0.6 mg/mL	• 500 mouse embryos were divided into three groups and incubated with either AD 0.005 mg/mL, H_2O_2 500 mmol/L, or TNF-α 500 ng with and without LC 0.3 or 0.6 mg/mL • For anti-apoptotic effect: All groups were incubated at 37C in 5%CO_2 for 4 h and transferred to HTF medium and incubated until 48 h for formation of the blastocyst stage. • For anti-oxidant and anti-proliferative effect on TNF-α: All groups were incubated at 37C in 5% CO_2 for 72 h until the formation of blastocyst stage. • Embryo staining by TUNEL was done to detect blastomere DNA damage	• Significant improvement in percentage BDR was seen at LC 0.3 mg/mL compared with the control ($p < 0.006$) • L-Carnitine at 0.3 and 0.6 mg/mL significantly reduced the blocking effect of AD, H_2O_2, and TNF-α and significantly decreased the level of DNA damage	[6]
LC on oocyte cytoskeleton and apoptosis in peritoneal fluid from patients with endometriosis	0.6 mg/mL of LC	• Peritoneal fluid was collected from 23 women suffering from endometriosis and 15 patients with tubal ligation who underwent laparoscopy • LC was diluted 1:1 with peritoneal fluid and cryopreserved mouse embryos were matured in that medium	Significantly improved microtubule and chromosome structure and decreased embryo apoptosis	[38]
LC on oocyte maturation and parthenogenetic embryos in pigs	0.25, 0.5, 1.0 and 2.0 mg/mL of LC in IVM medium	• Porcine ovaries were collected from prepubertal gilts and matured in medium containing various concentrations of LC. • LC was added in IVC medium to examine developmental competence of parthenogenic embryos	LC addition during IVM improved developmental potential of oocytes, and also quality of parthenogenic embryos by improving nuclear maturation and preventing OS and apoptosis	[14]
LC on lipid metabolism and in vitro maturation of porcine oocyte	0.3 to 10 mg/mL of LC	Ovaries from prepubertal cross-bred gilts were collected and IVF and IVC was performed in media containing LC	Enhanced mitochondrial functions, lipid metabolism for nuclear and cytoplasmic maturation of porcine oocytes	[54]
LC on oocyte maturation and embryo development	10 mM of LC in IVM medium	• Porcine ovaries were collected from 6 to 7 months old prepubertal gilts • Comparison of GSH, ROS levels and developmental gene expression in LC supplemented and non-supplemented group	• Reduced OS with increased GSH synthesis in LC supplemented group • Increased expression of developmental genes	[23]
LC on maturation rate of buffalo embryos	0.3, 0.6 and 1.2 mM/mL of LC	Oocytes were collected from Swamp buffalo and treated with various concentrations of LC	Significantly higher metaphase II oocytes than control group with faster maturation rate	[66]
LC on bovine embryo development and their cryotolerance	1.1518 mM and 3.030 mM of LC	• Oocytes were collected from bovine ovaries • IVF and IVC was performed in media containing LC	Improved cryotolerance, lipid metabolism in embryos	[68]

Table 2 In vitro studies with carnitine supplementation to improve oocyte quality, maturation and embryo development *(Continued)*

Study aim	Carnitine dose	Study design/Subjects	Outcomes	Reference
LC on vitrification of mouse germinal vesicle stage-oocytes and their in vitro maturation	3.72 mM (0.6 mg/mL) of LC in IVM medium	• B6.DBA cross-bed mice were superovulated and oocytes were collected • Oocytes grown in LC-supplemented IVM medium	Increased number of metaphase II oocytes and improved mitochondrial distribution in oocytes	[55]
ALC on lamb oocyte blastocyst rate, mitochondrial DNA copy number	2 mM of ALC in IVM medium	Prepubertal lamb oocytes were collected and matured in medium containing LC	Increased cytoplasmic volume of oocyte with more lipid droplets, but no alteration in mitochondrial volume, number or DNA copy number	[22]
LC on maturation of mouse embryos	0.3 and 0.6 mg/mL of LC	• Immature oocytes were collected from NMRI mice ovaries and treated with LC • Cleavage rate, BDR and GSH were evaluated	Improved implantation developmental competence and nuclear maturation of oocytes and increased GSH	[64]
LC on bovine blastocyst development	0.1, 0.5 and 1.0 mg/mL of LC in IVM medium	• Oocytes were collected from bovine ovaries and matured in medium containing LC • These oocytes were then subjected to IVF with fresh semen • Number of embryos and total cell count was performed	Improved developmental potential: increased number of oocytes and embryos with higher total cell count	[70]
LC in OS and antioxidant profile in sheep embryos produces in vitro	2.5, 5, 7.5 and 10 mM of LC in maturation medium	Oocytes were collected from sheep ovaries and matured in medium containing LC. These oocytes were then subjected to IVF with fresh semen.	• Oocyte maturation, embryo development increased • LC reduced OS and ROS production, increased antioxidant enzyme activities	[56]
LC on in vitro maturation of ZP and development of mouse embryos	0.5, 1, 2 and 4 mg/ml of LC	• Mice were superovulated and mating was carried out with males • 2-cell embryos were flushed from oviduct and cultured in LC containing medium • BDR, ZP thickness were measured	Increased number of blastocyst cells, ZP thickness and improved antioxidant activity	[71]

AD Actinomycin-D, *ALC* Acetyl-L-carnitine, *BDR* Blastocyst development rate, *GSH* Glutathione, *HTF* Human tubular fluid, H_2O_2 Hydrogen peroxide, *IVC* in vitro embryo culture, *IVF* in vitro fertilization, *IVM* in vitro maturation, *LC* L-Carnitine, *OS* Oxidative stress, *ROS* Reactive oxygen species, TNF-tumor necrosis factor, *ZP* Zona pellucida the resultant MII oocytes without increasing the ATP levels in MII oocytes [55].

Ghanem and co-workers reported similar observations of increased antioxidant activity and improved blastocyst quality by way of higher embryo development rate and fewer number of apoptotic cells after supplementing LC (1.5 mM, equivalent to 0.3 mg/mL) in culture media of bovine blastocyst during the pre-implantation stage [67]. Similar studies conducted earlier have also shown higher counts of total cells [68, 69] and lower apoptotic cells [69] in bovine embryos cultured in 0.3 mg/mL L-carnitine.

Manzano's group investigated the role of L-carnitine supplementation in the maturation of bovine oocytes and pre-implantation development of embryos. They reported improved developmental potential up to the blastocyst stage with higher blastocyst formation rate and increased total cell count and activity when the oocytes were matured in culture media added with 0.1–0.5 mg/mL LC. In a subsequent experiment, supplementation of the resulting zygotes with the same dose of LC in modified synthetic oviductal fluid medium displayed a higher blastocyst total cell count, but similar blastocyst formation rates as that of control [70].

Khanmohammadi and colleagues evaluated the effect of LC (0.5 mg/mL) supplementation on several indicators of embryo development and blastocyst quality such as thickness of zona pellucida, hatching rate and number of blastocyst cells. At a concentration of 0.5 mg/mL, LC exerted antioxidant properties, along with an enhancement of mitochondrial lipid metabolism to increase blastocyst cell number, blastocyst expansion and zona pellucida thinning, all of which promotes blastocyst quality leading to successful hatching and implantation. Conversely, LC at high concentrations (4 mg/ml) had a toxic effect on in vitro embryo development and blastocyst quality [71].

Possible mechanisms of action of LC

Direct effects

LC has been reported to maintain cellular energy [34], reduce oxidative stress [72] and minimize cell death by apoptosis [33], which are necessary for proper oocyte growth and maturation of blastocyst. As discussed earlier, the cumulus-oocyte complex (COC) and its lipid metabolism are one of the prime regulators of oocyte maturation [73]. LC helps in the metabolism of COC lipids by transferring fatty acids into the mitochondria and by facilitating β-oxidation [30]. LC is taken up by the tissues via the electrogenic force of the voltage-gated Na^+-channels. It uses the Na^+-driven LC / organic cation transporter-2 (OCTN-2) for its transport into the oocytes [74].

In the oocytes, LC gets converted to ALC by carnitine palmitoyltransferase-I (CPT-I) in the outer mitochondrial membrane and CPT-II helps in the regeneration of carnitine from acyl-carnitine after the translocation of long chain fatty acids into the mitochondrial matrix [31]. Within the oocyte, LC plays a significant role in ER, mitochondria as well as in the ooplasm. In the mitochondria, LC is converted to ALC, and balances the acetyl CoA/CoA ratio to maintain glucose metabolism through the TCA cycle, yielding a higher energy production [34]. LC helps in minimizing the concentration of pyruvate which prevents entry into the TCA cycle to curtail energy production (Fig. 2).

In the mitochondria, LC also scavenges ROS through its antioxidant property. It transports palmitate and other long chain fatty acids to the mitochondria to facilitate their utilization through β-oxidation [5]. In the ER, it decreases the concentration of palmitate by transferring it to the mitochondria or by eliminating it from which it may cause lipotoxicity of the oocytes through oxidative stress [34]. It is reported that higher ROS levels decrease maturation by affecting the COC, and also decreases embryo development and blastocyst fragmentation [75]. LC also promotes cellular proliferation and decreases apoptosis by inhibiting TNF-α and other anti-proliferative agents [33]. In endometriosis, LC has been claimed to possess dual effects through the uterine secretion of prostaglandins. LC treatment has been shown to increase the production of both PGE_1 and PGE_2. It was suggested that PGE_1 confers protection against endometriosis by attenuating the secretion of TNF-α, IFN-γ and interleukins (IL-2, IL-4 and IL-6), while PGE_2 induces cytokine release and thus endometriosis through its apoptotic and inflammatory functions [19, 46]. However, further robust studies are required to corroborate the findings regarding the role of LC on endometriosis.

Thus, in summary, free LC or ALC serves three important functions in oocytes through its direct action: first, it increases energy production by transferring palmitate into mitochondria and maintaining acetyl CoA/CoA ratio; secondly, it reduces oxidative stress and lipotoxicity by scavenging free radicals and removing excess palmitate from the ER, and finally it promotes oocyte growth and maturation by decreasing the rate of apoptosis.

Indirect effects

LC and ALC have also been reported to affect the HPG axis to promote reproductive hormone secretion [16, 17, 76]. It has been known that among the neural centers, LC's concentration is highest is in the hypothalamus [77]. In the hypothalamus, LC has been reported to decrease neuronal cell death and damage associated with aging [78] by its

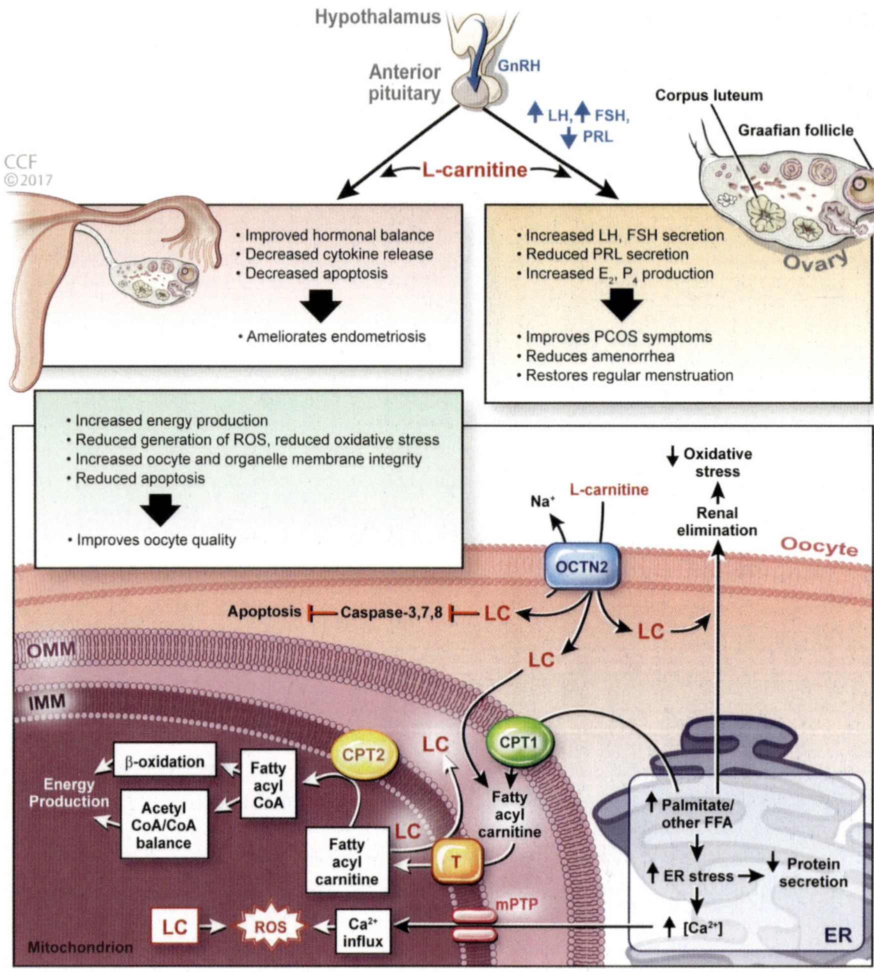

Fig. 2 Mechanism of L-carnitine action on female fertility. LC enters the oocyte through OCTN2 and through its direct action on oocyte quality, it increases energy production by β-oxidation, eliminates excess palmitate from ER to reduce ER stress, scavenges free radicals to reduce oxidative damage and inhibits caspases to prevent apoptosis. It implies its indirect action through HPG axis by regulating the reproductive hormone levels and thus mitigates reproductive disorders such as PCOS and amenorrhea. In endometriosis, it improves hormonal balance, decreases the release of cytokines as well as apoptosis and thus ameliorates endometriosis. CPT1, carnitine palmitoyltransferase-1; CPT2, carnitine palmitoyltransferase-2; T, CoA, coenzyme-A; ER, endoplasmic reticulum; FFA, free fatty acid; FSH, follicle stimulating hormone; GnRH, gonadotropin releasing hormone; IMM, inner mitochondrial membrane; LC, L-carnitine; LH, luteinizing hormone; mPTP, mitochondrial permeability transition pore; OCTN2, organic cation transporter-2; OM, oocyte membrane; OMM, outer mitochondrial membrane; PCOS, polycystic ovary syndrome; PRL, prolactin; ROS, reactive oxygen species; T, translocase

cholinomimetic activity [79]. It is reported that LC increases GnRH secretion from the hypothalamus by acting on the HPG axis [16, 17] and causing K^+-induced depolarization in hypothalamic neuronal cells to increase its secretory activity [80, 81]. They have shown that treatment with ALC increases serum levels of other reproductive hormones, like estradiol, progesterone, LH and decreases prolactin in the usual fashion with different phases of estrous in animal [16, 17]. Through its indirect endocrine effect, it prevents PCOS, amenorrhea and other problems related to the female reproductive cycle.

Costa and Stevenson (1984) with the administration of equine chorionic gonadotropin (eCG) and pregnant mare's serum gonadotropin (PMSG) showed that these components increases ovarian concentration of free LC and ALC, which shows the interaction between the direct and indirect mechanisms through cellular and hormonal regulations [82].

Combination effects with other supplements

LC or ALC has not only been supplemented individually, in many experiments researchers have supplemented it in combination with other nutrients [20, 21, 44, 83–88] (Table 3). The results of combination treatments i.e. LC and/or ALC with other nutrients are not very well documented in female fertility, but in the last two decades, scientists have started applying LC and/or ALC with other nutrients to improve fertility [84]. It has been

Table 3 Studies using a combination of carnitine and other nutrient supplementation to improve reproductive parameters

Study aims	Dosage and duration	Study design/Subjects	Relevant study outcomes	Reference
Effects of LC and CrNic on ovulation and fertilization rates in gilts	200 ppm LC + 200 ppb CrNic for 2 weeks prior to expected estrus	105 gilts Positive controls were fed 11 lbs./day of complete diet (flushing) Treatment group was fed 4 lbs./day of diet with/without various treatments	Increased ovulation and fertilization rate	[20]
Effects of dietary supplementation of LC and ascorbic acid in productive, reproductive, physiological and immunological performances of Golden Montazah aged breeder hens	100 and 200 mg LC/kg diet + 1 g ascorbic acid for 4 weeks	180 Golden Montazah hens + 18 cocks of 50 weeks old were randomly chosen. Birds were divided into 6 groups (each of 30 hens + 3 cocks), during the entire experimental period (from 50 to 70 weeks of age).	All groups fed diets of LC levels of 100 and 200 mg /kg diet alone and with 1 g ascorbic acid / kg diet were improved and recorded the best values of fertility and hatchability percentages. This improvement was increased with increasing LC level compared with the hens fed 1 g ascorbic acid /kg diet alone and the control group at the end of the experimental period.	[87]
CoQ10 and LC co-treatment in ovulatory response in rabbits	10 mg/kg CoQ10 + 40 mg/kg LC for 21 days	New Zealand White female rabbits of 5.3 months old	Higher ovulate rate, number of follicles, corpus luteum and increased number of embryos	[85]
LC and vegetable oil supplementation in broiler breeder fertility	60 ppm (females), 500 ppm (males)	–	In 5th and 6th week, egg production is increased with more cholesterol in egg yolk	[44]
Dietary LC and choline chloride on reproductive indices in Holstein Dairy Cattle	50 g/day	From 1-week pre-calving to 4-weeks after parturition	Decreased SCC and improved other immune indices	[21]
Both LC and ALC supplementations on ovulation and oocyte quality in CD1 mice	0.4 mg LC and 0.12 mg ALC/mouse/day for 3 weeks	Female CD1 mice of 8 weeks old	Decreased percentage of oocyte degeneration with more developing oocytes	[47]
NAC and LC on prevention of oocyte damage in women with mild endometriosis	1.5 mM of NAC with 0.6 mg/mL LC in follicular fluid	In follicular fluid sample from infertile women with endometriosis aged less than 38 years who underwent ICSI and induced in bovine oocytes	LC and NAC combination prevented oocyte damage in mild endometriosis	[84]
Effect of oral antioxidant and LC combination on IVF-ICSI outcomes	Vitamin C (180 mg), vitamin E (30 mg), zinc (15 mg), selenium (50 mg), LC tartarate (400 mg), folic acid (200 μg) and CoQ_{10} (40 mg) for 2 to 5 months at a daily dose of 2 capsules	Semen was taken for IVF and ICSI	• Enhanced semen quality • Improved sperm DNA integrity, fertilization rate, pregnancy rate, implantation rate, embryo quality as well as blastocyst development rate	[88]
LC plus ALC on neuroendocrine control of hypothalamic functions in FHA	LC fumerate (863 mg), ALC (250 mg), vitamin-C (90 mg), N-acetyl cysteine (50 mg), vitamin E (30 mg), iron (7 mg), pantothenic acid (6 mg), zinc (5 mg), vitamin B6 (2 mg), copper (0.5 mg), β-carotene (4.8 mg), folic acid (200 μg), vitamin-D3 (5 μg), selenium (27.5 μg), vitamin B12 (2.5 μg)	27 patients (aged 26.5 ± 2 years) with FHA for the last 6 months were subdivided into 2 groups: Group A (hypogonadotropic patients, plasma LH levels ≤3 mIU/ml, $n = 15$) Group B (normogonadotropic patients, plasma LH levels > 3 mIU/ml, $n = 12$)	• Carnitine administration significantly increases LH secretion in patients • Carnitine decreases cortisol and plasma amylase levels	[89]

ALC Acetyl-L-carnitine, *CoQ10* Coenzyme-Q10, *CrNic* Chromium nicotinate, *FHA* Functional hypothalamic amenorrhea, *LC* L-Carnitine, *ICSI* Intracytoplasmic sperm injection, *IVF* in vitro fertilization, *NAC* N-Acetyl cysteine previously reported that LC (150 mg/kg/day) while combined with ginger extract (100 mg/kg/day) improves hormonal levels as well as reproductive performance in male rats [83]. It is also known that obestatin and LC co-treatment improves fat metabolism and obesity-induced male infertility [86].

The role of LC in combination with other nutrients on female fertility is also demonstrated by various reports. As discussed earlier, Samland et al. (1998) have recorded the effect of LC supplementation on fertilization rate of gilts; they have not only recorded the effect of individual supplementation of LC (200 ppm), they have also combined it with chromium niconitate (CrNic) (200 ppb), an insulin promoter which increases insulin uptake by the cells. They have compared the outcomes of both cases in ovulation and fertilization rate and noted that LC individually potentiates ovulation, but when LC was combined with CrNic, it showed no alteration. They concluded that perhaps LC does not interact with CrNic to cause improvement in reproductive parameters [20].

In 2006, Adabi et al. in contrast, reported the supplementation of LC (60 ppm for females and 500 ppm for males) with vegetable fat powder (1.5%) and high lysine and methionine (0.3%) has increased fertility and hatchability in broilers. They also reported about their interaction as well as their role in lipid metabolism [44]. In 2011, Pirestani et al. supplemented LC individually (50 g/day/cow), as discussed earlier, as well as with choline chloride (60 g/day/cow) on SCC and reproductive indices of Holstein dairy cattle. They have reported choline chloride and LC co-administration has beneficial effects on SCC and reproductive indices, and that is better than individual LC supplementation [21].

In 2011, Hassan et al. supplemented different doses of LC (100 and 200 mg/kg diet) with vitamin C (1 g/kg diet) for 3 weeks and noted the reproductive performance of Golden Montahza laying hens, and reported increased egg production rate (2.1 and 2.7%) and egg quality [87]. In 2014, Kacem et al. formulated a special combination of vitamin C (180 mg), vitamin E (30 mg), zinc (15 mg), selenium (50 mg), LC tartarate (400 mg), folic acid (200 μg) and coenzyme-Q10 (40 mg). They have supplemented this formulation to male participants of a clinical trial of this drug for 2 to 5 months at a daily dose of 2 capsules before their semen has taken for IVF and intra-cytoplasmic sperm injection (ICSI). They have noted that the formulation has not only enhanced semen quality, it also improved sperm DNA integrity, fertilization rate, biochemical and clinical pregnancy rate, implantation rate, embryo quality as well as blastocyst development rate [88].

Cavallini et al. (2012), in their study, reported that 22 out of 33 male patients with severe idiopathic oligoasthenoteratozoospermia (OAT) of infertile couples whose partners had undergone at least one ICSI cycle, showed reduced sperm aneuploidy levels (assessed using fluorescent in situ hybridization performed on chromosomes X, Y, 13, 15, 16, 17, 18, 21 and 22) and improved sperm morphology after 3 months of treatment with LC 2×1 g/day, ALC $2 \times$ 500 mg/day and cinnoxicam (a lipophilic NSAID) $1 \times$ 30 mg/every 4 days [89]. Men with OAT have been reported to have elevated prostaglandin levels. NSAIDs act by reversibly inhibiting cyclooxygenase, which then inhibits the generation of prostaglandins and thromboxanes. Cinnoxicam and carnitines appear to have complementary mechanistic pathways, which facilitate the suppression of excess prostaglandin production, which could lead to improvement in sperm quality. The men with reduced sperm aneuploidy and improved sperm morphology as a result of the combination therapy in this study had significantly higher biochemical pregnancies, clinical pregnancies and live births after the treatment, despite having similar numbers of oocytes fertilized and embryos transferred [89].

In 2015, Abdel-Khalek et al. reported that coenzyme Q10 (10 mg/kg) and LC (40 mg/kg) for 21 days improved ovulatory response in rabbits, as well as embryo recovery and embryo vitrification in in vitro study [85]. Lastly, Virmani et al. (2015) combined both LC (0.4 mg/mouse) and ALC (0.12 mg/mouse) with micronutrients like zinc (4 ng/mouse), copper (0.8 ng/mouse) and iron (7 ng/mouse) and treated mice for 3 weeks daily to check the ovulation rate and oocyte quality. They have noted when LC and ALC are given in combination, its actions were better. Similarly, even when carnitines were given in combination with micronutrients, it showed better improvement in oocyte quality and quantity. They have also noted decreased rate of oocyte degeneration as well as increased rate of ovulation while supplemented with microelements. When they have tried this combination for IVF, they observed a better fertilization rate, 2-cell embryo development as well as birth rate [47].

Recently Genazzani et al. (2017) have repeated their experiment of combined LC and ALC effects on female fertility with a formulation containing LC fumerate (863 mg), ALC (250 mg), vitamin C (90 mg), N-acetyl cysteine (50 mg), vitamin E (30 mg), iron (7 mg), pantothenic acid (6 mg), zinc (5 mg), vitamin B6 (2 mg), copper (0.5 mg), β-carotene (4.8 mg), folic acid (200 μg), vitamin D3 (5 μg), selenium (27.5 μg), vitamin B12 (2.5 μg). They have reported that this formulation improves the condition of FHA and increases LH. They have also been shown to decrease stress-related cortisol and amylase levels [90].

Most of these reports pointing towards better interactions of LC and/or ALC with other nutrients and antioxidants to enhance fertility rate in female, including vitamin C [87, 88], vitamin E [88], zinc [47, 88], selenium [88], folic acid [88], coenzyme-Q_{10} [47, 88], vegetable oil containing high lysine [44] and many others [21, 47, 88].

Combination therapies involving other antioxidants in female fertility

The female reproductive system is vulnerable to oxidative damage and without antioxidant interventions, the copious chain of oxidative reactions would continue to damage the system [58, 91]. Apart from LC and ALC, as discussed earlier, in conserving and regulating female reproductive functions, there are several groups of antioxidants known to quench free radicals to keep it healthier. These include vitamins (C, E, and β-carotene), some metallo-enzymes including glutathione peroxidase (GPx, containing selenium), catalase (CAT, containing iron), superoxide dismutase (SOD, containing copper, manganese and zinc). Dietary intake of these antioxidant vitamins and minerals prejudice the coordinated functioning of the total antioxidant system [92].

Within the ovary, various antioxidant systems (consisting of CAT, carotenoids, vitamin E, and glutathione) work to keep ROS under strict regulation. SOD catalyzes the superoxide decomposition into H_2O_2 and oxygen, and it has its effects in the theca interna cells of antral follicles. The theca interna cells in turn protect oocyte during its maturation phase from getting damaged by excess ROS. One more antioxidant factor imperative for healthy development of the ovarian follicle is transferrin (iron-chelating glycoprotein) that impedes the generation of ROS [91]. The connection of OS with endometrial cyclical alterations is well accepted and the SOD levels are demonstrated to rise in response to such oxidative changes during the end of the secretory phase, just prior to menstruation [93].

Vitamin C, one of the most commonly used antioxidant, is found in the cytosol of oocyte and extracellular fluid. Its supplementation to infertile women is in practice to treat luteal phase defects and recurrent abortions [58]. It is a versatile vitamin with antioxidant as well as collagen-stimulating properties. Studies revealed that when vitamin C is ingested through diet, the mature ovarian follicles actively take it up leading to its sequestration in the follicles rather than in the serum [58].

During in vitro fertilization (IVF) embryo transfer, vitamin C supplementation is provided to the patients during hormonal stimulation to ensure higher concentration of vitamin C in the follicular fluid [94]. It effectively breaks the chain of oxidative reactions to stop the promulgation of the peroxidative damage to the oocyte [91]. It is also claimed to elevate the chance of ovulation and protect oocyte from DNA alterations owing to oxidative damage. It helps to regenerate Vitamin E and glutathione. As discussed earlier, Hassan et al. supplemented vitamin C with LC and found improved reproductive performance in hens. This combination has been shown to increase egg production and egg quality thus attributing to reduced OS and improved lipid metabolism following LC-vitamin C co-treatment. Vitamin E (α-tocopherol) is found in the cell membrane of the oocyte and is evidently the first line of defense recruited to disrupt the chain of fatty acid peroxidation protecting the oocyte from further oxidative damage [92]. The follicular and tubular fluid contains taurine, hypotaurine and transferrin which protects the embryo from OS [95]. Glutathione has a role in the improvement of zygote development after the morula or blastocyst gains 2-cell blocks and it is also present in the oocyte as well as in the tubal fluid [96].

Hence, the interplay of antioxidants and their combined effort to combat free radicals, are constantly protecting the delicate organs belonging to the female reproductive system. Antioxidants take charge of their own regeneration as lipoic acid aids in the regeneration of Vitamin C, glutathione, vitamin E as well as of itself, glutathione recycles vitamin C which in turn recycles vitamin E that is also regenerated via CoQ_{10}. This battalion of antioxidants, individually or in combination, if associated with LC or ALC, may lead to excellent results in improving female fertility. This can be suggested from the fact that the free radical quenching properties of the above-mentioned antioxidants as well as that of carnitines, when combined with the additional features of the carnitines, such as aiding fatty acid metabolism and energy production, would make the reproductive organs of female more robust.

Conclusions

This review has summarized the information procured from various research works about the implications of LC and/or ALC upon female fertility. These carnitines, either individually or in combination with other nutrients and antioxidants, are potent to improve and/or restore female reproductive functions. This review has also proposed a mechanism of LC- and ALC-induced enhancement of female fertility, (a) directly by increasing energy production in oocytes and effectively quenching free radicals to provide protection against oxidative damage to the reproductive cells, and also (b) indirectly, by imposing their beneficial effects through HPG axis to ameliorate serum levels of hormones. Thus, considering the substantial qualities of these carnitines in female reproduction, they can be used both as reproductive biomedicines to treat female infertility as well as fertility boosters to improve the reproductive performance in humans and animals.

Abbreviations

ALC: Acetyl L-Carnitine; ART: Assisted reproductive technology; BCB: Brilliant cresyl blue; CoA: Coenzyme-A; COC: Cumulus-oocyte complex; CPT: Cartinitine palmitoyltransferase; DHEA: Dehydroepiandrosterone; eCG: Equine chorionic gonadotropin; ER: Endoplasmic reticulum; FHA: Functional hypothalamic amenorrhea; FISH: Fluorescent in situ hybridization; GABA: γ-amino butyric acid; GnRH: Gonadotropin releasing hormone; HPG: Hypothalamo-pituitary gonadal axis; IFN: Interferon; IVF: In vitro fertilization; LC: L-carnitine; LDL: Low density lipoprotein; LH: Luteinizing hormone; MII: Metaphase-II; NO: Nitric oxide; OCTN: Organic cation transporter; OS: Oxidative stress; PCOS: Polycystic ovarian syndrome; PG: Prostaglandin; PLC: Propionyl L-carnitine; PMSG: Pregnant mare's serum gonadotropin; ROS: Reactive oxygen species; SCC: Somatic cell count; TNF: Tumor necrosis factor

Acknowledgements

Authors want to thank American Centre of Reproductive Medicine for providing support for the study.

Funding

None

Authors' contributions

PS (writing and revising the manuscript), DD (writing and revising the manuscript), AA (revising the manuscript). All authors read and approved the final manuscript.

Competing interests

The authors declare that they have no competing interests.

Author details

[1]American Center for Reproductive Medicine, Cleveland Clinic, Glickman Urological and Kidney Institute, Mail Code X-11, 10681 Carnegie Avenue, Cleveland, OH 44195, USA. [2]Department of Physiology, Faculty of Medicine, MAHSA University, Jalan SP2, Bandar Saujana Putra, 42610 Jenjarum, Selangor, Malaysia. [3]Faculty of Medicine, Universiti Teknologi MARA, Sungai Buloh Campus, Jalan Hospital, 47000 Sungai Buloh, Selangor, Malaysia.

References

1. Rutkowski M, Grzegorczyk K. Adverse effects of antioxidative vitamins. Int J Occup Med Environ Health. 2012;25:105–21.
2. May-Panloup P, Chretien MF, Malthiery Y, Reynier P. Mitochondrial DNA in the oocyte and the developing embryo. Curr Top Dev Biol. 2007;77:51–83.
3. Bentov Y, Esfandiari N, Burstein E, Casper RF. The use of mitochondrial nutrients to improve the outcome of infertility treatment in older patients. Fertil Steril. 2010;93:272–5.
4. Binienda Z, Virmani A. The Mitochondriotropic effects of L-carnitine and its esters in the central nervous system. Curr Med Chem - Cent Nervous Sys Agents. 2003;3:275–82.
5. Dunning KR, Robker RL. Promoting lipid utilization with l-carnitine to improve oocyte quality. Anim Reprod Sci. 2012;134:69–75.
6. Abdelrazik H, Agarwal A. L-carnitine and assisted reproduction. Arch Med Sci. 2009;1A:S43–7.
7. Aliabadi E, Soleimani Mehranjani M, Borzoei Z, Talaei-Khozani T, Mirkhani H, Tabesh H. Effects of L-carnitine and L-acetyl-carnitine on testicular sperm motility and chromatin quality. Iran J Reprod Med. 2012;10:77–82.
8. Cheng HJ, Chen T. Clinical efficacy of combined L-carnitine and acetyl-L-carnitine on idiopathic asthenospermia. Zhonghua Nan Ke Xue. 2008;14: 149–51.
9. Brooks DE. Carnitine, acetylcarnitine and the activity of carnitine acyltransferases in seminal plasma and spermatozoa of men, rams and rats. J Reprod Fertil. 1979; 56:667–73.
10. Dokmeci D. Oxidative stress, male infertility and the role of carnitines. Folia Med (Plovdiv). 2005;47:26–30.
11. Ismail AM, Hamed AH, Saso S, Thabet HH. Adding L-carnitine to clomiphene resistant PCOS women improves the quality of ovulation and the pregnancy rate. A randomized clinical trial. Eur J Obstet Gynecol Reprod Biol. 2014;180:148–52.
12. Samimi M, Jamilian M, Ebrahimi FA, Rahimi M, Tajbakhsh B, Asemi Z. Oral carnitine supplementation reduces body weight and insulin resistance in women with polycystic ovary syndrome: a randomized, double-blind, placebo-controlled trial. Clin Endocrinol. 2016;84:851–7.
13. Dunning KR, Russell DL, Robker RL. Lipids and oocyte developmental competence: the role of fatty acids and beta-oxidation. Reproduction. 2014;148:R15–27.
14. Wu GQ, Jia BY, Li JJ, Fu XW, Zhou GB, Hou YP, Zhu SE. L-carnitine enhances oocyte maturation and development of parthenogenetic embryos in pigs. Theriogenology. 2011;76:785–93.
15. Liu J, Head E, Kuratsune H, Cotman CW, Ames BN. Comparison of the effects of L-carnitine and acetyl-L-carnitine on carnitine levels, ambulatory activity, and oxidative stress biomarkers in the brain of old rats. Ann N Y Acad Sci. 2004; 1033:117–31.
16. Krsmanovic LZ, Virmani MA, Stojilkovic SS, Catt KJ. Actions of acetyl-L-carnitine on the hypothalamo-pituitary-gonadal system in female rats. J Steroid Biochem Mol Biol. 1992;43:351–8.
17. Genazzani AD, Lanzoni C, Ricchieri F, Santagni S, Rattighieri E, Chierchia E, Monteleone P, Jasonni VM. Acetyl-L-carnitine (ALC) administration positively affects reproductive axis in hypogonadotropic women with functional hypothalamic amenorrhea. J Endocrinol Investig. 2011;34:287–91.
18. Latifian S, Hamdi K, Totakneh R. Effect of addition of l-carnitine in polycystic ovary syndrome (PCOS) patients with clomiphene citrate and gonadotropin resistant. Int J Curr Res Acad Rev. 2015;3:469–76.
19. Dionyssopoulou E, Vassiliadis S, Evangeliou A, Koumantakis EE, Athanassakis I. Constitutive or induced elevated levels of L-carnitine correlate with the cytokine and cellular profile of endometriosis. J Reprod Immunol. 2005;65:159–70.
20. Samland CJ, Musser RE, Peters JK, Sawyer JT, Owen KQ, Davis DL. Ovulation and fertilization rate of gilts provided additional L-carnitine and chromium nicotinate. In: Kansas Agricultural Experiment Station Research Reports, editor, Swine Day. Manhattan: Agri Exp Station Cooper Ext Service; 1998. p. 25–7.
21. Pirestani A, Aghakhani M, Tabatabaei SN, Ghalamkari G, Baharlo F. Effects of dietary L-carnitine and choline chloride compound on reproduction indices and udder immune system in Holstein dairy cattle. In: Proceedings of international conference on life Science and Technology; 2011. p. 59–61.
22. Reader KL, Cox NR, Stanton JA, Juengel JL. Effects of acetyl-L-carnitine on lamb oocyte blastocyst rate, ultrastructure, and mitochondrial DNA copy number. Theriogenology. 2015;83:1484–92.
23. You J, Lee J, Hyun SH, Lee E. L-carnitine treatment during oocyte maturation improves in vitro development of cloned pig embryos by influencing intracellular glutathione synthesis and embryonic gene expression. Theriogenology. 2012;78:235–43.
24. Gulewitch VS, Krimberg R. Zur Kenntnis der Extraktivstoffe der Muskeln. II. Mitteilung: Über das Carnitin. Zeits für Physiol Chem. 1905;45:326–30.
25. Bremer J. Carnitine–metabolism and Functions. Physiol Rev. 1983;63:1420–80.
26. Shug AL, Schmidt MJ, Golden GT, Fariello RG. The distribution and role of carnitine in the mammalian brain. Life Sci. 1982;31:2869–74.
27. Rebouche CJ. Carnitine function and requirements during the life cycle. FASEB J. 1992;6:3379–86.
28. Marzo A, Arrigoni Martelli E, Mancinelli A, Cardace G, Corbelletta C, Bassani E, Solbiati M. Protein binding of L-carnitine family components. Eur J Drug Metab Pharmacokinet. 1991;3:364–8.
29. Vassiliadis S, Athanassakis I. A "conditionally essential" nutrient, L-carnitine, as a primary suspect in endometriosis. Fertil Steril. 2011;95:2759–60.
30. Dunning KR, Cashman K, Russell DL, Thompson JG, Norman RJ, Robker RL. Beta-oxidation is essential for mouse oocyte developmental competence and early embryo development. Biol Reprod. 2010;83:909–18.
31. Mingorance C, Rodriguez-Rodriguez R, Justo ML, Herrera MD, de Sotomayor MA. Pharmacological effects and clinical applications of propionyl-L-carnitine. Nutr Rev. 2011;69:279–90.
32. Arduini A, Denisova N, Virmani A, Avrova N, Federici G, Arrigoni-Martelli E. Evidence for the involvement of carnitine-dependent long-chain acyltransferases

in neuronal triglyceride and phospholipid fatty acid turnover. J Neurochem. 1994; 62:1530–8.
33. Abdelrazik H, Sharma R, Mahfouz R, Agarwal A. L-carnitine decreases DNA damage and improves the in vitro blastocyst development rate in mouse embryos. Fertil Steril. 2009;91:589–96.
34. Infante JP, Tschanz CL, Shaw N, Michaud AL, Lawrence P, Brenna JT. Straight-chain acyl-CoA oxidase knockout mouse accumulates extremely long chain fatty acids from alpha-linolenic acid: evidence for runaway carousel-type enzyme kinetics in peroxisomal beta-oxidation diseases. Mol Genet Metab. 2002;75:108–19.
35. Varnagy A, Bene J, Sulyok E, Kovacs GL, Bodis J, Melegh B. Acylcarnitine esters profiling of serum and follicular fluid in patients undergoing in vitro fertilization. Reprod Biol Endocrinol. 2013;11:67.
36. Fenkci SM, Fenkci V, Oztekin O, Rota S, Karagenc N. Serum total L-carnitine levels in non-obese women with polycystic ovary syndrome. Hum Reprod. 2008;23:1602–6.
37. Christiana K, George T, George F, Margarita T, Anna T, Costas F, Irene A. L-carnitine alters lipid body content in pre-implantation embryos leading to infertility. J Reprod Immunol. 2014;101-102:18–39.
38. Mansour G, Abdelrazik H, Sharma RK, Radwan E, Falcone T, Agarwal A. L-carnitine supplementation reduces oocyte cytoskeleton damage and embryo apoptosis induced by incubation in peritoneal fluid from patients with endometriosis. Fertil Steril. 2009;91:2079–86.
39. Center SA, Warner KL, Randolph JF, Sunvold GD, Vickers JR. Influence of dietary supplementation with (L)-carnitine on metabolic rate, fatty acid oxidation, body condition, and weight loss in overweight cats. Am J Vet Res. 2012;73:1002–15.
40. Jamilian H, Jamilian M, Samimi M, Afshar Ebrahimi F, Rahimi M, Bahmani F, Aghababayan S, Kouhi M, Shahabbaspour S, Asemi Z. Oral carnitine supplementation influences mental health parameters and biomarkers of oxidative stress in women with polycystic ovary syndrome: a randomized, double-blind, placebo-controlled trial. Gynecol Endocrinol. 2017;33:442–7.
41. Meczekalski B, Katulski K, Czyzyk A, Podfigurna-Stopa A, Maciejewska-Jeske M. Functional hypothalamic amenorrhea and its influence on women's health. J Endocrinol Investig. 2014;37:1049–56.
42. MBMR F, Flayyih NK. Effect of L-carnitine administration to pregnant mice on some reproductive hormones and organs. Iraqi J Vet Med. 2012;36:68–74.
43. Zhai W, Neuman SL, Latour MA, Hester PY. The effect of male and female supplementation of L-carnitine on reproductive traits of white leghorns. Poult Sci. 2008;87:1171–81.
44. Adabi SG, Moghaddam G, Taghizadeh A, Nematollahi A, Farahvash T. Effect of L-carnitine and vegetable fat on broiler breeder fertility, hatchability, egg yolk and serum cholesterol and triglyceride. Int J Poult Sci. 2006;5:970–4.
45. Tselekidou A, Athanassakis I. PGE1 versus PGE2: protective rather than inducing agent for endometriosis. Eur J Immunol. 2009;81:165.
46. Dionyssopoulou E, Anagnostaki E, Tselekidou A, Vassiliadis S, Athanassakis I. Establishment or aggravation of endometriosis-induction process. In: Arici A, Matalliotakis I, editors. Endometriosis-adenomyosis. Greece: PM Publications; 2011.
47. Virmani MA, Zerelli S, Vitullo P, Cossetti C. Effect Of nutrients on ovulation and oocytes quality in mice. In: Proceedings of 11th congress of the European Society of Gynecology. Roma: Edizioni Internazionali; 2015. p. 212–4.
48. Virmani MA, Virtullo P, Cossetti C. Improving Oocyte and Sperm Quality by L-Carnitine, Acetyl-L-carnitine and Other Nutrients as Major Determinant in Pregnancy Success. Journal of Perinatal Medicine. 45 Supplement. 2017;1:3.
49. Canbolat EP, Sagsoz N, Noyan V, Yucel A, Kisa U. Effects of l-carnitine on oxidative stress parameters in oophorectomized rats. Alex J Med. 2017;53: 55–60.
50. Corduk M, Sarica S. Effects of L-carnitine in layer diets containing different fat sources and energy levels on hen performance and egg quality. South Afr J Anim Sci. 2008;38:260–70.
51. Ramanau A, Kluge H, Spilke J, Eder K. Reproductive performance of sows supplemented with dietary L-carnitine over three reproductive cycles. Arch Tierernahr. 2002;56:287–96.
52. Musser RE, Dritz SS, Davis DL, Tokach MD, Nelssen JL, Goodband RD, Owen KQ. Effects of L-carnitine in the gestating sow diet on fetal muscle development and carcass characteristics of the offspring. J Appl Anim Res. 2007;31:105–11.
53. Scholz H, Heimendahl EV, Menn F, Ahrens A. Application of Protected L-Carnitine in Dairy Cows during Transition and High Lactation Period. Global J Sci Front Res. 2014;XIV:41–6.
54. Somfai T, Kaneda M, Akagi S, Watanabe S, Haraguchi S, Mizutani E, Dang-Nguyen TQ, Geshi M, Kikuchi K, Nagai T. Enhancement of lipid metabolism with L-carnitine during in vitro maturation improves nuclear maturation and cleavage ability of follicular porcine oocytes. Reprod Fertil Dev. 2011;23:912–20.
55. Moawad AR, Xu B, Tan SL, Taketo T. L-carnitine supplementation during vitrification of mouse germinal vesicle stage-oocytes and their subsequent in vitro maturation improves meiotic spindle configuration and mitochondrial distribution in metaphase II oocytes. Hum Reprod. 2014;29:2256–68.
56. Mishra A, Reddy IJ, Gupta PS, Mondal S. L-carnitine mediated reduction in oxidative stress and alteration in transcript level of antioxidant enzymes in sheep embryos produced in vitro. Reprod Domest Anim. 2016;51:311–21.
57. Pillich RT, Scarsella G, Risuleo G. Reduction of apoptosis through the mitochondrial pathway by the administration of acetyl-L-carnitine to mouse fibroblasts in culture. Exp Cell Res. 2005;306:1–8.
58. Agarwal A, Gupta S, Sharma RK. Role of oxidative stress in female reproduction. Reprod Biol Endocrinol. 2005;3:28.
59. Carlberg M, Nejaty J, Froysa B, Guan Y, Soder O, Bergqvist A. Elevated expression of tumour necrosis factor alpha in cultured granulosa cells from women with endometriosis. Hum Reprod. 2000;15:1250–5.
60. Bedaiwy MA, Falcone T. Peritoneal fluid environment in endometriosis. Clinicopathological implications. Minerva Ginecol. 2003;55:333–45.
61. Gupta S, Goldberg JM, Aziz N, Goldberg E, Krajcir N, Agarwal A. Pathogenic mechanisms in endometriosis-associated infertility. Fertil Steril. 2008;90:247–57.
62. Glabowski W, Kurzawa R, Wiszniewska B, Baczkowski T, Marchlewicz M, Brelik P. Growth factors effects on preimplantation development of mouse embryos exposed to tumor necrosis factor alpha. Reprod Biol. 2005;5:83–99.
63. Whiteside EJ, Boucaut KJ, Teh A, Garcia-Aragon J, Harvey MB, Herington AC. Elevated concentration of TNF-alpha induces trophoblast differentiation in mouse blastocyst outgrowths. Cell Tissue Res. 2003;314:275–80.
64. Zare Z, Masteri Farahani R, Salehi M, Piryaei A, Ghaffari Novin M, Fadaei Fathabadi F, Mohammadi M, Dehghani-Mohammadabadi M. Effect of L-carnitine supplementation on maturation and early embryo development of immature mouse oocytes selected by brilliant cresyle blue staining. J Assist Reprod Genet. 2015;32:635–43.
65. Bareh GM. The effect of endometriosis on the DNA integrity of different stages of Embryos' development and the role of L- carnitine in preventing damage to early stages. J Minimal Inv Gynecol. 2010;17:S51.
66. Phongmitr T, Liang Y, Srirattana K, Panyawai K, Sripunya N, Treetampinich C, Parnpai R. Effects of L-carnitine supplemented in maturation medium on the maturation rate of swamp buffalo oocytes. Buffalo Bulletin. 2013;32:613–6.
67. Ghanem N. L-carnitine improved bovine blastocyst rate and quality when supplemented at different preimplantation stages. Egypt J Anim Prod. 2015; 52:89–99.
68. Takahashi T, Inaba Y, Somfai T, Kaneda M, Geshi M, Nagai T, Manabe N. Supplementation of culture medium with L-carnitine improves development and cryotolerance of bovine embryos produced in vitro. Reprod Fertil Dev. 2013;25:589–99.
69. Ghanem N, Ha AN, Fakruzzaman M, Bang JI, Lee SC, Kong IK. Differential expression of selected candidate genes in bovine embryos produced in vitro and cultured with chemicals modulating lipid metabolism. Theriogenology. 2014;82:238–50.
70. Manzano PCVJ, Ocampo MB, Ocampo LC, Maylem ERS, Lazaro JV. Improved bovine blastocyst developmental potential by L-carnitine supplementation. Int J Sci Res Knowledge. 2015;3:021–9.
71. Khanmohammadi N, Movahedin M, Safari M, Sameni HR, Yousefi B, Jafari B, Zarbakhsh S. Effect of L-carnitine on in vitro developmental rate, the zona pellucida and hatching of blastocysts and their cell numbers in mouse embryos. Int J Reprod Biomed (Yazd). 2016;14:649–56.
72. Vanella A, Russo A, Acquaviva R, Campisi A, Di Giacomo C, Sorrenti V, Barcellona ML. L -Propionyl-carnitine as superoxide scavenger, antioxidant, and DNA cleavage protector. Cell Biol Toxicol. 2000;16:99–104.
73. Stojkovic M, Machado SA, Stojkovic P, Zakhartchenko V, Hutzler P, Goncalves PB, Wolf E. Mitochondrial distribution and adenosine triphosphate content of bovine oocytes before and after in vitro maturation: correlation with morphological criteria and developmental capacity after in vitro fertilization and culture. Biol Reprod. 2001;64:904–9.
74. Tamai I, Ohashi R, Nezu J, Yabuuchi H, Oku A, Shimane M, Sai Y, Tsuji A. Molecular and functional identification of sodium ion-dependent, high affinity human carnitine transporter OCTN2. J Biol Chem. 1998;273: 20378–82.
75. Bedaiwy MA, Falcone T, Mohamed MS, Aleem AA, Sharma RK, Worley SE, Thornton J, Agarwal A. Differential growth of human embryos in vitro: role of reactive oxygen species. Fertil Steril. 2004;82:593–600.

76. Virmani MA, Krsmanovic LZ, Stojilkovic SS, Catt KJ. Stimulatory effects of L-acetyl carnitine on the pituitary-gonadal axis in female rats. In: Advances in human female reproduction. New York: Sereno Symposium Publication, Raven Press; 1991. p. 291–6.
77. Bresolin N, Freddo L, Vergani L, Angelini C. Carnitine, carnitine acyltransferases, and rat brain function. Exp Neurol. 1982;78:285–92.
78. Amenta F, Cavallotti C, De Rossi M, Bossoni G, Carpi C. Effect of acetyl-L-carnitine treatment on some behavioural, histochemical and histological parameters of methylazoxymethanol microencephalic rats. Int J Tissue React. 1986;8:513–26.
79. Bodis-Wollner I. Physiological effects of acetyl-levo-carnitine in the central nervous system. Int J Clin Pharmacol Res. 1990;10:109–14.
80. Bigdeli H, Snyder PJ. Gonadotropin releasing hormone release from the rat hypothalamus: dependence on membrane depolarization and calcium influx. Endocrinology. 1978;103:281–6.
81. Krsmanovic LZ, Virmani MA, Stojilkovic SS, Catt KJ. Stimulation of gonadotropin-releasing hormone secretion by acetyl-L-carnitine in hypothalamic neurons and GT1 neuronal cells. Neurosci Lett. 1994;165:33–6.
82. Costa ND, Stevenson PM. Changes in coenzyme a and carnitine concentrations in superovulated rats. Biochim Biophys Acta. 1984;792:130–4.
83. Abo-Ghanema II, El-Nasharty MA, El-Far AH, Ghonium HA. Effect of ginger and L-carnitine on the reproductive performance of male rats. World Acad Sci Eng Technol. 2012;64:980–6.
84. Giorgi VS, Da Broi MG, Paz CC, Ferriani RA, Navarro PA. N-acetyl-cysteine and l-carnitine prevent meiotic oocyte damage induced by follicular fluid from infertile women with mild endometriosis. Reprod Sci. 2016;23:342–51.
85. Abdel-Khalek AE, El-Ratel IT, Wafa WM, El-Nagar HA, Younan GE, Fouda SF. Effect of pre-conception coenzyme Q10 and L-carnitine treatments on ovulatory response, genital characteristics and in vitro embryo characteristics in rabbits. Asian J Anim Vet Adv. 2015;11:53–9.
86. El-Damarawi MA, Salama ME. Obestatin and L-carnitine as a defensive strategy against fertility disorders induced by obesity in male rats. Tanta Med J. 2014;42: 103–11.
87. MSH H, Youssef SF, El-bahy MA. Effects of L-carnitine and ascorbic acid supplementation on productive, reproductive, physiological and immunological performance of golden montazah laying hens. Egypt Poult Sci. 2011;31:557–78.
88. Kacem O, Harzallah M, Zedini C, Zidi I, Meddeb S, Fekih M, Saidi H, Chaib A, Boughizane S, Ali HB, et al. Beneficial effect of an oral antioxidant supplementation (Fertimax2) on IVF-ICSI outcomes: a preliminary clinical study. Adv Reprod Sci. 2014;2:47–56.
89. Cavallini G, Magli MC, Crippa A, Ferraretti AP, Gianaroli L. Reduction in sperm aneuploidy levels in severe oligoasthenoteratospermic patients after medical therapy: a preliminary report. Asian J Androl. 2012;14:591–8.
90. Genazzani AD, Despini G, Czyzyk A, Podfigurna A, Simoncini T, Meczekalski B. Modulatory effects of l-carnitine plus l-acetyl-carnitine on neuroendocrine control of hypothalamic functions in functional hypothalamic amenorrhea (FHA). Gynecol Endocrinol. 2017:1–5.
91. Sekhon LH, Gupta S, Kim Y, Agarwal A. Female infertility and antioxidants. Curr Women's Health Rev. 2010;6:84–95.
92. McDowell LR, Wilkinson N, Madison R, Felix T. Vitamins and minerals functioning as antioxidants with supplementation considerations. In: Florida Ruminant Nutrition Symposium. Gainesville, FL: Best Western Gateway Grand; 2007. p. 30–1.
93. Sugino N, Karube-Harada A, Taketani T, Sakata A, Nakamura Y. Withdrawal of ovarian steroids stimulates prostaglandin F2alpha production through nuclear factor-kappaB activation via oxygen radicals in human endometrial stromal cells: potential relevance to menstruation. J Reprod Dev. 2004;50: 215–25.
94. Crha I, Hruba D, Ventruba P, Fiala J, Totusek J, Visnova H. Ascorbic Acid and infertility treatment. Cent Eur J Public Health. 2003;11:63–7.
95. Guerin P, El Mouatassim S, Menezo Y. Oxidative stress and protection against reactive oxygen species in the pre-implantation embryo and its surroundings. Hum Reprod Update. 2001;7:175–89.
96. de Matos DG, Furnus CC. The importance of having high glutathione (GSH) level after bovine in vitro maturation on embryo development effect of beta-mercaptoethanol, cysteine and cystine. Theriogenology. 2000;53:761–71.

Excessive nerve growth factor impairs bidirectional communication between the oocyte and cumulus cells resulting in reduced oocyte competence

Yiwen Zhai[1,2], Guidong Yao[3], Faiza Rao[1,2], Yong Wang[1,2], Xiaoyuan Song[1,2] and Fei Sun[1,2*]

Abstract

Background: Excessive nerve growth factor (NGF) is commonly found in the follicular fluid of patients with polycystic ovary syndrome (PCOS). Furthermore, oocytes from PCOS patients exhibit lower developmental competence. The purpose of this study was to explore the association between excessive NGF and low oocyte competence in vitro.

Methods: Excessive NGF was added to mouse cumulus oocyte complexes (COCs) cultured in vitro to investigate meiotic maturation of the oocyte. After culture, mRNA expression levels of *Pfkp* and *Ldha* genes in cumulus cells (CCs) and *Gdf9*, *Bmp15* and *Fgf8* genes in oocytes, were determined by real-time quantitative polymerase chain reaction (qPCR). We also investigated the mRNA content of *Pfkp* and *Ldha* in CCs from PCOS and non-PCOS patients.

Results: Excessive NGF significantly inhibited oocyte meiotic maturation. The inhibitory effect was mediated by the NGF high-affinity receptor, NTRK1. mRNA content of *Pfkp* and *Ldha* genes in CCs was significantly reduced by excessive NGF stimulation. Moreover, the expression levels of *Gdf9*, *Bmp15* and *Fgf8* were also decreased in oocytes, and was induced by excessive NGF-stimulated CCs. In addition, lower expression levels of *Pfkp* and *Ldha* in CCs were identified in Chinese PCOS patients with excessive NGF (PCOS, 22 ± 2.63 ng/ml, $n = 13$; non-PCOS, 7.18 ± 2.42 ng/ml, $n = 9$; $p < 0.01$) in the follicular fluid, suggesting a potential association between excessive NGF and decreased glycolysis in the CCs of women with PCOS.

Conclusions: Excessive NGF impairs bidirectional communication between oocyte and cumulus cells, which might be related to low oocyte competence.

Keywords: Polycystic ovary syndrome, NGF, Oocyte-derived paracrine factors, Bidirectional communication, Glycolysis

Background

Nerve growth factor (NGF) is a member of the neurotrophin family [1]. While originally reported to exert functionality in the nervous system, NGF has been found to play important roles in the reproductive system [1, 2]. Various types of cells in the mammalian ovary, including theca cells, granulosa cells and cumulus cells (CCs) have been reported to produce NGF [1, 3]. Consistent with its local production in the ovary, NGF is also known to participate in the regulation of folliculogenesis and ovulation [1, 2, 4–6]. The deficiency of NGF in mice is known to lead to a significant reduction of primary and secondary follicles, implying that NGF is necessary for the preantral-follicle stage [2, 4]. Furthermore, the preovulatory increase of NGF in the follicular fluid of rats, golden hamsters and sheep indicated the involvement of NGF in ovulation [1, 5]. Other studies reported that single nucleotide polymorphism of the NGF gene in goats might be associated with litter size, which also emphasized the importance of NGF in reproduction [7, 8]. NGF has also been reported to play roles in oocyte maturation [9]. The addition of NGF to the in vitro medium promoted the resumption of

* Correspondence: feisun@ustc.edu.cn
[1]School of Life Sciences, University of Science and Technology of China, Hefei, Anhui, People's Republic of China
[2]Hefei National Laboratory for Physical Sciences at Microscale, Hefei, Anhui, People's Republic of China
Full list of author information is available at the end of the article

meiosis in murine oocytes [10], and improves cleavage rate in sheep embryos [11]. However, NGF failed to enhance oocyte maturation and developmental competence in pigs and cows [9, 12]. Thus, the function of NGF in the process of oocyte maturation remains rather controversial and is in need of further elucidation.

Interestingly, an increasing number of studies are providing evidence to show that NGF is associated with ovarian diseases, such as polycystic ovary syndrome (PCOS) [1, 13–15]. PCOS, heterogeneously characterized by polycystic ovaries, hyper-androgenism and chronic anovulation, is a common ovarian disease which causes infertility or sub-fertility in 6–8% of women in reproductive age [16]. The presence of excessive NGF in follicular fluid is a clinical manifestation of PCOS patients [13, 15, 17]. Research has shown that transgenic mice expressing excessive NGF exhibit PCOS-like symptoms, such as the formation of follicular cysts, hyperandrogenemia, increased granulosa cell apoptosis, reduced ovulation and fertility and perturbed reproductive and metabolic features [13, 14]. Nevertheless, the mechanism underlying excessive NGF in the follicular fluid of patients with progressive PCOS remains unclear.

PCOS patients consistently suffer from the poor quality of oocytes [16, 18, 19] and this represents a major cause of sub-fertility or infertility [16, 18, 20]. Although a series of extra- and intra-ovarian factors have been identified and linked to abnormal oocyte maturation [16], the underlying mechanisms still require further clarification. Bidirectional communication between oocytes and the surrounding CCs plays an essential role in oocyte maturation [21–24]. During maturation, oocytes are deficient in synthesizing glucose metabolic enzymes; they use pyruvate as an energy substrate, which is transported from companion CCs [25–27]. Glycolysis in the CCs is dominated by oocyte-derived paracrine factors (ODPFs) [21], of which two families have been identified: the transforming growth factor β superfamily, including growth differentiation factor 9 (GDF9) and bone morphogenetic protein 15 (BMP15); and the fibroblast growth factor (FGF) family, including FGF8 and other members [28–30]. Deficiency of these genes in vivo, such as in $Gdf9^{-/-}$ and $Gdf9^{-/-}Bmp15^{-/-}$ mice, leads to reproductive defects [23]. The addition of BMP15 and FGF8 to in vitro cultured CCs has been shown to promote glycolysis [31]. Despite the fact that bidirectional communication is important to oocyte maturation, its role in the pathogenesis of PCOS remains undefined.

In the present study, we aimed to clarify the role of excessive NGF in the follicular fluid of PCOS patients and investigated the effect of excessive NGF on oocyte maturation in the mouse model. To mimic excessive NGF in the follicular fluid and dissect it from other micro-environmental factors, we performed in vitro culture of isolated mouse COCs in the presence of excessive NGF. We found that excessive NGF inhibited oocyte maturation in mouse COCs, and that the inhibitory effect was mediated by the bidirectional communication between oocyte and CCs. Moreover, corresponding to the observation that mRNA expression of glycolytic enzymes reduced in mouse CCs when COCs were cultured with excessive NGF, mRNA expression of glycolytic enzymes significantly reduced in CCs isolated from PCOS patients with excessive NGF in the follicular fluid. These findings revealed a potential pathogenic role of excessive NGF in the progression of PCOS by impairing oocyte maturation.

Methods

Animals

ICR mice were bred and raised in the Animal Center, University of Science and Technology of China. Mice were adapted to a 12-h light/12-h dark cycle at room temperature (22–24 °C). All experiments involved 21-day-old female mice. The study was approved by the Institutional Review Board of the University of Science and Technology of China on the 18th May 2012 (Reference: USTCACUC1201054).

Subjects

Follicular fluid and CCs were collected from 22 Han Chinese women ($n = 9$, non-PCOS; $n = 13$, PCOS) during their first cycle of in vitro fertilization (IVF) or intracytoplasmic sperm injection (ICSI) at the First Affiliated Hospital of Zhengzhou University from January 2015 to May 2015. Written informed consent was obtained from all patients and the study was approved by the Ethics Review Board of the First Affiliated Hospital of Zhengzhou University on 20thNovember 2014 (Reference: 2014-LW-1217). All of the PCOS patients were selected according to the Revised 2003 Consensus on Diagnostic Criteria: Oligo- and/or Anovulation, Hyper-androgenism and Polycystic Ovary [32]. All of the non-PCOS patients had normal ovarian morphology and regular menstrual cycles with male factor infertility. Age, ratio of body weight/height, luteinizing hormone (LH), follicle stimulating hormone (FSH) and testosterone levels of both of PCOS patients and non-PCOS patients were measured and recorded.

Human follicular fluid and CCs collection

After ovarian stimulation with agonadotropin-releasing hormone agonist (Serono, Geneva, Switzerland) and recombinant FSH (Serono, Geneva, Switzerland), three or more follicles reached 17mmin diameter, and then 6000–10,000 IU of human chorionic gonadotropin (hCG, LizhuInc., Zhuhai, China) was administered. COCs were then retrieved from aspirated follicles 36 h after the hCG trigger. Follicular fluid was obtained from the first aspirated follicles and centrifuged at 450 *g* for 5 min; the clear supernatant was then stored at − 80 °C for subsequent NGF assessment. CCs were collected from 9 non-PCOS patients and 5 PCOS patients who received ICSI-embryo transfer, but not IVF-embryo transfer treatment as CCs from such patients would be contaminated with human sperm.

Measurement of NGF in human follicular fluid

Follicular fluid was first treated with acid as described previously [17, 33] to increase measurable NGF levels. In brief, all samples were diluted 1:15,000 in Dulbecco's phosphate-buffered saline (DPBS) and treated with 1 mol/L of HCl at pH 2.6 for 30 min. This was then neutralized by 1 mol/L of NaOH to pH 7.6. NGF was then measured using a human β-NGF Duoset ELISA Kit (R&D Systems, Minneapolis, USA) in accordance with the manufacturer's instructions. In brief, 96-well plates were coated with anti-NGF (human) monoclonal antibody and incubated overnight at 4 °C. All washing steps were conducted 4 times with wash buffer (360 μl/well). Assay plates were washed as above and incubated with blocking buffer for 2 h at room temperature to block non-specific binding. Follicular fluid samples (200 μl/well) and gradient standard NGF samples were added to the appropriate assay wells in duplicate and then incubated for 6 h at room temperature. After incubation, the plates were washed and then detection antibody was added and incubated for 2 h at room temperature. Afterwards, plates were washed and labeled with streptavidin-HRP for 20 min in the dark. Then, substrate solution and stop solution were added into the plates for absorbance measurement. The concentration follicular fluid was calculated using a standard curve.

Reagents and medium for cell culture

Mouse β-NGF (R&D Systems, Minneapolis, USA) and K252α (Sigma-Aldrich, St. Louis, USA) were prepared at a concentration of 100 ng/ml and 10 mM, as described previously [34]. We used α-MEM culture media (Gibco, Calsbad, USA) supplemented with 0.3% (wt/vol) bovine serum albumen (BSA, Sigma-Aldrich, St. Louis, USA), 0. 23 mM pyruvate (Sigma-Aldrich, St. Louis, USA), 75 mg/L penicillin G and 50 mg/L streptomycin sulfate (Gibco, Calsbad, USA).

Isolation and collection of COCs, oocytectomized cumulus cells (OOX-cumulus cells) and denuded oocytes

Follicle development was stimulated by an intraperitoneal injection of 5 IU pregnant mare serum gonadotropin (PMSG, Sigma-Aldrich, St. Louis, USA) 44–48 h before harvesting ovaries. Ovaries were removed and large antral follicles were punctured with fine hypodermic needles (number 5 grade) under a dissecting microscope. COCs and denuded oocytes were collected using a mouth-controlled, small-bore glass pipette. OOX-cumulus cells were generated by microsurgically removing oocytes from the COCs, but leaving the zonapellucida intact, as previously described [23]. In brief, each COC was held by negative pressure with a holding pipette, and most, or all of the oocyte, was removed by negative pressure when a lancing pipette was pushed through the COC. This lead to a spherical zonapellucida and the surrounding CCs are referred to as OOX-cumulus cells hereafter.

During the isolation progress, 10 mM milrinone (Sigma-Aldrich, St. Louis, USA) was used to maintain oocytes at the germinal vesicle (GV) stage. After collection, COCs, OOX-cumulus cells and denuded oocytes were washed in culture medium three times in order to remove milrinone. These cells were then ready for further study.

Cell culture and evaluation of oocyte meiotic maturation in vitro

COCs were plated in droplets at a density of 1 COC/μl [23, 35]. COCs were then cultured in medium with NGF gradients (1, 10, 100 and 1000 ng/ml) for 18 h, or in medium containing100ng/ml of NGF for 10, 12, and 18 h with or without 10 μM K252α. The proportion of first polar body (PB1) was calculated by removing CCs under a stereomicroscope and evaluating the status of oocyte meiotic maturation.

COCs, OOX-cumulus cells, denuded oocytes and OOX-cumulus cells co-cultured with denuded oocytes [31, 36] (referred as "OOX + DO") were cultured separately with or without NGF for 18 h, then CCs and oocytes were collected for target gene analysis.

To examine whether NGF-treated CCs inhibit oocyte meiotic maturation, OOX-cumulus cells were first stimulated with NGF for 24 h (1 or 2 OOX-cumulus cells per microliter of medium) and then removed [37]. Denuded oocytes were then added into the supernatants at a concentration of 1 DO/μl for 18 h and then collected for target gene analysis.

Immunofluorescence

Ovaries were harvested as described above and 20-μm cryosections were prepared and blocked with 5% BSA for 1 h, incubated with rabbit anti-neurotrophic receptor tyrosine kinase 1 (NTRK1) monoclonal antibody (Abcam, Cambridge, UK) overnight at 4 °C, and then labeled with Alexa Fluor 549 donkey anti-rabbit antibody (Jackson Immuno Research, West Grove, USA). Sections were then stained with DAPI (Solarbio, Beijing, China) before mounting with Gold Anti-fade Reagent (Invitrogen, Calsbad, USA). Images were then acquired with an LSM710 (Carl Zeiss, Milano, Italy).

Table 1 Primers for real-time qPCR

Gene name	GenBank accession number	Sequences of forward (F) and reverse (R) primers	Amplification size (bp)
m-Pfkp	NM_019703	F: 5′-GCCGTGAAACTCCGAGGAA-3′ R: 5′-GTTGCTCTTGACAATCTTCTCATCAG-3′	96
m-Ldha	NM_001136069.2	F: 5′-TGTGGCAGACTTGGCTGAGA-3′ R: 5′-CTGAGGAAGACATCCTCATTGATTC-3′	105
m-Gdf9	NM_008110.2	F: 5′-TCACCTCTACAATACCGTCCGG-3′ R: 5′-GAGCAAGTGTTCCATGGCAGTC-3′	139
m-Bmp15	NM_009757.4	F: 5′-GCACGATTGGAGCGAAAATG-3′ R: 5′-CGTACGCTACCTGGTTTGATGC-3′	123
m-Fgf8	NM_010205.2	F: 5′-CAGGTCTCTACATCTGCATGAACAA-3′ R: 5′-TCTCCAGCACGATCTCTGTGAATA-3′	96
m-Actin	NM_007393.5	F:5′-TGGCTCCTAGCACCATGAA-3′ R: 5′-CTCAGTAACAGTCCGCCTAGAAGCA-3′	186
h-PFKP	NM_002627.4	F: 5′-AGGCGATGGACGAGAGGAGAT-3′ R: 5′-TGATGGCAAGTCGCTTGTAG-3′	93
h-LDHA	NM_001165414.1	F: 5′-TGCACCCAGATTTAGGGACTGAT-3′ R: 5′-CCCAGGATGTGTAGCCTTTGAG-3′	111
h-ACTIN	NM_001101.3	F: 5′-TGGCACCCAGCACAATGAA-3′ R: 5′-CTAAGTCATAGTCCGCCTAGAAGCA-3′	186

m- mouse, *h-* human, *bp* base pair

Real-time qPCR

RNA was extracted using the Dynabeads mRNA DIRECT micro kit (Ambion, Carlsbad, USA). Real-time qPCR was performed using the PrimeScript RT reagent kit (Takara, Shiga, Japan) and the SYBR Premix Ex Taq II Kit (Takara, Shiga, Japan). Primers used for real-time qPCR were selected according to previous reports [31, 34, 38] and listed in Table 1. The specificity of these primers were validated by dissociation curve analysis. Target genes were normalized to *actin* gene. Data were analyzed using the comparative $2^{-\Delta\Delta Ct}$ method [34].

Statistical analysis

Statistical analysis was performed using the Student's *t*-test. $P < 0.05$ was considered to be statistically significant ($^{*}P < 0.05$; $^{**}P < 001$; $^{***}P < 0.001$).

Results

Excessive NGF is present in the follicular fluid of PCOS patients and inhibits oocyte maturation in vitro

We firstly detected NGF content in follicular fluid of Chinese PCOS patients. The clinical characteristics of PCOS and non-PCOS patients were shown in Table 2. The concentration of NGF in follicular fluid was significantly higher

Table 2 Clinical characteristics of PCOS and non-PCOS patients

	PCOS	non-PCOS	*P* value
Total (*n*)	9	13	
IVF-ET (*n*)	4	4	
ICSI-ET (*n*)	5	9	
Age (year)	29.53 ± 5.61	28.22 ± 2.42	0.46
BMI	24.36 ± 3.24	22.63 ± 2.46	< 0.001
LH (IU/ml)	10.47 ± 4.62	6.23 ± 3.29	< 0.0001
FSH (IU/ml)	5.27 ± 1.41	7.58 ± 2.13	< 0.0001
Testosterone (ng/dl)	52.62 ± 18.74	26.37 ± 11.92	< 0.0001
Antral follicle count (*n*)	34.51 ± 13.08	16.24 ± 5.36	< 0.0001
Starting Gn dose (IU)	152.81 ± 32.24	178.77 ± 36.69	0.0013
Gn stimulation duration (day)	12.43 ± 3.26	10.37 ± 2.17	0.0026
Total Gn administrated (IU)	1899.43 ± 579.52	1933.46 ± 627.41	0.54
E2 level on hCG day (pg/ml)	5768.27 ± 2843.32	4689.66 ± 1895.24	0.005
Follicles ≥14 mm (*n*)	16.43 ± 4.15	12.46 ± 3.53	< 0.0001
Oocytes retrieved (*n*)	18.62 ± 8.05	13.88 ± 4.95	< 0.0001

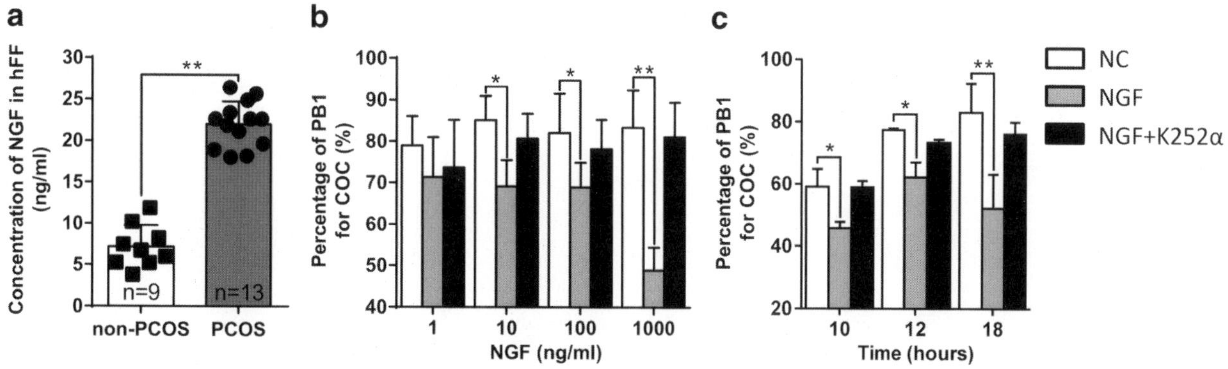

Fig. 1 Excessive NGF inhibited mouse oocyte maturation. **a** Excessive NGF in the follicular fluid of Chinese PCOS patients. Concentration of NGF in human follicular fluid (hFF) of Chinese non-PCOS patients ($n = 9$) and PCOS patients ($n = 13$) was determined by ELISA. **b–c** COCs were cultured with the indicated concentration of NGF for 18 h (**b**) or with 100 ng/ml NGF for the indicated times (**c**) in the presence or absence of 10 μM K252α. The proportion of PB1 extrusion was then calculated. The number of COCs for each group was ≥35. Representative data are presented as mean ± SEM. *, $p < 0.05$; **, $p < 0.01$

in the PCOS group (22 ± 2.63 ng/ml, $n = 13$) than that in the non-PCOS group (7.18 ± 2.42 ng/ml, $n = 9$) (Fig. 1a).

To observe the effect of NGF on oocyte maturation, mouse COCs from antral follicles were cultured with different concentrations of NGF. This showed that 10 and 100 ng/ml of NGF significantly suppressed PB1 extrusion, a hallmark of oocyte meiotic maturation, and that 1000 ng/ml of NGF had a stronger suppressive effect (Fig. 1b). Taking an overall consideration of both NGF concentrations in the follicular fluid of PCOS patients and their inhibitory effect in vitro, we chose 100 ng/ml as an excessive concentration of NGF that mimics excessive levels of NGF in the follicular fluid of PCOS patients and used this concentration in our subsequent experiments. The inhibitory effect of 100 ng/ml NGF on PB1 extrusion was observed at 10, 12, and 18 h after NGF treatment (Fig. 1c), indicating that the inhibitory effect existed throughout the progression of meiosis I.

NTRK1, the high affinity receptor for NGF, is expressed on CCs in antral follicles

To explore the mechanisms underlying the inhibitory effect of NGF, we analyzed the cellular expression of NTRK1, the high affinity receptor for NGF previously known as TrkA [1]. Intense expression of NTRK1 was detected on the surface of CCs in antral follicles (Fig. 2). Notably, expression of NTRK1 was not detected on oocytes in antral follicles (Fig. 2). Thus, in our in vitro cultured COCs, NTRK1 was exclusively expressed by CCs. To validate the role of NTRK1, we utilized K252α, the phosphorylation inhibitor of NTRK1, during in vitro culture of COCs. The addition of K252α into the culture medium of COCs abolished the suppressive effect of NGF, indicating that the inhibitory effect was mediated by NTRK1. Collectively, these results indicate that excessive NGF inhibit the meiotic maturation of oocytes in COCs via its high affinity receptor NTRK1 which is expressed on CCs.

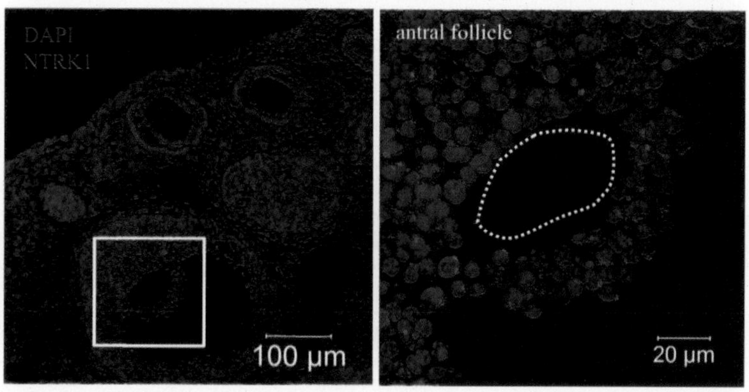

Fig. 2 Cellular localization of NTRK1 at the antral follicle stage. Left, representative overview confocal image of NTRK1 staining. Right, magnified image of an antral follicle. Dotted line shows the position of the oocyte. Representative images of three independent experiments are shown

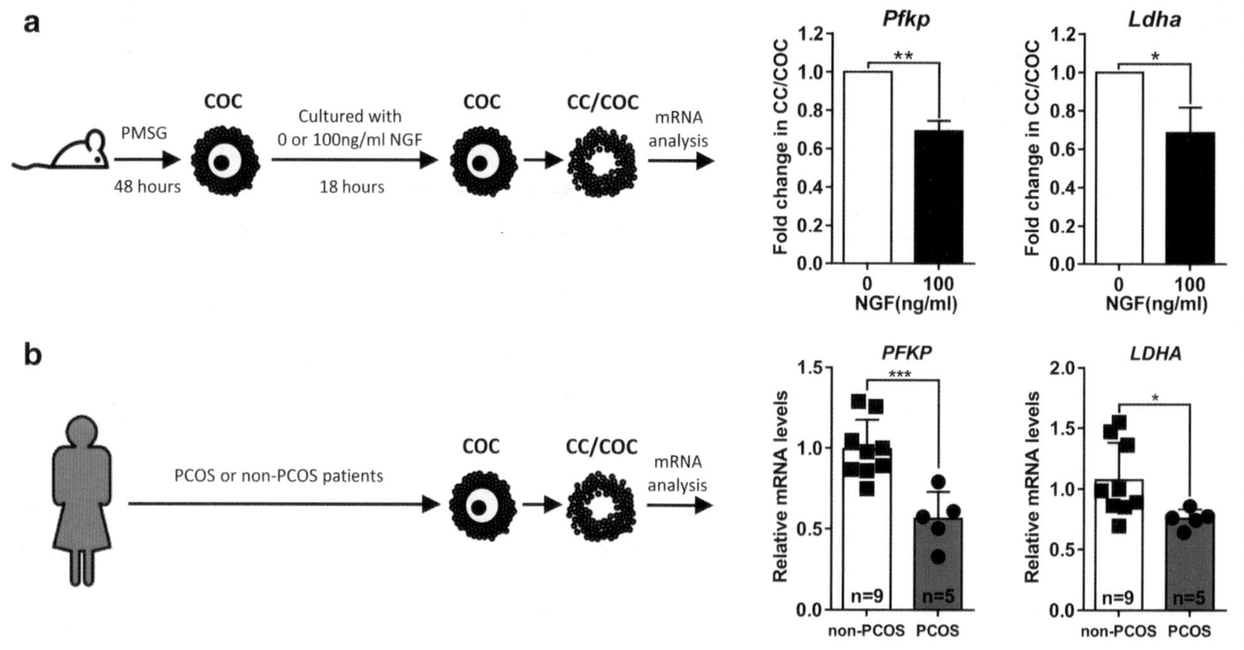

Fig. 3 Down-regulation of *Pfkp* and *Ldha* in CCs/COCs occurred in both mice and humans. **a** Relative mRNA levels of *Pfkp* and *Ldha* in mouse CCs/COCs were determined by real-time qPCR, after culturing with 100 ng/ml NGF for 18 h. ≥35 COCs in each group were used and experiments were repeated three times. **b** Relative mRNA levels of *PFKP* and *LDHA* in CCs from non-PCOS ($n = 9$) patients and PCOS patients ($n = 5$) were determined by real-time qPCR. Data are presented as mean ± SEM. The student's *t*-test was used for statistical analysis. *, $p < 0.05$; **, $p < 0.01$; ***, $p < 0.001$

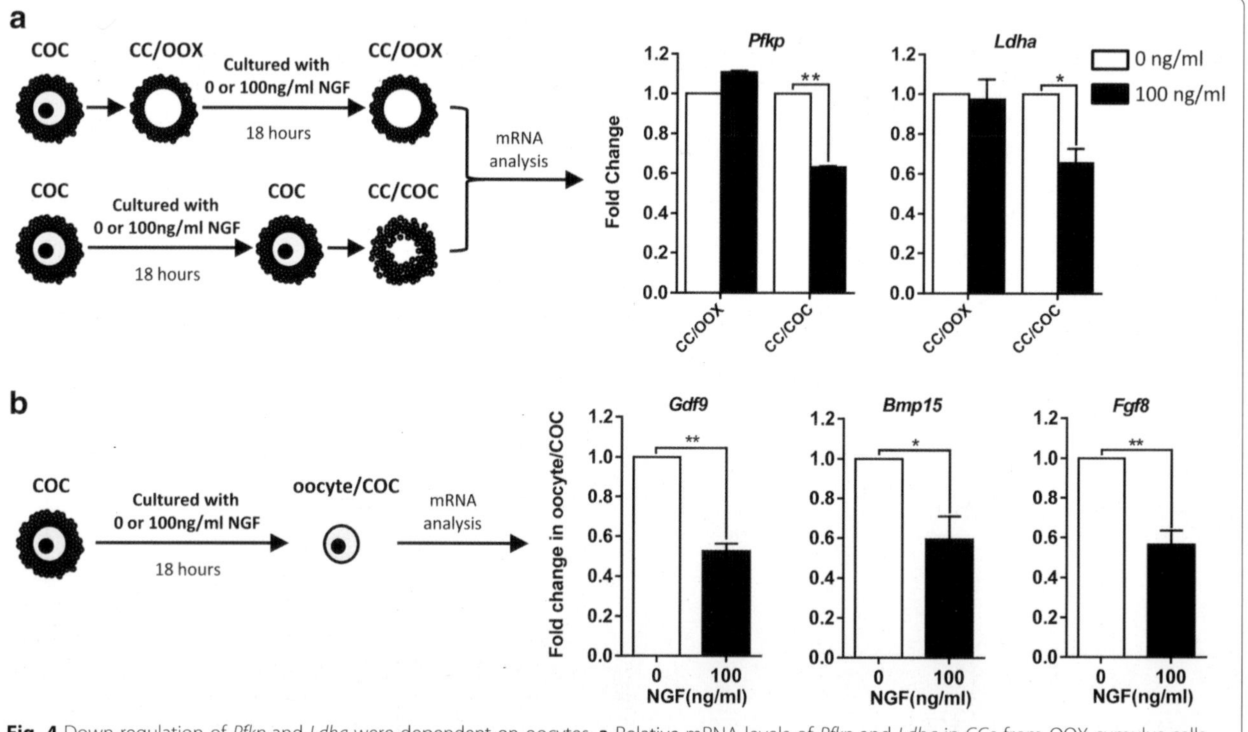

Fig. 4 Down-regulation of *Pfkp* and *Ldha* were dependent on oocytes. **a** Relative mRNA levels of *Pfkp* and *Ldha* in CCs from OOX-cumulus cells or CCs/COCs were determined by real-time qPCR in the presence or absence of NGF. CC/OOX, OOX-cumulus cells group; CCs/COC, cumulus cells from the COC group. **b** Relative mRNA levels of *Gdf9*, *Bmp15* and *Fgf8* in oocytes/COCs cultured with or without 100 ng/ml NGF for 18 h were determined by real-time qPCR. ≥35 samples were used in each group. Data of three independent experiments are presented as mean ± SEM. The student's *t*-test was used for statistical analysis *, $p < 0.05$; **, $p < 0.01$

The glycolysis of CCs from COCs is down-regulated in the presence of excessive NGF in both mice and humans

Because the inhibitory effect of excessive NGF was mediated by NTRK1 expressed on CCs and because glycolysis in the CCs produces the pyruvate that is essential for oocyte maturation, we next analyzed the effect of NGF on glycolysis in CCs. Mouse antral follicle-derived COCs were stimulated by excessive NGF and then CCs were collected to examine the expression of *Pfkp* and *Ldha*, genes encoding rate-limiting enzymes of glycolysis [31]; this allowed us to evaluate the process of glycolysis. The mRNA expression levels of *Pfkp* and *Ldha* decreased significantly in the presence of excessive NGF (Fig. 3a). Similar to the results in mice, the mRNA expression levels of *PFKP* and *LDHA* in CCs from PCOS patients were lower than that in non-PCOS patients (Fig. 3b). *PFKP* was down-regulated by 2-fold (Fig. 3b, left) while *LDHA* was reduced by 1.5-fold (Fig. 3b, right). Collectively, this data suggests that in the presence of excessive NGF, the expression levels of glycolytic rate-limiting enzymes in the CCs of COCs were down-regulated in both mice and humans.

NGF-induced down-regulation of glycolysis in CCs is dependent on oocytes

To observe the direct effect of excessive NGF on CCs, OOX-cumulus cells were treated with excessive NGF but no significant change of mRNA levels of *Pfkp* and *Ldha* was observed (Fig. 4a). Taking into account the significant inhibition of NGF on glycolysis in CCs from cultured COCs (Fig. 4b), it can be concluded that the inhibitory effect of NGF on glycolysis in CCs was dependent on oocytes. Consistent with the down-regulated glycolysis in CCs, the mRNA expression levels of *Gdf9*, *Bmp15* and *Fgf8*, which are three well-characterized ODPFs, were decreased in oocytes from COCs cultured with excessive levels of NGF (Fig. 4b). Levels of *Gdf9* and *Fgf8* were reduced by 2-fold and *Bmp15* was reduced by 1.5-fold. Therefore, the reduced production of ODPFs in oocytes might be responsible for the down-regulation of glycolysis in CCs.

NGF-stimulated CCs inhibited the production of ODPFs in oocytes

We further explored how excessive NGF caused a reduced production of ODPFs. As NTRK1 is expressed on CCs, but

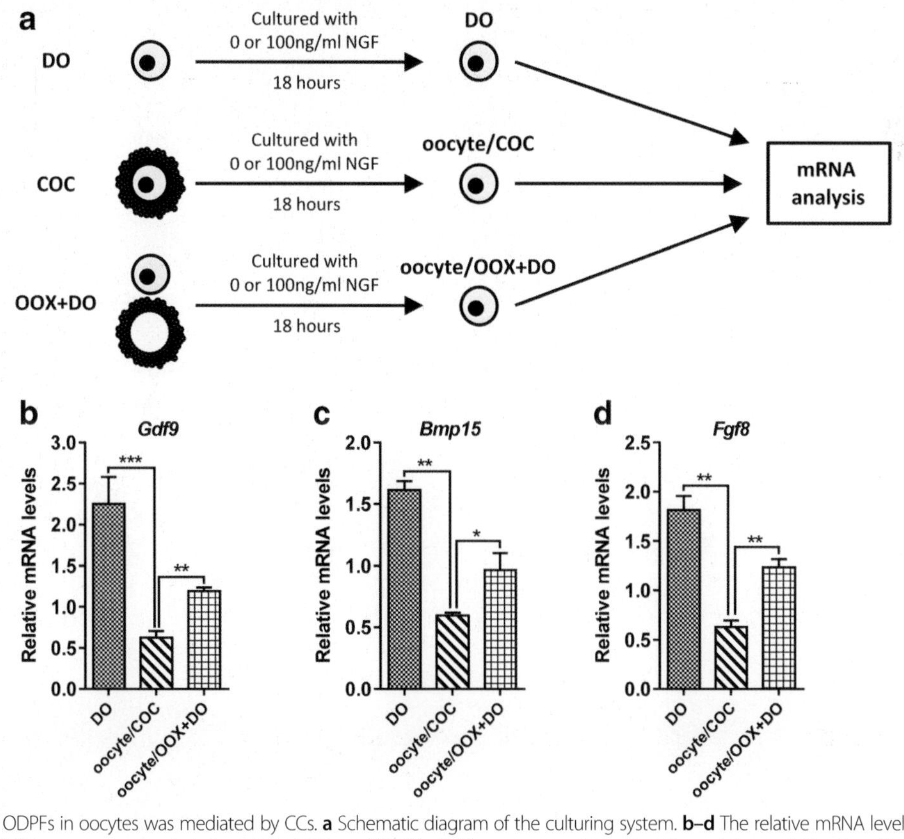

Fig. 5 Decrease of ODPFs in oocytes was mediated by CCs. **a** Schematic diagram of the culturing system. **b–d** The relative mRNA levels of *Gdf9* (**b**), *Bmp15* (**c**) and *Fgf8* (**d**) in oocytes respectively from DOs, COCs and "OOX + DO" group were determined by real-time q-PCR cultured in medium with 100 ng/ml NGF for 18 h. DO, denuded oocyte; oocyte/COC, oocytes from COC group; oocyte/OOX + DO, oocytes from the co-cultured OOX-cumulus cells and denuded oocytes group. ≥35 oocytes were used for RNA extraction in each group. Experiments were repeated at least three times independently. Data are presented as mean ± SEM. Student's two-tailed t-test was used for statistical analysis *, $p < 0.05$; **, $p < 0.01$, ***, $p < 0.001$

not on oocytes, the reduction in ODPF production in oocytes might be caused by NGF-stimulated CCs. Indeed, when stimulated with excessive NGF, oocytes cultured in the presence of CCs, either in the form of COCs or separately added OOX-cumulus cells to cultured denuded oocytes (referred as "OOX + DO"), expressed less ODPFs than denuded oocytes cultured alone (Fig. 5). These results also implied that the inhibitory effect upon the production of ODPFs was mediated by soluble factors derived from CCs. To validate this, OOX-cumulus cells were stimulated with excessive NGF for 18 h, and the culture supernatant was collected to culture denuded oocytes (Fig. 6a). The expression of ODPFs in denuded oocytes cultured in the supernatant of NGF-stimulated OOX-cumulus cells decreased significantly (Fig. 6b). The inhibitory effect of the supernatant was correlated with the concentration of cultured OOX-cumulus cells. The supernatant of OOX-cumulus cells cultured at a concentration of 2 OOXs/μl exhibited a stronger inhibitory effect than that cultured at a concentration of 1 OOX/μl. Overall, CCs stimulated by excessive NGF inhibited the production of ODPFs in oocytes.

Discussion

Previous studies have reported that NGF content is significantly increased in the ovarian follicular fluid of PCOS patients from Germany, Italy and Canada [13, 15, 17]. In the present study, we also observed excessive levels of NGF in the follicular fluid of Chinese PCOS patients. The increase of NGF in follicular fluid is associated with lower ovarian responses in aged women [39]. Studies in the rat have shown that the abnormally elevated production of NGF within the ovary increases androgen secretion, disrupts the estrous cycle and is sufficient to initiate several of the structural and functional alterations associated with the development of follicular cysts [40]. In the present study, by treating in vitro cultured COCs with excessive concentrations of NGF, we revealed an inhibitory role of excessive NGF on oocyte maturation. Furthermore, by using well-established models of OOX-cumulus cells, we proved that bidirectional communication between oocytes and CCs mediated the inhibitory function of NGF. Thus, excessive NGF inhibited oocyte maturation in a bidirectional communication dependent manner, indicating a potential pathogenic role of NGF in the progression of PCOS.

According to previous reports, the concentration of NGF in the follicular fluid of PCOS patients varies over a large range across different studies [13, 15, 17]. For example, Dissen et al. reported that the median concentration of NGF in 11 PCOS patients was 5–7 ng/ml [13].

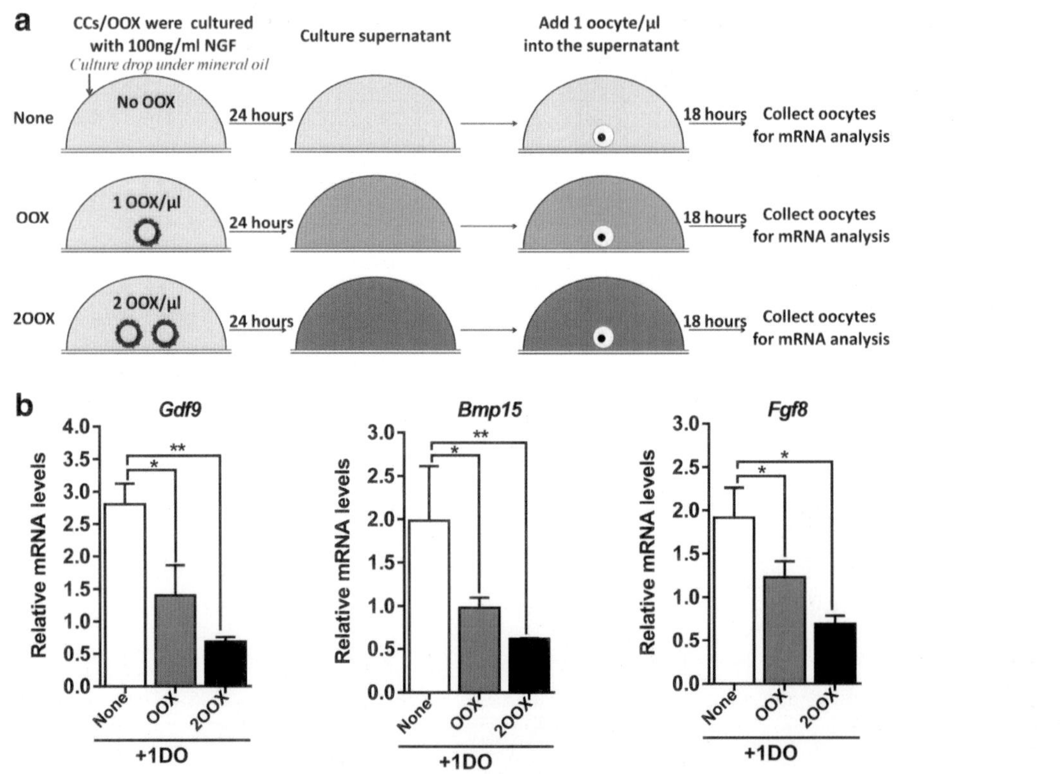

Fig. 6 NGF-stimulated CCs inhibited the production of ODPFs in oocytes. **a** Schematic diagram of the culturing system. **b** Relative mRNA levels of *Gdf9*, *Bmp15* and *Fgf8* in oocytes cultured as in (**a**) were determined by real-time qPCR. ≥35 oocytes were obtained for RNA extraction in each group. Data of three independent experiments are presented as mean ± SEM. The student's *t*-test was used for statistical analysis. $^{*}p < 0.05$; $^{**}p < 0.01$

Sadeu et al. further reported that NGF concentration in 16 PCOS patients ranged from 58.5 to 375 ng/ml [17]. In another study, Gulino et al. reported that the mean concentration of NGF in 32 PCOS patients was 2023.30 ± 587.09 pg/mL [15]. In our present study, the concentration of NGF in follicular fluid ranged from 18 to 26 ng/ml for the PCOS group. The differences in NGF concentrations across these studies might be caused by a variety of factors, such as geography, population, ethics and hormone levels [16]. Since the follicular fluid provides a micro-environment for oocyte development and maturation, it is valuable to explore the role of excessive NGF on oocyte maturation. In the present study, we cultured mouse COCs with different NGF concentrations, ranging from 1 to 1000 ng/ml, which covered the wide range of NGF concentrations reported in previous studies. Combining NGF concentration in the follicular fluid of PCOS patients and the effect of different NGF concentrations during in-vitro culturing, 100 ng/ml of NGF was considered as a moderate concentration to mimic excessive NGF because of its significant inhibitory effect and was therefore used for subsequent experiments throughout the present study.

To explore the mechanisms underlying the inhibitory effect of NGF, we analyzed the cellular expression of NGF receptors. Two different NGF receptors have been characterized: NTRK1, the high affinity receptor for NGF and previously known as TrkA; and p75, a pan-specific receptor for NT family members [1]. NTRK1 is expressed on mesenchymal cells, CCs and granulosa cells in mouse antral follicles, while p75 is only expressed on mesenchymal cells [1, 4]. Consistent with these previous reports, we detected NTRK1 expression on CCs but not on oocytes in mouse antral follicles. Thus, in our in vitro culturing system, CCs were the cells directly affected by excessive NGF. Moreover, the application of K252α abolished the inhibitory effect of excessive NGF, further validating the involvement of NTRK1. In human antral follicles, the expression of NTRK1 on CCs has been reported by several studies [1, 3], while its expression in oocytes remains controversial. Nevertheless, human CCs are also capable of being stimulated by NGF in the follicular fluid. Besides the uniform expression of NTRK1 on CCs in mice and humans, decreased glycolysis, indicated by the reduced expression of *Pfkp* and *Ldha*, was observed in both mouse CCs from COCs treated with excessive levels of NGF and human CCs from the COCs of PCOS patients. As it is very difficult to obtain human samples for research, their number was low. Be that as it may, these specimens strengthened the hypothesis that was initially observed by us in mice. Since the CCs of PCOS and non-PCOS patients were collected from patients who received ICSI treatment, the corresponding oocytes were used for embryo culturing and transfer, making it impossible to analyze the expression of ODPFs in human oocytes. However, previous reports showed that the expression of GDF9 and BMP15 in oocytes from PCOS patients was reduced compared to normal ovulatory women [41, 42]. Collectively, these results suggested that the mechanisms we found in mice were also applicable for PCOS patients.

Excessive NGF inhibited the meiotic maturation of COCs cultured in vitro, suggesting that NGF can contribute to the pathogenesis of PCOS by impairing the development of COCs. Although we proved that bidirectional communication between CCs and oocytes was necessary for the inhibitory effect of excessive NGF, further experiments need to be conducted in the future. Initially, experiments treating CC/COC with GDF9, BMP15 and FGF8 in the presence of NGF should be conducted to demonstrate that ODPFs can reverse the suppression of *Pfkp* and *Ldha* by excessive NGF. Secondly, how NGF-stimulated CCs down-regulate the production of ODPFs in oocytes is still unclear. Our results suggested the existence of CC-derived inhibitory factor(s). Further identification of these inhibitory factor(s) is therefore very valuable. On the other hand, in the antral follicles of both mice and humans, mesenchymal cells are also reported to express NGF receptors [1]. Thus, mesenchymal cells are also potential target cells for excessive NGF in

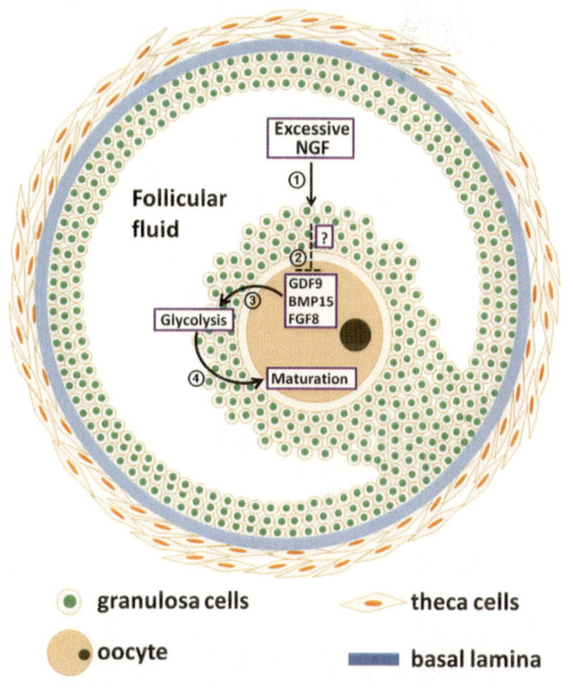

Fig. 7 Working model. ① Excessive NGF in the follicular fluid of PCOS patients. ② Stimulated-CCs secreted inhibitory factor(s) (undefined yet) and down-regulated the production of ODPFs in oocytes. ③ Down-regulation of ODPFs could reduce glycolysis in CCs. ④ Reduction of glycolysis in CCs impaired oocyte meiotic maturation at the antral follicle stage

PCOS patients. Overall, it is valuable to clarify the pathogenic roles of excessive NGF and therapies targeting NGF may be beneficial for patients suffering from PCOS.

Conclusions

The present study could be summarized as Fig. 7. It demonstrates that in vitro addition of excessive NGF inhibits glycolysis in CCs and maturation of oocytes in mouse COCs and the inhibition is dependent on bidirectional communication between oocytes and CCs. Pharmacological blocking of NGF-high affinity receptor NTRK1 by K252α abolished the inhibitory effect on oocyte maturation. Excessive NGF inhibits glycolysis in CCs of COCs, at least in part, by reducing the production of ODPFs in oocytes. Importantly, dysfunction of glycolysis in CCs was identified in PCOS patients with excessive NGF in the follicular fluid. Our findings revealed a pathogenic role of excessive NGF in PCOS.

Abbreviations

BMP15: Bone morphogenetic protein 15; BSA: Bovine serum albumin; CCs: Cumulus cells; COC: Cumulus-oocyte complex; ELISA: Enzyme linked immunosorbent assay; FGF: Fibroblast growth factor; FGF8: Fibroblast growth factor 8; GDF9: Growth differentiational factors 9; ICSI: Intracytoplasmic sperm injection; IVF: In vitro fertilization; LDHA: Lactate dehydrogenase A; NGF: Nerve growth factor; NTRK1: Neurotrophic receptor tyrosine kinase 1; ODPFs: Oocyte-derived paracrine factors; OOX-cumulus cells: Oocytectomized cumulus cells; PBS: Phosphate buffered saline; PCOS: Polycystic ovary syndrome; PFKP: Phosphofructokinase, platelet; PMSG: Pregnant mare serum gonadotropin

Acknowledgments

We thank Professor Youqiang Su (Nanjing, China), Mr. Guangping Yang (Nanjing, China) for assistance on producing OOX-cumulus cells from COCs and Professor Yunhai Zhang (Hefei, China) for providing assistance with the instrumentation.

Funding

This work was supported by grants from the National Natural Science Foundation of China (Grant No. 81430027 and 81671510 to F.S.) and the National Basic Research Program of China (973 Program) (No. 2014CB943100 to F.S.). The founding sponsors had no role in the present study.

Authors' contributions

YZ designed and performed the experiments and wrote the paper; FR revised the paper; GY, YW, and XS supplied reagents and materials. FS designed and supervised the experiments and wrote the manuscript. All authors read and approved the final manuscript.

Competing interests

The authors declare that they have no competing interests.

Author details

[1]School of Life Sciences, University of Science and Technology of China, Hefei, Anhui, People's Republic of China. [2]Hefei National Laboratory for Physical Sciences at Microscale, Hefei, Anhui, People's Republic of China. [3]Reproductive Medical Center, The First Affiliated Hospital of Zhengzhou University, Zhengzhou, Henan, People's Republic of China.

References

1. Streiter S, Fisch B, Sabbah B, Ao A, Abir R. The importance of neuronal growth factors in the ovary. Mol Hum Reprod. 2016;22(1):3–17.
2. Dissen GA, Romero C, Hirshfield AN, Ojeda SR. Nerve growth factor is required for early follicular development in the mammalian ovary. Endocrinology. 2001;142(5):2078–86.
3. Abir R, Fishc B, Jin S, Barnnet M, Ben-Haroush A, Felz C, Kessler-Icekson G, Feldberg D, Nitke S, Ao A. Presence of NGF and its receptors in ovaries from human fetuses and adults. Mol Hum Reprod. 2005;11(4):229–36.
4. Dissen GA, Romero C, Paredes A, Ojeda SR. Neurotrophic control of ovarian development. Microsc Res Tech. 2002;59(6):509–15.
5. Mayerhofer A, Dissen GA, Parrott JA, Hill DF, Mayerhofer D, Garfield RE, Costa ME, Skinner MK, Ojeda SR. Involvement of nerve growth factor in the ovulatory cascade: trkA receptor activation inhibits gap junctional communication between thecal cells. Endocrinology. 1996;137(12):5662–70.
6. Chaves RN, Alves AMCV, Duarte ABG, Araujo VR, Celestino JJH, Matos MHT, Lopes CAP, Campello CC, Name KPO, Bao SN, et al. Nerve growth factor promotes the survival of goat preantral follicles cultured in vitro. Cells Tissues Organs. 2010;192(4):272–82.
7. Naicy T, Venkatachalapathy RT, Aravindakshan TV, Radhika G, Raghavan KC, Mini M, Shyama K. Nerve Growth Factor gene ovarian expression, polymorphism identification, and association with litter size in goats. Theriogenology. 2016;86(9):2172–2178.e3.
8. Naicy T, Venkatachalapathy RT, Aravindakshan TV, Raghavan KC, Mini M, Shyama K. Relative abundance of tissue mRNA and association of the single nucleotide polymorphism of the goat NGF gene with prolificacy. Anim Reprod Sci. 2016;173:42–8.
9. Linher-Melville K, Li J. The roles of glial cell line-derived neurotrophic factor, brain-derived neurotrophic factor and nerve growth factor during the final stage of folliculogenesis: a focus on oocyte maturation. Reproduction. 2013; 145(2):R43–54.
10. Barboni B, Mattioli M, Gioia L, Turriani M, Capacchietti G, Berardinelli P, Bernabo N. Preovulatory rise of NGF in ovine follicular fluid: possible involvement in the control of oocyte maturation. Microsc Res Tech. 2002;59(6):516–21.
11. Crispo M, dos Santos-Neto PC, Vilariño M, Mulet AP, De León A, Barbeito L, Menchaca A. Nerve growth factor influences cleavage rate and embryo development in sheep. J Anim Sci. 2016;94(10):4447–51.
12. Papp AB, Somfai T, Tartaglione M, Varga E, JC G. The effect of nerve growth factor on nuclear progression of porcine oocytes during in vitro maturation and embryo development. Acta Vet Hung. 2005;53(1):91–101.
13. Dissen GA, Garcia-Rudaz C, Paredes A, Mayer C, Mayerhofer A, Ojeda SR. Excessive ovarian production of nerve growth factor facilitates development of cystic ovarian morphology in mice and is a feature of polycystic ovarian syndrome in humans. Endocrinology. 2009;150(6):2906–14.
14. Wilson JL, Chen W, Dissen GA, Ojeda S, Cowley MA, Garcia-Rudaz C, Enriori PJ. Excess of nerve growth factor in the ovary causes a polycystic ovary-like syndrome in mice, which closely resembles both reproductive and metabolic aspects of the human syndrome. Endocrinology. 2014;155(11):4494–506.
15. Gulino FA, Giuffrida E, Leonardi E, Marilli I, Palumbo MA. Intrafollicular nerve growth factor (NGF) concentration in patients with polycystic ovarian syndrome case-control study. Minerva Ginecol. 2016;68(2):110–6.
16. Qiao J, Feng HL. Extra- and intra-ovarian factors in polycystic ovary syndrome: impact on oocyte maturation and embryo developmental competence. Hum Reprod Update. 2011;17(1):17–33.
17. Sadeu JC, Doedée A, Neal MS, Hughes EG, Foster WG. Neurotrophins (BDNF and NGF) in follicular fluid of women with different infertility diagnoses. Reprod BioMed Online. 2012;24(2):174–9.

18. Dumesic DA, Abbott DH. Implications of polycystic ovary syndrome on oocyte development. Semin Reprod Med. 2008;26(1):53–61.
19. Wood JR, Dumesic DA, Abbott DH, Strauss JF 3rd. Molecular abnormalities in oocytes from women with polycystic ovary syndrome revealed by microarray analysis. J Clin Endocrinol Metab. 2007;92(2):705–13.
20. Heijnen E, Eijkemans MJC, Hughes EG, Laven JSE, Macklon NS, Fauser B. A meta-analysis of outcomes of conventional IVF in women with polycystic ovary syndrome. Hum Reprod Update. 2006;12(1):13–21.
21. Hussein TS, Thompson JG, Gilchrist RB. Oocyte-secreted factors enhance oocyte developmental competence. Dev Biol. 2006;296(2):514–21.
22. Eppig JJ. Oocyte control of ovarian follicular development and function in mammals. Reproduction. 2001;122:829–38.
23. Su Y-Q, Wu X, O'Brien MJ, Pendola FL, Denegre JN, Matzuk MM, Eppig JJ. Synergistic roles of BMP15 and GDF9 in the development and function of the oocyte-cumulus cell complex in mice: genetic evidence for an oocyte-granulosa cell regulatory loop. Dev Biol. 2004;276(1):64–73.
24. Matzuk MM, Burns KH, Viveiros MM, Eppig JJ. Intercellular communication in the mammalian ovary: oocytes carry the conversation. Science. 2002; 296(5576):2178–80.
25. Biggers JD, Whittingham DG, Donahue RP. The pattern of energy metabolism in the mouse oocyte and zygote. Proc Natl Acad Sci U S A. 1967;58:560–7.
26. Leese HJ, Barton AM. Production of pyruvate by isolated mouse cumulus cells. J Exp Zool A Ecol Genet Physiol. 1985;234(2):231–6.
27. Sugiura K, Pendola FL, Eppig JJ. Oocyte control of metabolic cooperativity between oocytes and companion granulosa cells: energy metabolism. Dev Biol. 2005;279(1):20–30.
28. Valve E, Penttilä TL, Paranko J, Härkönen P. FGF-8 is expressed during specific phases of rodent oocyte and spermatogonium development. Biochem Biophys Res Commun. 1997;232(1):173–7.
29. Elvin JA, Clark AT, Wang P, Wolfman NM, Matzuk MM. Paracrine actions of growth differentiation factor-9 in the mammalian ovary. Mol Endocrinol. 1999;13:1035–48.
30. Shimasaki S, Kelly Moore R, Otsuka F, Erickson GF. The bone morphogenetic protein system in mammalian reproduction. Endocr Rev. 2004;25(1):72–101.
31. Sugiura K, Su YQ, Diaz FJ, Pangas SA, Sharma S, Wigglesworth K, O'Brien MJ, Matzuk MM, Shimasaki S, Eppig JJ. Oocyte-derived BMP15 and FGFs cooperate to promote glycolysis in cumulus cells. Development. 2007; 134(14):2593–603.
32. Wei D, Xie J, Yin B, Hao H, Song X, Liu Q, Zhang C, Sun Y. Significantly lengthened telomere in granulosa cells from women with polycystic ovarian syndrome (PCOS). J Assist Reprod Genet. 2017;34(7):861–8.
33. Zettler C, Bridges DC, Zhou XF, Rush RA. Detection of increased tissue concentrations of nerve growth factor with an improved extraction procedure. J Neurosci Res. 1996;46(5):581–94.
34. Wang Y, Liang N, Yao G, Tian H, Zhai Y, Yin Y, Sun F. Knockdown of TrkA in cumulus oocyte complexes (COCs) inhibits EGF-induced cumulus expansion by down-regulation of IL-6. Mol Cell Endocrinol. 2014;382(2):804–13.
35. Su Y-Q, Denegre JM, Wigglesworth K, Pendola FL, O'Brien MJ, Eppig JJ. Oocyte-dependent activation of mitogen-activated protein kinase (ERK1/2) in cumulus cells is required for the maturation of the mouse oocyte–cumulus cell complex. Dev Biol. 2003;263(1):126–38.
36. Zhang M, Su YQ, Sugiura K, Xia G, Eppig JJ. Granulosa cell ligand NPPC and its receptor NPR2 maintain meiotic arrest in mouse oocytes. Science. 2010; 330:366–9.
37. Wigglesworth K, Lee KB, O'Brien MJ, Peng J, Matzuk MM, Eppig JJ. Bidirectional communication between oocytes and ovarian follicular somatic cells is required for meiotic arrest of mammalian oocytes. Proc Natl Acad Sci. 2013;110(39):E3723–9.
38. Monti M, Redi C. Ologenesis specific genes (Nobox, Oct4, Bmp15, Gdf9, Oogenesin1 and Oogenesin2) are differentially expressed during natural and gonadotropin-induced mouse follicular development. Mol Reprod Dev. 2009;76(10):994–1003.
39. Palumbo MA, Giuffrida E, Gulino FA, Leonardi E, Cantarella G, Bernardini R. Nerve growth factor (NGF) levels in follicular fluid of infertile patients undergoing to in vitro fertilization (IVF) cycle. Gynecol Endocrinol. 2013; 29(11):1002–4.
40. Dissen GA, Lara HE, Leyton V, Paredes A, Hill DF, Costa ME, Martinez-Serrano A, Ojeda SR. Intraovarian excess of nerve growth factor increases androgen secretion and disrupts estrous cyclicity in the rat. Endocrinology. 2000; 141(3):1073–82.
41. Wei LN, Huang R, Li LL, Fang C, Li Y, Liang XY. Reduced and delayed expression of GDF9 and BMP15 in ovarian tissues from women with polycystic ovary syndrome. J Assist Reprod Genet. 2014;31(11):1483–90.
42. Teixeira de Resende LO, Vireque AA, Santana LF, Moreno DA, de Sa Rosa e Silva AC, Ferriani RA, Scrideli CA, Reis RM. Single-cell expression analysis of BMP15 and GDF9 in mature oocytes and BMPR2 in cumulus cells of women with polycystic ovary syndrome undergoing controlled ovarian hyperstimulation. J Assist Reprod Genet. 2012;29(10):1057–65.

Permissions

All chapters in this book were first published in RBE, by BioMed Central; hereby published with permission under the Creative Commons Attribution License or equivalent. Every chapter published in this book has been scrutinized by our experts. Their significance has been extensively debated. The topics covered herein carry significant findings which will fuel the growth of the discipline. They may even be implemented as practical applications or may be referred to as a beginning point for another development.

The contributors of this book come from diverse backgrounds, making this book a truly international effort. This book will bring forth new frontiers with its revolutionizing research information and detailed analysis of the nascent developments around the world.

We would like to thank all the contributing authors for lending their expertise to make the book truly unique. They have played a crucial role in the development of this book. Without their invaluable contributions this book wouldn't have been possible. They have made vital efforts to compile up to date information on the varied aspects of this subject to make this book a valuable addition to the collection of many professionals and students.

This book was conceptualized with the vision of imparting up-to-date information and advanced data in this field. To ensure the same, a matchless editorial board was set up. Every individual on the board went through rigorous rounds of assessment to prove their worth. After which they invested a large part of their time researching and compiling the most relevant data for our readers.

The editorial board has been involved in producing this book since its inception. They have spent rigorous hours researching and exploring the diverse topics which have resulted in the successful publishing of this book. They have passed on their knowledge of decades through this book. To expedite this challenging task, the publisher supported the team at every step. A small team of assistant editors was also appointed to further simplify the editing procedure and attain best results for the readers.

Apart from the editorial board, the designing team has also invested a significant amount of their time in understanding the subject and creating the most relevant covers. They scrutinized every image to scout for the most suitable representation of the subject and create an appropriate cover for the book.

The publishing team has been an ardent support to the editorial, designing and production team. Their endless efforts to recruit the best for this project, has resulted in the accomplishment of this book. They are a veteran in the field of academics and their pool of knowledge is as vast as their experience in printing. Their expertise and guidance has proved useful at every step. Their uncompromising quality standards have made this book an exceptional effort. Their encouragement from time to time has been an inspiration for everyone.

The publisher and the editorial board hope that this book will prove to be a valuable piece of knowledge for researchers, students, practitioners and scholars across the globe.

List of Contributors

Jiayi Zheng, Haiping Wang and Wenhui Zhou
Medical Center for Human Reproduction, Beijing Chaoyang Hospital, Capital Medical University, Beijing 100020, People's Republic of China

Andreas N. Kavazis
School of Kinesiology, Auburn University, 301 Wire Road, Auburn, Alabama36849, USA

Yufeng Zhang and Wendy R. Hood
Department of Biological Sciences, Auburn University, Auburn, AL, USA

Jing Zhao, Xi Huang, Bin Xu, Yi Yan, Qiong Zhang and Yanping Li
Reproductive Medicine Center, Xiangya Hospital, Central South University, 87 Xiang Ya Road, Changsha, Hunan 410008, People's Republic of China

Meng Rao and Li Tang
Department of reproduction and genetics, the First Affiliated Hospital of Kunming Medical University, No. 295 Xi Chang road, Kunming 650032, China

Zhengyan Zeng
Department of Neurology, the First Affiliated Hospital of Kunming Medical University, Kunming 650032, China.

Yuying Wang, Yi Zhang, Tzuchun Lin, Yun Sun, Wei Liu and Tao Tao
Department of Endocrinology and Metabolism, Renji Hospital, School of Medicine, Shanghai Jiaotong University, 160 Pujian Road, Shanghai 200127, China.

Wei Liu
Department of Endocrinology and Metabolism, Renji Hospital, School of Medicine, Shanghai Jiaotong University, 160 Pujian Road, Shanghai 200127, China
Shanghai Key laboratory forAssisted Reproduction and Reproductive Genetics, Center for Reproductive Medicine, Renji Hospital, School of Medicine, Shanghai Jiaotong University, 160Pujian Road, Shanghai 200127, China

Wei Zhou
Department of Emergency, South Campus, Renji Hospital, School of Medicine, Shanghai Jiaotong University, Shanghai, China.

Chunhua Wu
Division of Ultrasonography, Department of Radiology, Renji Hospital, School of Medicine, Shanghai Jiaotong
University, 160 Pujian Road, Shanghai 200127, China

Yun Sun and Wei Liu
Shanghai Key laboratory forAssisted Reproduction and Reproductive Genetics, Center for Reproductive Medicine, Renji Hospital, School of Medicine, Shanghai Jiaotong University, 160Pujian Road, Shanghai 200127, China

Luyang Zhao, Chenglei Gu, Mingxia Ye, Zhe Zhang, Li'an Li, Wensheng Fan and Yuanguang Meng
Department of Gynecology and Obstetrics, People's Liberation Army (PLA) Medical School, Chinese PLA General Hospital, Beijing 100853, China

Luyang Zhao
Department of Gynecology and Obstetrics, People's Liberation Army (PLA) Medical School, Chinese PLA General Hospital, Beijing 100853, China
Department of Gynecology and Obstetrics, Peking University People's Hospital, Beijing, China

Chenglei Gu
Department of Gynecology and Obstetrics, People's Liberation Army (PLA) Medical School, Chinese PLA General Hospital, Beijing 100853, China
Department of Gynecology and Obstetrics, the 309th Hospital of Chinese PLA, Beijing, China

Xiaodan Cao, Yun Cui, Xiaoxia Zhang, Jiangtao Lou, Jun Zhou, Huafeng Bei and Renxiong Wei
Department of Clinical Laboratory, Ningbo Municipal Hospital of Traditional Chinese Medicine, Ningbo 315000, China

Stacy Colaco and Deepak Modi
Department of Molecular and Cellular Biology, ICMR-National Institute for Research in Reproductive Health, JM Street, Parel, Mumbai, Maharashtra 400012, India

Erica Silvestris, Raffaele Rosania and Giuseppe Loverro
Interdisciplinary Department of Medicine, Section of Obstetrics and Gynecology, University of Bari Aldo Moro, P.za G.Cesare, 11-70124 Bari, Italy

Giovanni de Pergola
Departmentof Biomedical Sciences and Human Oncology, Section of Internal Medicine and Clinical Oncology, University of Bari Aldo Moro, P.za G.Cesare, 11-70124 Bari, Italy

Tetsuro Hanada, Shunichiro Tsuji, Shiro Wakinoue1, Kyoko Kasahara, Fuminori Kimura, and Takashi Murakami
Department of Obstetrics and Gynecology, Shiga University of Medical Science, Seta Tsukionowa-cho, Otsu, Shiga 520-2192, Japan

Misako Nakayama and Misako Nakayama
Department of Pathology, Division of Pathology and Disease Regulation, Shiga University of Medical Science, Seta Tsukionowa-cho, Otsu, Shiga 520-2192, Japan

Takahide Mori
Academia for Repro-Regenerative Medicine, Nonprofit Organization, 394-1 Higashi-Hinodono-cho, Ichijo-Shinmachi-Higashiiru, Kamigyo-ku, Kyoto 602-0917, Japan

Sandeep K. Rajput, Joseph K. Folger and George W. Smith
Laboratory of Mammalian Reproductive Biology and Genomics, Michigan State University, East Lansing, MI 48824, USA
Department of Animal Science, Michigan State University, East Lansing, MI 48824, USA

Mohamed Ashry
Laboratory of Mammalian Reproductive Biology and Genomics, Michigan State University, East Lansing, MI 48824, USA
Department of Animal Science, Michigan State University, East Lansing, MI 48824, USA
Department of Theriogenology, Faculty of Veterinary Medicine, Cairo University, Giza, Egypt

Jason G. Knott
Developmental Epigenetics Laboratory, Michigan State University, East Lansing, MI 48824, USA
Department of Animal Science, Michigan State University, East Lansing, MI 48824, USA

Nabil A. Hemeida and Refaat S. Ragab
Department of Theriogenology, Faculty of Veterinary Medicine, Cairo University, Giza, Egypt

Omaima M. Kandil
Department of Animal Reproduction and Artificial Insemination, Veterinary Research Division, National Research Center, Giza, Egyp

Kylie Beck and Muhammad Anzar
Agriculture and Agri-Food Canada, Saskatoon Research and Development Center, Canadian Animal Genetic Resource Program, S7N OX2, Saskatoon, SK, Canada
Departmnet of Veterinary Biomedical Sciences, Western College of Veterinary Medicine, University of Saskatchewan, Saskatoon, SK S7N 5B4, Canada

Jaswant Singh
Departmnet of Veterinary Biomedical Sciences, Western College of Veterinary Medicine, University of Saskatchewan, Saskatoon, SK S7N 5B4, Canada

Mohammad Arshud Dar
Vaccination and Infectious Disease Organization, University Saskatchewan, Saskatoon S7N 5E3, Canada

Huan-Chin Tseng, Jhih-Jie Yu and Ling-Yu Yeh
Department of Medical Research, Mackay Memorial Hospital, Tamsui District, New Taipei City 251, Taiwan

Sheng-Hsiang Li
Department of Medical Research, Mackay Memorial Hospital, Tamsui District, New Taipei City 251, Taiwan
Mackay Junior College of Medicine, Nursing, and Management, Beitou District, Taipei City 112, Taiwan

Robert Kuo-Kuang Lee
Department of Medical Research, Mackay Memorial Hospital, Tamsui District, New Taipei City 251, Taiwan
Department of Obstetrics and Gynecology, Mackay Memorial Hospital, Taipei City 104, Taiwan
Department of Obstetrics and Gynecology, Taipei Medical University, Taipei City 110, Taiwan

Yuh-Ming Hwu
Department of Obstetrics and Gynecology, Mackay Memorial Hospital, Taipei City 104, Taiwan

Mackay Medical College, Sanzhi District, New Taipei City 252, Taiwan
Mackay Junior College of Medicine, Nursing, and Management, Beitou District, Taipei City 112, Taiwan

Ming-Huei Lin
Department of Obstetrics and Gynecology, Mackay Memorial Hospital, Taipei City 104, Taiwan
Mackay Junior College of Medicine, Nursing, and Management, Beitou District, Taipei City 112, Taiwan

Chi-Chen Fan
Office of Superintendent, Mackay Memorial Hospital, Taipei City, Taiwan
Department of Medical Laboratory Science andBiotechnology, Yuanpei University, Hsinchu 300 Taiwan

Andrea Sansone, Carla Di Dato, Carlotta Pozza, Andrea Isidori and Daniele Gianfrilli
Department of Experimental Medicine, Section of Medical Pathophysiology, Food Science and Endocrinology, Sapienza - University of Rome, Viale ReginaElena 324, 00161 Rome, Italy

Cristina de Angelis
I.O.S.& COLEMAN Srl, Naples, Italy
Dipartimento di Medicina Clinica e Chirurgia, Sezione di Endocrinologia, Università "Federico II" di Napoli, Naples, Italy

Davide Menafra and Rosario Pivonello
Dipartimento di Medicina Clinica e Chirurgia, Sezione di Endocrinologia, Università "Federico II" di Napoli, Naples, Italy

Anja Baufeld and Jens Vanselow
Institute of Reproductive Biology, Leibniz Institute for Farm Animal Biology (FBN), Wilhelm-Stahl-Allee 2, 18196 Dummerstorf, Germany

Ashok Agarwal
American Center for Reproductive Medicine, Cleveland Clinic, Glickman Urological and Kidney Institute, Mail Code X-11, 10681 Carnegie Avenue, Cleveland, OH 44195, USA

Pallav Sengupta
Department of Physiology, Faculty of Medicine, MAHSA University, Jalan SP2, Bandar Saujana Putra, 42610 Jenjarum, Selangor, Malaysia

Damayanthi Durairajanayagam
Faculty of Medicine, Universiti Teknologi MARA, Sungai Buloh Campus, Jalan Hospital, 47000 Sungai Buloh, Selangor, Malaysia

Ya-Li Yang, Tian-Xia Xiao, Bao-Bei Wang, Pei-Gen Ren and Jian V. Zhang
Research Laboratory for Reproductive Health, Shenzhen Institutes of Advanced Technology, Chinese Academy of Sciences, Shenzhen 518055, China

Li-Feng Sun
Research Laboratory for Reproductive Health, Shenzhen Institutes of Advanced Technology, Chinese Academy of Sciences, Shenzhen 518055, China
University of Chinese Academy of Sciences, Beijing 100049, China

Shasha Qi and Lei Yan
Center for Reproductive Medicine, Shandong Provincial Hospital Affiliated to Shandong University, Jinan 250021, People's Republic of China
National Research Center for Assisted Reproductive Technology and Reproductive Genetics, Jinan 250021, People's Republic of China
The Key laboratory for Reproductive Endocrinology, Shandong University, Ministry of Education, Jinan 250021, People's Republic of China

Zi-Jiang Chen
Center for Reproductive Medicine, Shandong Provincial Hospital Affiliated to Shandong University, Jinan 250021, People's Republic of China
National Research Center for Assisted Reproductive Technology and Reproductive Genetics, Jinan 250021, People's Republic of China
The Key laboratory for Reproductive Endocrinology, Shandong University, Ministry of Education, Jinan 250021, People's Republic of China
Shanghai Key Laboratory for Assisted Reproduction and Reproductive Genetics, Shanghai 200030, People'sRepublic of China
Center for Reproductive Medicine, Ren Ji Hospital, Schoolof Medicine, Shanghai Jiao Tong University, Shanghai 200030, People's Republic of China

Zhao Liu
Department of Urology, Qilu Hospital of Shandong University, 107 Wenhua Xi Road, Jinan 250012, People's Republic of China

Yu-lan Mu, Mingjiang Li, Xingbo Zhao and Hui Zhang
Department of Obstetrics and Gynecology, Shandong Provincial Hospital Affiliated to Shandong University, 324 Jingwu Road, Jinan 250021, People's Republic of China

Ashok Agarwal
American Center for Reproductive Medicine, Cleveland Clinic, 10681 Carnegie Avenue, Desk X11, Cleveland, OH 44195, USA

Luna Samanta
American Center for Reproductive Medicine, Cleveland Clinic, 10681 Carnegie Avenue, Desk X11, Cleveland, OH 44195, USA
Redox Biology Laboratory, Department of Zoology, School of Life Sciences, Ravenshaw University, Cuttack, Odisha 753003, India

Rajeshwari Parida
Redox Biology Laboratory, Department of Zoology, School of Life Sciences, Ravenshaw University, Cuttack, Odisha 753003, India

Tania R. Dias
American Center for Reproductive Medicine, Cleveland Clinic, 10681 Carnegie Avenue, Desk X11, Cleveland, OH 44195, USA
Universidade da Beira Interior, 6201-001 Covilhã, Portugal
Department of Microscopy, Laboratory of Cell Biology, Institute of Biomedical Sciences Abel Salazar and Unit for Multidisciplinary Research in Biomedicine, University of Porto, 4050-313 Porto, Portugal
LAQV/REQUIMTE - Laboratory of Bromatology and Hydrology, Faculty of Pharmacy, University of Porto, 4050-313 Porto, Portugal

Wei Xia, Duo Zhang, Jing Ouyang, Yan Liang, Huiyu Zhang, Zhen Huang, Guiling Liang, Qian Zhu and Jian Zhang
Department of Obstetrics and Gynaecology, International Peace Maternity and Child Health Hospital, School of Medicine, Shanghai Jiaotong University, Shanghai, China
Institute of Embryo-Fetal Original Adult Disease Affiliated to School of Medicine, Shanghai Jiaotong University, Shanghai, China

Xiaoming Guan
Department of Obstetrics and Gynaecology, Baylor College of Medicine, Houston, TX, USA

Rosemary Foster and Leah W. Gatune
Vincent Center for Reproductive Biology, Vincent Department of Obstetrics and Gynecology, Massachusetts General Hospital, 55 Fruit Street, Yaw 10A, Boston, MA 02114, USA

Anatte E. Karmon, Amy E. Lee and Aaron K. Styer
Vincent Center for Reproductive Biology, Vincent Department of Obstetrics and Gynecology, Massachusetts General Hospital, 55 Fruit Street, Yaw 10A, Boston, MA 02114, USA
Department of Obstetrics, Gynecology, and Reproductive Biology, Harvard Medical School, Boston, MA 02115, USA

Eden R. Cardozo
Vincent Center for Reproductive Biology, Vincent Department of Obstetrics and Gynecology, Massachusetts General Hospital, 55 Fruit Street, Yaw 10A, Boston, MA 02114, USA
Department of Obstetrics, Gynecology, and Reproductive Biology, Harvard Medical School, Boston, MA 02115, USA
Women and Infants Fertility Center, Brown University Warren Alpert Medical School, 90 Plain Street, Providence, RI 02905, USA

Akin Usta, Cagla Bahar Bulbul and Ertan Adali
Department of Obstetrics and Gynecology, School of Medicine, Balıkesir University Faculty of Medicine, Cagis Yerleskesi, Bigadic yolu 17. km, 10145 Balikesir, Turkey

Eyup Avci and Hasan Kadi
Department of Cardiology, School of Medicine, Balikesir University, Balikesir, Turkey

Fangrong Wu, Xiaoyan Chen, Yingyu Liu, Bo Liang, Hui Xu and Tin Chiu Li
Department of Obstetrics and Gynaecology, The Chinese University of Hong Kong, Shatin, Hong Kong

Chi Chiu Wang
Department of Obstetrics and Gynaecology, The Chinese University of Hong Kong, Shatin, Hong Kong
Li Ka Shing Institute of Health Sciences, Faculty of Medicine, The Chinese University of Hong Kong, Shatin, Hong Kong
School of Biomedical Sciences, Faculty of Medicine, The Chinese University of Hong Kong, Shatin, Hong Kong

Yiwen Zhai, Faiza Rao, Yong Wang, Xiaoyuan Song and Fei Sun
School of Life Sciences, University of Science and Technology of China, Hefei, Anhui, People's Republic of China
Hefei National Laboratory for Physical Sciences at Microscale, Hefei, Anhui, People's Republic of China

Guidong Yao
Reproductive Medical Center, The First Affiliated Hospital of Zhengzhou University, Zhengzhou, Henan, People's Republic of China

Index